ANALGETICS

MEDICINAL CHEMISTRY
A Series of Monographs

EDITED BY

GEORGE deSTEVENS

CIBA Pharmaceutical Company
Division of CIBA Corporation
Summit, New Jersey

ANALGETICS

EDITED BY

George deStevens

CIBA Pharmaceutical Company
Divison of CIBA Corporation
Summit, New Jersey

1965

ACADEMIC PRESS   New York and London

ACADEMIC PRESS INC.
111 Fifth Avenue, New York, New York 10003

United Kingdom Edition published by
ACADEMIC PRESS INC. (LONDON) LTD.
Berkeley Square House, London W. 1

LIBRARY OF CONGRESS CATALOG CARD NUMBER: 65-15524

PRINTED IN THE UNITED STATES OF AMERICA.

List of Contributors

Numbers in parentheses indicate the pages on which the authors' contributions begin.

WILLIAM T. BEAVER, *Division of Clinical Investigation, The Sloan-Kettering Institute for Cancer Research, New York, New York* (75)

H. BESENDORF, *Research Department, F. Hoffmann-LaRoche & Co., AG, Basle, Switzerland* (281)

A. BROSSI, *Research Department, Hoffmann-LaRoche, Inc., Nutley, New Jersey* (281)

ALFRED BURGER, *Department of Chemistry, University of Virginia, Charlottesville, Virginia* (1)

GEORGE DEStevens, *CIBA Pharmaceutical Company, Division of CIBA Corporation, Summit, New Jersey* (405)

ROBERT A. HARDY, JR., *Lederle Laboratories, A Division of American Cyanamid Co., Pearl River, New York* (179)

RAYMOND W. HOUDE, *Division of Clinical Investigation, The Sloan-Kettering Institute for Cancer Research, New York, New York* (75)

M. GERTRUDE HOWELL, *Lederle Laboratories, A Division of American Cyanamid Co., Pearl River, New York* (179)

WALTER KROHS,* *Formerly Research Chemist of Farbwerke Hoechst AG, Germany* (331)

EVERETTE L. MAY, *National Institutes of Health, Bethesda, Maryland* (123)

L. A. PIRK, *Research Department, Hoffmann-LaRoche, Inc., Nutley, New Jersey* (281)

A. RHEINER, JR., *Research Department, F. Hoffmann-LaRoche & Co., AG, Basle, Switzerland* (281)

LEWIS J. SARGENT, *National Institutes of Health, Bethesda, Maryland* (123)

STANLEY L. WALLENSTEIN, *Division of Clinical Investigation, The Sloan-Kettering Institute for Cancer Research, New York, New York* (75)

CHARLES A. WINTER, *Merck Institute for Therapeutic Research, West Point, Pennsylvania* (9)

Present address: Bad Soden im Taunus, Hessen, Germany

Foreword

The many advances made in medicinal chemistry within the past quarter-century have done much to further our knowledge of the relationship between chemical structure and biological activity. This relationship has led to a tremendous collaborative effort between chemists and biologists, and this has been evidenced further by the considerable number of reviews which have appeared on various aspects of medicinal chemistry. For the most part, these have been confined to single chapters on selected topics. Of necessity, in such a format, it has been difficult to cover a particular area very broadly.

The purpose of this series is to present a series of monographs, each dealing with a specific field in medicinal chemistry. Thus, these edited or authored volumes will make available to the medicinal chemist and biologist an opportunity to review critically a topic; consequently, a broader perspective of a subject can be realized.

GEORGE DESTEVENS

Preface

It is hoped that this volume on the chemistry and pharmacology of analgetics will satisfactorily fill an important gap in the literature of medicinal chemistry. It is addressed to all those interested in the interdisciplinary aspects of analgetic research, i.e., organic chemists, biochemists, pharmacologists, physiologists, and clinicians.

The arrangement of the subject matter follows a plan to reduce repetition to a minimum. The opening chapter is a general introduction to the volume. Discussions of the physiology and pharmacology of pain as presented in Chapter II and the clinical measurement of pain in Chapter III are considered by the Editor to be necessary prerequisites for full appreciation of the subsequent chapters.

The ensuing chapters follow a chronological development, with the exception of Chapter VIII on general synthetics. The literature records many compounds which allegedly show analgetic activity. The author of this chapter has selected those compounds which have been introduced in clinical medicine and also some compounds which appear to offer a different approach to the design of new types of analgetics. The inclusion of a few compounds from his own laboratory made possible the use of data not published heretofore.

Summit, New Jersey   George deStevens
January 1965

ix

Contents

CHAPTER I   Introduction

Alfred Burger

CHAPTER II   The Physiology and Pharmacology of Pain and Its Relief

Charles A. Winter

CHAPTER III   Clinical Measurement of Pain

Raymond W. Houde, Stanley L. Wallenstein, and William T. Beaver

CHAPTER VII Pyrazole Derivatives

Walter Krohs

CHAPTER VIII General Synthetics

George deStevens

Introduction

ALFRED BURGER

DEPARTMENT OF CHEMISTRY, UNIVERSITY OF VIRGINIA,
CHARLOTTESVILLE, VIRGINIA

Pain is a syndrome of sensations with which all humans become inevitably familiar. From the moment of birth and the tearful response to the slap of the obstetrician, one suffers through the subsequent humiliating educational and corrective measures of one's elders, and through the traumatic experiences at the hands and kicks of one's youthful peers. After the diseases of childhood, one emerges into adult life with ample experience of pain and distaste for this feeling. Nobody escapes minor pain on many occasions, and few are as lucky as not to be plagued by some major pain off and on. Some individuals have a higher pain threshold than others and may be better equipped psychologically to cope with pain. However, at one time or another virtually every human being seeks medical help for the alleviation of pain. As every physician can attest, pain is the most common reason for a visit to a doctor's office.

In some cases, it is possible to remove the cause of the pain, and thereby to remove the pain sensation. In many other instances, relief from pain is all the physician has to offer. In all cases, rapid symptomatic relief from pain is wanted, and drugs which can provide such relief are among the most sought-after medicines. The tremendous demand for such substances is attested by the large number of advertisements in the professional and lay press announcing pain-relieving drugs, and the number of radio and television programs sponsored by manufacturers of such materials. Research on the chemistry, metabolism, pharmacological actions, and clinical efficacy and selectivity of analgetics constitutes a considerable and continuing share of medicinal inquiry.

The term analgesia derives from the Greek, ἄνα (without) and ἄλγος (pain). It is used in medicine and pharmacology to describe a state without pain, usually brought about during or in anticipation of a pain stimulus by

1

ALFRED BURGER

administration of a drug or procedure which relieves pain. A drug which depresses pain without causing loss of consciousness is called an analgetic agent.[1]

Analgetics have been sought by man at all times. Tribal medicine men and witches stewed herbal brews which were administered to injured or sick patients with proper incantations and exorcisms. Refinements in these techniques were elaborated by physician-priests of all faiths. They combined the releasing, tranquilizing, and hypnotic power of prayers with soothing concoctions made of herbs which they collected, tried, and if successful, grew in the gardens of monasteries and temples. In traumatic emergencies, wines and other alcoholic liquors were also used extensively to obtund pain and divert the attention of the patient from even an extremely painful operation. In such acute therapeutic applications, the undesirable and toxic side-effects of the medicines could be disregarded, and possible long-range damages resulting from the development of tolerance and addiction[2] could be overlooked. This attitude is still held for modern analgetics used in the treatment of postoperative pain.

It is a witness to the conservatism of the medical profession that the most ancient pain-relieving product, opium, still furnishes the most widely used potent clinical analgetic agents. The opium alkaloids are in turn the structural prototypes of the more widely accepted modern synthetics which are classified as potent analgetics. The use of opium goes back in antiquity. The Sumerians seem to have used it 5500 years ago, and it is mentioned in the *Ebers Papyrus* (ca. 1550 B.C.). Opium is the condensed sap of the unripe seed and capsule of the opium poppy, *Papaver somniferum*. Originally native to the Middle East, the opium poppy was collected by the Assyrians and worked up by a method not unlike the present one; it seems to have been used to produce sleep. Theophrastus (3rd century B.C.) gives an account

[1] The term *analgesic* is wide-spread in the U.S.A. and Canada. It is grammatically incorrect, and constitutes a hang-over from early days when a short medical curriculum did not allow for time to acquire a knowledge of etymology. Because of the general acceptance of this term, it will be used along with and in place of the term *analgetic* throughout this treatise. Curiously, the terms *anesthesia* ($\dot{\alpha}\nu+\dot{\alpha}\iota\sigma\vartheta\eta\sigma\iota\varsigma$: absence of sensibility) and *anesthetic* have always been used correctly.

[2] The widely accepted term "drug addiction" has been used in this and subsequent chapters to implicate situations arising from the continued use of potent analgetics, and involving severe symptoms upon withdrawal of the drug. The Committee on Drug Addiction and Narcotics of the National Academy of Sciences—National Research Council "concurred in the recommendation of the Expert Committee on Addiction-Producing Drugs of the World Health Organization that the term drug dependence be substituted for the terms drug addiction and drug habituation" (*see* Bulletin, Drug Addiction and Narcotics, National Academy of Sciences—National Research Council, Division of Medical Sciences, Washington 25, D. C., February 1964).

2

of these early activities (*1*). The Arabs appear to have exported opium to the Far East; the Chinese used it for dysenteries first but later began to smoke it. Addiction to opium dates back to the Middle Ages. The use of opium continued also in Europe, and from the times of Hippocrates and other Greek and Roman physicians its acceptance expanded into the Renaissance. There was not much progress in the purification of opium, Paracelsus' (1490–1540) "laudanum" being essentially an aqueous dispersion of the tarry material. Interestingly, addiction remained mild because morphine is decomposed thermally during the smoking. Even when opium eating (or rather drinking of an aqueous-alcoholic solution) became fashionable, addiction was not much of a problem because morphine is not too well absorbed from the gastrointestinal tract. Nevertheless, serious cases of addiction were recorded, and the situation became more serious after Christopher Wren invented and first used a crude hypodermic "syringe" consisting of a quill and a bladder, and injected opium intravenously. The euphoria following these injections led to misuse and the establishment of a group of opium addicts in the West.

The isolation of morphine by Sertüner (1803), of other opium alkaloids by subsequent investigators, and the synthesis (Wright, 1884) and clinical use and abuse (Dreser and Floret, 1898) of morphine diacetate (heroin) will be described in Chapter IV. These events heralded the modern age of potent analgetics with all its advantages, dangers, and medical and social problems. A final quantitative evaluation of the effects of potent analgetics in man may be hard to perform. The type of pain to be dulled, and the individual and psychological factors permit a distinction of analgetic and placebo only on a biostatistical basis.

It is a coincidence that Dreser who first studied heroin also introduced aspirin into clinical practice (*2*). It is almost as if he had been guided from a highly potent but also highly addicting drug, to a low-grade analgetic to which at least addiction has not become known. Aspirin (acetylsalicylic acid) arose from studies on salicylic acid and its esters. Salicylic acid, extractable from the essential oil of *Spiraea ulmaria*, had been used for almost a century for the relief of pain and as an antipyretic. Its excellent action in reducing swelling and relieving pain in rheumatic fever was discovered by Stricker in 1876. In the form of its methyl ester which occurs in several other essential oils, it can be used as a topical minor antineuralgic agent. The acetate ester of the phenolic hydroxyl group of salicylic acid, was first prepared in 1859 (*3*); forty years later it started its popular career as an antipyretic and for "the relief of minor pains." The sheer fact that aspirin has passed the 10^6 kg mark annually in the United States alone, is a commentary on the type of pain most widely combatted with nonprescription

3

drugs. It is worth remembering that the low-grade analgetic effect of aspirin is hard to assay in laboratory animals.

Aspirin has been used as much as an antipyretic agent in fever as for its analgetic effects. At the time of the discovery of these properties, two other types of antipyretic analgetics had already made their appearance by chance observations. They were the pyrazolone derivatives, especially antipyrine and aminopyrine, first synthesized by Knorr (4), and several p-aminophenol derivatives, particularly acetophenetidine (phenacetin) (5). In spite of their rather minor analgetic activity, these compounds have enjoyed a long-lived use. Quite recently, phenacetin has been withdrawn from several "triple-action" headache nostrums (APC: aspirin-phenacetin-caffeine) which had been promoted extensively for many years. The reason is the increased awareness of methemoglobinemia attributable to p-aminophenol derivatives, and now observed more frequently even with p-acetamidophenyl alkyl ethers. Neither the older pyrazolone derivatives or the newer pyrazolidine-diones (phenylbutazone), nor the compounds of the aminophenol series have rivaled aspirin in the obtusion of low-grade pains, perhaps because of their smaller degree of effectiveness, and because of more frequent annoying and even dangerous side effects. Had some of the older compounds been discovered 75 years later, they would not have had much chance to stand up to the regulations for new drugs of the U.S. Food and Drug Administration. It is even doubtful whether aspirin could have passed this hurdle.

Hope has not been abandoned that medium-potent analgetics with a minimum of side effects will be found in analogs of these drugs, or in other structural types. A selection of the hundreds of experimental compounds tested has been reviewed in a monograph (6a, b). The discovery of such an analgetic would be a comfort to millions of people, and its sale a commercial success to its manufacturer. The properties of "the" ideal—and probably unattainable—analgetic have been outlined by Pfeiffer (7). It should be effective against all types of pain, but not alter other sense receptors; it should have a large therapeutic margin of safety, a rapid onset and a long duration of action. It should not depress the cardiovascular and respiratory systems; should not affect the gastrointestinal tract; should be effective orally and parenterally; should not act as an antidiuretic; should be inexpensive to manufacture, and chemically stable; and, above all, should not lose its effectiveness through the development of tolerance which in turn may lead to habit formation or addiction. Even though such a drug may never be found, these goals have been the mainspring for continued research on analgetics over many decades. So many examples of dichotomy in therapeutic agents are known, and so often has a separation of activities been achieved adequately, that most medicinal chemists cannot believe that high

4

analgetic potency and at least addiction liability should not be separable. The possibility of sharply reducing or eliminating addiction liability opens a world wide vista of abolishing deep human misery and its attending criminality.

In medicinal chemistry, one must have a suitable lead compound which may be varied or dissected structurally to upgrade potency and discard unwanted side effects. In a search for a potent analgetic agent with less or no addiction liability, morphine offered the best point of departure. Obviously, potency could be increased as it was in heroin, but alas, this was accompanied by a high increase in addiction liability. The two properties fall sharply by methylation to codeine; here one-tenth of the analgetic potency of morphine is retained while addiction liability also decreases sharply. It seemed then that further structural variation was justified. A ten-year experimental program was instituted in 1929 by the National Research Council of the United States. A team of chemists at the University of Virginia (L. F. Small, E. Mosettig, A. Burger, and co-workers), and a similar team of pharmacologists at the University of Michigan under the leadership of N. B. Eddy, prepared and tested over 450 compounds for analgetic and other morphine-like activities. Approximately 125 of them were derived chemically from the naturally occurring alkaloids—morphine, codeine, or thebaine (Chapter IV). The rest of the substances were model compounds obtained by synthesis and containing some of the ring systems present in the morphine skeleton, equipped with various functional groups.

It has been remarked that "the fact that Vongerichten distilled morphine with zinc dust and isolated phenanthrene from the distillate, condemned a generation of organic chemists to hard labor making phenanthrene derivatives as model compounds for morphine-like activity." Although the chemical synthesis of the phenanthrene derivatives comprised a considerable amount of fun and interest, much truth can be read into that statement in retrospect. The most active derivative in that series was about one-tenth as active as codeine and was toxic (*8*).

The breakthrough came from an observation by Schaumann when he examined a compound prepared by Eisleb for *in vivo* antispasmodic activity (*9*). The substance, ethyl 1-methyl-4-phenylpiperidine-4-carboxylate hydrochloride, was an amino ester conceived to imitate the structure of traditional atropine-type antispasmodics. During the test Schaumann observed a Straub tail reaction, a phenomenon one usually associates with the centrally exciting component of opiate activity. This led him to subject the animals to a standard test for analgesia, and the potent analgetic activity of the material was thus revealed. The compound became known as meperidine. An inspection of its structure then revealed that meperidine has certain

5

features in common with morphine, most importantly, a quaternary carbon atom attached to an aromatic nucleus, and an aminoalkyl moiety. An electron-withdrawing group is needed in 4-arylpiperidines.

Variation of these structural characteristics even over a wide range, furnished evidence that other potent analgetics may be constructed along these lines. Details of these findings will be found in Chapter V. Although it is true that broad adherence to these basic structural concepts permits a fair measure of predictability of analgetic properties, all these structural requirements are not essential to produce such properties. The emergence of N-methylmorphinan (10) and its phenolic 3-hydroxy derivative (11) as pronounced analgetics have demonstrated the acceptability of this generalization. Indeed, May and his co-workers (11–13) have been able to strip down the structure of morphine in other ways, replacing the entire third ring of the phenanthrene skeleton by small alkyl groups. The resulting 5,9-dialkyl-6,7-benzomorphans and related types show a definite dissociation of strong analgetic activity and addiction liability (13).

In the course of work on N-allylnormorphine (nalorphine) and similar compounds as antagonists to morphine and other potent analgetics (for a brief review, see references 6b, p. 334), the species specificity of the analgetic properties of these substances was discovered. Moderately potent to potent analgetics were found among derivatives of 6,7-benzomorphan in which the nitrogen was substituted by less common alkyl groups [dimethylallyl, cyclopropylmethyl (14)]. Some of these compounds exhibit considerable dissociation of addiction liability and analgetic action; the clinically most acceptable of them (α-5,9-dimethyl-2-dimethylallyl-2'-hydroxy-6,7-benzomorphan, pentazocine) has been reported as causing no more addiction liability than a placebo. It remains to be seen whether the lack of euphoria which distinguishes pentazocine, its clinically undesirable property of respiratory depression, and the high cost of production will permit this otherwise near-ideal analgetic to rival morphine in a statistically significant relief from deep pain.

A less potent (15) analgetic, 4-dimethylamino-1,2-diphenyl-3-methyl-3-propionoxybutane (propoxyphene) (16) with very little demonstrable addiction liability in man and few side effects, has been in clinical use successfully for some time.

In these asymmetric molecules, configuration and conformation are of great importance for strong analgetic activity. Doubts have been expressed that stereospecificity constitutes an absolute requirement in all such cases. Many compounds lacking molecular asymmetry are known to possess moderate analgetic properties (Chapters VI–VIII).

Hypotheses proposed to explain potent morphine-type analgetic activity range from an examination of structural and steric features of the drug molecules, to implications of the metabolic fate of the compounds or their interaction with enzyme systems, as the causes of analgetic actions. In structurally related series, one can often point to a balance of the effect of several molecular moieties, but this becomes much more difficult if one compares less obviously related compounds. The very high activity of 1-diethylaminoethyl-5-nitro-2-(4-ethoxybenzyl)benzimidazole and other similar benzimidazole derivatives (17) (up to $1500 \times$ morphine, ED_{50} is $1 \mu g/kg$) (18) and with addiction potentials comparable to that of morphine makes it appear as if several molecular features of a macromolecular bioreceptor, with different receptive moieties, must be involved in triggering analgetic effects.

The compounds discussed in Chapters VI–VIII may be only a prelude to more selective and potent analgetics of the near future. If the physiology of pain (Chapter II) could be classified more concisely, and if perhaps a simpler assay of experimental and clinical pain could be developed, then the physician might be offered a choice of analgetic drugs for pain of different severity, origin, and permanence. Such physiological and analytical concepts are still in the formative stage. Almost every meeting of therapists and pharmacologists sponsors extensive discussions on the etiology of pain, the search for anatomical sites of pain reception and analgesia, and all sorts of chemical, electrical, mechanical, and psychopharmacological methods by which responses to, and relief from pain may be measured more reproducibly and more significantly (19). Even if analgetic tests could be unified and understood better in laboratory animals only, a decisive step toward more useful drugs would have been taken. With the steadily increasing refinement of pharmacological and electrophysiological technique and theory, one may hope that new and meaningful biological improvements in the study of analgetic drugs may be found soon. This all-important development would enable a chemist to plan more graded and selectively active compounds on the basis of structure-activity comparisons. Labeling of many representative drugs with tracer elements, and following their absorption, distribution, and excretion, would provide a further badly needed guide to chemical planning of new agents. The study of the metabolites of active as well as of inactive agents would help to explain why some of the drugs are inactive and would aid in avoiding similar failures in the future. Finally, as the biochemical theory of transmission and interruption of painful stimuli is perfected, the interaction of various chemicals with the macromolecular bioreceptors or enzyme systems should become more amenable to experimentation. Progress in this area will be the capstone of our understanding of pain and analgesia.

REFERENCES

1. Quoted from D. I. Macht, *J. Am. Med. Assoc.* **64**, 477 (1915).
2. H. Dreser, *Arch. Ges. Physiol.* **76**, 306 (1899).
3. H. v. Gilm, *Ann.*, **112**, 180 (1859).
4. L. Knorr, *Ber.* **16**, 2597 (1883); **17**, 2037 (1884); *Ann.* **238**, 137, 160, 203 (1887).
5. V. Hinsberg and A. Kast, *Centr. Klin. Med.* **25**, 145 (1887).
6a. A. Burger, *in* "Medicinal Chemistry" (A. Burger, ed.) pp. 341–356. Wiley (Interscience), New York, 1960.
6b. E. L. May, in "Medicinal Chemistry" (A. Burger, ed.), pp. 332–333. Wiley (Interscience), New York, 1960.
7. C. C. Pfeiffer, *Mod. Hosp.* **76**, 100 (1951).
8. N. B. Eddy, *J. Pharmacol. Exptl. Therap.* **45**, 518 (1932); E. Mosettig and A. Burger, *J. Am. Chem. Soc.* **57**, 2189 (1935); A. Burger and E. Mosettig, *ibid.*, **58**, 1570 (1936).
9. O. Eisleb and O. Schaumann, *Deut. Med. Wochschr.* **65**, 967 (1939).
10. R. Grewe, *Angew. Chem.* **59**, 194 (1947).
11. E. L. May and J. G. Murphy, *J. Org. Chem.* **20**, 257 (1955), and references 4, 5, and 6, cited therein.
12. S. E. Fullerton, E. L. May, and E. D. Becker, *J. Org. Chem.* **27**, 2144 (1962).
13. J. H. Ager, S. E. Fullerton, and E. L. May, *J. Med. Chem.* **6**, 322 (1963).
14. S. Archer, N. F. Albertson, L. S. Harris, A. K. Pierson, and J. G. Bird, *J. Med. Chem.*, **7**, 123 (1964); see also M. Gates and T. A. Montzka, *ibid.*, **7**, 127 (1964).
15. C. M. Gruber, Jr., *J. Pharmacol. Exptl. Therap.* **113**, 25 (1955).
16. A. Pohland and H. R. Sullivan, *J. Am. Chem. Soc.* **75**, 4458 (1953).
17. A. Hunger, J. Kebrle, A. Rossi, and K. Hoffmann, *Experientia* **13**, 400 (1957); *Helv. Chim. Acta* **43**, 800, 1032, 1046, 1298, 1727 (1960).
18. N. B. Eddy, *Chem. & Ind.* (*London*) p. 1462 (1959).
19. See, for example, *Abstr. Federation Meeting, Atlantic City, New Jersey, April, 1963* Sect. 48ff.

CHAPTER II

The Physiology and Pharmacology of Pain and Its Relief

CHARLES A. WINTER

MERCK INSTITUTE FOR THERAPEUTIC RESEARCH,
WEST POINT, PENNSYLVANIA

I. Introduction

"If I can ease one life the aching,
Or cool one pain, ...
I shall not live in vain."
Emily Dickinson, Part I, *Life*

The relief of pain has been a chief goal of the physician since antiquity. The complaint of pain brings more people to seek his aid than do all other causes.

Analgesia is therefore a matter of prime importance to the practicing physician and to his patients. However, in spite of the primal urgency of pain, its universality, its importance in medical practice, and the volumes devoted to its discussion, the physiology of pain is still not well understood. The spectacular advances that have been made in many fields of medical science do not have their counterpart in the field of analgesia.

It is a matter of common knowledge that some two-thirds of all the prescriptions written by American physicians are for drugs that did not exist a decade or two ago. The tranquilizers, antibiotics, corticosteroids, antihistaminics, new diuretics, antihypertensive agents, and many others now bring relief to the victims of many ills that could scarcely be dreamed of by our fathers. But all of these do not lessen the demand for relief of pain. In contrast to all this array of new drugs, the analgesics most widely used—codeine, morphine, phenacetin, aspirin—were all developed before this century.

This relative lack of progress has not been for want of trying. An acceptable substitute for the opium alkaloids is the subject of an intensive search. There is scarcely a laboratory engaged in the testing of new compounds for pharmacological activity that does not include an examination of at least some of them for analgesic action.

These efforts have permitted the introduction of a number of new compounds including pethidine[1] (*281*), methadone (*206*), *d*-propoxyphene (*97–99*), phenazocine (*67, 73, 205, 235, 242*), anileridine (*190*), and many others. However, none of these can be considered as the ideal analgesic agent. Only one of them, *d*-propoxyphene, is officially considered to be nonaddicting, and it lacks the therapeutic potency of the opium alkaloids in severe pain. An ideal agent would be effective against either mild or severe pain, it would be free from respiratory depressant or other distressing side effects, and it would be nonaddicting. None of these or other new

---

[1] The term "pethidine" is employed instead of "meperidine" because it is in more common international usage and has been proposed as the international nonproprietary name (*164*).

agents fulfill all these criteria. The search for those which will meet these exacting requirements will be facilitated as we increase our understanding of the physiology of pain, and as we develop better methods of testing new compounds.

A breakthrough in this field may come at any time, even before this review appears in print. It is possible that the recent reports on the use of narcotic antagonists as analgesics (*4, 5, 63, 110, 131, 132, 133, 144, 146, 236*) (see Chapter IV) may be the beginning of a new era in pain relief, but at the moment it is too early to be certain.

II. The Nature of Pain

A. PAIN AS A SUBJECTIVE PHENOMENON

Progress in the field of analgesia is hampered by lack of knowledge of the fundamental physiology of pain and of the mechanism by which analgesic drugs can relieve pain. Everybody knows what pain is from personal acquaintance, but none of us can define it. It is such a subjective and intimate experience that it has defied all attempts by anyone to define it to the satisfaction of others. Many have attempted to define it, as Beecher (*24*) has discussed in some detail. We come to know pain as an unpleasant experience, a punishing affliction. Yet, it is one of our most useful sensations; indeed, painful perception is essential if we are to avoid the threats of bodily injury which are ever present. This becomes evident when we consider the rare cases of individuals who lack the ability to perceive pain. Such persons have great difficulty in learning not to injure themselves—not only by exposure to external causes of trauma, but even by such simple acts as chewing food.

B. THE "STIMULUS-RESPONSE" CONCEPT

Receptors for pain are present in most areas of the body—in skin, viscera, blood vessels, skeletal muscles, the cornea, and other organs. Stimuli activating these receptors give rise to sensory impulses which must be properly integrated and translated into a perception or sensation. This is a simple "stimulus-response" concept. If pain perception involved nothing more than this, the understanding of pain mechanisms and the actions of drugs might be simpler than it has proven to be. Instead, the concept of pain involves various levels of complexity and meaning (*232*). A patient presenting a complaint of "pain" may not have any structural or functional injury threatening the organism, but the symptom may be a symbolic transformation of a threat of a different nature. Pain in this context belongs to the realm of psychiatry and will not be discussed in detail in this review.

Even "physical" pain is a complex phenomenon. Many discussions of

11

the problem of pain include only that which arises from sensory stimuli due to trauma or disease of a peripheral structure. But it should not be forgotten that a painful lesion can exist at any level of the central nervous system. Even lesions of the cerebrum may give rise to painful sensations. These may be projected by the patient to a peripheral structure, and present a difficult diagnostic problem (*26, 50*). Perhaps thorough study of such cases in the clinic, in the physiological laboratory, and at the histopathological bench would yield dividends in the furtherance of our understanding of the central mechanisms of pain.

C. THE PSYCHIC COMPONENT

Even the "stimulus-response" type of pain is more complex than is sometimes recognized. In this context, we may include pain resulting from wounds or other damage to the periphery, as well as experimental pain. If pain were merely a response to a stimulus—to a wound, for example—one might expect that a severe wound would always produce pain, and that the intensity of the pain would be related to the severity of the stimulus which caused it. Beecher (*19, 23*) has shown that in men wounded in battle, this was not the case. He was astonished to find that three-fourths of the seriously wounded did not need analgesic medication, and even refused it when offered. The degree of pain was not related to the severity of the wound. A similar blocking of pain perception has often been remarked in athletes suffering injuries during the excitement of competition.

On the other hand, post-operative patients with incisions similar to those of the wounded soldiers usually complain of severe pain and need analgesic medication. Though the condition of the wounded tissues may be similar in the two cases, the response to the stimulus is altered by the different psychic state. The soldier is relieved and happy to be away from the battle front, while the postoperative patient has been subjected to the shattering experience of major surgery. In Beecher's view the pain for which medication is needed is a combination of a response to a physical stimulus and a psychic modification of the sensation, which could better be called "suffering," in distinction from simple "pain" as a response to a stimulus, as one sees in experimental pain in man (*20*).

These observations are really not new, as the following quotations attest:

> "The history of a soldier's wound beguiles the pain of it."
> Laurence Sterne in *Tristram Shandy*, Book I (1760)
> "The labour we delight in physics pain."
> William Shakespeare in *Macbeth*

The perception of pain is modified not only by the psychic state at the moment, but also by the individual's previous history. A complete response to painful stimuli is, to some extent at least, an example of learned behavior. The experiments reported by Melzack (*174, 175*) are instructive. Dogs were reared from puppyhood to maturity in isolation. The animals were deprived of normal sensory and social experiences from the age of four weeks (weaning) to eight months. They could not see out of their cages, or come into contact with people or other dogs. Their only disturbance was the daily removal of a sliding partition to allow them to enter the freshly cleaned half of their two-compartment cage. Various tests of painful stimuli were made beginning three to five weeks after they were released into a normal environment. The restricted dogs learned only slowly or not at all to avoid a toy car which was maneuvered by the experimenter; when the car touched the animal, an electric shock was delivered. Normal litter mates learned quickly not to let the car touch them.

The restricted animals did not even withdraw from a flame touching the nose and would repeatedly sniff at it. They similarly did not give an indication of "feeling" the pain of a pin prick though localized reflex twitches were elicited. The authors concluded that behavior related to pain can not be regarded simply in terms of frequency and intensity of stimulation or of reflex responses. Perception and response to pain also involve earlier perceptual experience.

It should be clear, then, that for the response to a noxious stimulus to be perceived as pain or suffering, certain conditions have to be fulfilled. The stimulus may invoke a sensation; it may induce withdrawal or other skeletal muscle responses; it may produce reactions mediated by the autonomic nervous system. But in the sense that pain is a complaint demanding the use of medication for its relief, further processing by the central nervous system is required. This factor, which Beecher (*24*) has called "psychic reaction component" converts a simple sensation to an unsettling experience. Wolff and Goodell (*278*) also point out the dissociation of pain perception and the reaction pattern. Keats and Beecher (*130*) noted that barbiturates relieve many cases of severe pain, and related this effect to the inhibition of the psychic phase of pain experience. They compared this action to that of frontal lobotomy.

Since the reports by Gardner on the analgesic effects of auditory stimuli in dental surgery (*88, 89*), several investigators have attempted to study the mechanism underlying these observations. Gardner and his co-workers were not satisfied with the assumption that impulses in the sensory pain pathway were directly inhibited within the brain stem by the auditory impulses, but they also considered that psychological factors contributed to the effect seen. These included reduction of anxiety, distraction of attention, and suggestion by the operator.

13

When experimental pain thresholds were studied in the laboratory, auditory stimuli were found to be without effect on the threshold or upon intensity discrimination when pain was induced by the Hardy-Wolff-Goodell (*108*) procedure in human subjects (*38*). Nor did noise affect the threshold for sensation induced by electric stimuli to the teeth (*39*). The pain produced by immersion of the fingers in ice water was also not significantly affected by auditory stimuli unless accompanied by suggestion (*176*). Hence, it appears that intense auditory stimulation alone does not affect pain thresholds as measured by a variety of techniques, yet under proper conditions it is capable of obtunding (in some subjects) the rather severe pain of dental drilling and extraction. When the sound stimuli were supplemented by a strong suggestion that it would abolish the pain, the threshold rose (*176*).

In experiments by Melzack and collaborators (*176*) one can not say that at any time the effect of pure auditory stimuli was studied. The subjects "concentrated on the music by tracking it with the noise-volume knob, keeping time by tapping their feet, singing out loud and so forth." So, in addition to the sound stimulation, there was a strong element of attention to divert the subject from the painful stimuli. This combination was still not enough to raise the pain threshold, unless accompanied by suggestion. On the other hand, the combination of suggestion, distraction or attention, and auditory stimulation was more effective than suggestion alone. These workers also pointed out that the results were obtained on a slowly rising pain. When painful stimuli were employed which induced an intensity of sensation rising suddenly and sharply, the pain could not be "controlled" by distraction or other means.

D. THE PAIN THRESHOLD

Sharp pain of sudden onset is a feature of cutaneous pain induced by the Hardy-Wolff-Goodell dolorimeter, and by the other means that have been commonly employed in the laboratory to produce experimental pain in man. The principal methods used have been radiant heat, electric shock, ischemic arm pain with hand clenching, and mechanical stimulation with von Frey hairs. After an exhaustive review of the relation between the analgesic action of drugs and their effect upon pain threshold in man, Beecher (*24*) concluded that "no dependable relationship has been established." A large number of studies has claimed such a relationship, but Beecher pointed out that they were all open to criticism of one sort or another, and an equally impressive number failed to demonstrate it. According to Kornetsky (*139*) the attitude of the experimenter toward the subject is an important factor. Studies on the effect of analgesic drugs upon the threshold to the "slowly rising pain" as described by Melzack (*176*) seem not to have been done.

It seems clear that the principal effect of any analgesic agent in relieving pain in man is upon the "psychic reaction component" rather than on the sensation itself. This applies whether the analgesic agent is a drug, a distracting stimulus (e.g., a strong auditory stimulus), or psychic excitement (as in an athletic contest, for example). This has been pointed out by other reviewers, but deserves restatement, for it is too often ignored by those who speak of "analgesia" and "pain threshold elevation" as though they were synonymous terms.

If this is true, one may well ask, "Is it of any value to study the responses of animals to analgesic drugs?" It is pertinent to compare the responses of human subjects and of animals as subjects in experiments on experimental pain and its modification by drugs. Powerful analgesic drugs such as morphine and pethidine relieve pain of pathological origin. They do not reliably raise pain threshold in man, but they do raise the reaction threshold in animals. The human subject exposed to experimental pain realizes that the experience poses no real threat to him, while with pathological pain the consequences are potentially serious, possibly even threatening to life itself.

An animal, on the other hand, can scarcely be expected to make such a distinction. When a potentially painful stimulus is given to an animal, the experimenter commonly takes as an end point a reflex movement of some sort. Although it can not be said with assurance that the animal "feels pain" at this point, and Benjamin (*29*) viewed threshold pain as scarcely disagreeable, the stimuli are of such a nature that if applied at sufficient intensity or for a long enough time, they presumably would cause pain. The point at which the animal responds is therefore more properly referred to as a "reaction threshold" rather than as a "pain threshold." Nevertheless, the animal makes the sort of response (tail flick, skin twitch, etc.) we might expect him to make if he *did* feel pain.

It is not unreasonable to assume that a sensation is evoked; if this sensation is a perceptual response to a stimulus that can be characterized as "nociceptive," a distinction between it and "pain" is uncertain and arbitrary. Since the animal has no way of knowing that this stimulus is any different from one which is really threatening, the same reaction factors may be involved in experimental and pathological pain. As Beecher (*24*) puts it, "Pain is pain to an animal, presumably, and all pain serious and significant."

Elevations in reaction thresholds in animals may therefore be regarded as very different from those in man, and as corresponding more closely to pathological pain. This may account for the fact that, although there has been much criticism of the work claiming that potent analgesics raise the

15

pain threshold in man, there is general agreement that these drugs do raise reaction thresholds in animals. A difficulty in accepting this concept arises from a common failure to show in animals analgesic effects of the salicylates and similar compounds, and of narcotic antagonists such as nalorphine. This will be discussed in a later section.

III. Stimulation of Pain Receptors

A. THE "ADEQUATE STIMULUS"

Most sensory receptors are adapted to respond most readily to a particular form of energy; e.g., the retina is far more sensitive to light than to pressure, the warmth end organs of the skin are most readily stimulated by radiant heat, etc. The form of energy to which a receptor is most responsive is termed the "adequate stimulus" for that particular organ. Pain receptors, unlike the more specialized end organs, may be activated by a variety of stimuli, including radiant heat, extreme cold, electrical impulses, cutting or tearing of certain tissues, stretching or other deformations, pressure, and chemical insult. In general, painful sensations are elicited by all these means in healthy tissues only if the stimulus is relatively strong: for example, weak pressure elicits a sensation of touch, and strong pressure is required to produce pain; the warmth end organs of the skin are some 2000 times as sensitive to heat as are the pain receptors.

The stimuli which evoke pain have one thing in common: they threaten damage to the organism. Hence, the pain receptors are called "nociceptors" —a term introduced by Sherrington (211). A nociceptive stimulus is therefore the "adequate stimulus" for the pain receptors.

Most of the research on pain has been done with cutaneous pain. Most cutaneous sensations are punctiform in distribution; that is, there are spots that respond to a warm stimulus but not to cold, others to cold but not to warmth, still others to pressure, etc. Pain, on the other hand, can be elicited from almost every point in the skin, although there are some "analgesic areas." For this reason, it is often questioned whether pain is actually a separate modality of sensation. If by sensory modality we mean "a subjectively distinctive response to stimulation" (204), pain can well be classified as a separate modality.

Pain receptors are generally considered to be fine free nerve endings without specialized structures. Sensitivity to pain is present not only in the skin, but in the mucous membranes lining the external orifices, in blood vessels, skeletal muscles, joints, the cornea, peritoneum, and many other structures. The axons of pain fibers are richly branched, and the branches of a single axon interconnect to form a net. Branches from different axons overlap and interlace, but do not form a syncytium; i.e., there is no protoplasmic connection between different axons.

Although we have spoken of pain as a sensory modality, and of potentially damaging assault as the stimulus for pain, it must not be concluded that all pain has the same quality, or that pain receptors in different organs are equally sensitive to the same sort of stimuli. Cutting the skin is usually painful, but not cutting the intestine; on the other hand, the skin will stand considerable traction without pain, but traction on the intestine is painful (57). Even though cutaneous and visceral pain may differ in quality, experimentally induced pain of either type is said to show the same relationship between intensity of stimulus and duration required to produce a response (156).

Pressure on nerves is commonly supposed to be a common cause of spontaneous pain in various disease states, and such pains as those experienced in sciatic pains are often attributed to "pressure on nerve roots." Kelly (135) argues, however, that this has not been proven. He points out that tumors of nerve trunk or cord are often painless; rather, pressure is a secondary factor which operates only when tissues are already hyperalgesic. Regardless of the merit of the contention that pathological processes may cause pain by pressure on nerves, there is no doubt that pain receptors in many areas may be stimulated by strong pressure externally applied. Pressure on deep fascia and periosteum is painful, but the extreme pressure of clamping the gut is not. De Jong and Cullen (62) noted that on rare occasions clamping, cutting, and ligation of the sciatic nerve during amputation leads to pain even in the presence of an otherwise satisfactory spinal block. Sufficiently strong stimuli can stimulate nerve trunks, though the nerve endings are probably more sensitive.

B. Qualities of Pain

It is clear that receptors for pain in different areas are differentially sensitive to diverse types of stimuli. The quality of the pain engendered is also varied. Indeed, the quality and time course of pain depends not only upon the region or organ stimulated, but sometimes upon intensity or duration of stimulus, and upon what other sensory structures are simultaneously stimulated. So varied are the qualities of pain that many words have been used to describe them, and a number of different classifications have been proposed. A needle prick on the skin produces a brief flash of pain aptly called "pricking." If it seems to go deeper, it may be referred to as "stabbing." The same stimulus applied over a longer time may be referred to as "burning," though no heat is involved. Cutaneous pain may be "bright" or "dull" depending upon whether it is brief and superficial, or

17

is a more diffuse type elicited by stimulation of the deeper layers by prolonged pinching, for example.

Pain of this kind is usually localized and involves relatively little emotional concern or affect. If the pain is deeper, or if there is visceral pain, it is frequently accompanied by autonomic responses—sweating, fall in blood pressure, nausea. It may then be diffuse or vaguely localized, and strongly tinged with affect. These two manifestations have long been termed "epicritic" and "protopathic," respectively—terms that are not in general favor now, though some modern authors still find them useful (90). Pfeiffer (193) suggested that pain be classified in three categories: the superficial epicritic pain he termed "supain"; the duller aching protopathic type he called "deepain"; a third type with an all-or-nothing character, apparently mediated by fibers in the sympathetic system and exemplified by pain in the nail bed was designated "sympain." He illustrated the difference in these types by their differential responses to analgesic drugs when the pain was experimentally induced. This classification, though often cited, has not been widely adopted.

IV. The "Pain Substance"

Since pain receptors may be activated by a wide variety of stimuli—mechanical, thermal, electrical, or chemical—it has occurred to many investigators to inquire whether the actual stimulus to the receptor or nerve is a chemical substance formed or released by these various disturbances of the tissue.

One of the first of these was Lewis' classic analysis of ischemic muscle pain (152). When the circulation was occluded in the forearm of a subject gripping an ergograph once each second, pain soon appeared, and became severe in 60 to 90 seconds. The onset of the pain was remarkably constant. It remained between contractions, so muscle tension was not the direct cause. The pain continued undiminished after the exercise stopped if the occlusion remained, but disappeared within a few seconds when circulation was restored. Lewis thought that some pain factor, which he called "Factor P," arose in the muscle during the contraction process. It could stimulate pain endings only if accumulated in fairly large quantity, as it would with circulation stopped. The exercise increased the amount of Factor P until it reached a threshold level for causing pain. This pain was then continuous until the factor was eliminated by restoration of the blood supply.

These observations were further extended by Dorpat and Holmes (65). They found that pain identical in quality to ischemic muscle pain could be obtained with the circulation intact during sustained contractions, or even with intermittent contractions if continued long enough. Using muscle temperature as an index of blood flow, they found that contracted muscles exhibit a degree of ischemia proportional to the strength of the contraction. Recovery after cessation of exercise paralleled the rate of recovery from fatigue and was proportional to postcontraction blood flow. They concluded that Factor P could not be depression in muscle pH, or accumulation of carbon dioxide or lactic acid, since the time curve of their disappearance was different from that of the pain. From various considerations, they concluded that potassium released from muscle cells was Factor P.

Potassium chloride solution introduced into the skin produces pain, too, though Skouby thought that the concentrations required were so large that potassium can hardly be of significance as a mediator of pain under ordinary conditions (219). Histamine, on the other hand, was an effective pain inducer, especially if given with acetylcholine in concentrations of 10^{-8} to 10^{-5} of histamine and 10^{-6} to 10^{-5} of acetylcholine. Histamine is liberated from damaged cells, presumably occurs in areas giving rise to pain, is active in low concentrations, and "therefore may contribute in the chemical mediation of pain" (219). However, he did not conclude that histamine is the only mediator. It did not change the pain threshold for heat, nor did subliminal amounts of histamine summate with subliminal concentrations of potassium to produce pain. Small concentrations of acetylcholine, on the other hand, lowered the pain threshold for histamine, potassium, or heat. He concluded that neither histamine nor potassium is involved in the initiation of pain when heat is the stimulus.

Keele (134) also concluded, on the basis of a review of the literature, that there must be more than one chemical mediator for initiation of pain impulses. He postulated the existence of different types of receptors particularly sensitive to diverse chemical agents. "N receptors" sensitive to nicotine and acetylcholine could excite "C receptors." The C receptors could also be excited by bradykinin or serotonin, though these substances might also act without exciting C receptors. Potassium might excite all the receptors, and the nerve fiber as well. He thought it possible that all these mechanisms could be present on a single nerve fiber.

Lindahl (155), on the other hand, dismissed potassium, histamine, serotonin, acetylcholine, and a wide variety of organic metabolites as mediators of pain on the ground that the concentrations required for producing pain were invariably higher than those present in the tissues. Working with buffered acid solutions, on the other hand, he recorded pain reactions at pH values as high as 6.2, and increasing with lower pH. Since inflamed tissues may have pH as low as 5, he regarded hydrogen ions as the chemical factor in pain.

These relatively simple substances do not by any means complete the roll of chemical factors producing pain. Keele and collaborators (*6*) found that when either inflammatory exudate, whole blood, or plasma is in contact with glass, a substance soon appears which causes pain when applied to the exposed base of a cantharidin blister. This "pain-producing substance" appeared to be a polypeptide with biological and chemical properties resembling those of bradykinin, a polypeptide which Rocha e Silva (*202*) had described as a smooth muscle stimulating factor. Both Keele and Margolis (*160*) commented on the similarity between the formation of the plasma pain factor and the process of blood clotting. It was suggested (*6*) that the factor might play a role in the development of pathological pain. It might develop when plasma escapes from capillaries and makes contact with damaged tissues.

Keele's pain-producing substance was apparently considered by Lim and collaborators (*194*), to be the same as von Euler and Gaddum's substance P, though Lim seems merely to have inferred their identity, rather than proved it. Pain-producing properties were studied by injecting material intra-arterially and recording the pseudoaffective responses—vocalization, and changes in respiration and blood pressure—elicited by the injection in dogs or cats. Responses were elicited by injections into hindleg, heart, spleen, or other organs, and the preparation was considered to be analogous to visceral pain in man (*103*). Substance P and bradykinin were of nearly equal potency, requiring only about 1 μg to elicit the response. Other substance mentioned by various authors as possible pain factors—histamine, acetylcholine, serotonin, and potassium—required hundreds or thousands of times as much material to elicit comparable responses. Bradykinin was also found to be more potent than acetylcholine, histamine, or serotonin as a nociceptive when injected intradermally in guinea-pigs (*54*).

The above discussion is merely a sampling of the vast literature on the subject of a chemical mediator for the initiation of the pain impulse. More extensive bibliographies appear in the references cited, and in references *44* and *153*. It is clear that a wide variety of substances have been investigated. Tissue damage, whether by impact, cutting, burning, or more insidious pathological processes, is accompanied not only by nociception, but by vasodilatation, increased capillary permeability, edema, flare, hyperesthesia, and increased sensitivity to both nociceptive and nonnociceptive stimuli. Some of these have long been regarded as chemically mediated (e.g., Lewis' H substance). It seems not unreasonable that a pain-producing substance could be liberated under these conditions. Perhaps it need not always be the same substance. Chapman *et al.* (*44*) expressed the view that several "pain substances" may participate in initiating activity in nerve endings, though they emphasized the activity of a bradykinin-like substance which, because of its association with neurogenic vasodilatation, they called "neurokinin."

The hypothesis that a bradykinin-like substance is the chemical mediator for visceral pain would, perhaps, stand on firmer ground if intra-arterial injections of such materials produced signs of pain more reliably. In the laboratory where much of this work has been done (103), as many as one-third the animals were unaffected by the injections. This is not necessarily a fatal flaw in the hypothesis, provided it can be explained.

It may be concluded that the idea of a peripheral chemical mediator for pain has much to commend it, but it has not been proven that there is any one unique substance which has been proven to be *the* mediator.

V. Neurophysiology of Pain and Analgesia

A. PAIN RECEPTORS

The skin in some areas contains, in addition to the bare nerve endings, a variety of specialized encapsulated endings. It was long assumed that the bare endings were specific receptors for noxious stimuli and that the encapsulated endings served the other cutaneous senses. It can no longer be confidently asserted that this is true. The investigations of Weddell and collaborators (149, 150, 216, 217) demonstrated that a wide range of sensory experience including cold, heat, touch, as well as pain, could be elicited by appropriate stimulation of free nerve endings in the skin and in the cornea. Adjacent areas of the skin having different types of endings do not exhibit differential sensitivity.

These findings offer difficulties for the theory that there are specific receptors for each modality of cutaneous sensibility. The work of the Weddell group is an excellent example of carefully controlled critical experiments with well-reasoned conclusions. Their evidence led them to conclude that all the sensory qualities reported as the result of warming or cooling the skin, including pain, are the result of the activity of groups of unencapsulated nerve endings initiating action potentials which reach the central nervous system in different tempero-spatial patterns. They reject the view that the various receptors merely lower the threshold of excitability of the nerve fibers for one kind of stimulus; instead, the skin has "universal receptors." The pattern of action potentials for which these receptors are responsible is related to the way in which the stimulus affects the skin. Their findings could not support either the "law" of specific irritability of nerve fibers or the thesis that specific nerve terminals subserve specific cutaneous sensory modalities.

21

Many years before these investigations, Adrian [quoted by Sweet (231)] had noted a difference in the duration of volleys of discharges in a sensory nerve induced by strong (painful) and weak mechanical stimulation and thought it would "make for economy if one and the same nerve fiber could be used to signal nonpainful stimulation by a brief discharge and painful stimulation by a much longer one." At the time Adrian wrote (1928), it was supposed that the bare nerve endings were exclusively pain receptors. Pain, according to the newer ideas, is not represented in the periphery by its own neural apparatus as distinctive in its way as, for example, the structures for sight and hearing; as Haugen (112) puts it, the concept of specific cutaneous modalities "is held by some neurophysiologists to be a manner of speaking rather than an actuality."

B. Peripheral Nerves

Noxious stimuli applied to the skin are generally held to stimulate small myelinated A-δ fibers and the still smaller unmyelinated C fibers. These conduct at different rates, 10 meters per second or more for the former and about 0.5 to 2 meters per second for the latter. The evidence for these fibers as pain conductors has been reviewed by Sweet (231). Evidence from nerve block studies indicated that the A fibers were concerned with touch and the C fibers with pain, but this concept has also been questioned. Sinclair (217) showed that almost any order of sensory block could be obtained depending upon the subject, the site of stimulation, and the nature of the stimulus.

Many investigators have thought that a single stimulus produced an immediate pain followed by lack of sensation, then a "second pain" or "double pain." The view that two types of fibers with different velocities of conduction seem to be involved apparently provided a neural basis for double pain. This concept has also been challenged. Sinclair (217) concluded that the idea of two sets of pain fibers rests upon work which is not immune to criticism, and thought that the question of double pain has not been settled. Jones (128), using a calibrated, rigidly mounted needle algesimeter could not demonstrate double pain in normal subjects (much of the work on double pain had been done under abnormal conditions) so long as the stimulus was prevented from stimulating the same receptors more than once.

Sweet (231), after reviewing the evidence, clearly did not favor the double pain concept, and, indeed, believed the whole subject of pain conduction by nerve fibers of specific size to be worthy of careful review. Similar questions were also raised by Barber (8).

Fibers belonging to different modalities seem to be distributed throughout the various fiber sizes. But there is unquestionably a differential subjective response to various stimuli. Hence, either pain, touch, cold, and warmth may be each *separately* represented by fibers of more than one size, or, as an alternative hypothesis, each type of stimulus sets off a distinctive pattern of impulses depending upon the relative number of activated fibers of various sizes. The latter hypothesis has been suggested by a number of investigators (references in *8*, p. 431).

It has been demonstrated (*248*) that stimulation of a single hair in the rabbit ear resulted in impulses passing up several different fibers. The fibers involved were of different sizes and different rates of conduction. Hence, even the simplest kind of stimulation results in a complex pattern of nerve volleys. Weddell (*248*) pointed out that stimulation of a single hair is an unnatural occurrence and the pattern from a more physiological stimulus must be even more complex.

From this discussion it is clear that von Frey's classical codification of cutaneous sensibility, which has found its way into textbooks, has not held up under critical examination. Instead of four primary modalities—cold, warmth, touch, and pain—each ascribed specifically to the end apparatus of a particular nerve, the revised concept is that a "complex spatially and temporally dispersed pattern of impulses" (*217*) determines the subjective response. Nowhere has this been made clearer than in Lele and Weddell's study (*150*) of the cornea. All the nerves to the cornea end in fine filaments morphologically indistinguishable from one another, but all four modalities could clearly be elicited.

Somatic pain arising from deeper structures, such as muscles and tendons, apparently arises in similar endings; there are also larger C fibers present. These deep sensibilities are carried in the sensory components of the muscular nerves, and may or may not enter the cord by the same dorsal root as the fibers from the overlying skin (*282*).

Although the autonomic nervous system is generally regarded as an efferent system, there is abundant evidence of pain fibers in both sympathetic and parasympathetic nerves (*231*). DeJong and Cullen (*62*) pointed out that pain is sometimes present after low spinal anesthesia, mediated by pain fibers carried by the sympathetic trunk and entering the cord by way of a dorsal root above the level of spinal block. Pain fibers in the sympathetic trunks may arise from extremities as well as from the viscera.

C. SPINAL CORD

The delineation of the pathways followed by nociceptive impulses through the cord and the brain is complex and the reader is referred for details to standard textbooks of neuroanatomy and neurophysiology, to such reviews as those of Sweet (*231*), Barber (*8*), and Wikler (*256*), and to specialized papers such as those of White (*254*), Kennard (*136*), Yoss (*282*), Collins and Nulsen (*55*), and Bowsher (*36*).

The afferent fibers enter the cord by way of the dorsal roots and synapse in the dorsal horn. Information about the pathway from that point has been obtained by several methods, including degeneration studies after sectioning various tracts, special staining techniques, recording of action potentials during peripheral stimulation with and without interruption of pathways, and relief of pain by cordotomy.

It is commonly stated that the fibers activated by noxious stimuli cross the cord in the anterior commisure and ascend in the lateral spinothalamic tract on the opposite side. The situation is more complex than this indicates, for sectioning the lateral spinothalamic tract does not always produce analgesia as expected, and, indeed, with appropriate stimuli pain may still be elicited [literature reviewed by Barber (*8*)]. Some of the pain fibers ascend ipsilaterally, and nociceptive stimuli can, in some instances at least, activate fibers outside the anterolateral quadrant. The situation is further complicated by the fact that there are species differences, so that findings in animals are not necessarily applicable to man.

In the cat, for example, according to Kennard (*136*) transmission is chiefly by bilateral pathways, mostly in the dorsolateral region of the cord, but some in the ventral columns. Hemicordotomy or anterolateral cordotomy are said not to abolish responses to painful stimuli in the cat, dog, or monkey (cf. references cited in *163*, p. 279).

Surgical incision of the spinothalamic tract for the relief of intractable pain is often successful, or partly so, but because of the existence in many individuals of other nociceptive pathways, relief is often sought in vain (*8*, *254*). It has been suggested that sometimes when an existing pathway is interrupted, hitherto unused ones are employed (*32*, *157*).

D. Brain Stem

The spinothalamic fibers carry impulses to the nucleus ventralis posterolateralis in the thalamus; this is their classical ending, but the majority of the fibers have collaterals terminating at lower levels. Many functional systems of the brain are affected by connections in the centre median, the reticular formation, and other centers. Stimulation of the reticular activating system affects wide areas of the cerebral cortex and results in many physiological changes. The activity of this system alters synaptic transmission in sensory relays, and produces activation of the electroencephalogram, behavioral arousal, and autonomic activity. Hence, this system helps to regulate sensory transmission; it is active in the integration of the body's responses to painful stimuli; and it alerts the cerebral cortex.

At what point in this complex system the subject becomes consciously aware of pain is difficult to say. The above description is oversimplified, and much is omitted; the possible pathways at the brain stem level are multiple. Yoss (282) concluded that in the monkey, deep pain reaches consciousness at subcortical levels, presumably in the dorsal thalamus. The question is probably not solvable, and the answer is one of interpretation. As discussed above (see Section V, A), a full appreciation of "pain" depends not merely on a perception of a nociceptive stimulus, but requires integration of the highest centers.

Kerr *et al.* (137) found that when the canine tooth of the cat was stimulated, impulses could be recorded not only in the spinothalamic and reticular formation, but in central gray, central tegmental tract, and in the lemniscal tract. Both the spinothalamic and the lemniscal tracts sent projections to the cortex, and the latter could not be blocked by an analgesic mixture of nitrous oxide and oxygen. Perhaps the widespread projection of nociceptive impulses accounts for the fact that pain is not a simple sensory experience like sight or hearing, but has strong affective dimensions. One can not speak of a "pain center" in the brain. Prefrontal lobotomy is sometimes performed for intense pain; patients often report after such an operation that the sensory component of pain is still present, but it no longer bothers them [literature reviewed by Barber (8)].

E. Neural Mechanisms in Analgesia

Morphine and related drugs have very complex effects upon the spinal cord, brain stem, and cerebral cortex. Although these effects have been examined in a large number of publications, the neural mechanisms involved in analgesia are not known. The dissociation between sensory perception and affect noted after prefrontal lobotomy is also seen after treatment with opiates. Wikler (256) has commented on the similarity of effects of prefrontal lobotomy and morphine, and he suggested that opiates may interfere with reverberating activity between the frontal lobe and the diencephalon. He also suggested that these drugs may diminish the cortical excitatory state below the optimal level for precise discrimination.

In these two activities, there would be mechanisms both for obtunding the affective aspects of pain and for raising the threshold for pain at the cerebral level. Vernier's results (241) indicated that the aversive thresholds for electrical stimulation of the brain stem nuclei associated with the pain pathway were elevated by morphine in conscious monkeys. Whether this was due to decrease in electrical excitability of the regions stimulated or to depression of the activity of their connections was not determined.

Wikler (256, 258) has reviewed in detail the complex actions of morphine on the central nervous system. The effects on spinal cord reflexes vary somewhat with dose, and with the preparation used, i.e., whether the spinal cord was sectioned or intact, whether section was at a high level (e.g., C-1) or low (e.g., L-2, L-3); when the cord was intact, lesions in the brain stem also affected the result. In general, simple reflexes (e.g., the knee jerk) were little affected by the drug, but there were profound effects on multineurone reflex discharges.

Most of these studies have been performed on hind limb reflexes. In the intact animal or human in everyday life, a nociceptive stimulus to the leg may involve a very complex, well-organized withdrawal response affecting several joints. Such withdrawal responses are characterized by late asynchronous discharges superimposed on a prolonged ventral root potential. In general, flexor, cross extensor, and Philippson's reflexes are depressed by morphine in spinal animals (cf. references cited in 258, p. 171).

The considerable number of spinal reflexes depressed by opiates seems to indicate a certain nonspecificity of action. Koll et al. (138) thought that this nonspecificity was due to the use of doses higher than those required for analgesia. At low doses (0.3 to 0.4 mg/kg in spinal or decerebrate cats) a selective depressant action of morphine on spinal nociceptive pathways could be demonstrated. With only slightly larger doses (0.5 to 0.6 mg/kg) reflex arcs not specifically related to the nociceptive systems were affected.

According to Wikler and Frank (255) in the chronic spinal dog the reflexes most markedly and consistently depressed by opiates are those characterized by marked after-discharge; those unaffected or enhanced were those having little after-discharge. They interpreted this as indicating an internuncial neurone system as the locus of depressant action.

Morphine, then, may produce a direct effect on the spinal cord both by depressing activation of the nociceptive pathways and by inhibiting reflex expression of noxious stimulation. Spinal cord activity is also affected indirectly through augmentation of inhibitory mechanisms in the brain stem. Irwin et al. (118) thought that their data on the tail flick response in rats suggested an augmentation of supraspinal inhibitory mechanisms as well as a direct effect upon the reflex arc. An increase in high spinal and supraspinal inhibitory activity by morphine has also been suggested by others (163, 258, 259).

In most of these experiments, morphine was the only drug studied. Cook and Bonnycastle (56) questioned whether the action of analgesic drugs on the spinal cord was of importance in the relief of pain. They studied a number of opiates and nonopiates and found that drugs having similar analgesic actions differed in their spinal effects.

Studies of the effects of morphine and other analgesic drugs upon various regions of the brain have been more concerned with what might be considered "side effects" rather than attempting to analyze the responses of the brain to nociceptive stimuli and their modification by drugs. These include respiratory depression, blood pressure effects, bradycardia, emetic action, miosis, body temperature changes, release of pituitary hormones, both anterior and posterior, and others. These are all interesting and important activities of the compounds, and have been often reviewed (*163, 256, 259*). There is no reason to suppose that they are related directly to analgesia, and, indeed, part of the effort in finding better therapeutic agents has been spurred by the hope that such effects could be avoided.

The existence of such a wide variety of central activities of morphine and similar compounds has made the analysis of central actions very difficult. There seems to be a mixture of depressant and stimulant properties, varying with different species and with different methods of study. Neither the electrical excitability of the cortex nor its threshold for convulsant drugs seems to be altered by moderate doses of morphine (*256*, p. 446). Monnier *et al.* (*182*) found that a narcotic (pethidine) and nonnarcotic (aminopyrine) analgesic had the same effects upon nicoceptive threshold to electrodental stimulation, but opposite effects upon the midbrain reticular system. Hence, they suggested that the analgesic action of neither compound is directly related to this system. Carroll and Lim (*42*) suggested that morphine first blocks synapses in the thalamic sensory relay, with larger doses required to block those in the brain stem and spinal column.

Morphine seems not to affect primary cortical responses evoked by stimulation of the sciatic nerve, or the amplitude or latency of responses in the primary afferent pathway following toothpulp stimulation (*47*), but recruiting responses are enhanced (*47, 87*).

Sinitsin (*218*) recorded cortical and subcortical potentials of the afferent system evoked in cats by contralateral sciatic nerve stimulation. Morphine, trimeperidine, and methadone were studied—all gave similar results. The drugs did not affect conduction in the classical sensory paths. In the thalamus, potentials evoked in the lemniscus medialis and the nucleus ventralis posterolateralis were not altered, even by large doses (15 to 20 mg/kg). On the other hand, relatively small doses (0.5 to 3 mg/kg) markedly depressed responses in the associative thalamocortical projection system and in associative areas of the cortex. Sinitsin stated that analgesics did not depress the general reticular neuron system, but selectively blocked the connection of this system with the classical afferent somatosensory pathways.

Studies of this kind are difficult to perform and to interpret, but they might eventually offer some explanation for the ability of analgesic agents to relieve the anguish of pain without abolishing its perception. The effects described by Sinitsin, if confirmed, demonstrate a fundamental difference between the action of morphine-like drugs and such depressants as barbiturates and volatile anesthetics.

VI. Methods of Testing Analgesic Drugs in Animals

A. INTRODUCTION

A very large number of laboratories test new compounds for analgesic activity. When one reads the literature on analgesic testing, it sometimes seems that scarcely two workers use identical methods to elicit a response from the animals and to evaluate the data obtained. The methods employed can be classified into relatively few categories, but each procedure differs in detail from others.

Many of the papers to be mentioned in this discussion contain references to other methods, and testing procedures were especially reviewed and discussed by Goetzl *et al.* (*92*), Miller (*177*) and Beecher (*24*); hence, no attempt will be made to cover the literature completely. These authors list certain criteria which a method should fulfill if it is to meet the ideal of yielding information that can be expressed in quantitative terms on the relation between intensity of stimulus and intensity of pain experience, and hence on the extent to which a drug reduces pain. Among the criteria which have been suggested are the following.

The method should permit quantitative determination of the threshold value of the nociceptive stimulus. In man, this would usually be the lowest stimulus intensity leading to a verbal report by the subject. In animals, it would be the reaction threshold. This can be determined either by applying graded intensities of stimulation, each one for a predetermined time, or by applying a constant intensity until a response occurs. In the latter case, one obtains a reaction time or response time, but essentially it is still a threshold, obtained by temporal summation. It is important not only that threshold be obtained, but that intensities greatly in excess of the threshold should not be used, because nociceptive stimuli at threshold values approach those which cause tissue damage. On the other hand, there should be sufficient margin of safety that the increase in threshold or response time produced by moderate doses of drug can be measured.

The method should also yield quantitative information on differences in intensities of stimuli and should discriminate between graded doses of drug and between drugs of different potencies.

It has been suggested that the ideal method should be applicable to both man and animals. To the present author, this seems to be an unrealistic requirement. It needs merely to be pointed out that most workers have not been able to demonstrate reliably an increase in pain threshold after morphine in man when using a thermal method of inducing pain, but an average student in the laboratory has no difficulty doing so in animals. It is necessary, however, that the method selected for animal experiments have some predictive value in pathological pain in man. For new series of compounds, this may present difficulties, but surely a difference in response to drugs from one species to another is not unique to analgesic drugs.

Goetzl thought that a method should also be able to make a quantitative determination of the different qualities of pain. Miller pointed out that no one method could meet this criterion, since each is based on a single type of nociceptive stimulus. If the effects of drugs upon different qualities of pain were to be investigated, we might have to test a drug by a separate method for each quality.

The method should be sufficiently sensitive to reveal low grades of effect if one is not to overlook leads for new types of compounds. There is the additional practical consideration in a large screening program that there is often an insufficient supply of a new and untried compound to test by any but a sensitive method. Miller (*177*) pointed out that no method measured up well in this respect; several attempts have been made since to improve sensitivity, but much remains to be done.

A quantitative relationship between intensity of stimulus and intensity of the pain experienced is a criterion that is completely unworkable in animals, and as Beecher (*24*) points out, is of dubious value in man, since the reaction factor can not be held constant.

Most authors have been careful to designate the reactions they observe as response threshold, reaction threshold, or nociceptive threshold. There are, however, many papers which speak of "pain reaction" or even " pain sensation." In the interest of accurate terminology, this practice is to be discouraged.

Methods for testing analgesic drugs are usually classified according to the type of nociceptive stimulus used. Thus, we have thermal, electrical, mechanical and chemical methods. With the recent development of behavioral techniques, a special category for them seems warranted.

B. THERMAL METHODS

According to Beecher (*24*) the first use of heat to produce experimental pain was by Goldscheider in 1884. But the greatest impetus to the use of thermal procedures, and indeed to quantitative measurement of pain threshold in general, was the introduction of the method of Hardy, Wolff, and Goodell (*107*) in 1940. Not only has an extensive series of papers come from their own laboratory based on this method, but their work has inspired many other workers to devise their own methods and modifications. Hardy, Wolff, and Goodell used human subjects (mainly themselves) but the general principal of applying sharply localized heat to elicit a response from animals has been more widely adopted than any other form of nociceptive stimulus. These have been so thoroughly reviewed and discussed by Beecher (24) that no more than a general survey will be attempted here.

The use of thermal stimuli permits quantitative determination of threshold values. The amount of energy delivered by the apparatus to produce the heat can be readily measured and easily varied, but the actual stimulus, which is the energy absorbed by the mechanism initiating the response of the organism, can not be measured. The relation of energy delivered by the apparatus to the surface of the skin and that reaching the reactive site will vary somewhat depending upon the homeostatic mechanisms (e.g., local circulation) of the area. The energy delivered to the skin can be measured by a radiometer (107), and if one can assume that rise in skin temperature is a function of the radiant energy absorbed and that there is a linear transfer of heat from the skin surface to the receptors, then it follows that barring changes in circulation in the area, the stimulus to the receptors will be a function of the wattage input into the heat lamp (27).

The threshold value is a function of the energy produced by the apparatus, and the effect of an analgesic drug is to increase the amount of energy required to attain the raised threshold. In a properly designed test procedure, the amount of energy delivered to the test area does not damage the tissue noticeably, so that the stimulation can be repeated upon identical areas with reproducible results.

To attain the reaction threshold, the skin temperature must be elevated to a point where a response is induced. Factors which may influence this point are: (i) the absolute temperature attained; (ii) the degree of rise above the resting level; (iii) the rate of temperature change; (iv) the temperature gradient across the skin to the level of the receptors; and (v) the temperature difference between adjacent areas. Not all of these factors have been thoroughly studied, but Hardy (109) found that the pain threshold in man was the same regardless of the rate of temperature increase. The mean threshold temperature was 45.5° C for rates of increase which gave rise to reports of pain within a range of about 3.5 to 30 seconds. At slower rates, this temperature was not attained and pain was not reported.

Furthermore, the same relationship held for the pain threshold in normal human subjects, for reaction threshold in a paraplegic subject, for the rat tail-flick, and for the contraction of the cutaneous maximus muscle in the guinea pig. This critical skin temperature for nociception is the same as the minimal temperature for gross tissue damage, with the important difference that the latter requires maintenance of this temperature for several hours.

Analgesic drugs of the morphine class produce changes in skin temperature which vary with the species. In the dog, moderate doses lower skin temperature, and much of the rise in reaction threshold after drug can be accounted for by this change (274). In the rat, on the other hand, the tail skin temperature is elevated by analgesic doses of morphine, so the prolongation of reaction time is entirely due to the increased temperature of reaction induced by the drug (274).

The original Hardy-Wolff-Goodell procedure used radiant heat from a lamp at a fixed duration of 3 seconds. The intensity was increased until the subject felt a sharp stab of pain at exactly the end of the 3-second exposure. This was the "threshold pain." Some of the modifications of the method have applied heat by conduction instead of radiation. Some have used fixed intensity with variable duration.

Among the first to apply these findings to the study of analgesic drugs were D'Amour and Smith (58) in rats and Andrews and Workman (3) in dogs. Some modification of the D'Amour-Smith method is still probably the most widely used technique for testing new compounds.

D'Amour and Smith focused the light rays from a light bulb on the tip of a rat's tail, and the intensity was adjusted so that a sudden flick of the tail occurred in about 5 seconds. The criterion for the action of an analgesic drug was failure of the animal to move the tail. In a subsequent paper (224) this was modified by the use of a point system so that graded effects of a drug could be expressed. Although three determinations were made after drug administration, only one—the highest—was used to determine an animal's score. These authors introduced the use of a "cut-off" time, and any animal not responding in 10 seconds was judged to have complete analgesia. This practice has been generally followed since then, and is a necessary precaution if repeated measurements are to be made, for tissue damage produced by longer exposure affects subsequent readings.

Although the necessity for having some sort of cut-off time has been recognized by all those using the fixed-intensity variable-duration technique, not all have used the 10-second cut-off. For example, Bavin et al. (12), using the same 5-second predrug average response time, used 12 seconds for the cut-off, while Davies et al. (59) used 15 seconds. Davies further modified the procedure by using a red hot wire $\frac{1}{8}$ inch below the tail as the source of heat instead of a lamp. Even a cut-off time as long as 30 seconds has been used (168). Most workers have felt that this would be too long a duration; and in our own laboratory we adopted a cut-off time of 10 seconds (with predrug reaction time of 4–5 seconds) after finding that a 15-second cut-off time introduced undesired irregularities in subsequent responses. Bonny-castle and Ipsen (*34*) determined the mean pre-drug reaction time and set a cut-off time 2.3 standard deviations above that. The extra labor involved in this refinement does not seem to add a proportionately greater precision to the assay. Carroll (*41*) thought that any thermal stimulus which induced a response would inevitably produce tissue injury, and that the best one could do was to adopt a cut-off time which would permit drug evaluation.

The D'Amour-Smith method has also been used in mice, with a normal reaction time 3.4 ± 0.7 seconds and a cut-off time three times the predrug reading for each animal, essentially the same as in the original method (*104*).

Hart's modification (*111*) consisted of applying a warmth stimulus to the rat's tail before applying the stimulus producing the response. This was done by keeping the lamp burning at reduced intensity and warming the tail before short-circuiting the resistance and applying the high intensity stimulus. He thought that this modification increased the reliability of the results by permitting the rat to become adapted to the sensation of warmth. However, data were not presented to demonstrate the improved reliability; indeed, he stated that his variability was greater than that reported by D'Amour and Smith.

Hart reported that consecutive observations on the same rat may vary as much as 1.7 seconds, while Bonnycastle and Leonard (*35*) recorded control reaction times ranging from 5 to 14 seconds in a single group of 18 rats. Other workers have not reported such wide variability of control data. In our own laboratory, control data from 19 groups of 6 rats each, with three successive readings about an hour apart, showed that the highest and lowest figures obtained for any rat was within 0.7 second of the average for the group in approximately 90% of the cases.

Winter and Flataker (*273*) pointed out that the observer's reaction time is an increasingly greater part of the response time recorded as stimuli of greater intensity are used. Bass and Vanderbrook (*11*) sought to eliminate this factor by installing a photocell below the tip of the rat's tail, so that the flick of the tail automatically stopped the timing circuit. This modification has been adopted by a number of workers. The results obtained appear to be no better and no worse than those achieved without this refinement.

Rat tail-flick methods more closely approaching the original Hardy-Wolff-Goodell procedure, are those employing the fixed-time variable-intensity technique, in which the threshold is obtained. Thorp (*237*) measured the threshold in terms of watts input into the lamp, with a 2-second exposure time. Criterion of response was any movement of the rat, even if the tail did not twitch. Tye and Christensen (*238*) counted the number of rats failing to respond by a tail-flick at a stimulus of 320 mcal/second/cm^2 applied for 3 seconds.

For routine use where large numbers of tests must be done, Thorp's method has the disadvantage of being more time-consuming than the simpler reaction time determination. The doses of drugs required, and the relative order of activity of various drugs, are not essentially different.

Both Tye and Thorp emphasize the necessity of "training" the rats by exposing the tail to repeated stimuli of relatively high intensity to establish the desired behavioral pattern of removing the tail within the time limit when the fixed-time variable intensity technique is used. Tye repeated this "reminder" before each determination. This seems to be a disadvantage because of the risk of tissue damage. With the reaction-time procedure, a single preliminary test of each animal's response is all the "training" necessary in most instances, in our experience.

A further modification of the tail-flick procedure employing conducted rather than radiant heat was described by Ben-Massat et al. (25) in mice and Janssen et al. (124) in rats. This consisted of dipping the tail in hot water and timing the withdrawal reaction. This method has not been widely used, so it is difficult to judge its advantages or disadvantages over the D'Amour-Smith technique, but in general it appears to be sensitive to the same drugs at about the same dose levels. A possible exception is Ben-Bassat's finding of a relatively high degree of analgesic potency for nalorphine—one-third that of morphine. This is much closer to the clinical reports by Lasagna and Beecher (144) and by Keats and Telford (131) of activity of this compound than the usual results obtained by radiant heat methods. Winter et al. (275) detected no effect of nalorphine on the response of dogs to radiant stimuli, and less than one-tenth the activity of morphine in rats (276).

The method of Andrews and Workman (3), which determined the threshold value of radiant stimuli required to produce a "skin-twitch" in the dog, has not found application as a screening procedure. If for no other reason, the expense of the animal subjects and the relatively large amount of drug needed would invalidate its routine use for this purpose. It has, however, been used in broader studies of evaluation of narcotic analgesics (189, 272, 274, 275). The skin-twitch method has been used in rats (233), and its application to guinea pigs has been thoroughly explored by Winder in a number of carefully analyzed experiments described in considerable detail in a series of articles (263–266).

The method as described by Winder seems to be less sensitive to morphine than is the D'Amour-Smith procedure. It is stated that 9 mg/kg of morphine intraperitoneally are required for a 25% rise in threshold (267, 270). With the D'Amour-Smith procedure, on the other hand, reaction time has been

33

reported to approach or attain cut-off time with only 4 mg/kg of morphine sulfate subcutaneously (*189, 272, 273*). Using a fixed-time variable-intensity modification of the D'Amour-Smith method, Thorp (*237*) obtained about 43% rise in threshold with 3.3 mg/kg of morphine subcutaneously, while Basil *et al.* (*10*) recorded 33% rise with 2.5 mg/kg subcutaneously. Part of this difference may be due to the route of administration; several authors (*53, 169, 215*) have reported morphine to be more effective when injected subcutaneously than when given intraperitoneally, a finding in agreement with data in our own laboratory. Whatever the method used or the species employed, the majority of workers who have injected morphine intraperitoneally used larger doses than most of those administering it subcutaneously.

Another method of measuring analgesic drug action by noting the response to thermal stimuli is the one generally called the "mouse hot plate" method, introduced by Woolfe and Macdonald (*280*). Mice were placed in a cylinder on a metal plate maintained at a constant temperature $\pm 0.5°$ C. Temperatures from 55° to 70° C were used in 5° steps. The animal's first sign of discomfort was to sit on its hind legs and lick or blow on its forepaws. A few seconds later, the animals would kick with the hind paws or attempt to jump out of the cylinder. Only the hind paw reaction was used for evaluation since normal mice often groom their forepaws. The criterion of the effect of an analgesic drug was the number of mice of groups of 10 which did not respond within 30 seconds exposure on the hot plate.

This method was used by Eddy and associates (*71, 72*) for testing a large number of compounds. As adapted by Eddy, the plate temperature was maintained first by a light bulb, but later by a constant temperature boiling mixture of ethyl formate and acetone at 55.8° C as described by Chen and Beckman (*46*). Reaction times were determined 5, 10, 20, 30, 45, and 60 minutes after subcutaneous injection of drug, and the area of the time-effect curve was plotted. The percentage of animals exhibiting plotted areas in excess of twice the standard deviation above an undrugged group was determined for several dose levels and the ED_{50} calculated by probit analysis. The sensitivity of this method for narcotic analgesics compares favorably with that of the D'Amour-Smith method in rats, with morphine exhibiting an ED_{50} on the order of 3 mg/kg.

C. ELECTRICAL METHODS

The use of electrical shock for producing pain in man and nociceptive responses in animals has given rise to many difficulties and inconsistencies. Beecher (*24*) has reviewed these critically and he concludes, in agreement with Hill *et al.* (*115*), that while electrical shock is easy to apply, it is most difficult to control. Even if voltage and amperage are known, biological tissues offer impedance which can not be controlled. Goetzl *et al.* (*92*) considered electrical stimulation of the tooth pulp as the nearest approach to the "ideal" algesimetric method, but they did not present data on its usefulness for demonstrating analgesic activity, and others (see reference *24*) have deemed it not sufficiently sensitive or reliable.

Thorp (*237*) attempted to use an electronic stimulator, with electrodes on the scotal sacs of rats. The intensity of the stimulus could be measured with a peak voltmeter, but the contact resistance of the electrodes was so variable that the method proved to be unreliable. More recently, Monjé and Ritter (*181*) found wide differences in pain sensitivity among subjects stimulated by induction currents on the skin, on different points, on different days, and in different test series. Nevertheless, they consider the method satisfactory for testing drugs, though they admit that reverse effects were sometimes seen and "a single series may yield fallacious results."

In spite of the irregularities in the results reported by electrical methods, reports of their use in testing drugs in animals continue to appear. Most of these relate to stimuli applied either to the tooth pulp or to the tail. The tooth pulp method is based on the often asserted proposition that pain is the only sensation arising from stimulation of the tooth. This is, at best, a doubtful assumption. It has frequently been remarked that other sensations are evoked at lower intensities than those required for pain (cf. references cited in *24*). Scott and Tempel (*207*) have recently demonstrated single unit potentials from receptors sensitive to heat, cold, and touch in the canine tooth of the cat. Warmth receptors were sensitive to a rise of $1.2°$ C. Larger thermal increments (degree not specified) sometimes led to a reflex motor response involving aversive tongue movement. Whether this latter response ("pain"?) was a result of more intense stimulation of the thermal receptors, or of specific pain receptors, was not determined. It is probably true that pain may be evoked in the tooth by a variety of stimuli if sufficiently intense, but as pointed out above, this is true of pain receptors in many areas, and is not sufficient proof that the tooth pulp is a unique pain system as is often assumed, even by such careful workers as Chin and Domino (*47*).

The tooth pulp method has also recently been applied to other species, including the guinea pig (*261*). Leaders and Keasling (*148*) compared oral and subcutaneous potencies of a number of analgesic drugs by a tooth pulp procedure in rabbits. The method seems to lack sensitivity, since the subcutaneous doses of morphine, for example, required for their study were on the order of 16 to 32 mg/kg, as judged from Fig. 1 of the paper.

A number of workers have used electrical stimulation of the tail of mice as described by Grewal (*96*). Shocks were applied once each second, and the number of shocks counted which caused the mouse to squeak. If a drugged

35

mouse required more than 3 shocks above the predrug number in the same mouse, he was rated as having analgesia. This method, also, was not very sensitive, and required "not less than 60 mice" for each dose of drug. The determination was made 15 minutes after subcutaneous injection. This is well before the peak of action of most morphine-like drugs in moderate doses, which may partly account for the irregular results.

When Charpentier (45) applied electrical shocks to the tails of rats, results were so variable that although 8 mg/kg of morphine intraperitoneally raised the threshold by 78%, the change was not statistically significant.

Some recent workers seem to have achieved fairly good results with electrical stimuli applied to the tails of mice, though in most cases it is not clear that the apparatus and technique were any different from others who had obtained less satisfactory data. Maxwell (164), for example, used a method like that of Grewal mentioned above (which had also previously been described by Burn et al., referred to by Maxwell). He obtained parallel log dose-response lines for morphine and codeine, with ED_{50} for morphine on the order of 2 mg/kg. It is not clear how many mice were required to achieve these results.

McKenzie and Beechey (169) obtained responses related to log dose, though with considerable scatter, with electrical stimuli to the tail of mice, using a 4-dose level assay and using only 6 or 7 mice per point. Each mouse was treated as an individual. The voltage was adjusted until successive pulses evoked squeak responses; the increment in this "repetition threshold" was designated as "analgesic effect." This method permitted relative potency assays between drugs, but lacked sensitivity; it is rather puzzling why these authors required 10 mg/kg or morphine subcutaneously to obtain a barely detectable response.

Nilsen (185) inserted the electrodes in the mouse's tail beneath the skin. But even though this might be expected to decrease variability, evidently it did not, as he commented on the extreme individual variation. Significant changes in threshold were found in different parts of the tail, with sensitivity increasing toward the base. Significant, and in many cases very large, threshold differences were also associated with age, sex, and the strain of mouse. Mice also became more sensitive after the first stimulation of the day, but thereafter remained relatively constant. Responses to analgesic drugs varied greatly with the predrug threshold, those with lower thresholds being more sensitive. It is difficult to judge the practicability of this method, since the data listed were obviously pooled from a large and variable number of experiments (e.g., the dose-response curve for codeine was obtained from responses to 3 doses, with 70, 1267, and 35 animals, respectively).

It is apparent that there are a great many variables to be controlled, that there has not been uniform success in controlling them, and that no electrical stimulation technique has been proved to be the "ideal" testing method for analgesic drugs.

D. MECHANICAL METHODS

The deformation of tissue by pressure dependably induces pain responses. In the skin, this may be done by fine needle-like points or by gross pressure; in the hollow viscera, it takes the form of distention by balloon. All of these methods have been used with many modifications in man, but in animals most of the observations have been done with gross pressure (see Beecher's review, 24).

Methods using pressure on the tails of animals such as the classical Haffner (105) and Eddy (69) techniques were in use before the Hardy-Wolff-Goodell procedure gave such prominence to the employment of thermal stimuli. They were hampered by lack of precision, and some of the more recent modifications have attempted to improve the methods in this respect. Another drawback is that pressure sufficient to attain the nociceptive threshold sometimes renders the tail tender so that subsequent determinations are affected. A pressure method, to be of general usefulness, should be designed with this in mind.

The criterion of having attained the nociceptive threshold is usually vocalization. In rats, this takes the form of a brief, just audible squeak, and the procedure is sometimes called the "squeak threshold" method. The neural mechanisms involved in vocalization are different from those in the heat-induced tail-flick. The latter can be elicited in spinal rats (118), although there are differences in tail flicks of spinal and intact animals (273). Vocalization, on the other hand, disappears after midbrain section; Guzman et al. (103) regarded vocalization as the most specific central indicator of pain in animals. Benjamin (28) regarded all the usual endpoints used in animals—skin twitch, tail-flick, or withdrawal reaction—as side effects of pain because they are spinal reflexes, and undesirable side effects at that, for an ideal analgesic agent should eliminate pain without affecting reflex activity. It does not necessarily follow that a drug eliminating the squeak response must act on higher centers. Drugs acting peripherally at the site of stimulation might equally well raise or abolish the squeak threshold.

Two rather similar ways of using the rat squeak threshold for assaying analgesic drugs were described by Eagle and Carlson (66) and Green et al. (95). The former used a metal rod with a sharp tip directed to a point 1 cm from the base of the tail. This was connected to a scale graduated in grams of pressure in 10-g intervals. As the end point, they used the squeak, or other evidence of discomfort. Green et al. used a blunt tip, and measured

37

the pressure in centimeters of mercury to elicit a struggle or a squeak. They found the squeak threshold to be about 1.6 cm Hg higher than struggle threshold; for evaluation of drugs, they used the mean of the two thresholds. The tip of the tail was found to be more sensitive than either the middle or the base, and was used in drug evaluation. Way and his collaborators used modifications of these procedures (37, 245), as did Winder et al. (269).

There was general agreement among these authors that the method lacks precision unless young rats are used. Green et al. observed minimum variation in rats 4 to 5 weeks old, and Way specifies that the rats should weigh no more than 80 gm. Our own experience confirms this restriction. Presumably, the increasing cornification of the skin of the tail of the animal as it approaches sexual maturity renders the tail less sensitive.

If threshold determinations are to be made repeatedly with pressure at the same place on the tail, a cut-off pressure is as important as in the D'Amour-Smith procedure and for the same reason. Eagle and Carlson used 500 gm of pressure as the cut-off point, while Way, using a similar apparatus, set the cut-off at 25 gm (245) or 50 gm (37) above predrug levels, which ranged from 10 to 30 gm. There is a very large difference between these two modifications of the same procedure. Green et al. (95), using a blunt rather than a sharp point, observed that in morphinized rats a pressure 8 times threshold (cut-off pressure) caused bruising, and that repeated stimulation after morphine led to a depressed threshold after recovery from the drug. Since their control squeak thresholds were about 85 mm Hg, and the cut-off was on the order of 680 mm Hg, this is not surprising.

From these widely divergent figures for threshold and cut-off values used by different authors, it is clear that no comparison between them can be given in terms of the actual pressure used at the tissue level to initiate a response from the animal. What is missing in them, and indeed in all the pressure methods published, is an estimate of the amount of pressure actually applied to the rat's tail [or the foot in the Randall-Selitto method (see below)]. Another factor in determining threshold is the rate at which pressure is increased, and this has not been uniform among different laboratories.

In an apparatus constructed in our laboratory for testing the Green procedure with pressure exerted on about 12 sq mm of tail surface and increased at the rate of 3 mm Hg/sec, we estimated that the tissue was sustaining a pressure of 20.8 gm/sq mm of tail surface when the squeak threshold was reached. At a cut-off of 100 mm Hg, pressure was estimated to be 47.5 gm/sq mm (unpublished observations). Data are not available to compare these figures with others, since no other similar calculations have been made.

Green et al. (95) stated that when rats were tested five times at 20-minute intervals, variance between trials was not significantly greater than that between rats. Hence, there was no advantage in using a rat as his own control. Most authors have, however, compared predrug and postdrug thresholds. For predrug determinations to be valid as controls, the investigator should determine whether under his conditions the threshold remains constant. We conducted an experiment to test this. When observations were made at the same point—20 mm from the tip of the tail—at 30-minute intervals, the squeak threshold was significantly ($P = 0.05$) below control level by the third reading, and only 50% of control by the third hour. Even when a different point was used for each determination, there was nearly as marked a downward trend in threshold values (unpublished data). Hence, the decrement was due to conditioning of the animals rather than to tissue injury. However, if only two predrug readings were taken two to three hours apart, they agreed quite well, and if no more than two preinjection and two postinjection determinations were made (for example, 30 and 90 minutes after injection), the threshold was sufficiently stable for testing drugs. Indeed, the pressure method seems to be more responsive to nonnarcotic agents in our hands than is the D'Amour-Smith procedure, and it is quite rapid. Winder thoroughly established the usefulness of a thermal method in guinea pigs for the assay of analgesic drugs, but in his more recent papers, he has put major emphasis on results with the squeak threshold in rats (*270, 271*).

Collier *et al.* (*53*) applied artery clips to each toe of guinea pigs or rats and counted the squeaks. Although no threshold was obtainable since pressure was not graded, the doses of narcotic drugs needed to reduce the squeaks by 50% was not much different from doses found effective by other methods.

A modification of the pressure method that has received considerable attention is that of Randall and Selitto (*197*). An apparatus similar to that of Green *et al.* was employed, but pressure was applied to the hind paw of the rat instead of the tail. The sensitivity of the foot was increased by injection of 0.1 ml of 20% suspension of brewer's yeast. The yeast produced an inflammatory reaction, and the threshold for a struggle response from the animal was markedly reduced in the inflamed foot. Thresholds in inflamed feet were increased not only by narcotic drugs, but also by sodium salicylate and phenylbutazone. The latter are antiinflammatory drugs, and presumably reduced the amount of inflammation (though the authors did not measure foot volume). However, they expressed the opinion that the analgesic effect of these compounds could not be fully explained by the presumed antiinflammatory action, since the threshold of the inflamed foot was increased above the normal threshold of the control foot.

Salicylate and phenylbutazone did not alter the threshold of the normal foot, and Randall postulated that the drugs might have accumulated in the edema fluid and exerted a peripheral analgesic effect. Drugs such as morphine and aminopyrine also increased threshold in the normal foot, presumably due to central action.

In a subsequent study, Randall and his group (198) showed that salicylate reduced the temperature of the yeast-inflamed paw, but that this effect was not essential to the change in reaction threshold produced by the drug. This method has been further analyzed by Gilfoil et al. (91), who measured foot volume as well as reaction threshold. By injecting varying concentrations of yeast, they found a lack of strict correlation between the amount of edema and degree of hyperesthesia in the inflamed foot. The lowest concentration used, 0.1 ml of 2.5% suspension, produced an increase in foot volume as great as that of 5% suspension, but the former produced no hyperesthesia, while the latter gave a marked reduction in threshold. Aspirin in doses having no significant effect on foot volume markedly raised the reaction threshold for struggle or squeak response compared to that of the inflamed foot of the animals not receiving drug. They did not find, as Randall and Selitto (197) reported, that aspirin could increase the threshold of the inflamed foot above the normal threshold of the control foot.

One modification in the apparatus which Gilfoil et al. introduced seems to merit an investigation by others, whether using the foot or the tail for determining reaction threshold to pressure. The rat was placed in a position so that the hind legs extended over the edge of a table or platform, and hung in a vertical position in contact with a block. The plunger exerting pressure was in a horizontal position. Hence, the only pressure applied by the piston was that measured by the manometer; the weight of the plunger itself did not impinge on the tissue. Perhaps if there were better standardization of equipment in different laboratories, the wide divergences in the amount of pressure needed to reach a reaction threshold, as mentioned above, would not occur, and it would be easier to compare results from different laboratories.

It must be said, however, that all these various modifications of the pressure method yield data with potent analgesics that are not widely divergent. Morphine seems to be about as effective whether it is tested by one of these mechanical methods, by thermal procedures, or by some of the electrical stimulation procedures. The Randall-Selitto and Gilfoil et al. modifications seem to have advantages for drugs of the salicylate class, though Eagle and Carlson (66) and Way et al. (245) reported small effects for such compounds without inducing inflammation. Indeed, a few authors have made such reports using thermal stimuli, but most investigators regard thermal methods as inadequate for this class of drugs.

E. Behavioral Methods

An element of behavioral response may be present in many testing procedures, and the effect of conditioning upon results obtained has not commonly been taken into account. The "flinch-jump" method recently described by Evans (81) relies upon behavioral observations. Several procedures based upon Skinnerian operant behavior have recently yielded interesting information.

The use of operant behavioral techniques for testing analgesic drugs is relatively new. In essence, this approach consists of administering a nociceptive stimulus to the animal which can be graded in intensity from subthreshold levels to a level which becomes aversive. The animal can then reduce the intensity by an appropriate behavioral response, such as pressing a lever, to a nonaversive level. Intensity is then again gradually increased until the threshold is reached again, and the cycle is repeated. Thus, by recording the intensity of the stimulus and the responses of the animal, a record is obtained of the "aversive threshold."

This sort of behavioral schedule should not be confused with the more widely used avoidance schedules. The latter may be a "conditioned avoidance" in which, if the animal makes a behavioral response to a warning signal, the aversive stimulus does not occur. Alternatively, the warning signal may be absent but the stimulus can still be avoided; this modification was introduced by Sidman (212). In most variations of the avoidance procedure, if shock is not avoided, it is repeated until the subject presses a lever to turn off the current; if he does so, he escapes the shock.

In the aversive threshold determination, there is no warning signal, and the shock reaches an aversive level more or less insidiously. Once it is reached, it can be escaped by lever pressing. Generally, the schedule is arranged so that a number of presses (e.g twenty) are required. The stimulus can be escaped but not avoided.

A number of studies on the effect of morphine on behavior have appeared, but relatively few which have direct bearing on the antinociceptive action of the drug. Hill et al. (116) proposed that the effect of morphine on a "conditioned anxiety" response in rats might form the basis of a test for analgesic activity. Hungry rats working for food rewards by bar-pressing were given an unavoidable aversive shock after being warned by an auditory stimulus. The rats became conditioned to "expect" the shock whenever the tone sounded. After conditioning was established, the operant behavior (bar-pressing) ceased whenever the tone sounded, then resumed after the shock. Pretreatment of animals with morphine in doses below those exhibiting hypnotic and neuromuscular effects partially restored operant behavior during the tone-shock interval. The degree of restoration was related to dose within the range of 4 to 8 mg/kg of morphine subcutaneously (lower doses not tested).

An effect of morphine such as that described by Hill *et al.* could be the result of several different theoretically possible actions of the drug. It might weaken perception of the nociceptive stimulus, or in effect, reduce its effective intensity; it might suppress the psychic reaction component so that even if the subject were fully aware of the stimulus, it might be less aversive. A third alternative would be a general depression of the animal's behavior. These possibilities were examined by Milligan and Kalman (*179*). Rats were placed in two different kinds of operant situations. In the first, the animal received a cue stimulus; a press of the lever after the cue was rewarded with food. In one group the cue was electric shock; in the other group, it was a light. The aversiveness of the shock was irrelevant to the subject, who had only to distinguish whether it was given or not. In the second experiment, rats trained with shock as the cue were subjected to shocks of varying intensities.

In both experiments, a high dose of morphine, 15 mg/kg, acted as a general depressant. In the first experiment, lower doses also produced an over-all reduction when light was the cue, but an increase in nonreinforced responding (i.e., responses outside the period when food would be delivered). In the second experiment, the lower doses (5 and 10 mg/kg) permitted the animals to perform more effectively at higher shock levels than without drug. These stimuli of greater intensities had apparently lost some of their aversiveness.

The lowest dose of morphine used in these experiments was higher than those required to demonstrate antinociceptive action of the drug. It would be interesting to see what the effects would be at lower doses. The antinociceptive action of morphine in rats, as tested by the usual methods, has a relatively brief duration depending on dose. These authors did not mention how long after drug administration the effects lasted. For example, would the time of the apparent reduction of effective intensity of an aversive stimulus coincide with that of the antinociceptive action of the drug?

According to Lauener (*147*) the conditioned emotional response (CER) of rats, similar to that studied by Hill *et al.* (*116*), was unaffected by morphine in doses which did not lower over-all behavioral activity as measured by lever pressing rate. The same was true of chlorpromazine. The most effective drug in suppressing the CER, according to Lauener, was chlordiazepoxide, which is not an analgesic agent. Domino *et al.* (*64*) suggested that morphine does not depress conditioned avoidance responses, in doses not producing general depression of the organism, if responses are used which are highly resistant to extinction.

42

Although the avoidance schedules described above do not seem suitable for testing a compound specifically for the possession of antinociceptive properties, they are useful in delineating part of the behavioral activity of drugs. A modification of the avoidance schedule which may better fulfill the criteria for analgesic testing was called "fractional escape" by Weiss and Laties (*250*). Rats received brief shocks at regular intervals through a grid floor. In the absence of a behavioral response, each shock was stronger than the preceding one. Each lever press between shocks reduced shock intensity by one step. In an alternative method, shock above the aversive level was continuously applied, but lever presses reduced the intensity to a level tolerated by the animal. In a subsequent paper (*251*) the authors studied the effects of varying the interval between shocks and of changing the number of responses required to reduce the shock. The technique was applied to the study of drugs (*252*). It was found that salicylates in doses of 62.5 to 250 mg/kg or morphine in doses of 2.5 mg/kg raised the level at which the rats would maintain the intensity of the shock. Ordinary escape behavior was not affected by these doses, and sodium pentobarbital, 10 mg/kg (intraperitoneal), did not affect the shock level. The authors did not feel, however, that their data were sufficient to prove that the observed effect was an analgesic one.

The effect of drugs on the fractional escape procedure was also studied in rats by McConnell (*167*) and in monkeys by Vernier (*241*), Weitzman and Ross (*253*), and Malis (*159*). McConnell did not find a qualitative difference between morphine and chlordiazepoxide, since with both compounds the minimum effective dose raising the threshold for fractional escape also depressed continuous avoidance. Malis reported qualitative differences between morphine, meperidine, codeine, and aspirin on the one hand, and chlorpromazine and pentobarbital on the other hand.

Weitzman and Ross (*253*) presented shocks to monkeys through electrodes implanted in the trigeminal ganglion. Stimuli applied once a second were increased in intensity each 5 seconds. A response on the lever decreased the intensity by one step. The animals maintained a rather constant level of stimulation for many hours. The preparation was highly sensitive to morphine; dose-related increases in threshold were obtained with 0.125 to 0.5 mg/kg (intravenous) the latter raising the stimulus to the highest level permitted by the observer—the cut-off voltage. Although other drugs, such as sodium pentobarbital, chlorpromazine, methamphetamine, and procaine also affected performance, the effects were qualitatively different from those obtained with morphine.

Weitzman and Ross advanced the hypothesis that this procedure may have an important bearing on the study of pain threshold and its control by drugs. They point out that stimulation of the trigeminal ganglion is known to produce pain in man, and the untrained monkey's responses—withdrawal and avoidance reactions, grimacing, vocalization, and increased motor activity—appear to be nonverbal responses to "pain." When the animal permitted the stimulus to reach its maximum under the influence of the high dose of morphine, gross contractions of the facial muscles occurred with each stimulus; the animal was fully alert and reactive, but gave no evidence of discomfort. It is impossible, of course, to know what subjective sensory experience was present, so it can not be determined whether under the influence of morphine the animal did not perceive pain, or whether pain had lost its aversiveness.

The experiments by Vernier (241), also in monkeys, were similar except that electrodes were implanted in a number of subcortical areas, including nucleus ventroposteriolateralis, nucleus ventroposteriomedialis, nucleus centre median, the reticular formation, and the trigeminal ganglion. Electrical stimuli in all of these proved to be aversive when increased stepwise, and the animals turned off the current by lever pressing when the aversive threshold was reached. Morphine and anileridine raised the aversive thresholds, and the effects were qualitatively different from those of chlorpromazine and pentobarbital. The authors related the former to analgesia and the latter to a general depressant effect. The action of morphine could be reversed by nalorphine.

It is tempting to speculate that by means of such investigations, much information can be gained on the site of action of various analgesic drugs within the central nervous system. Much remains to be done before this hope can be realized. More information is also needed on the specificity of these reactions for drugs whose primary action is considered to be antinociceptive. Many different kinds of drugs should be tested. At present, the principal usefulness of behavioral techniques in the study of analgesic drugs appears to be as a tool for investigating physiological mechanisms, rather than as a primary screen for rapid evaluation of large numbers of unknown compounds.

F. TESTING OF NONNARCOTIC ANALGESICS

The proliferation of methods for testing compounds classed as "potent analgesics" attests to the difficulties that have attended the development of reliable techniques. It has been even more difficult to devise procedures to measure the antinociceptive activities of compounds which do not share the properties associated with the opium alkaloids and their synthetic substitutes.

The nonnarcotic analgesics differ greatly in their chemical structure and pharmacological activities. Many possess antipyretic and antiinflammatory properties, but these do not seem to account for their antinociceptive abilities. As Randall (*199*) points out, the pharmacological properties of these compounds overlap, so they are usually classified by chemical structure. They include aspirin and its analogs, aniline derivatives such as acetophenetidin, pyrazole derivatives including aminopyrine and phenylbutazone, *d*-propoxyphene, and various muscle relaxants and tranquilizers.

To this group probably should be added the narcotic antagonists which have recently been reported to be analgesic in man (*63, 110, 131, 132, 133, 144, 146*). These compounds are chemically related to narcotic analgesics, such as morphine and phenazocine, but their analgesic activity was discovered in man, not in animals, and testing methods adequately demonstrating antinociceptive activity of these compounds in animals have not appeared in the literature.

Aminopyrine and *d*-propoxyphene are compounds which give positive results with some of the testing methods mentioned above, but it has been more difficult to devise methods that will dependably demonstrate activity of compounds of the salicylate class. Winder (*268*) has given a thorough review of attempts to do so. As he points out, small antinociceptive effects of salicylates have been seen when radiant heat techniques or the rat tail-pinch squeak threshold procedure have been employed. But the doses required are relatively large, and not only are the effects small but frustratingly uncertain. One can observe what seems to be a response one day, and fail the next day by what seems to be an identical procedure. A common experience is illustrated by the finding of Way *et al.* (*245*), who could demonstrate an effect of aspirin by the squeak threshold method, but the effective dose for 50% of the animals was the same as the LD_{50}.

Winder (*268*) has expressed the view that analgesics of this class depend for their clinical effectiveness not on an antinociceptive action alone, but on a combination of such activity to a mild degree together with an adjunctive activity. In the case of aspirin, he proposes a suppression of the early phases of inflammation—a "preinflammatory" action—as the adjunctive property. Other adjunctive properties possessed by other mild analgesics might be antipyretic, sedative, or relaxing properties. In this view, then, if one were looking for a "super-aspirin," one might test for a compound with superiority in both antinociceptive and antiinflammatory (or antipreinflammatory) activities. Such a compound might then presumably have both central and peripheral pain-relieving properties.

In the methods most commonly used, whether thermal, mechanical, or electrical, the criterion of effectiveness is a rise in threshold of a suddenly induced pain. Most pathological pains are of more insidious origin than that;

45

many of them have inflammation of some sort as an accompanying phenomenon, perhaps largely responsible for the stimulation of the pain endings.
The Randall-Selitto technique (see Section VI, D, above) of superimposing
a pressure stimulus upon an already established inflammatory process
might well be considered as possibly antinociception with an adjunctive
antiinflammatory activity.

Winder (268) pointed out that the relative activities of various nonnarcotic analgesics reported by Randall and Selitto were close to their
clinical potencies, except for aminopyrine. Their report of a dose-related
effect of sodium salicylate within a range of 25 to 100 mg/kg, is in contrast
to the very high doses required by most methods. Essentially the same dose
range of aspirin was found effective by Williams (262) using their method.
As noted above (Section VI, D), a possible fault of the Randall-Selitto
method is that the effect of a compound on local circulation and edema
might give a false picture of the effectiveness of a compound; this objection
has been at least partly met by Gilfoil et al. (91).

Another method which has been advocated for testing nonnarcotic analgesics is based on inhibition of a "writhing syndrome." This was introduced
by Vander Wende and Margolin (239) and by Siegmund et al. (213). The
latter observed that intraperitoneal injection of 2-phenyl-1,4-benzoquinone
into mice (0.25 ml of 0.02% solution) gave rise to intermittent contractions
of the abdominal muscles, with extension of the hind legs and twisting of the
trunk. Most mice show this syndrome only occasionally, and with enormous
variation in frequency (113), so the animals require careful monitoring.
A similar syndrome can be induced by intraperitoneal injection of a variety
of other substances (68, 142, 239), and in other species (40, 142, 239).

The syndrome can be abolished or prevented by local anesthetics (213,
239) so that is probably initiated by a local action of the injected compound,
but beyond that, little is known of its mechanism. It seems not to be associated with intestinal spasm, since anticholinergic and antispasmodic drugs
will not block it (213). Nor does it seem to be due to release of serotonin or
histamine (68). According to Carroll and Lim (40) brain stem mechanisms
are involved; spinal section or decerebellation blocks the syndrome, but not
midbrain section.

The relationship of the "writhing syndrome" to nociceptive reactions
requiring analgesic drugs for their relief is questionable. It seems to be
distressingly nonspecific in its response to pharmacological agents. Although
it responds to a variety of nonnarcotic and narcotic analgesics in mice (213),
the dose of aminopyrine and of morphine effective in mice is ineffective in
rats (68). LSD, on the other hand, is effective in rats but not in mice (68).
Some antihistaminic drugs—tripelennamine (113, 213) and diphenhy-

dramine (*213*)—are reported to be active, but not chlorpheniramine (*68*). Indeed, a number of compounds of various pharmacological classes will protect against the syndrome (*113*).

The relative activities of the various nonnarcotic analgesics as tested by the writhing method often do not correspond to their clinical effectiveness. There is a large discrepancy in the relative potencies of sodium salicylate, aspirin, and salicylamide as reported by different laboratories (*113, 142, 213*). And by one method of evaluating the results (*113*), phenylbutazone is more potent than any of these. This suggests the possibility that the writhing syndrome may be in some way related to an inflammatory (or preinflammatory) state, a suggestion also made by Winder (*268*). Phenylbutazone is a potent antiinflammatory agent, but is not notable as an analgesic except in inflammatory diseases.

Emele and Shanaman (*78, 79*) sought to meet some of these objections by using bradykinin as the writhe-inducing agent, and they claim better specificity than that obtained by the use of phenylquinone. However, they tested only one species (mice), and their modification seems to exaggerate the analgesic effectiveness of phenylbutazone and imipramine, while *d*-propoxyphene was inactive by their procedure.

It may be concluded, then, that the place of the writhing test in the assay of analgesic drugs is yet to be established.

The morphine antagonists which have recently come into prominence as non-addicting analgesics present a special challenge to the pharmacologist. As mentioned above (Section VI,B), most workers have failed to demonstrate more than a slight antinociceptive action for nalorphine, though it is a potent analgesic in man.

Among the compounds of special interest in this connection are Win 20,740 and Win 20,228; these are, respectively, 2-cyclopropylmethyl-2′-hydroxy-5,9-dimethyl-6,7-benzomorphan, also known as cyclazocine, and 2-(3,3-dimethylallyl)-2′-hydroxy-5,9-dimethyl-6,7-benzomorphan, or pentazocine. A number of other similar compounds have also been studied (*5, 110, 132,* see also Chapter IV in this volume). As little as 0.25 mg of cyclazocine by mouth or by injection was found to be equal to 10 mg of morphine subcutaneously in postpartum pain (*146*) but the compound had the disadvantage of producing dysphoria and other mental effects. Pentazocine, given by injection to postoperative patients, was reported to be an analgesic in the potency range of morphine (*133*). These compounds, though they produce some morphine-like side effects, are said to be essentially nonaddicting (*110*).

Harris and Pierson (*110*) studied the antinociceptive activity of these compounds by the D'Amour-Smith technique in rats and by the Eddy-Leimbach hot plate procedure in mice. Pentazocine was inactive in the former test, and active in the latter only within the toxic range. Cyclazocine was active in both tests, but required doses which produced flaccid paralysis. Both compounds antagonized morphine, cyclazocine being more potent, and pentazocine less potent, than nalorphine.

From these and other findings, it was concluded (5, 110) that thermal methods of testing analgesic drugs have better predictive ability for addiction liability than for analgesic activity in man. It has also been postulated by Keats (132) that there is a correlation between potency as narcotic antagonists and the production of psychotomimetic effects in man.

The failure of thermal methods of testing to predict analgesic activity for these compounds, and the apparent correlation between effectiveness in such tests and addictive liability, may mean that in the future, other types of assays will prove to be more generally useful. No studies have appeared in which these compounds have been tested for antinociceptive activity in animals except by thermal methods, other than that of Evans (81) who found nalorphine to be effective in doses of 0.5 to 2 mg/kg using "flinch" and "jump" responses of rats to electrical shocks. It might be instructive to test these compounds by several different methods.

VII. Mode of Action of Analgesic Drugs

A. DISTRIBUTION OF ANALGESIC DRUGS IN THE BRAIN

More than a decade ago, Beckett (14) pointed out that theories regarding the mode of action of the potent analgesics were highly speculative, and that "a clear picture . . . is, as yet, a distant goal, despite the multitudinous array of facts which have been collected." There seems to be no reason for revising this statement, but a summary of some of the suggestions that have been made may be in order.

Van Rossum (240) has outlined the basic steps in drug action. First, the drug has to reach the direct vicinity of the receptors in adequate concentration. Second, there must be a drug-receptor interaction. Third, is the reaction of the tissue. This seems obvious, but the analysis of how these reactions occur is not easy.

In the case of morphine, for example, there seems to be no doubt that its analgesic action is exerted primarily in the brain, and probably as a result of access to relatively small regions of the brain. Extremely small amounts of morphine must be involved. Adler et al. (1) found that one hour after injection of 2 mg/kg of C^{14}-labeled morphine in rats, cerebral levels were on the order of 0.07 μg per gram of tissue, and Way and Adler (247) pointed out that even this was probably too high by several fold. Intracerebral injection of as little as 0.5 μg of morphine 2 mm under the surface of the brain prolonged the reaction time of mice on a hot plate (*170*) and Adler reported an ED_{50} of 10 $\mu g/kg$ for morphine by intraventricular injection in mice, tested by the tail-flick procedure (*2*).

The levels of several strong analgesics in the brain were very low compared to those in other tissues (*247*); a partial blood-brain barrier develops rather early in life (*143*). Some morphinan compounds, on the other hand, are said to attain concentrations in the brain much higher than in plasma (*172*). There seems to be no evidence on the question of whether or not transfer from blood to brain is achieved by an active transport system, as Davson and Pollay have suggested for some other substances (*60, 61*).

Morphine, codeine, levorphanol, methadone, and nalorphine seem to achieve rather quickly a widespread distribution in the brain (*117, 171, 178, 183, 184*). Analyses of a large number of different regions of the brain gave no indication that morphine (*183, 184*) or nalorphine (*117*) tended to concentrate in areas commonly considered as "pain pathways." Perhaps this should not be expected, for the distribution pattern is much like that described for other organic bases. These compounds have many activities in the central nervous system (CNS) besides analgesia, and must have affinities for receptors in many areas. Nor are all the binding sites necessarily concerned with physiological activity. The marked differences in pharmacological activity of the *d-* and *l-*forms of some analgesic drugs (e.g., methadone) are well known. This suggests a different receptor affinity for the isomers, but intimate details regarding differential distribution within the central nervous system are lacking.

It has been remarked that the rise and decline in CNS concentration of labeled morphine, codeine, methadone (*178*), and nalorphine (*117*) correspond in time with rise and fall in their analgesic (or antagonist) activity. On the other hand, several observations indicate that there is not always a correlation between free drug concentration in the CNS and pharmacological activity. Hug and Woods (*117*) commented on the apparent extreme rapidity with which nalorphine enters into and disappears from brain tissue. Mulé *et al.* (*184*) noted that in animals receiving both morphine and nalorphine there was a lack of correlation between the quantities of free morphine in the CNS and morphine-like pharmacological activity. Apparently the nalorphine antagonized morphine without displacing it from the CNS, though there is no certainty that displacement from specific receptor sites had not occurred. Discrepancy between brain level and pharmacological activity is also apparent from the reduction by adrenocorticotrophic hormone (ACTH) of drug-induced prolongation of the tail-flick response in rats (*273*) and the failure of ACTH to affect brain levels of drug (*1*).

Much has been learned about the distribution and metabolism of analgesic

49

agents from such studies, but we are still far from a knowledge of the specific sites of concentration of the drugs which are responsible for the desirable pharmacological properties. Quantification of drug effects at the actual receptor sites and at the molecular level is still a project for the future. Accumulation of a drug in the brain or in other tissue implies some form of binding or interaction between drug and tissue (203), but much of the binding may be nonspecific with respect to pharmacological activity.

B. THE RECEPTOR SITE

An analgesic receptor may be assumed to be a configuration of atoms, either in the cellular membrane or within the cell, arranged in such a way as to complement the structure of the analgesic drug. The receptor may be an enzyme (173). Some of the physical and chemical properties which a binding site for potent analgesics may possess have been postulated by Beckett (15–18). These have been critically discussed by others, most recently by Mellett and Woods (173). The receptor is presumed to be a charged anionic site with dimensions on the order of 6.5×8.5 Å separated from a flat surface by a cavity. The aromatic portion of the drug molecule is postulated to be attracted to the flat surface by van der Waal's forces. The basic group of the drug is attracted to the anionic site, while the cavity provides a third dimension for additional attraction.

Although these concepts may not fit all drugs with potent analgesic action, they have stimulated considerable research and form a basis for design of new drugs. Many questions remain unanswered; the specific anatomical localization of the sites which account for the response we call "analgesic" is unknown. Nor do we know whether the same sort of receptors are responsible for analgesia and for the many other pharmacological actions of morphine. The series of events in the cell which are initiated as a result of the drug-receptor interaction remains to be discovered.

C. BIOCHEMICAL CONSEQUENCES OF DRUG-RECEPTOR INTERACTION

Attempts to explain analgesic effects on the basis of such actions as changes in cholinergic mechanisms, or effects on catecholamines or oxidative enzymes, have not proven to be very fruitful. Some of the literature has been reviewed by Beckett (14) and Mellett and Woods (173).

Investigations and speculations regarding the possible role of either cholinergic or adrenergic mechanisms of pain and its relief have emerged from a number of observations, such as evidence of autonomic activation during severe pain, interactions between analgesics and autonomic agents, and the ability of morphine and other analgesics to inhibit cholinesterase (31).

Slaughter and Munsell (220) found that the action of morphine on the response threshold to tail-pinch in the cat was potentiated by prostigmine and antagonized by atropine, and they suggested possible clinical utility for prostigmine-morphine combinations. These findings were extended to man (48). Clinical advantages have also been claimed for morphine-d-amphetamine combination (82).

From such observations as those of Bernheim and of Slaughter, and others of similar nature (83), there has been a tendency for some to emphasize autonomic mechanisms in pain and in analgesia (86, 93, 94), as is exemplified by the statement, "Every modification of the neurovegetative tonus provokes a diminution of the painful perception" (86). Not all the investigators who have combined atropine and morphine have agreed with Slaughter and Munsell's results (74, 114, 151). Doses employed have varied widely, and various investigators have used different endpoints for determining morphine activity—including death (74), which can scarcely be said to have any relation to analgesia.

Compounds which have been reported to increase the activity of morphine either on response threshold of animals to nociception, or on clinical pain in man, or both, embrace a wide variety of pharmacological agents. They include central depressants and central stimulants, anticholinergics, adrenergics, ganglionic blocking agents, a variety of amines, and other kinds of drugs (74, 82, 83, 86, 93, 102, 114, 151, 158, 191, 214, 220).

Such a variety of drug interactions do not support a simple hypothesis, such as "pain is cholinergic, analgesia is adrenergic"—attributed to Pero (see reference 14)—or that analgesics are substances which antagonize acetylcholine in certain areas of the brain—attributed to Burn (see reference 14). Slomka and Schueler (223) postulated that for the morphine type of analgesia, both a sympathomimetic and a parasympathomimetic moiety must be present in the same molecule, and yet their presence does not assure activity of a given unknown compound. Blohm and Willmore (33) concluded that cholinesterase inhibition has nothing to do with morphine-like analgesia, though it might be related to side effects, since nalorphine is at least as potent an inhibitor as morphine; since the publication of their paper, it has been discovered that nalorphine is a potent analgesic in man (131).

Young et al. (283) in an attempt to find evidence for the frequent suggestion that analgesia may be related to some phase of acetylcholine metabolism, studied a number of compounds of various structures, analgesics, analgesic antagonists, and related structures, and found no correlation among central, peripheral, and anticholinesterase activities. Beecher (24, p. 130) has critically examined the evidence for participation of the autonomic nervous system in analgesia. One point which he made and which is not generally appreciated is that factors other than analgesia may be involved in a determination of pain threshold (see Section II, D). A demonstration that pain threshold is apparently elevated by physostigmine or by epinephrine, for example, is not necessarily the equivalent of proving that these compounds have a general analgesic effect.

Other biochemical changes that have been linked with the action of strong analgesics include effects on oxidative enzymes and catecholamines. Although some earlier workers reported that analgesics inhibited the uptake of oxygen by brain tissue (cf. references cited in *14*), the concentrations used were too high to be of practical significance, and Elliott *et al.* (*76*) pointed out that there is general agreement that morphine has little effect on the metabolism of brain tissue in ordinary Ringer-type solutions. They did find, however, that slices of cerebral cortex respiring in calcium-deficient solution were stimulated by potassium, and this stimulation was inhibited by morphine; morphine did not inhibit the potassium-stimulated oxygen uptake if the usual amount of calcium was present. Their results were partially at variance with those reported by Takemori (*234*), but if, indeed, these electrolytes are important for morphine action, it could indicate possible activity at the cell surface. The concentrations of morphine used by these workers were high compared to those present in the brain during analgesia.

Wang and Bain (*243, 244*) could demonstrate an action of morphine on cytochrome enzymes, but expressed their disappointment in not finding a specific step in the chain sufficiently sensitive to account for analgesic activity. During the stage of excitation in morphinized mice, brain coenzyme A and hexokinase activity are said to be increased, and the effect counteracted by levallorphan (*80*).

An implication that epinephrine or norepinephrine may be a mediator in analgesia has received some support, and sympathomimetic amines have been said to produce analgesia. References to some of the earlier work were listed by Ivy *et al.* (*123*) who reported epinephrine to be analgesic in dogs and in man. Similar reports are occasionally found in the more recent literature (*129*). Brain levels of catecholamines are said to be variously affected by analgesics (*84, 100, 195, 210, 221*).

D. N-DEALKYLATION AND ANALGESIA

Many related compounds, such as morphine, codeine, pethidine, nalorphine, and anileridine are metabolized partly by N-dealkylation. Conjugation and hydrolysis also occurs, and for those compounds with an ether linkage at the 3-position, O-dealkylation has been described. N-dealkylation has a special significance in a discussion of analgesia because of the attention which has been accorded to the hypothesis advanced by Beckett and co-workers (*17*). They postulated that the N-dealkylated product is the actual analgesic compound, and the analgesic response is initiated after the drug (morphine, for example) is adsorbed on the receptor surface and the alkyl group is removed (producing normorphine, for example).

This hypothesis has been so thoroughly reviewed and discussed by Way and Adler (*247*) that there is little to add to their discussion (in addition, they review the other metabolic pathways of morphine and its surrogates in equally thorough fashion); in the main, references listed by Way and Adler will be omitted. Beckett's hypothesis is in accord with the fact that as the size of the alkyl group increases from methyl to allyl, analgesic activity as judged from animal experiments decreases, to be replaced by morphine antagonism; the hypothesis states that larger alkyl groups are more strongly adsorbed, but less readily dealkylated.

However, nalorphine *in man* is as potent an analgesic as morphine (*131, 144*). And, according to Way and Adler, normorphine has been recovered as a biotransformation product after morphine administration only in the rat. Furthermore, it has been shown (*276*) that when a still larger alkyl group—amyl or larger—is attached to the N-position, potent analgesics are obtained according to the results of animal experiments. According to the hypothesis, these should be antagonists. Normorphine itself is antagonized by nalorphine.

Nor-compounds in general are less potent analgesics than their corresponding N-methyl congeners when injected intraperitoneally, but normorphine is highly potent when injected intracisternally. If one accepts the explanation that blood-borne normorphine gains access to the brain less readily than does the methylated compound, these observations are in accord with the hypothesis, but this is conjecture. Recently, Jóhannesson and Milthers (*126*) reported that when morphine or normorphine were given by subcutaneous or intraperitoneal route, the former induced a higher concentration in the brain, but when they were given intravenously they were found in the same concentrations in the brain. The difference in potency ratio, then, found after intraperitoneal as compared to intracisternal administration, might be due to difference in absorption rather than in transport from blood to brain. Elison *et al.* (*75*) found that when deuterium was substituted for *N*-methyl hydrogen in morphine, the compound was less readily N-demethylated than ordinary morphine, and it was less potent. However, it was also more basic, so the difference in potency could have been due to a difference in receptor affinity rather than to rate of N-demethylation.

Evidence has been obtained by Milthers (*180*) that morphine and nalorphine are dealkylated in the brain of rats. In eviscerated rats given morphine, the ratio of normorphine to morphine was higher in the brain than in the blood. On the other hand, the rat brain can also methylate normorphine to morphine. Clouet (51) administered C^{14}-labeled methionine as a methyl donor intracisternally, followed by normorphine. Labelled morphine was then isolated from the brain.

It may be concluded that although there are a number of observations in accord with Beckett's hypothesis, there are also difficulties in accepting it without alteration. It has stimulated much investigation, but the role of N-dealkylation in the mechanism of action of potent analgesics is still uncertain.

E. NONNARCOTIC ANALGESICS

The nonnarcotic analgesics are sometimes referred to as "mild" analgesics. Though they are effective in relieving pain in many instances, they seem to have a lower "ceiling" of effectiveness than the drugs of the morphine type. The distinction between "strong" and "mild" analgesics is not to be confused with distinctions in potency in terms of size of the dose required, but rather in the severity of pain which they will control. The nonnarcotic analgesics are synthetic compounds which do not induce euphoria or physical dependence such as to place them under the control of narcotic laws.

Examples of this class are the salicylates, especially acetylsalicyclic acid, acetophenetidin, aminopyrine, and phenylbutazone. These compounds are not only analgesic, but also antipyretic and antiinflammatory. Two compounds recently described, mefenamic acid (43, 271) and indomethacin (277), might be added to this group, but these are at this writing still in the experimental stage. Other nonnarcotic drugs which are sometimes used as analgesics but which lack antipyretic and antiinflammatory activity include the phenothiazine tranquilizing agents, and the newer synthetic compounds—carisoprodol (30) and phenyramidol (186). d-Propoxyphene has some properties of both narcotic and nonnarcotic analgesics; its analgesic effectiveness resembles that of the latter type and it is generally considered to be nonaddicting, though one case of addiction has been reported (77). A discussion of numerous compounds employed as nonnarcotic analgesics and a general survey of their pharmacological properties has recently been published by Randall (199). A number of reviews of salicylates have appeared including those by P. K. Smith (227, 228) and M. J. H. Smith (226).

The mechanism by which these compounds relieve pain is not clear, and the different nonnarcotics do not necessarily employ the same mechanism. Aspirin is chiefly effective against headache, rheumatic and muscular pains, and the vague discomfort accompanying minor febrile illness. Myalgia and arthralgia are frequently associated with inflammation and edema. The antiinflammatory and antiedema activity of aspirin may account in large part for the analgesic activity in such cases. The cause of the pain may be removed. It is possible that pain relief by phenylbutazone is almost entirely by such a mechanism; as pointed out by Winder (268), recent clinical literature regards phenylbutazone as an antiinflammatory agent rather than as an analgesic.

Aspirin almost certainly has analgesic effectiveness beyond that which can be accounted for by its antiinflammatory activity. It has been demonstrated to provide relief in postoperative (22), postpartum (97, 145), and chronic pain in man (192). There is much evidence that aspirin acts at a peripheral site, but it is not proven that it does not also affect to some degree the psychic reaction component of pain.

The antipyretic analgesics relieve fever, but usually have no effect on normal body temperature in moderate doses; toxic doses of salicylates induce fever, probably because of the large increase in metabolic rate which they stimulate. The occurrence of antipyresis and analgesia together has led to the suggestion that aspirin may affect the hypothalamus, but there is no evidence for such a site of action for the analgesia, and there is evidence that aspirin may have antipyretic activity independently of the hypothalamic thermoregulatory center (199, pp. 319–320).

The nonnarcotic analgesics in general exhibit a bewildering variety of pharmacological activities. O'Dell (187) sought to characterize the properties which might be helpful in giving a drug the ability to relieve pain. Though he studied a number of drugs, the parameters tested were too limited to allow conclusions as to the optimal activity profile a desirable analgesic should have. Of the drugs studied by him, phenyramidol was favored because it was said to have little "central dulling" effect; this conclusion was based upon the finding that doses required to decrease motor activity in mice were greater than those required to increase response time in mice exposed to a nociceptive thermal stimulus. On the other hand, the compound was said to have "marked centrally-induced muscle relaxant action," though the doses required for this activity were higher than those depressing voluntary activity (interpreted as "central dulling"). Hence it is not clear why central depression is said not to play an important role in the analgesic effectiveness of phenyramidol (187), while muscle relaxation resulting from interneuronal blockade is said to contribute importantly to the analgesic effect (186). The compound is also stated to be devoid of antiinflammatory activity (186), but it has been reported to relieve pain in rheumatic disorders (9). It seems reasonable to conclude that whatever the analgesic effectiveness of this compound turns out to be in the long run, its mechanism of action is still to be determined.

O'Dell did not include aspirin in his study. Possibly this was because many workers have found it difficult to demonstrate antinociceptive activity of aspirin by the techniques he used. The pharmacological effects of aspirin are many and varied (*199, 226, 227, 228*), and it probably has greater therapeutic versatility than is generally realized. Reid (*200*) relates this variety of therapeutic aptitudes to the diverse physiological effects which the compound exhibits; many of these activities appear to be peripheral and can be demonstrated *in vitro*. Unfortunately, many of these therapeutic features appear at relatively high levels of serum salicylate, with a concomitant risk of unwanted side effects.

Frommel *et al.* (*85*) have recently sought to establish aspirin as a psychopharmacological agent, with actions in various animal tests ranging all the way from chlorpromazine-like to amphetamine-like; in some tests, results after acute and subacute administration differed. The conclusions, however, are based mainly upon interactions with other psychoactive drugs, chiefly depressants; no behavioral measurements were made.

The importance of the antiinflammatory and antiedema action of aspirin as part of its analgesic effect was mentioned above. Lim (*153, 154*) views the action of nonnarcotic analgesics (or "antalgics") as being due entirely to a peripheral mechanism. The receptors for the type of pain which responds to these drugs are considered to be a part of the plexus in the blood vessels walls. The vascular receptors presumably are stimulated by the release of sensitizing substances. Aspirin and similar drugs perhaps inhibit the formation of such substances by an antiinflammatory action, and in addition, evidence has been sought by cross-circulation experiments (*154*) that response of the experimental subject to a painful substance is also blocked. Strom and Coffman (*229*) have recently described in human subjects alterations by aspirin therapy of vascular reactivity to catecholamines in skin and muscle. It is not certain that there is a relationship between these observations and Lim's hypothesis, but if they are related, it is interesting to note that Strom and Coffman observed effects in skin vessels, though Lim (*153*) regarded aspirin as ineffective in cutaneous nociception.

Winder's hypothesis (*268*) that a peripheral "antipreinflammatory" property is essential for the action of aspirin-like drugs was mentioned above (Section VI,F). In this view, the early stages of the reaction by tissue to injury are suppressed. Winder, however, does not regard this as the sole explanation for the analgesic action. He terms it an "adjunctive" action, and considers aspirin to have some central antinociceptive activity as well. This seems to be a reasonable view, when one considers other evidences that aspirin has central activities and, furthermore, compounds even more active than aspirin peripherally as antiinflammatory or antipreinflammatory agents (e.g., phenylbutazone, cortical steroids) are not notable for their analgesic activity. At least some compounds related to nonnarcotic analgesics can cross the blood-cerebrospinal fluid barrier (196), and it may be not unreasonable to assume that their analgesic activity is a combination of central and peripheral effects.

Salicylates and similar compounds have a variety of metabolic effects, besides their striking stimulation of over-all metabolic rate. Some of these have been reviewed by Smith (225). The picture, however, is rather confused since some of the compounds with similar antiinflammatory and analgesic properties have diverse biochemical effects (see also, Tables III and VIII in reference 199). Some of the enzymatic activities that have been described include inhibition of fibrinolysin, uncoupling of oxidative phosphorylation, interference with transaminase reactions, stimulation of intermediary carbohydrate metabolism, effects on sulfhydryl levels, and others. Although attempts have been made to correlate one or another of these properties with drug action, Smith (225) pointed out, quite properly, that there are many conflicting observations, and that no unifying concept has yet appeared to give an adequate explanation of the activities of salicylates or other drugs of this class.

VIII. Tolerance and Physical Dependence

This chapter is concerned with pain and its relief; hence, it is not the place to discuss tolerance, physical dependence, or the other phenomena of addiction in detail. A brief account of some aspects of these phenomena is pertinent, particularly as related to the problems encountered in the search for new antinociceptive drugs. For fuller details, the reader is referred to the many reviews of the subject, such as those of Wikler (256), Isbell and Fraser (122), Reynolds and Randall (201), Seevers and Deneau (209), and Halbach and Eddy (106). A number of shorter discussions are also available (120, 208, 257, 260).

The term *addiction* is a rather inclusive one, embracing desire for the drug, tendency to increase the dose, psychological and/or physical dependence, and detrimental effect on the individual and society [see the World Health Organization definition, quoted by Halbach and Eddy (106) and by Isbell and White (120)].[1] The production of the phenomena of addiction is

[1] Since this was written, the Expert Committee on Addiction-Producing Drugs, World Health Organization, has recommended changes in the definition (see Chapter I).

characteristic of all the "potent analgesics" whether of natural or synthetic origin, with the exception of the narcotic antagonists.

Not all the phenomena of addiction are readily subjected to quantitative measurement in animals. Tolerance and physical dependence can be determined. Demonstration of psychic dependence is more complex and difficult, but Beach (13) equated morphine-seeking behavior in morphine-dependent rats with true addiction. The behavioral technique of Weeks (249) may also prove to be useful in studying a possible "psychic" dependence in animals. In man, all the narcotic analgesics produce the entire syndrome labeled "addiction", and it is generally assumed that any compound including both tolerance and physical dependence is probably addicting in the full sense.

Compounds with chemical structures related to the narcotic analgesics but which are morphine antagonists are nonaddicting (119). On the other hand, some totally unrelated compounds such as alcohol and barbiturates are addicting, and physical dependence as exhibited by an abstinence syndrome upon withdrawal has been demonstrated (121, 122). Such drugs are outside the scope of this discussion.

Tolerance and dependence, though often linked and produced by the same drugs, are distinct phenomena, and in some respects are not interdependent (209). Tolerance refers to a decrease in effect of a drug upon repeated administration, with a requirement for larger doses to achieve the initial effect. Dependence is a latent condition, becoming manifest only when drug administration is stopped or an antagonist is given. There ensues a set of specific symptoms and signs called the abstinence syndrome or withdrawal syndrome. It is highly drug specific, and can be relieved only by administration of a drug having pharmacological properties similar to those of the drug which produced the dependence. According to Seevers and Deneau (209), dependence can be induced in only one type of cell, the neuron.

Although dependence is a central nervous system phenomenon, tolerance can be shown not only to CNS effects, but to some of the peripheral actions. Morphine tolerance does not occur to the direct stimulant and convulsant effects, and only partially to bradycardia and pupillary actions, but develops rather readily to narcosis, euphoria, analgesia, respiratory depression, emetic action, and hypothermia.

Seevers and Deneau (209) speak of acute tolerance as exemplified by the resistance to the hypotensive action of morphine in a dog which has received a single large dose an hour before the experiment. This and similar phenomena are included in the term tachyphylaxis, and is observed with many drugs. These studies were concerned with peripheral actions of the drug. Others have described acute tolerance to a variety of effects and even to the unmasking of acute physical dependence by nalorphine after single injections or infusions of morphine in the dog (*161*) and the cat (*162*). Acute tolerance is not generally observed when the usual single dose or short term therapy is given to man (*21*).

Seevers and Deneau (*209*) have pointed out that studies of acute tolerance and acute cross tolerance have no predictive value with respect to addiction liability of compounds in man. It is probably safe to say that all addicting compounds will give positive results in such tests, but so will some non-addicting substances.

Of greater interest in the present context is chronic tolerance. This can be demonstrated by relatively low repeated doses properly spaced, but more dramatically if the dose is increased as rapidly as possible. The first manifestation is a decrease in duration of action of the drug, followed by a diminished maximal response. An approximation of the initial response requires a higher dose, and as the cycle is repeated, almost complete tolerance is developed to the depressant action of a dose which would be fatal to the nontolerant individual. It is never quite complete, and massive doses can still cause death.

Tolerance and physical dependence are most readily elicited if the subjects (human or animal) are injected 1 to 4 times daily. It has been observed in the rat with only a single weekly injection; this was possibly noted by Simon and Eddy (*215*), has been observed in our laboratory (unpublished data), and is apparent to some degree in the data in D'Amour and Smith's paper (*58*). Man, monkey, and the dog exhibit tolerance most readily; with somewhat greater difficulty it can be demonstrated in the mouse, guinea pig, rabbit, and even the cat (*209*).

For a discussion of the mechanism of tolerance, the reader is referred to the reviews mentioned above, especially those by Reynolds and Randall (*201*) and Seevers and Deneau (*209*). One may summarize by saying that there appears to be a change in the cells of the nervous system, but the nature of the change is unknown. It can not be accounted for by differences in distribution or fate of the drug in the tolerant and nontolerant individual (*230, 279*). Indeed, even though equal amounts of morphine may be present in the tissues of tolerant and nontolerant animals, the latter may be deeply narcotized while the former are relatively unaffected.

Evidence is strongly against the formation of an antimorphine substance by subjects exposed to the drug; indeed, recent evidence indicates that a morphine potentiating factor may be present (*49, 140, 141*).

Axelrod (*7*) postulated that the liver enzymes which N-demethylate morphine may serve as models for analgesic drug receptors. They are inactivated by prolonged drug exposure. Reduction of enzyme activity and development of tolerance occurred in parallel fashion (*52*). It was suggested that tolerance developed because receptor sites were no longer available. This concept has been critically examined by Way and Adler (*246, 247*), and Seevers and Deneau (*209*) pointed out the limited value of peripheral tissue models in defining the characteristics of tolerance or dependence in the central nervous system.

If access to the receptors by morphine is denied by simultaneous (*188*) or prior (*209*, p. 607) administration of an antagonist, manifestations of tolerance and physical dependence are inhibited. Morphine appears to be less readily N-demethylated in the brains of tolerant than of nontolerant rats according to the results of Jóhannesson and Milthers (*127*) but this does not necesssarily prove that the receptors for N-dealkylation were not available, since nalorphine was dealkylated to the same extent in both groups of animals.

Brain cholinesterase remains unchanged by tolerance (*125*), as does serotonin and γ-aminobutyric acid (*166*). The findings reported with brain catecholamines are more complicated. During chronic morphinism, in which tolerance was induced to large doses for a prolonged period, brain catecholamines were elevated in rats (*101, 222*) but not in dogs (*101, 165*). Precipitation of abstinence signs by withdrawal or by injection of nalorphine reduced the concentration of catecholamines in the brains of dogs (*101, 165*) but not in rats (*101, 165, 222*). It has been suggested (*101, 165*) that this species difference in brain catecholamine metabolism may be related to the difference in the abstinence syndrome exhibited. The signs in dogs are predominantly excitatory, while those in rats are a mixture of excitatory and depressant phenomena. Reduction in brain dopamine also seemed to be correlated with abstinence signs in dogs (*101*).

These biochemical studies of tolerance and physical dependence have not succeeded in elucidating all the mechanisms involved in the phenomena, but they are important steps toward our eventual understanding. The final hypothesis should be able to settle once and for all whether or not tolerance and physical dependence are inextricably linked. Studies on brain biochemistry must be confined primarily to animals. Interspecies comparisons are, therefore, of importance.

Halbach and Eddy (*106*) have prepared an excellent summary of tests for physical dependence in mice, rats, rabbits, cats, dogs, monkeys, and man. The reader is referred to their review for a comparison of the responses of the various species, so far as it is known, and especially for a detailed description of the important studies in monkeys at the University of Michigan and of the methods used in man at the Addiction Research Center in Lexington, Kentucky. One of the important conclusions of these studies is that no drug has yet been found in these two centers which will suppress morphine abstinence phenomena, or which will prevent the morphine withdrawal syndrome, except those drugs which themselves will produce physical dependence.

As a result of the efforts of these groups, there are now methods which permit judgments to be made regarding the addiction liability of new compounds as they become available for study. Although the methods are expensive and time-consuming they are less so than the former requirement of years of practical use of a drug before such a judgment could be made. Perhaps as better methods are devised in lower species, they can become more useful as links in the chain, and reasonably valid predictions can be made regarding which compounds should be submitted to those centers. And, finally, if the mechanism of physical dependence were fully known, perhaps nonaddicting drugs could be designed for the relief of pain without the risk of the human waste involved in addiction.

REFERENCES*

1. T. K. Adler, H. W. Elliott, and R. George, Some factors affecting the biological disposition of small doses of morphine in rats. *J. Pharmacol. Exptl. Therap.* **120**, 475–487 (1957).
2. T. K. Adler, The comparative potencies of codeine and its demethylated metabolites after intraventricular injection in the mouse. *J. Pharmacol. Exptl. Therap.* **140**, 155–161 (1963).
3. H. L. Andrews and W. Workman, Pain threshold measurements in the dog. *J. Pharmacol. Exptl. Therap.* **73**, 99–103 (1941).
4. S. Archer, N. F. Albertson, L. S. Harris, A. K. Pierson, and J. G. Bird, Narcotic antagonists as analgesics. *Science* **137**, 541–542 (1962).
5. S. Archer, N. F. Albertson, L. S. Harris, A. K. Pierson, and J. G. Bird, Pentazocine: strong analgesics and analgesic antagonists in the benzomorphan series. *J. Med. Chem.* **7**, 123–127 (1964).
6. D. Armstrong, C. A. Keele, J. B. Jepson, and J. W. Stewart, Development of a pain-producing substance in human plasma. *Nature*, **174**, 791–792 (1954).
7. J. Axelrod, Possible mechanism of tolerance to narcotic drugs. *Science* **124**, 263–264 (1956).
8. T. X. Barber, Toward a theory of pain: relief of chronic pain by prefrontal leucotomy, opiates, placebos, and hypnosis. *Psychol. Bull.* **56**, 430–460 (1959).
9. R. C. Batterman, Utilization of phenyramidol hydrochloride for clinical analgesia. *Ann. N.Y. Acad. Sci.* **86**, 203–207 (1960).
10. B. Basil, N. D. Edge, and G. F. Somers, The pharmacology of phenadoxone or *dl*-6-morpholino-4,4-diphenyl-heptan-3-one hydrochloride. *Brit. J. Pharmacol.* **5**, 125–141 (1950).
11. W. B. Bass and M. J. Vanderbrook, A note on an improved method of analgetic evaluation. *J. Am. Pharm. Assoc. Sci. Ed.* **41**, 569–570 (1952).

* References in this chapter are listed in alphabetical order.

12. E. M. Bavin, F. J. Macrae, D. E. Seymour, and P. D. Waterhouse, The analgesic and antipyretic properties of some derivatives of salicylamide. *J. Pharm. Pharmacol.* **4**, 872–878 (1952).
13. H. D. Beach, Morphine addiction in rats. *Can. J. Psychol.* **11**, 104–112 (1957).
14. A. H. Beckett, Analgesics—a general survey. *J. Pharm. Pharmacol.* **4**, 425–447 (1952).
15. A. H. Beckett, Analgesics and their antagonists: some steric and chemical considerations. Part I. *J. Pharm. Pharmacol.* **8**, 848–859 (1956).
16. A. H. Beckett, A. F. Casy, N. J. Harper, and P. M. Phillips, Analgesics and their antagonists: some steric and chemical considerations. Part II. *J. Pharm. Pharmacol.* **8**, 860–873 (1956).
17. A. H. Beckett, A. F. Casy, and N. J. Harper, Analgesics and their antagonists: some steric and chemical considerations. Part III. *J. Pharm. Pharmacol.* **8**, 874–884 (1956).
18. A. H. Beckett, Stereochemical factors in biological activity. *Proc. Intern. Union Physiol. Sci.* **1**, Part II, 805–818 (1962).
19. H. K. Beecher, Pain in men wounded in battle. *Ann. Surg.* **123**, 96–105 (1946).
20. H. K. Beecher, Pain and some factors that modify it. *Anesthesiology* **12**, 633–641 (1951).
21. H. K. Beecher, Analgesic power and the question of "acute tolerance" to narcotics in man. *J. Pharmacol. Exptl. Therap.* **108**, 158–167 (1953).
22. H. K. Beecher, A. S. Keats, F. Mosteller, and L. Lasagna, The effectiveness of oral analgesics (morphine, codeine, acetylsalicylic acid) and the problem of placebo "reactors" and "non-reactors." *J. Pharmacol. Exptl. Therap.* **109**, 393–400 (1953).
23. H. K. Beecher, Relationship of significance of wound to the pain experienced. *J. Am. Med. Assoc.* **161**, 1609–1613 (1956).
24. H. K. Beecher, The measurement of pain. *Pharmacol. Rev.* **9**, 59–209 (1957).
25. J. Ben-Bassat, E. Peretz, and F. G. Sulman, Analgesimetry and ranking of analgesic drugs by the receptacle method. *Arch. Intern. Pharmacodyn.* **122**, 434–447 (1959).
26. M. B. Bender and R. Jaffe, Pain of cerebral origin. *Med. Clin. N. Am.* **42**, 691–700 (1958).
27. F. B. Benjamin, Pain reaction to locally applied heat. *J. Appl. Physiol.* **4**, 907–910 (1952)
28. F. B. Benjamin, Effect of aspirin on suprathreshold pain in man. *Science* **128**, 303–304 (1958).
29. F. B. Benjamin and W. M. Helvey, Iontophoresis of potassium for experimental pain endurance in man. *Proc. Soc. Exptl. Biol. Med.* **113**, 566–568 (1963).
30. F. M. Berger, M. Kletzkin, B. J. Ludwig, and S. Margolin, The history, chemistry and pharmacology of carisoprodol. *Ann. N.Y. Acad. Sci.* **86**, 90–107 (1960).
31. F. Bernheim and M. L. C. Bernheim, Action of drugs on the choline esterase of the brain. *J. Pharmacol. Exptl. Therap.* **57**, 427–436 (1936).
32. G. H. Bishop, The peripheral unit for pain. *J. Neurophysiol.* **7**, 71–80 (1944).
33. T. R. Blohm and W. G. Willmore, Effects of N-allylnormorphine on cholinesterase. *Proc. Soc. Exptl. Biol. Med.* **77**, 718–721 (1951).
34. D. D. Bonnycastle and J. Ipsen, A study of the qualitative differences in response to analgetic drugs. *Acta Pharmacol.* **6**, 333–353 (1950).
35. D. D. Bonnycastle and C. S. Leonard, An estimation of the activity of analgetic materials. *J. Pharmacol. Exptl. Therap.* **100**, 141–145 (1950).
36. D. Bowsher, Termination of the central pain pathway in man: the conscious appreciation of pain. *Brain* **80**, 606–624 (1957).
37. D. C. Brodie, E. L. Way, and G. E. Smith, Jr., A note on a modification of a method for evaluating salicyl-type analgetics. *J. Am. Pharm. Assoc. Sci. Ed.* **41**, 48–49 (1952).

38. W. Camp, R. Martin, and L. F. Chapman, Pain threshold and discrimination of pain intensity during brief exposure to intense noise. *Science* **135**, 788–789 (1962).
39. S. Carlin, W. D. Ward, A. Gershon, and R. Ingraham, Sound stimulation and its effect on dental sensation threshold. *Science* **138**, 1258–1259 (1962).
40. M. N. Carroll, Jr. and R. K. S. Lim, Mechanism of phenylquinone writhing. *Federation Proc.* **17**, 357 (1958).
41. M. N. Carroll, Jr., The effect of injury in nociceptive tests employed in analgetic assays. *Arch. Intern. Pharmacodyn.* **123**, 48–57 (1959).
42. M. N. Carroll, Jr. and R. K. S. Lim, Observations on the neuropharmacology of morphine and morphinelike analgesia. *Arch. Intern. Pharmacodyn.* **125**, 383–403 (1960).
43. L. J. Cass and W. S. Frederick, Experiments in relief of clinical pain with N-(2,3-xylyl)anthranilic acid (CI-473; mefenamic acid). *J. Pharmacol. Exptl. Therap.* **139**, 172–176 (1963).
44. L. F. Chapman, A. O. Ramos, H. Goodell, and H. G. Wolff, Neurohumoral features of afferent fibers in man. *Arch. Neurol.* **4**, 617–650 (1961).
45. J. Charpentier, Analyse de l'action de la morphine chez le rat par une nouvelle méthode quantitative. *Compt. Rend. Acad. Sci.* **255**, 2285–2287 (1962).
46. J. Y. P. Chen and H. Beckman, A satisfactory apparatus for study of analgesia in mice. *Science* **113**, 63 (1951).
47. J. H. Chin and E. F. Domino, Effects of morphine on brain potentials evoked by stimulation of the tooth pulp of the dog. *J. Pharmacol. Exptl. Therap.* **132**, 74–86 (1961).
48. E. M. Christensen and E. G. Gross, Analgesic effects in human subjects of morphine, meperidine and methadon. *J. Am. Med. Assoc.* **137**, 594–599 (1948).
49. J. Clift, J. Roush, and G. Kiplinger, Further studies on the morphine-potentiating factor (MPF) in sera of morphine-tolerant animals. *Pharmacologist* **5**, 250 (1963).
50. G. L. Clinton and M. J. Fox, Central pain syndrome. *Wisconsin Med. J.* **57**, 169–174 (1958).
51. E. H. Clouet, The methylation of nomorphine in rat brain in vivo. *Biochem. Pharmacol.* **12**, 967–972 (1963).
52. J. Cochin and J. Axelrod, Biochemical and pharmacological changes in the rat following chronic administration of morphine, nalorphine and normorphine. *J. Pharmacol. Exptl. Therap.* **125**, 105–110 (1959).
53. H. O. J. Collier, B. T. Warner, and R. J. Sherry, A multiple toe-pinch method for testing analgesic drugs. *Brit. J. Pharmacol.* **17**, 28–40 (1961).
54. H. O. J. Collier and I. R. Lee, Nociceptive responses of guinea pigs to intradermal injections of bradykinin and kallidin-10. *Brit. J. Pharmacol.* **21**, 155–164 (1963).
55. W. F. Collins and F. E. Nulsen, Studies on sensation interpreted as pain: central nervous system pathways. *Clin. Neurosurgery* **8**, 271–281 (1962).
56. L. Cook and D. D. Bonnycastle, An examination of some spinal and ganglionic actions of analgetic materials. *J. Pharmacol. Exptl. Therap.* **109**, 35–44 (1953).
57. K. B. Corbin, What is pain ? *Proc. Mayo Clinic* **31**, 205–208 (1956).
58. F. E. D'Amour and D. L. Smith, A method for determining loss of pain sensation. *J. Pharmacol. Exptl. Therap.* **72**, 74–79 (1941).
59. O. L. Davies, J. Raventós, and A. L. Walpole, A method for the evaluation of analgesic activity using rats. *Brit. J. Pharmacol.* **1**, 255–264 (1946).
60. H. Davson and M. Pollay, Influence of various drugs on the transport of ^{131}I and PAH across the cerebrospinal-fluid-blood barrier. *J. Physiol. (London)* **167**, 239–246 (1963).

61. H. Davson and M. Pollay, The turnover of ^{24}Na in the cerebrospinal fluid and its bearing on the blood-brain barrier. *J. Physiol.* (*London*) 167, 247–255 (1963).
62. R. H. De Jong and C. S. Cullen, Theoretical aspects of pain: bizarre pain phenomena during low spinal anesthesia. *Anesthesiology* 24, 628–635 (1963).
63. T. J. DeKornfeld and L. Lasagna, Win 20740, a potent new analgesic agent. *Federation Proc.* 22, 248 (1963).
64. E. F. Domino, A. J. Karoly, and E. L. Walker, Effects of various drugs on a conditioned avoidance response in dogs resistant to extinction. *J. Pharmacol. Exptl. Therap.* 141, 92–99 (1963).
65. T. L. Dorpat and T. H. Holmes, Mechanisms of skeletal muscle pain and fatigue. *Arch. Neurol. Psychiat.* 77, 628–640 (1955).
66. E. Eagle and A. J. Carlson, Toxicity, antipyretic and analgesic studies on 39 compounds including aspirin, phenacetin and 27 derivatives of carbazole and tetrahydrocarbazole. *J. Pharmacol. Exptl. Therap.* 99, 450–457 (1950).
67. J. E. Eckenhoff, Phenazocine, a new benzomorphan narcotic analgesic. *Anesthesiology* 20, 355–358 (1959).
68. E. T. Eckhardt, F. Cheplovitz, M. Lipo, and W. M. Govier, Etiology of chemically induced writhing in mouse and rat. *Proc. Soc. Exptl. Biol. Med.* 98, 186–188 (1958).
69. N. B. Eddy, Studies on morphine, codeine and their derivatives. I. General methods. *J. Pharmacol. Exptl. Therap.* 45, 339–359 (1932).
70. N. B. Eddy and B. Ahrens, Studies of morphine, codeine, and their derivatives. VI. The measurement of the central effect of codeine, dihydrocodeine, and their isomers by the use of maze-trained rats. *Am. J. Psychol.* 47, 614–623 (1935).
71. N. B. Eddy, C. F. Touchberry, and J. E. Lieberman, Synthetic analgesics. I. Methadone isomers and derivatives. *J. Pharmacol. Exptl. Therap.* 98, 121–137 (1950).
72. N. B. Eddy and D. Leimbach, Synthetic analgesics. II. Dithienylbutenyl- and dithienylbutylamines. *J. Pharmacol. Exptl. Therap.* 107, 385–393 (1953).
73. N. B. Eddy, J. G. Murphy, and E. L. May, Structures related to morphine. IX. Extension of the Grewe morphinan synthesis in the benzomorphan series and pharmacology of some benzomorphans. *J. Org. Chem.* 22, 1370–1372 (1957).
74. R. Eerola, The combined action of morphine and atropine. *Ann. Med. Exptl. Biol. Fenniae* 40, 83–90 (1962).
75. C. Elison, H. Rapoport, R. Laursen, and H. W. Elliott, Effect of deuteration of N—CH$_3$ group on potency and enzymatic N-demethylation of morphine. *Science* 134, 1078–1079 (1961).
76. H. W. Elliott, N. Kokka, and E. L. Way, Influence of calcium deficit on morphine inhibition of QO$_2$ of rat cerebral cortex slices. *Proc. Soc. Exptl. Biol. Med.* 113, 1049–1052 (1963).
77. A. Elson and E. F. Domino, Dextro propoxyphene addiction. *J. Am. Med. Assoc.* 183, 482–485 (1963).
78. J. F. Emele and J. Shanaman, Bradykinin writhing: a new analgesic testing method. *Federation Proc.* 22, 248 (1963).
79. J. F. Emele and J. Shanaman, Bradykinin writhing: a method for measuring analgesia. *Proc. Soc. Exptl. Biol. Med.* 114, 680–682 (1963).
80. C. J. Estler, Änderungen der Hexokinaseaktivität im Gehirn weisser Mäuse unter der Einwirkung zentral erregander Pharmaka. *Arch. Exptl. Pathol. Pharmakol.* 243, 292–293 (1962).
81. W. O. Evans, A new technique for the investigation of some analgesic drugs on a reflexive behavior in the rat. *Pyschopharmacologia* 2, 318–325 (1961).

82. W. O. Evans, The synergism of autonomic drugs on opiate or opiod-induced analgesia: a discussion of its potential utility. *Military Med.* **127**, 1000–1003 (1962).
83. S. Flodmark and T. Wrammer, The analgetic action of morphine, eserine and prostigmine studied by a modified Hardy-Wolff-Goodell method. *Acta Physiol. Scand.* **9**, 88–96 (1945).
84. D. X. Freedman, D. H. Fram, and N. J. Giarman, The effect of morphine on the regeneration of brain norepinephrine after reserpine. *Federation Proc.* **20**, 321 (1961).
85. E. Frommel, C. Fleury, I. von Ledebur, M. Beguin, and S. Family, The place of acetylsalicylic acid in psychopharmacology. *Arzneimittel-Forsch.* **13**, 851–856 (1963).
86. E. Frommel, D. Vincent, C. Fleury, and J. Schmidt-Ginzkey, Analgesia, neurovegetative system, cholinesterase and monoaminoxydase. *Arch. Intern. Pharmacodyn.* **139**, 470–475 (1962).
87. H. Gangloff and M. Monnier, The topical action of morphine, levorphanol (levorphan) and the morphine antagonist levallorphan on the unanesthetized rabbit's brain. *J. Pharmacol. Exptl. Therap.* **121**, 78–95 (1957).
88. W. J. Gardner and J. C. R. Licklider, Auditory analgesia in dental operations. *J. Am. Dental Assoc.* **59**, 1144–1149 (1959).
89. W. J. Gardner, J. C. R. Licklider, and A. Z. Weisz, Suppression of pain by sound. *Science* **132**, 32–33 (1960).
90. R. W. Gerard, The physiology of pain. *Ann. N. Y. Acad. Sci.* **86**, 6–12 (1960).
91. T. M. Gilfoil, I. Klavins, and L. Grumbach, Effects of acetylsalicylic acid on the edema and hyperesthesia of the experimentally inflamed rat's paw. *J. Pharmacol. Exptl. Therap.* **142**, 1–5 (1963).
92. F. R. Goetzl, D. Y. Burrill, and A. C. Ivy, A critical analysis of algesimetric methods with suggestions for a useful procedure. *Quart. Bull. Northwestern Univ. Med. School* **17**, 280–291 (1943).
93. T. Gordonoff, Pain and the vegetative nervous system. *Arch. Intern. Pharmacodyn.* **122**, 208–220 (1959).
94. T. Gordonoff, Pain and the inhibition of cholinesterase. *Farmaco (Pavia) Ed. Sci.* **17**, 364–373 (1962).
95. A. F. Green, P. A. Young, and E. I. Godfrey, A comparison of heat and pressure analgesiometric methods in rats. *Brit. J. Pharmacol.* **6**, 572–585 (1951).
96. R. S. Grewal, A method for testing analgesics in mice. *Brit. J. Pharmacol.* **7**, 433–437 (1952).
97. C. M. Gruber, Jr., E. P. King, M. M. Best, J. F. Schieve, F. Elkus, and E. J. Zmolek, Clinical bio-assay of oral analgesic activity of propoxyphene (Lilly), acetylsalicylic acid, and codeine phosphate, and observations on placebo reactions. *Arch. Intern. Pharmacodyn.* **104**, 156–166 (1956).
98. C. M. Gruber, Jr., C. L. Miller, J. Finneran, and S. M. Chernish, The effectiveness of d-propoxyphene hydrochloride and codeine phosphate, as determined by two methods of clinical testing for relief of chronic pain. *J. Pharmacol. Exptl. Therap.* **118**, 280–285 (1956).
99. C. M. Gruber, Jr., Codeine phosphate, propoxyphene hydrochloride, and placebo. *J. Am. Med. Assoc.* **164**, 966–969 (1957).
100. L. M. Gunne, Catecholamine metabolism in morphine withdrawal in the dog. *Nature* **195**, 815–816 (1962).
101. L. M. Gunne, Catecholamines and 5-hydroxytryptamine in morphine tolerance and withdrawal. *Acta Physiol. Scand.* **58**, Suppl. 204 (1963).

102. G. P. Gupta and B. N. Dhawan, Potentiation of morphine analgesia by mecamylamine. *Arch Intern. Pharmacodyn.* **134**, 54–60 (1961).

103. F. Guzman, C. Braun, and R. K. S. Lim, Visceral pain and the pseudaffective response to intra-arterial injection of bradykinin and other analgesic agents. *Arch. Intern. Pharmacodyn.* **136**, 353–384 (1962).

104. H. Haas, E. Hohagen, and G. Kollmannsperger, Vergleichende Untersuchungen mit Analgeticis. *Arzneimittel-Forsch.* **3**, 238–247 (1953).

105. F. Haffner, Experimentelle Prüfung schmerzstillender Mittel. *Deut. Med. Wochschr.* **55**, 731–733 (1929).

106. H. Halbach and N. B. Eddy, Tests for addiction (chronic intoxication) of morphine type. *Bull. World Health Organ.* **28**, 139–173 (1963).

107. J. D. Hardy, H. G. Wolff, and H. Goodell, Studies on pain. A new method for measuring pain threshold: observations on spatial summation of pain. *J. Clin. Invest.* **19**, 649–657 (1940).

108. J. D. Hardy, H. G. Wolff, and H. Goodell, "Pain Sensations and Reactions." Williams & Wilkins, Baltimore, Maryland, 1952.

109. J. D. Hardy, Pharmacodynamics of human disease. 3. The pain threshold and the nature of pain sensation. *Postgraduate Med.* **34**, 579–589 (1963).

110. L. S. Harris and A. K. Pierson, Some narcotic antagonists in the benzomorphan series. *J. Pharmacol. Exptl. Therap.* **143**, 141–148 (1964).

111. E. R. Hart, The toxicity and analgetic potency of salicylamide and certain of its derivatives as compared with established analgetic-antipyretic drugs. *J. Pharmacol. Exptl. Therap.* **89**, 205–209 (1947).

112. F. P. Haugen, Recent advances in the neurophysiology of pain. *Anesthesiology* **16**, 490–494 (1955).

113. L. C. Hendershot and J. Forsaith, Antagonism of the frequency of phenylquinone-induced writhing in the mouse by weak analgesics and non-analgesics. *J. Pharmacol. Exptl. Therap.* **125**, 237–240 (1959).

114. A. Herz, Über die Beeinflussung zentral dämpfender und erregender Morphinwirkung durch Anticholinergica, Nicotinolytica und Antihistaminica an der Ratte. *Arch. Exptl. Pathol. Pharmakol.* **241**, 236–253 (1961).

115. H. E. Hill, H. G. Flanary, C. H. Kornetsky, and A. Wikler, Relationship of electrically induced pain to the amperage and the wattage of shock stimuli . *J. Clin. Invest.* **31**, 464–472 (1952).

116. H. E. Hill, R. E. Belleville, and A. Wikler, Reduction of pain-conditioned anxiety by analgesic doses of morphine in rats. *Proc. Soc. Exptl. Biol. Med.* **86**, 881–884 (1954).

117. C. C. Hug, Jr. and L. A. Woods, Tritium-labeled nalorphine: its CNS distribution and biological fate in dogs. *J. Pharmacol. Exptl. Therap.* **142**, 248–256 (1963).

118. S. Irwin, R. W. Houde, D. R. Bennett, L. C. Hendershot, and M. H. Seevers, The effects of morphine, methadone and meperidine on some reflex responses of spinal animals to nociceptive stimulation. *J. Pharmacol. Exptl. Therap.* **101**, 132–143 (1951).

119. H. Isbell, Attempted addiction to nalorphine. *Federation Proc.* **15**, 442 (1956).

120. H. Isbell and W. M. White, Clinical characteristics of addictions. *Am. J. Med.* **14**, 558–565 (1953).

121. H. Isbell, H. F. Fraser, A. Wikler, R. E. Belleville, and A. J. Eisenman, An experimental study of the etiology of "rum fits" and delirium tremens. *Quart. J. Studies Alc.* **16**, 1–33 (1955).

122. H. Isbell and H. F. Fraser, Addiction to analgesics and barbiturates. *Pharmacol. Rev.* **2**, 355–397 (1950).

123. A. C. Ivy, F. R. Goetzl, S. C. Harris, and D. Y. Burrill, The analgesic effect of intra-carotid and intravenous injection of epinephrine in dogs and of subcutaneous injection in man. *Quart. Bull. Northwestern Univ. Med. School* **18**, 298–306 (1944).

124. P. A. J. Janssen, C. J. E. Niemegeers, and J. G. H. Dony, The inhibitory effect of Fentanyl and other morphine-like analgesics on the warm water induced tail withdrawal reflex in rats. *Arzneimittel-Forsch.* **13**, 502–507 (1963).

125. T. Jóhannesson, Morphine as an inhibitor of brain cholinesterases in morphine-tolerant and non-tolerant rats. *Acta Pharmacol. Toxicol.* **19**, 23–25 (1962).

126. T. Jóhannesson and K. Milthers, Morphine and normorphine in the brain of rats. A comparison of subcutaneous, intraperitoneal and intravenous administration. *Acta Pharmacol. Toxicol.* **19**, 241–246 (1962).

127. T. Jóhannesson and K. Milthers, The lethal action of morphine and nalorphine given jointly to morphine tolerant and non-tolerant rats. *Acta Pharmacol. Toxicol.* **20**, 80–89 (1963).

128. M. H. Jones, Second pain: fact or artifact. *Science* **124**, 442–443 (1956).

129. T. Kameyama, Studies on analgesics. VI. Analgesic activity of sympathomimetic amines and other drugs. *J. Pharm. Soc. Japan* **81**, 215–221 (1961).

130. A. S. Keats and H. K. Beecher, Pain relief with hypnotic doses of barbiturates and a hypothesis. *J. Pharmacol. Exptl. Therap.* **100**, 1–13 (1950).

131. A. S. Keats and J. Telford, Nalorphine, a potent analgesic in man. *J. Pharmacol. Exptl. Therap.* **117**, 190–196 (1956).

132. A. S. Keats and J. Telford, Narcotic antagonists as analgesics—clinical aspects. *Am. Chem. Soc. Symposium* in press.

133. A. S. Keats and J. Telford, Studies of analgesic drugs: VIII. A narcotic antagonist analgesic without psychotomimetic effects. *J. Pharmacol. Exptl. Therap.* **143**, 157–164, (1964).

134. C. A. Keele, The common chemical sense and its receptors. *Arch. Intern. Pharmacodyn.* **139**, 547–557 (1962).

135. M. Kelly, Does pressure on nerves cause pain? *Med. J. Australia* **47**, 118–121 (1960).

136. M. A. Kennard, The course of ascending fibers in the spinal cord of the cat essential to the recognition of painful stimuli. *J. Comp. Neurol.* **100**, 511–524 (1954).

137. D. I. B. Kerr, F. P. Haugen, and R. Melzack, Responses evoked in the brain stem by tooth stimulation. *Am. J. Physiol.* **183**, 253–258 (1955).

138. W. Koll, J. Haase, G. Block, and B. Mühlberg, The predilective action of small doses of morphine on nociceptive spinal reflexes of low spinal cats. *Intern. J. Neuropharmacol.* **2**, 57–65 (1963).

139. C. Kornetsky, Effects of anxiety and morphine on the anticipation and perception of painful radiant thermal stimuli. *J. Comp. Physiol. Psychol.* **47**, 130–132 (1954).

140. C. Kornetsky and G. F. Kiplinger, Potentiation of a depressant effect of morphine by sera from morphine-tolerant animals. *Federation Proc.* **21**, 418 (1962).

141. C. Kornetsky and G. F. Kiplinger, Potentiation of an effect of morphine in the rat by serum from morphine-tolerant and abstinent dogs and monkeys. *Psychopharmacologia* **4**, 66–71 (1963).

142. R. Koster, M. Anderson, and E. J. DeBeer, Acetic acid for analgesic screening. *Federation Proc.* **18**, 412 (1959).

143. H. J. Kupferberg and E. L. Way, Pharmacological basis for the increased sensitivity of the newborn rat to morphine. *J. Pharmacol. Exptl. Therap.* **141**, 105–112 (1963).

144. L. Lasagna and H. K. Beecher, The analgesic effectiveness of nalorphine and nalorphine-morphine combinations in man. *J. Pharmacol. Exptl. Therap.* **112**, 356–363 (1954).

145. L. Lasagna, The clinical measurement of pain. *Ann. N. Y. Acad. Sci.* **86**, 28–37 (1960).

146. L. Lasagna, T. J. DeKornfeld, and J. W. Pearson, The analgesic efficacy and respiratory effects in man of a benzomorphan "narcotic antagonist". *J. Pharmacol. Exptl. Therap.* **144**, 12–16, (1964).

147. H. Lauener, Conditioned suppression in rats and the effect of pharmacological agents thereon. *Pyschopharmacologia* **4**, 311–325 (1963).

148. F. E. Leaders and H. H. Keasling, Oral vs. subcutaneous potency of codeine, morphine levorphan, and anileridine as measured by rabbit toothpulp changes. *J. Pharm. Sci.* **51**, 46–49 (1962).

149. P. P. Lele, G. Weddell, and C. M. Williams, The relationship between heat transfer, skin temperature, and cutaneous sensibility. *J. Physiol. (London)* **126**, 206–234 (1954).

150. P. P. Lele and G. Weddell, The relationship between neurohistology and corneal sensibility. *Brain* **79**, 119–154 (1956).

151. B. Levy and L. D. Edwards, The influence of various agents upon the intensity and duration of morphine analgesia in rats. *J. Am. Pharm. Assoc. Sci. Ed.* **45**, 797–800 (1956).

152. T. Lewis, "Pain." Macmillan, New York, 1942.

153. R. K. S. Lim, Visceral receptors and visceral pain. *Ann. N. Y. Acad. Sci.* **86**, 73–89 (1960).

154. R. K. S. Lim, F. Guzman, K. Goto, C. Braun, and D. W. Rodgers, Evidence establishing central and peripheral sites of action for narcotic and non-narcotic analgesics respectively. *Federation Proc.* **22**, 249 (1963).

155. O. Lindahl, Pain: a chemical explanation. *Acta Rheumatol. Scand.* **8**, 161–169 (1962).

156. M. Lipkin and M. H. Sleisenger, Studies on visceral pain: measurements of stimulus intensity and duration associated with the onset of pain in esophagus, ileum and colon. *J. Clin. Invest.* **37**, 28–34 (1958).

157. W. K. Livingston, "Pain Mechanisms." Macmillan, New York, 1943.

158. S. G. Macris, J. S. Gravenstein, C. W. Reichle, and H. K. Beecher, Drug synergism (potentiation) in pain relief in man: papaverine and morphine. *Science* **128**, 84–85 (1958).

159. J. L. Malis, Effects of drugs on the regulation of an aversive stimulus in the monkey. *Federation Proc.* **21**, 327 (1962).

160. J. Margolis, Plasma pain-producing substance and blood clotting. *Nature* **180**, 1464–1465 (1957).

161. W. R. Martin and C. G. Eades, Demonstration of tolerance and physical dependence in the dog following a short-term infusion of morphine. *J. Pharmacol. Exptl. Therap.* **133**, 262–270 (1961).

162. W. R. Martin and A. J. Eisenman, Interactions between nalorphine and morphine in the decerebrate cat. *J. Pharmacol. Exptl. Therap.* **138**, 113–119 (1962).

163. W. R. Martin, Strong analgesics. *In* "Physiological Pharmacology" (W. S. Root and F. G. Hofmann, eds.), Vol. I, pp. 275–312. Academic Press, New York, 1963.

164. D. R. Maxwell, H. T. Palmer, and R. W. Ryall, A comparison of the analgesic and some other central properties of methotrimeprazine and morphine. *Arch. Intern. Pharmacodyn.* **132**, 60–73 (1961).

165. E. W. Maynert and G. I. Klingman, Tolerance to morphine. I. Effects on catecholamines in the brain and adrenal glands. *J. Pharmacol. Exptl. Therap.* **135**, 285–295 (1962).

166. E. W. Maynert and G. I. Klingman, Tolerance to morphine. II. Lack of effects on brain 5-hydroxytryptamine and γ-aminobutyric acid. *J. Pharmacol. Exptl. Therap.* **135**, 296–299 (1962).

167. H. J. McConnell, Analgesic activity of Versidyne[T.M.] HCl, *d*-propoxyphene and morphine sulfate as measured by a "fractional escape" procedure. *Federation Proc.* **21**, 418 (1962).

168. A. McCoubrey, Antagonism of analgesia by *p*-cyclohexyloxy-α-phenylethylallylamine and some observations on hyperalgesia. *Brit. J. Pharmacol.* **9**, 289–294 (1954).

169. J. S. McKenzie and N. R. Beechey, A method of investigating analgesic substances in mice, using electrical stimulation of the tail. *Arch. Intern. Pharmacodyn.* **135**, 376–392 (1962).

170. M. Medaković and B. Banić, The effects of two phenylacetic acid derivatives on the analgesic action of morphine in mice. *J. Pharm. Pharmacol.* **15**, 660–665 (1963).

171. L. B. Mellett and L. A. Woods, The intracellular distribution of N—C¹⁴-methyl levorphanol in brain, liver and kidney tissue of the rat. *J. Pharmacol. Exptl. Therap.* **125**, 97–104 (1959).

172. L. B. Mellett, Plasma levels and brain concentrations of radioactive morphinan isomers in dogs and rats. *Pharmacologist* **5**, 251 (1963).

173. L. B. Mellett and L. A. Woods, Analgesia and addiction. *In* "Progress in Drug Research" (E. Jucker, ed.), Vol. 5. Birkhäuser, Basel, Switzerland, 1963.

174. R. Melzack and T. H. Scott, The effects of early experience on the response to pain. *J. Comp. Physiol. Psychol.* **50**, 155–161 (1957).

175. R. Melzack, The perception of pain. *Sci. Am.* **204**, 41–49 (April, 1961).

176. R. Melzack, A. Z. Weisz, and L. T. Sprague, Strategems for controlling pain: contributions of auditory stimulation and suggestion. *Exptl. Neurol.* **8**, 239–247 (1963).

177. L. C. Miller, A critique of analgesic testing methods. *Ann. N. Y. Acad. Sci.* **51**, 34–50 (1948).

178. J. W. Miller and H. W. Elliott, Rat tissue levels of carbon-14 labeled analgetics as related to pharmacological activity. *J. Pharmacol. Exptl. Therap.* **113**, 283–291 (1955).

179. M. M. Milligan and G. Kalman, A selective method for the study of drug effects on behavior. *Proc. Western Pharmacol. Soc.* **6**, 7–8 (1963).

180. K. Milthers, N-Dealkylation of morphine and nalorphine in the brain of living rats. *Nature* **195**, 607 (1962).

181. M. Monje and O. Ritter, Untersuchungen über die Bestimmung der Schmerzempfindlichkeit und ihrer Beeinflussung durch Medikamente. *Arzneimittel-Forsch.* **9**, 753–757 (1959).

182. M. Monnier, G. Nosal, and C. Radouco-Thomas, Action of analgesics on electrical brain activity, behaviour and nociceptive reaction. *Intern. J. Neuropharmacol.* **2**, 217–229 (1963).

183. S. J. Mulé and L. A. Woods, Distribution of N—C¹⁴-methyl labeled morphine. I. In central nervous system of nontolerant and tolerant dogs. *J. Pharmacol. Exptl. Therap.* **136**, 232–241 (1962).

184. S. J. Mulé, L. A. Woods, and L. B. Mellett, Distribution of N—C¹⁴-methyl labeled morphine. II. Effect of nalorphine in the central nervous system of nontolerant dogs and observations on metabolism. *J. Pharmacol. Exptl. Therap.* **136**, 242–249 (1962).

185. P. L. Nilsen, Studies on algesimetry by electrical stimulation of the mouse tail. *Acta Pharmacol. Toxicol.* **18**, 10–22 (1961).

186. T. B. O'Dell, Pharmacology of phenyramidol (IN511) with emphasis on analgesic and muscle-relaxant effects. *Ann. N.Y. Acad. Sci.* **86**, 191–202 (1960).

187. T. B. O'Dell, Experimental parameters in the evaluation of analgesics. *Arch. Intern. Pharmacodyn.* **134**, 154–174 (1961).

188. P. D. Orahovats, C. A. Winter, and E. G. Lehman, The effect of N-allylnormorphine upon the development of tolerance to morphine in the albino rat. *J. Pharmacol. Exptl. Therap.* **109**, 413–416 (1953).

189. P. D. Orahovats, C. A. Winter, and E. G. Lehman, Pharmacological studies of mixtures of narcotics and N-allylnormorphine. *J. Pharmacol. Exptl. Therap.* **112**, 246–251 (1954).

190. P. D. Orahovats, E. G. Lehman, and E. W. Chapin, Pharmacology of ethyl-1-(4-amino-phenethyl)-4-phenylisonipecotate, anileridine, a new potent synthetic analegesic. *J. Pharmacol. Exptl. Therap.* **119**, 26–34 (1957).

191. P. D. Orahovats, E. G. Lehman ,and E. W. Chapin, Potentiating effects of quinine. I. Analgesics and hypnotics. *Arch. Intern. Pharmacodyn.* **110**, 245–258 (1957).

192. L. R. Orkin, S. I. Joseph, and M. Helrich, Effects of mild analgesics on postpartum pain: a method for evaluating analgesics. *N.Y. State Med. J.* **57**, 71–73 (1957).

193. C. C. Pfeiffer, R. R. Sonnenschein, L. Glassman, E. H. Jenney, and S. Bogolub, Experimental methods for studying analgesia. *Ann. N.Y. Acad. Sci.* **51**, 21–33 (1948).

194. G. D. Potter, F. Guzman, and R. K. S. Lim, Visceral pain evoked by intra-arterial injection of substance P. *Nature* **193**, 983–984 (1962).

195. G. P. Quinn, B. B. Brodie, and P. A. Shore, Drug-induced release of norepinephrine in cat brain. *J. Pharmacol. Exptl. Therap.* **122** 63A (1958).

196. D. P. Rall, J. R. Stabenau, and C. G. Zubrod, Distribution of drugs between blood and cerebrospinal fluid: general methodology and effects of pH gradients. *J. Pharmacol. Exptl. Therap.* **125**, 185–193 (1959).

197. L. O. Randall and J. J. Selitto, A method for measurement of analgesic activity on inflamed tissue. *Arch. Intern. Pharmacodyn.* **111**, 409–419 (1957).

198. L. O. Randall, J. J. Selitto ,and J. Valdes, Anti-inflammatory effects of xylopropamine. *Arch. Intern. Pharmacodyn.* **113**, 233–249 (1957).

199. L. O. Randall, Non-narcotic analgesics. *In* "Physiological Pharmacology" (W. S. Root and F. G. Hofmann, eds.) Vol. I, pp. 313–416. Academic Press, New York, 1963.

200. J. Reid, Therapeutic properties of salicylate and its mode of action. *Ann. N.Y. Acad. Sci.* **86**, 64–72 (1960).

201. A. K. Reynolds and L. O. Randall, Tolerance, I, 14, and Opiate Addiction, I, 16. *In* "Morphine and Allied Drugs". Univ. of Toronto Press, Toronto, Canada, 1957.

202. M. Rocha e Silva, W. T. Beraldo, and G. Rosenfeld, Bradykinin, a hypotensive and smooth muscle stimulating factor released from plasma globulin by snake venoms and by trypsin. *Am. J. Physiol.* **156**, 261–273 (1949).

203. L. J. Roth and C. F. Barlow, Drugs in the brain. *Science* **134**, 22–31 (1961).

204. T. C. Ruch, *In* "Medical Physiology and Biophysics" (T. C. Ruch and J. F. Fulton, eds.),Chapter 13. 18th ed. Saunders, Philadelphia, Pennsylvania, 1960.

205. M. S. Sadove, M. J. Schriffrin, and R. Heller, Jr., A clinical comparison of two new narcotic analgesics. *Current Therap. Res.* **1**, 109–114 (1959).

206. C. C. Scott and K. K. Chen, The actions of 1,1-diphenyl-1-(dimethylaminoisopropyl)-butanone-2, a potent analgesic agent. *J. Pharmacol. Exptl. Therap.* **87**, 63–71 (1946).

207. D. Scott, Jr. and T. R. Tempel, Receptor potentials in response to thermal and other excitation. *In* " Sensory Mechanisms in Dentine ". (D. J. Anderson, ed.), pp. 27–46. Pergamon Press, New York, 1963.

208. M. H. Seevers and L. A. Woods, The phenomena of tolerance. *Am. J. Med.* **14**, 546–557 (1953).

209. M. H. Seevers and G. A. Deneau, Physiological aspects of tolerance and physical dependence. *In* "Physiological Pharmacology" (W. S. Root and F. G. Hofmann, eds.), Vol. I, pp. 565–640. Academic Press, New York, 1963.

210. M. Segal and G. A. Deneau, Brain levels of epinephrine (E), norepinephrine (N), dopamine (D) and 5-HT during administration and withdrawal of morphine in monkeys. *Federation Proc.* **21**, 327 (1962).

211. C. S. Sherrington, "The Integrative Action of the Nervous System." Yale Univ. Press, New Haven, Connecticut, 1906.

212. M. Sidman, Avoidance conditioning with brief shock and no exteroceptive warning signal. *Science* **118**, 157–158 (1953).

213. E. Siegmund, R. Cadmus, and G. Lu, A method for evaluating both non-narcotic and narcotic analgesics. *Proc. Soc. Exptl. Biol. Med.* **95**, 729–731 (1957).

214. E. B. Sigg, G. Carpio, and J. A. Schneider, Synergism of amines and antagonism of reserpine to morphine analgesia. *Proc. Soc. Exptl. Biol. Med.* **97**, 97–100 (1958).

215. A. K. Simon and N. B. Eddy, Studies of morphine, codeine, and their derivatives. V. The use of maze-trained rats to study the effect on the central nervous system of morphine and related substances. *Am. J. Psychol.* **47**, 597–613 (1935).

216. D. C. Sinclair, G. Weddell, and E. Zander, The relationship of cutaneous sensibility to neurohistology in human pinna. *J. Anat.* **86**, 402–411 (1952).

217. D. C. Sinclair, Cutaneous sensation and the doctrine of specific energy. *Brain* **78**, 584–614 (1955).

218. L. N. Sinitsin, Effect of analgesics on the evoked potentials of the afferent systems in the brain. (In Russian.) *Farmakol. i Toksikol.* **24**, 259–267 (1961).

219. A. P. Skouby, The influence of acetylcholine, curarine and and related substances on the threshold for cutaneous pain. *Acta Physiol. Scand.* **29**, 340–352 (1953).

220. D. Slaughter and D. W. Munsell, Some new aspects of morphine action effects on pain. *J. Pharmacol. Exptl. Therap.* **68**, 104–112 (1940).

221. J. Sloan, A. J. Eisenman, J. W. Brooks, and W. R. Martin, Catecholamine and serotonin levels in tissues of morphine-addicted rats following abrupt withdrawal. *Federation Proc.* **21**, 326 (1962).

222. J. W. Sloan, J. W. Brooks, A. J. Eisenman, and W. R. Martin, The effect of addiction to and abstinence from morphine on rat tissue catecholamine and serotonin levels. *Psychopharmacologia* **4**, 261–270 (1963).

223. M. B. Slomka, and F. W. Schueler, Chemical constitution and analgetic action. *J. Am. Pharm. Assoc. Sci. Ed.* **41**, 618–624 (1952).

224. D. L. Smith, M. C. D'Amour, and F. E. D'Amour, The analgesic properties of certain drugs and drug combinations. *J. Pharmacol. Exptl. Therap.* **77**, 184–193 (1943).

225. M. J. H. Smith, Salicylates and metabolism. *J. Pharm. Pharmacol.* **11**, 705–720 (1959).

226. M. J. H. Smith,, Some recent advances in the pharmacology of salicylates. *J. Pharm. Pharmacol.* **5**, 81–93 (1953).

227. P. K. Smith, Certain aspects of the pharmacology of the salicylates. *Pharmacol. Rev.* **1**, 353–382 (1949).

228. P. K. Smith, The pharmacology of salicylates and related compounds. *Ann. N.Y. Acad. Sci.* **86**, 38–63 (1960).

229. E. A. Strom and J. D. Coffman, Effect of aspirin on circulatory responses to catecholamines. *Arthritis Rheumat.* **6**, 689–697 (1963).
230. C. Y. Sung, E. L. Way, and K. G. Scott, Studies on the relationship of metabolic fate and hormonal effects of *d, l*-methadone to the development of drug tolerance. *J. Pharmacol. Exptl. Therap.* **107**, 12–23 (1953).
231. W. H. Sweet, Pain. *In* "Handbook of Physiology", Section 1: Neurophysiology, Vol. 1, Am. Physiol. Soc., Washington, D.C., 1959.
232. T. S. Szasz, The nature of pain. *Arch. Neurol. Psychiat.* **74**, 174–181 (1955).
233. M. L. Tainter and O. H. Buchanan, A comparison of certain actions of Demerol and methadone. *Calif. Med.* **70**, 1–9 (1949).
234. A. E. Takemori, Cross-cellular adaptation to methadone and meperidine in cerebral cortical slices from morphinized rats. *J. Pharmacol. Exptl. Therap.* **135**, 252–255 (1962).
235. D. H. Tedeschi, R. E. Tedeschi, and E. J. Fellows, Analgesic and other neuropharmacologic effects of phenazocine (NIH 7519, Prinadol) compared with morphine. *J. Pharmacol. Exptl. Therap.* **130**, 431–435 (1960).
236. J. Telford, C. N. Papadapoulos, and A. S. Keats, Studies of analgesic drugs. VII. Morphine antagonists as analgesics. *J. Pharmacol. Exptl. Therap.* **133**, 106–116 (1961).
237. R. H. Thorp, The assessment of analgesic activity in new synthetic drugs. *Brit. J. Pharmacol.* **1**, 113–126 (1946).
238. A. Tye and B. V. Chistensen, The estimation of some analgetic potencies. *J. Am. Pharm. Assoc., Sci. Ed.* **41**, 75–77 (1952).
239. C. Vander Wende and S. Margolin, Analgesic tests based upon experimentally induced acute abdominal pain in rats. *Federation Proc.* **15**, 494 (1956).
240. J. M. van Rossum, The relation between chemical structure and biological activity. *J. Pharm. Pharmacol.* **15**, 285–316 (1963).
241. V. G. Vernier, J. J. Boren, P. G. Knapp, and J. L. Malis, Effect of depressant drugs on thresholds for aversive pain stimulation. *Federation Proc.* **20**, 323 (1961).
242. S. L. Wallenstein, A. Rogers, and R. W. Houde, Relative analgesic potency of phenazocine and morphine. *Pharmacologist* **1**, 78 (1959).
243. R. I. H. Wang and J. A. Bain, Cytochrome enzymes in the brain and liver of the chronically morphinized rat. *J. Pharmacol. Exptl. Therap.* **108**, 349–353 (1953).
244. R. I. H. Wang and J. A. Bain, Analgesics and enzymes of the cytochrome chain. *J. Pharmacol. Exptl. Therap.* **108**, 354–361 (1953).
245. E. L. Way, A. E. Takemori, G. E. Smith, Jr., H. H. Anderson, and D. C. Brodie, The toxicity and analgetic activity of some congeners of salicylamide. *J. Pharmacol. Exptl. Therap.* **108**, 450–460 (1953).
246. E. L. Way and T. K. Adler, The pharmacologic implications of the fate of morphine and its surrogates. *Pharmacol. Rev.* **12**, 383–446 (1960).
247. E. L. Way and T. K. Adler, "The Biological Disposition of Morphine and Its Surrogates." World Health Organ., Geneva, Switzerland, 1962; also published as installments *Bull. World Health Organ.* **25**, 227–262 (1961); **26**, 51–66 (1962); **26**, 261–284 (1962); **27**, 359–394 (1962).
248. G. Weddell, D. A. Taylor, and C. M. Williams, Studies on the innervation of skin. III. The patterned arrangement of the spinal sensory nerves to the rabbit ear. *J. Anat.* **89**, 317–342 (1955).
249. J. R. Weeks, Self-maintained morphine "addiction"—a method for chronic programmed intravenous injections in unrestricted rats. *Federation Proc.* **20**, 397 (1961).

250. B. Weiss and V. G. Laties, Fractional escape and avoidance on a titration schedule. *Science* **128**, 1575–1576 (1958).

251. B. Weiss and V. G. Laties, Titration behavior on various fractional escape programs. *J. Exptl. Anal. Behavior* **2**, 227–248 (1959).

252. B. Weiss and V. G. Laties, Changes in pain tolerance and other behavior produced by salicylates. *J. Pharmacol. Exptl. Therap.* **131**, 120–129 (1961).

253. E. D. Weitzman and G. S. Ross, A behavioral method for the study of pain perception in the monkey. *Neurology* **12**, 264–272 (1962).

254. J. C. White, Conduction of pain in man. Observations on its afferent pathways within the spinal cord and visceral nerves. *Arch. Neurol. Psychiat.* **71**, 1–23 (1954).

255. A. Wikler and K. Frank, Hindlimb reflexes of chronic spinal dogs during cycles of addiction to morphine and methadone. *J. Pharmacol. Exptl. Therap.* **94**, 382–400 (1948).

256. A. Wikler, Sites and mechanisms of action of morphine and related drugs in the central nervous system. *Pharmacol. Rev.* **2**, 435–506 (1950).

257. A. Wikler, Psychiatric aspects of drug addiction. *Am. J. Med.* **14**, 566–570 (1953).

258. A. Wikler, "The Relation of Psychiatry to Pharmacology." Williams & Wilkins, Baltimore, Maryland, 1957.

259. A. Wikler, Opiates and opiate antagonists. A review of their mechanism of action in relation to clinical problems. U.S. Public Health Monograph No. **52** (1958).

260. A. Wikler, Narcotics. *Proc. Assoc. Res. Nerv. Diseases* **37**, 334–355 (1959).

261. A. E. Wilder-Smith, E. Frommel, and S. Radouco-Thomas, Preliminary screening of some new oxadiazol-2-ols with special reference to their antipyretic, analgesic and anti-inflammatory properties. *Arzneimittel-Forsch.* **13**, 338–341 (1963).

262. M. W. Williams, Analgesic effects of APC combination in rat. *Toxicol. Appl. Pharmacol.* **1**, 447–453 (1959).

263. C. V. Winder, C. C. Pfeiffer, and G. L. Maison, The nociceptive contraction of the cutaneous muscle of the guinea pig as elicited by radiant heat. *Arch. Intern. Pharmacodyn.* **72**, 329–359 (1946).

264. C. V. Winder, Distribution of resting pain-reaction thresholds in guinea pigs, with a statistical concept of gradation of biological effect. *Yale J. Biol. Med.* **19**, 289–310 (1947).

265. C. V. Winder, A preliminary test for analgetic action in guinea pigs. *Arch. Intern. Pharmacodyn.* **74**, 176–192 (1947).

266. C. V. Winder, Quantitative evaluation of analgetic action in guinea pigs. Morphine, ethyl-1-methyl-4-phenylpiperidine-4-carboxylate (Demerol) and acetylsalicylic acid. *Arch. Intern. Pharmacodyn.* **74**, 219–232 (1947).

267. C. V. Winder, An experiment in analgesimetry. *Ann. N.Y. Acad. Sci.* **52**, 838–854 (1950).

268. C. V. Winder, Aspirin and algesimetry. *Nature* **184**, 494–497 (1959).

269. C. V. Winder, E. M. Jones, J. K. Weston, and J. Gajewski, 14-Hydroxymorphinone and 8,14-dihydroxydihydromorphinone. *Arch. Intern. Pharmacodyn.* **122**, 301–311 (1959).

270. C. V. Winder, J. Wax, B. Serrano, L. Scotti, S. P. Stackhouse, and R. H. Wheelock, Pharmacological studies of 1,2-dimethyl-3-phenyl-3-propionoxypyrrolidine (CI-427), an analgetic agent. *J. Pharmacol. Exptl. Therap.* **133**, 117–128 (1961).

271. C. V. Winder, J. Wax, L. Scotti, R. A. Scherrer, E. M. Jones, and F. W. Short, Anti-inflammatory, antipyretic and antinociceptive properties of N(2,3-xylyl)-anthranilic acid (mefenamic acid). *J. Pharmacol. Exptl. Therap.* **138**, 405–413 (1962).

272. C. A. Winter and L. Flataker, Studies on heptazone (6-morpholino-4,4-diphenyl-3-heptanone hydrochloride) in comparison with other analgesic drugs. *J. Pharmacol. Exptl. Therap.* **98**, 305–317 (1950).

273. C. A. Winter and L. Flataker, The effect of cortisone, desoxycorticosterone and adrenocorticotrophic hormone upon the responses of animals to analgesic drugs. *J. Pharmacol. Exptl. Therap.* **101**, 93–105 (1951).

274. C. A. Winter and L. Flataker, The relation between skin temperature and the effect of morphine upon the response to thermal stimuli in the albino rat and the dog. *J. Pharmacol. Exptl. Therap.* **109**, 183–188 (1953).

275. C. A. Winter, P. D. Orahovats, L. Flataker, E. G. Lehman, and J. T. Lehman, Studies on the pharmacology of N-allylnormorphine. *J. Pharmacol. Exptl. Therap.* **111**, 152–160 (1954).

276. C. A. Winter, P. D. Orahovats, and E. G. Lehman, Analgesic activity and morphine antagonism of compounds related to nalorphine. *Arch. Intern. Pharmacodyn.* **110**, 186–202 (1957).

277. C. A. Winter, E. A. Risley, and G. W. Nuss, Antiinflammatory and antipyretic activities of indomethacin 1-(p-chlorobenzoyl)-5-methoxy-2-methylindole-3-acetic acid. *J. Pharmacol. Exptl. Therap.* **141**, 369–376 (1963).

278. H. G. Wolff and H. Goodell, The relation of attitude and suggestion to the perception of and reaction to pain. *Proc. Assoc. Res. Nerv. Diseases* **23**, 434–448 (1943).

279. L. A. Woods, Distribution and fate of morphine in non-tolerant and tolerant dogs and rats. *J. Pharmacol. Exptl. Therap.* **112**, 158–175 (1954).

280. G. Woolfe and A. D. Macdonald, The evaluation of the analgesic action of pethidine hydrochloride (Demerol). *J. Pharmacol. Exptl. Therap.* **80**, 300–307 (1944).

281. F. F. Yonkman, Pharmacology of Demerol and its analogs. *Ann. N.Y. Acad. Sci.* **51**, 59–82 (1948).

282. R. E. Yoss, Studies of the spinal cord. Part 3. Pathways for deep pain within the spinal cord and brain. *Neurology* **3**, 163–175 (1953).

283. D. C. Young, R. A. vander Ploeg, R. M. Featherstone, and E. G. Gross, The interrelationships among the central, peripheral and anticholinesterase effects of some morphinan derivatives. *J. Pharmacol. Exptl. Therap.* **114**, 33–37 (1955).

CHAPTER III

Clinical Measurement of Pain[1]

RAYMOND W. HOUDE,
STANLEY L. WALLENSTEIN,
and WILLIAM T. BEAVER

DIVISION OF CLINICAL INVESTIGATION,
THE SLOAN-KETTERING INSTITUTE FOR CANCER RESEARCH,
NEW YORK, NEW YORK

[1] The authors' studies referred to in this chapter were supported in part by grants awarded by the Committee on Drug Addiction and Narcotics, National Academy of Sciences—National Research Council, from funds contributed by a group of interested pharmaceutical manufacturers, and in part by grant B-2649 from the National Institutes of Health.

75

I. Introduction

Our modern concepts of pain as a measurable phenomenon distinct from other sensations have their origins in the pioneering work of Weber and Fechner just over a century ago, and it is only in very recent times that systematic attempts to measure the reduction of pain by analgetics have been undertaken. Because of the subjective nature of pain and our incomplete understanding of its precise mechanisms, the ability to evaluate analgetic drugs of necessity must be based on observations in man. However, with the great mass of new synthetic drugs that are continually being developed, it is not practical or even desirable to screen all new drugs for potential analgetic power in man and, recognizing the possibility of false leads, laboratory animal screening procedures must be relied upon to provide the more likely candidates for clinical trial. Unfortunately, the correlation of analgetic performance in animals with that in man has left much to be desired. On the other hand, the clinical yardstick has not in itself been a completely reliable standard, for the medical literature is replete with conflicting reports of the efficacy of many of the analgetic drugs and there is still considerable division of opinion on many aspects of analgetic testing in man.

II. Pain and Pain Relief

A. SEMANTIC PROBLEMS

Although pain is a universal experience of mankind, and everyone appears to know what it means intuitively, pain is uncommonly difficult to define. The often repeated statement of Sir Thomas Lewis (1) that pain is "known to us by experience and described by illustration" succinctly expresses the dilemma. Pain has long been recognized as having no proper stimulus—for it can be induced by a wide variety of stimuli—and until the middle of the nineteenth century it was considered a "quale" or feeling state. The investigations of Weber, Fechner and later Müller, von Helmholtz, von Frey and many others led to the consideration of pain as a specific sensation subserved by a special neural apparatus. The concept of a dual aspect of pain is believed to have emerged from the writings of Marshall (*2*) and Strong (*3*), who felt that pain consisted of both cognitive and affective components. Subsequently, attempts were made to measure the original sensation and the reaction to pain as two distinct and separable phenomena. The systematic investigations of Wolff and Hardy (*4*) and their associates led them to the conclusion that the adequate stimulus for pain was the damaging of tissue; that the pain threshold in man is relatively uniform, stable, and independent of age, sex, various emotional states and fatigue; and that known analgetics raise the pain threshold. A number of subsequent investigators have been unable to confirm these results (*5*, *6*) and some have raised serious questions about the constancy of the experimental pain threshold and its applicability to the evaluation of analgetic drugs (*6*). Although the artificial dichotomy of the pain experience has proved useful in studying and understanding the phenomenon, it is doubtful that there is such a thing as a pure sensation of pain separate and distinct from the influence of reaction. Beecher (*6*) contends, "variations of great degree in the reaction part (of pain) are determined by the significance of the cause of the pain . . . the significance of the pain controls the field of usefulness for study of pain of a given origin."

Analgesia generally connotes the absence or diminished awareness of pain. However, the problem of categorizing a drug as an analgetic is somewhat more complex in that it involves other factors as well. Analgetics are commonly defined as those drugs which on systemic administration selectively act on the central nervous system or relieve pain without producing loss of consciousness. Difficulties arise in that the precise mechanisms by which even the commonly designated analgetics exert their effects are not known and, furthermore, selectivity of effect is at best a matter of degree. Although it is customary to exclude agents that act by removing the cause of pain and those that block pain impulses in peripheral nerves, there is reason to believe that some commonly designated analgetics such as the salicylates may, in fact, exert their analgetic effects in the periphery (*7*, *8*). With the increasing complexity of pharmaceutical agents being presented to the investigator for analgetic testing, it would appear that the difficulty in classifying drugs into arbitrary categories will be compounded and, in the long run, classification will simply be determined on the basis of their major therapeutic applications.

B. SUBJECTIVE AND OBJECTIVE INDICES

Just as the pain threshold is thought by some to be a measure of pain sensation or perception, so have behavioural and autonomic responses frequently associated with pain been considered by others to be measures of pain or pain reaction. The advantages of measuring objective responses are obvious; they are apparent as physical signs and most can be recorded or measured mechanically, whereas subjective experiences can only be measured introspectively and communicated to the onlooker by power of speech. Since a wide variety of reflex, autonomic and behavioural changes are frequently associated with the pain experience, there have been extensive investigations of a variety of these reactions of which the galvanic skin reflex, vasomotor responses, heart rate, respiratory rate and rhythmicity, pupil size, facial expression and overt behaviour are but a few. However, although these changes may occur in the presence of pain, they are associated as well with other subjective states, such as fear and anxiety, which may or may not accompany the pain experience so that although objective, these measures are generally not reliable indices of pain itself. In evaluating analgetic drugs, difficulties with such indices are compounded by the fact that they may be directly influenced by drugs which may or may not have appreciable effects on the subjective experience of pain. Experimentally induced pain techniques of measuring pain threshold or of matching existing clinical pain are frequently spoken of as "objective" although, in the final analysis, they are dependent upon the subjective report of subjects. What is "objective" about these techniques is the quantitation of the *stimulus* rather than the *response*.

Distinction must be made between an objective response and objectivity of an experiment. Objectivity in the latter sense is not unique to the laboratory; it can also be achieved by use of appropriate experimental designs and controls in the clinical situation. The most successful efforts to quantify pain in the clinical situation have been those that accepted the patient's own reports as appropriate indices of the pain experience (*9, 10*). To be sure, language in general tends to be imprecise and this tendency is perhaps most evident in the verbalization of subjective experiences. This presents serious problems to the investigator in converting verbal end points into meaningful measurement data, and what finally emerges as an analgetic response will represent, in large measure, the patient's own conception of his pain and the investigator's preconceptions of what constitutes satisfactory analgesia. There are many factors in the clinical setting which influence the choice of the most practical or meaningful yardsticks to be employed. These measures may be gross or fine and qualitative or quantitative. Some investigators appear to prefer quantal measures such as "at least 50% relief of pain" (*11, 12*), "complete relief of pain" (*13*), "presence or absence of comfort" (*11*), or "better," "no change," or "worse" days (*14*). Others have used measurement scales of "pain intensity" (*10, 15–18*) degrees of "pain relief" (*18, 19*), or a composite of "pain intensity" and "pain relief" (*20*). Finally, still others have employed "therapeutic indices" which confound analgesia with side effects (*21*). The fact that each investigator is speaking a different language has made inter-investigator comparisons difficult and has resulted in some confusion in evaluating the literature.

C. EVALUATION OF ANALGETICS

The clinical evaluation of the merits of any putative analgetic obviously involves more than the mere assessment of its analgetic effects. Untoward side effects and addiction liability, for example, are as important determinants of the therapeutic usefulness or relative advantages of drugs as is their analgetic efficacy. However, the evaluation of clinical analgetic power is material in its own right for, in this way, the clinician is best able to provide leads to the medicinal chemist and pharmacologist in developing new classes of analgetics whose spectrum of activity may be more desirable than those of the standard analgetics.

In spite of the relative convenience and more rigorous controls which can be applied in the laboratory, the controlled drug study in the clinical setting is now more than ever the crucial test of any new analgetic. This is true for several reasons. Most obviously, the only conclusive proof of the value of a drug in the therapy of a disease or the alleviation of a symptom lies in successful therapeutic trials in patients with that particular disease or symptom. Of equal importance, however, is the fact that no experimental model has yet been developed which will reliably predict the response to analgetics of patients with pain due to disease or injury. Beecher (*9*) has reviewed this subject in great detail and applied the terms "experimental pain" and "pathological pain" to distinguish what is conveyed in the two situations, and admonishes the proponents of the experimental approach for focusing their inventive powers on the machine to be used rather than the man to be tested. Indeed, an increasing number of investigators in the past decade or so have been able to show that controlled clinical experimentation can provide results which are reproducible and valid in the sense that they have held up well under the test of subsequent, more extensive clinical experience.

III. General Considerations in Analgetic Testing

A. SURVEYS AND EXPERIMENTS

Any study intended as a drug assay assumes a causal relationship between the drugs being tested and the results obtained. However, not all drug studies are so designed that causal inferences can be drawn with any degree of confidence. As Mainland (*22*) points out: "Causation in medicine is like an iceberg, mostly hidden from view, but we often behave as though what we can see now is all that matters, and we disregard the submerged mass that may wreck our causal inferences." In clinical studies of analgetic drugs, the problem of causal relationships is indeed formidable for, as mentioned in preceding paragraphs, we have at best an incomplete knowledge of how analgetics exert their effects, and pain, the object of measurement, is a subjective state influenced by a complexity of factors which are extremely difficult to assess. The extent to which all these known or unknown quantities are unequally distributed among treatments constitutes bias and the manner in which one contends with bias determines whether or not he conducts a meaningful experiment (23). Bias is thus something more than the conscious or unconscious prejudices of the investigator, observer, or subjects.

The distinctive features of an experiment in the strict sense are that the investigator comparing the effects of two or more factors assigns them himself to the individuals that comprise this test population and he can assign the factors in such way as to reduce the risk of bias to a predetermined degree (22). Reducing the risk of bias involves more than the mere matching of attributes known to be capable of influencing results, for in the clinical setting for testing analgetics this alone would not insure that the complexity of *hidden* variables are randomly distributed. Only deliberate randomization insures the chance occurrence of hidden bias. If this is done and if chance can be ruled out as the likely cause of observed treatment difference (in terms of the "null" hypothesis), then the cause of the differences can reasonably be attributed to the treatments.

On the other hand, in a survey the investigator does not assign the factors under test at will. In this case, the differences, even when not attributable to chance, may be due either to the treatments or to the bias. A survey may demonstrate an *association* between treatments and effects, but it does not provide a substantial basis for inferring causal relationships between the two.

The distinction between a survey and an experiment is meaningful in that it helps us to define the limits of the inferences that we can draw from our results. Only when an experiment is well controlled are we justified in inferring causal drug-effect relationships. In this respect, an uncontrolled experiment is, for all practical purposes, no different than a survey. The attributes of a sound analgetic drug assay are essentially those enumerated by Denton and Beecher (11). They include the use of the double blind technique, randomized allocation of treatments, and the inclusion of standard and placebo drug controls.

B. PATIENT VARIABLES

The actions of analgetics are virtually always reported in terms of the patient population in which they have been studied and it is recognized that the type or cause of pain, and clinical setting, are potential sources of patient variability. However no patient population is truly homogeneous and one means of attempting to contend with variation within the study population is by selecting or matching patients according to certain attributes on the assumption that controlling these variables will increase the sensitivity and reliability of analgetic assays.

1. *Age*

Children and the aged are usually excluded from analgetic assays and this may, in itself, account for the apparent inconsequential effects of age on controlled studies of analgetics as they are customarily done. In any event, the limitations of communicating with children, and the more complex and variable interrelationships of age, size, and organ function in both the young and elderly, make the results obtained in these patients difficult to interpret. Although analgetic studies have been carried out in the aged (*14*), and also in children (by utilizing indirect indices of pain such as crying and restlessness) (*24*), there is little substantial information on the subject of the effect of age *per se* on the relative effectiveness of analgetics.

2. *Sex and Race*

Some investigators continue to match their patients by sex and race but we know of no studies which have been appropriately designed to measure how significant these factors are in evaluating analgesia. Beecher (*6*) has cited a variety of reports, many contradictory, on the effect of sex and race upon experimental pain threshold, but he questions, in any case, how germane this type of measurement is to the clinical performance of analgetics. Most investigators currently engaged in clinical analgetic testing do not manipulate the sex and race distribution of their experimental population and, when reporting their results, often fail to specify its composition in respect to these factors.

3. *Body Weight*

That there is some relationship between body size and response to a given dose of a drug is common knowledge. However, the extent to which differences in *body weight* influence the results of analgetic studies in adults has been a subject of controversy. Although several investigators conventionally make adjustments for body weight in administering test drugs in their studies, there have been no convincing demonstrations that the conclusions, or the variability of the results, would have been substantially different if this were not done. The problem is again a complex one for, in the adult, body weight only roughly correlates with either the blood volume or the size of organs and, when dealing with sick patients, these relationships can be further confounded by trauma, surgery, or disease. Jackson and Smith (*25*) tried to determine from their data whether a correlation existed between response (per cent patients relieved; average length of relief) to a fixed dose of an analgetic and weight, and found none. Moreover, Sunshine (*26*) has also analyzed his data derived from the administration of fixed doses of aspirin and codeine by mouth to a large population of adults with pain of varied etiology and he, too, was unable to discern a consistent correlation of effect and weight.

4. *Psychological Variables*

Patients differ appreciably in terms of their attitudes towards their pain, their disease, and their physician; and these personality differences are crucial variables in the pain experience. Although they are commonly recognized as being capable of influencing the results of analgetic assays, they are not easily measurable or readily manipulated by the investigator and remain potential sources of hidden bias in any experiment. They are best coped with by procedures designed to distribute them randomly among treatment groups, or by means of crossover comparisons in which each patient serves as his own control.

C. DRUG VARIABLES

1. *Criteria for Drug Administration*

In studies of more or less acute pain, the drug is usually given on demand, and most investigators also specify that the pain intensity shall be at minimum value, such as moderate pain, because of the relatively poor ability of patients with slight pain to discriminate between analgetics (*27*). Studies in which the criterion of administration is something other than the complaint of pain (such as "restlessness"), are open to the question as to whether analgesia is really the drug effect being measured.

A second general approach is by-the-clock administration at specified intervals. This method is often used in chronic experiments and has the advantage of requiring a minimum of cooperation from ward personnel. The chief criticism which may be leveled at by-the-clock administration of drug is that many doses may be given when a patient has little or no pain. In the absence of pain, the patient is of course unable to discriminate between active drug and placebo, and between graded doses of drug. Data derived from the response to these doses is of questionable value and difficult to interpret (*20*). It will tend to dilute the rest of the data in the study, perhaps to a point where no difference can be demonstrated between any of the drugs, including placebo. When test medications are administered on demand, the minimum time interval between administration of the test drug and the next analgetic medication presents something of a dilemma to the investigator. Intervals ranging from as short as one-half hour (28) to 6 hours (20) have been used in various studies. A short time interval between doses increases the chance of carryover effects and it increases the danger that a second analgetic may be given before the test drug has had time to demonstrate its action. On the other hand, where the prescribed minimum interval is too long, the patient is not likely to take kindly to suffering for a prolonged period simply to provide a more accurate appraisal of a drug's time-action curve; and the investigator will have trouble justifying to himself, and to his associates engaged in the care of the patient, withholding medication under these circumstances. In the clinical situation, a practical solution obviously involves a compromise based on all these considerations.

2. *The Effect of Concurrent or Previous Therapy*

It is a truism that definitive therapy of any form given for the disease or the cause of pain may influence the response of the patient to the study drug. It is equally true that some drugs given for other symptoms may influence pain or potentiate analgetics. For example, Keats and Beecher (29) have reported that barbiturates are analgetics in their own right and Sadove *et al.* (30) and Jackson *et al.* (25) have reported that tranquilizers are capable of potentiating analgetics. Some claims have also been made that other drugs such as psychic stimulants, sympathomimetic amines, and cholinergic agents may relieve pain. While many of these claims have not been substantiated by well controlled studies, most investigators consider it wise to eliminate such medication during the course of the study or, where this is not possible, to design the experiment so as to balance out their effects.

The patient's previous experiences with analgetics are also capable of influencing responses to study drugs. His expectancy of relief or particular side effects, and his prejudices for or against a particular form of medication, be it pill, capsule, or injection, are all molded by what has happened to him in the past. Previous experience with narcotics also introduces the complications of physical dependence and tolerance which can affect the responses to the study medication. What effect this will have will depend largely on the drugs being tested. If the test medication does not support physical dependence and is administered over a period of time, withdrawal may occur and produce apparent diminution of analgesia or an apparent increase in side effects attributed to the test drug. If the test drug is a narcotic antagonist, withdrawal may be precipitated abruptly, with similar or more dramatic consequences. If the test medications are narcotics and cross-tolerance is not complete, the relative potency estimates may be biased as a result. However, if precautions are taken in selecting patients or in balancing the patients with prior narcotic experience among the test treatments, the relative potency estimates have been found not to differ significantly from those obtained in nontolerant patients with acute pain (see Section VII, A, Table II).

D. OBSERVER VARIABLES

1. *Methods of Collecting Data*

A wide variety of methods for collecting clinical data on the analgetic actions of drugs have been employed with varying degrees of success. Questionnaires or "pain charts" to be filled out by the patients themselves have been used to advantage by some investigators (*15, 31*). However, success would seem to depend on such factors as the motivation of the patient, his particular milieu, and his preoccupation with his disease. It has been our experience (*32*) that hospitalized patients with cancer tend to use such charts as a means of carrying to their physician their inner hopes, fears, and special personal problems. As a result, the data on pain or analgesia tends to become obscure or lost in the process. Others (*33, 34*) have also found that records kept by the patient himself can be inaccurate and misleading.

Some investigators have relied upon the nursing staff or other regular ward personnel for the making of observations. The disadvantages of this approach are that these people are busy with other duties and the reliability (and even validity) of their observations tends to be colored by their personal biases (*35*), various degrees of interest or disinterest, and acceptance or rejection of the study and the extra work involved.

The method of choice, wherever feasible, is the use of full-time, trained observers who can maintain an objective interest in carrying out the experiment (*11*). Although this may limit the length of time of the observation period to that of the working day of the observer, the amount of information gained far outweighs that lost. Some investigators have attempted to lengthen the period by the use of more than one observer. However, the effect of the observer-patient interaction on results has never been satisfactorily measured and it would seem wise to design the experiment in such a way as to balance this source of potential bias.

Observations have been made either for each dose of medication given, or in terms of retrospective evaluation of a number of doses given for periods of time ranging up to 3 weeks (*36*). Some investigators conduct weekly interviews, others obtain daily reports (*14*), and still others make multiple observations at short intervals after the administration of medication (*10, 37*).

Only when frequent observations are made after drug administration can such parameters of drug action as time of onset, peak action, duration, and other time-effect relationships be adequately defined.

2. *Anamnestic Interviews*

The data collected in any of the ways outlined above may be either on-the-spot reports of the current status of the patient or anamnestic reports covering periods varying from hours to weeks. Whether recorded on-the-spot or by an anamnestic interview, subjective reports of pain are always influenced by a wide variety of external factors. However, when there is any appreciable time lapse between the occurrence of pain, or the response to medication, and the reporting of the event, other outside influences and the vagaries of memory may further confound the results (*34*).

It should be borne in mind that all subjective reports in terms of "relief," even when intended to reflect the present status of the patient, are inherently anamnestic as they depend on recall of pain intensity prior to receipt of medication. When the time period involved is relatively short, recall may be sufficiently adequate so that no great damage is done to the data. However, when the time period involves days, or even weeks, considerable caution should be used in relating patients' responses to drug effects.

3. *Sleep and Analgesia*

A special problem associated with the collection of data is whether or not the observer should accept sleep as evidence of no pain or awaken the patient for his report. Swerdlow *et al.* (*38*) reported that patients often reported pain when awakened and Lasagna (*39*) found that 69% of his sleeping patients reported various degrees of pain on being aroused. He pointed out that sedative effects may well be confused with analgesia in equating sleep with no pain.

IV. The Study Regimen

A. CROSSOVER AND NONCROSSOVER STUDIES

Experiments in the clinical evaluation of analgetics have used two methods for the allocation of patients to treatments. The simplest method involves the random assignment of patients to two or more groups, the patients in each group receiving only a single treatment (i.e., a fixed dose of a particular drug, administered once or repeatedly). The alternative method of "crossover" comparison utilizes each patient as his own control by giving him sequentially more than one treatment. The crossover is complete or incomplete depending on whether the patient receives all or only some of the total number of treatments available.

The notable advantage of crossover design lies in eliminating the variation introduced into the experimental results by the unequal distribution of patient variables among treatment groups. This decreased variation yields an economy in the number of patients required to demonstrate a significant difference between treatments. It has been our regular experience, for example, to find highly significant differences among cancer patients in crossover comparisons while the variation between replications in the same patients is usually no greater than the residual experimental error.

Unfortunately, the use of the patient as his own control does not assure that the pain will return to the same baseline prior to each treatment. If the pain fluctuates with time in a relatively random way, this poses no greater source of variation in the crossover than in the noncrossover study. However, if there is a definite time trend in the pain severity, as has been demonstrated for postoperative pain by Meier *et al.* (*40*), and for postpartum pain by Free and Peeters (*13*), interpretation of the results of crossover studies becomes much more of a problem. These groups found, upon analyzing their data both by crossover comparison and by the use of the first dose only, that the latter gave more precise results in terms of drug discrimination. In respect to reaction to drug their patients were more like other patients at similar times after operation or delivery than they were like themselves at different times. Meier *et al.* found a further complication in crossover comparisons when drugs are administered in sequence with timing controlled by patient demand. The time of administration of the second drug is dependent on the effectiveness of the first medication and this can bias the results when pain is decreasing. In these two studies, unless the patient's pain continued long enough to require all four test medications, what data the patient contributed to the study was lost to an analysis based on crossover data only. Meier *et al.* lost data from over 25% of their patients due to this cause, and Free and Peeters lost data from about 70%. It is apparent from reports in the literature that the percentage of dropouts bears a direct relationship to the number of treatments in the crossover and an inverse relationship to the chronicity of the patient's pain. In our studies in cancer patients, the percentage of dropouts is considerably lower than those mentioned above and we have not observed significant time trends in studies using up to 6 doses of medication. Moreover, Lasagna (*41*), using alternate administration of a dose of morphine and a dose of normorphine in postoperative patients who received from 1 to 13 doses, saw no impressive difference between an analysis of the effects of all doses given and first-dose-only data, and neither Keats nor Beecher have reported difficulty with excessive dropouts in doing two dose crossover comparisons in patients with postoperative pain.

Crossover comparisons carry with them possible complications of carryover, order, or learning effects among doses within the study. This may represent pharmacologic potentiation or antagonism of the action of one drug by another. Lasagna (42), for example, noted that there was evidence that methotrimeprazine potentiated the effects of succeeding doses of morphine in a study in postoperative patients. Carryover may also be purely psychological and represent a positive or negative reinforcement of the following dose. Sunshine *et al.* (43) found in a crossover study that placebo was more effective than aspirin when both were given as a second dose although the reverse relationship held on considering first dose data. He attributed this anomaly to the fact that patients who recieved placebo as a second dose initially received an "effective" analgetic, and their anticipation of receiving another effective medication may have improved their reaction to placebo. Still another type of potential psychological carryover or learning effect is that patients may, on repeated presentation, discriminate between placebo and active drug on the basis of side effects rather than analgesia. While this problem may be overcome by the use of a placebo medication with side effects similar to those of the test medications, this introduces other variables into the experiment and, moreover, there is no substantial evidence that this type of learning effect has been a serious problem in analgetic testing.

The noncrossover study, while free from carryover effects within the study, is subject to errors inherent in the variability in patient groups, which in some clinical settings can be considerable. Noncrossover comparisons generally require relatively large or homogeneous patient groups. However, if the number of patients available for the study is expected to be small, or if the patients have more or less persistent pain, a great deal more information can usually be obtained by resorting to a crossover design.

In summary then, the crucial assumption presupposed in the decision to use crossover experimental design is that the variation between the responses of different patients will be greater than the variation of responses at different times in the same patient. Whether the crossover or noncrossover design will yield the better results in a given experimental setting, where both are feasible on the basis of other considerations, can only be settled empirically.

B. Oral and Parenteral Drug Studies

Some analgetics, particularly the narcotics, are significantly less potent when administered orally than parenterally, and the sparse data available indicates that oral-parenteral potency ratios vary from compound to compound. It is uncertain what part of this discrepancy in potency is due to failure of absorption by the gastrointestinal tract and what portion is due to differences in rate of biotransformation, since orally administered drugs would be expected to enter the portal blood and pass through the liver before entering the systemic circulation. In spite of the considerable practical as well as theoretical significance of these potency ratios, suitably controlled experiments to provide this data have been few because of the methodological problems inherent in this type of study.

Potency relationships derived by comparing the results of separate experiments in different patient populations are *ipso facto* subject to bias. However, patient populations which are suitable for the evaluation of parenteral analgetics often are not suitable for oral studies, and the converse is also true. Oral analgetic administration may be contraindicated in the very ill patient, the patient in the immediate postoperative period, or the patient with severe acute pain who demands rapid relief. On the other hand, it may be difficult to persuade some patients with mild to moderate pain to accept injections, and if they are outpatients, it may be difficult to arrange for giving them injections.

The maintenance of double-blind conditions in oral-parenteral studies requires giving both forms of medication (e.g., a capsule and an injection) on each drug administration, with one form being a dummy. We have used this technique successfully for a number of such studies (*10, 44–46*). As can be seen from the results of the racemorphan study (see Section VI,B), the addition of a dummy given by the alternate route to a 5 mg dose of racemorphan given orally or parenterally had no significant effect on patient response to the drug in the circumstances of this study.

C. OUTPATIENT STUDIES

Although the hospital environment itself is quite variable, it is subject to much more control than can be exerted over an outpatient population. In the latter situation, observations are in general made at less frequent intervals; they are often retrospective or rely upon the patient's cooperation in filling out report cards. The situation offers no guarantee that the patient will not take interfering medications or that he will take the medications as prescribed. For these reasons, outpatient studies have proven to be less sensitive than studies carried out on hospitalized patients. Modell (*34*) attributes his inability to distinguish between aspirin and placebo in outpatients with arthralgic pain to these factors. On the other hand, meaningful outpatient data can be obtained using intelligent, well motivated subjects. For example, a study by Murray (*31*) showed that a population of medical and pharmacy students with headaches were able to distinguish not only between a placebo and aspirin but also between graded doses of aspirin.

D. LONG-TERM DRUG STUDIES

The understanding of the properties and potentialities of an analgetic requires a knowledge not only of the immediate effects of a single dose, but also information as to how these immediate effects are modified in the course of chronic administration. However, there are certain problems peculiar to long-term studies, and many of the difficulties inherent in analgetic studies utilizing a single or few doses become compounded on repeated drug administration. The long-term study of an analgetic is more expensive in funds, observer time, and use of patient material than a short-term study of the same drug, and the effects of pain trends and dropouts become a major problem. In view of the above difficulties, few investigators who conduct analgetic studies of acceptable scientific design have devoted their time and facilities to chronic drug studies. Since tolerance, cross-tolerance, and cumulative or toxic effects may influence the effectiveness of drugs when they are used therapeutically and the purpose of an analgetic assay is to predict what happens when drugs are employed in medical practice, there is an obvious need for studies comparing the analgetic effects of drugs on short-term administration with those of long-term administration. Up to the present, our knowledge of the effects of long-term administration is largely based either on uncontrolled studies of analgesia or experiments utilizing endpoints other than pain or pain relief (e.g., studies of addiction liability in post-addicts).

V.   Experimental Design

A. STUDIES TO DETERMINE ANALGETIC EFFECT

Experimental design will ultimately depend on what the investigator wishes to learn about the test drug. If it is not known whether the drug has analgetic action in man, a comparison of a single dose of the test medication, a standard agent, and a placebo may be sufficient to answer the question. However, some difficulties may well be encountered in selecting an appropriate dose for study. Clues as to the dose may come from the results of animal experimentation or from preliminary observations in man. However, these often may be misleading and there is an appreciable risk that a test drug may be prematurely dismissed as ineffective merely because the dose chosen was inappropriate. If the dose is too low, the results may well be indistinguishable from the placebo and, depending largely upon one's criteria of analgesia, if the dose is too high the analgetic effect may be obscured by untoward side effects. The acquisition of reasonably comprehensive knowledge about the properties and potentialities of a drug requires exploration of a fairly wide range of doses. This principle is *de rigueur* when

89

studying the animal pharmacology of a compound and it is no less necessary in the clinical experiment.

B. Drug Interaction Studies

If the purpose of the investigation is to determine the effects of a combination of drugs, a variety of experimental designs are available. Perhaps

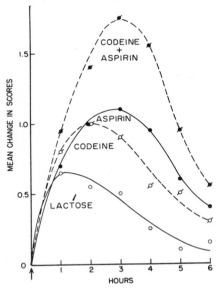

Fig. 1. Time-effect curves for lactose, 600 mg of aspirin, 32 mg of codeine, and a combination of 600 mg of aspirin and 32 mg of codeine. Changes in pain intensity (ordinate) are plotted against time after drug administration in hours (abscissa). Eleven patients with pain due to cancer received a total of twenty oral doses of each medication administered in a random order. Both drugs were significantly more effective than the placebo and the combination was significantly more effective than either drug alone. Combining the drugs produces effects that are statistically additive, indicating that the drugs do not interfere with or enhance each other's actions and supporting the hypothesis that their modes of action are different.

the simplest and most efficient of these is a factorial study in which each dose of drug is given alone and in combination, and compared with a placebo control. An example of a simple factorial experiment is shown in Fig. 1. In this study, 600 mg of aspirin and 32 mg of codeine were given alone and in combination, and lactose served as the placebo medication. Orthogonal treatment comparisons carried out on the results provide estimates of the effects of each drug alone and of the effects of combining them (in terms of whether they enhance or interfere with each other). The aspirin–codeine factorial study demonstrated a significant analgetic effect for each drug alone. No significant interaction of the two drugs in combination was found and the fact that their effects were additive suggests that their modes of action may be different.

On occasion, the effect of the drug combination will depend upon the proportions of the drugs in the combination, and a simple factorial experiment using only a single combination of doses will be inadequate. This type

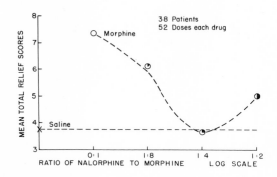

FIG. 2. Dose ratio-effect curves for various morphine-nalorphine combinations in patients with pain due to cancer. Changes in the hourly pain intensity scores summed for 6 hours after medication (ordinate) are plotted against the log-dose ratio of nalorphine to morphine on a logarithmic scale (abscissa). Each patient received a saline placebo medication, either 5 or 10 mg of morphine sulfate, and the same dose of morphine plus various proportions of nalorphine. The effect of the placebo medication is indicated by the horizontal line.

of effect has been encountered in studies of narcotic and narcotic antagonist combinations. An example of such a study is shown in Fig. 2. Various proportions of nalorphine were combined with either 5 or 10 mg of morphine and the analgetic effects of the combinations were compared with sterile saline and morphine alone. The combinations appear to have a biphasic curve. As the ratio of nalorphine to morphine in the mixture is increased progressively to 1:4, analgesia is decreased to placebo level. Further increases in the proportion of nalorphine in the mixture brought on a return of analgesia. A 1:1 combination of morphine and nalorphine produced an even greater increase in analgesia. This point is not included in the figure as it produced such a high incidence and severity of psychic and other side effects that it had to be discontinued, and the data for this point is incomplete. Since

Lasagna and Beecher (*47*) and Keats and Telford (*48*) found nalorphine to be an analgetic in its own right, we have hypothesized that, in the lower ratios, nalorphine interferes with the morphine effect while in the higher ratios it exerts its own analgetic action (*49*).

C. RELATIVE POTENCY ASSAYS

Most often, an investigator will be interested in comparing the effects of two analgetic agents in terms of their relative analgetic potency, relative ceiling effects, and relative side effect liability. Such comparisons depend

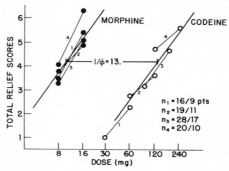

FIG. 3. Dose-effect curves for intramuscular morphine and codeine. The changes in the hourly pain intensity scores summed for 6 hours after medication (ordinate) are plotted against dose on a logarithmic scale (abscissa) for each of four sequential experiments carried out in patients with pain due to cancer. Each experiment consisted of a lower and upper dose of each drug and are plotted as the points connected by the fine lines. The number of doses and patients for each point are tabulated in the lower right hand corner of the figure. The heavy lines are the common drug slopes for the combined experiments plotted through the over-all mean effects for each drug. The horizontal line connects equi-effective doses of the two drugs indicating that 13 times as much codeine as morphine was required to produce the same total analgetic effect. In each experiment, 8 and 16 mg of morphine sulfate served as standards. Doses of codeine phosphate in the four sequential series covered a range of from 30 to 240 mg.

on the assumption that one drug is acting as a diluent of the other—for if they are not, a relative potency value means very little. The experimental design for a relative potency assay should include a built-in test of this assumption. This should include graded dose information on both the standard and the test drug in order to determine that the slopes of the straight-line portions of the dose-effect curves are parallel. Comparisons are best made in the range of approximate equi-analgetic effect to reduce errors due to extrapolation. With the aid of Dr. Irwin Bross, we have developed a method of carrying out such comparisons using a series of sequential experiments (*16*) and one such study is illustrated in Fig. 3, a relative potency comparison of intramuscular morphine and codeine. Each experiment consisted of two doses of the standard (8 and 16 mg of morphine) and two doses of the test drug, codeine. The doses of codeine were adjusted in each experiment, based on the results in the previous experiment, in order to bring them into the same effect range with the morphine standard. In this way, points along the dose-effect curve for the test medication are obtained, with a high concentration of data in the area of equal effect with the standard medication. This study revealed that codeine is indeed able to produce effects equivalent to ordinary doses of morphine, but about 13 times the dose of codeine is required to do so. Tests of high doses of each drug showed some evidence that the codeine effect tends to level off, but only above this range of doses.

When a series of graded doses is used in an experiment in the clinical evaluation of analgetics, it is most efficient to space the doses at logarithmic intervals, and to plot the dose-response curves in terms of effect against the logarithm of the dose. This is advisable because the relationship between stimulus and response in most biologic systems is not a simple arithmetic one, but may be thought of most conveniently in terms of the response of a population with a lognormal distribution of sensitivites to a stimulus. Therefore, a plot of effect versus log dose will lead to the characteristic sigmoid curve of a cumulative normal distribution, the middle portion of which is sufficiently similar to a straight line to be treated as such mathematically (50). Plotting effect against dose on an arithmetic scale tends to produce an apparent leveling off of effect and has misled some investigators into making erroneous estimates of the ceiling effect of some analgetics (16).

If one drug is indeed acting as a diluent of another and their time-effect curves are similar, a single number can adequately reflect their relative potency relationship and this relationship will hold true regardless of whether the estimate is made in terms of peak action or in terms of a calculation of total effect based on the area under the time-effect curves. On the other hand, when the time-effect curves of the two drugs are not similar, no single number can express the potency ratios of the two drugs adequately. This may well be the case in comparing the curves after oral and parenteral administration of narcotics and is illustrated by the comparisons of morphine given orally and intramuscularly in Fig. 4. The length of time to the onset of peak action of the oral drug is longer, as is the duration of analgetic effect. Our estimates of relative potency based on these data indicate that intramuscular morphine is about six times as potent as oral morphine in terms of total effect and considerably more than that in terms of peak effect. Presentation of time-effect curves in graphic form gives the best expression of the complex potency relationships. Reporting relative potency in terms of *both* "peak" and "total" also contributes to our understanding of the drugs

93

and both end points are clinically useful. These data also illustrate the serious errors of interpretation which could arise were observation made at only one arbitrary time after administration.

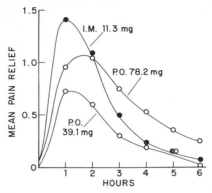

FIG. 4. Time-effect curves for oral (P.O.) and intramuscular (I.M.) morphine. Changes in pain intensity (ordinate) are plotted against time after drug administration in hours (abscissa). The oral doses represent the logarithmic means of the upper and lower oral doses from a series of sequential experiments. The intramuscular dose represents the mean of an 8 and 16 mg standard used in the same experiments. All drugs were administered in a random order to 25 patients with pain due to cancer. Differences in the configuration of the time effect curves indicate that the orally administered drug cannot be considered as acting merely as a diluent of the parenterally administered drug, and that estimates of relative potency will vary depending on which criterion one uses: peak effect, duration of effect, or total effect.

VI. Standards and Controls

Because of the subjective nature of pain and analgesia, our assurance that the response that we are measuring is in fact related to the drug effect that we are attempting to assay must come from within the study itself. Although some investigators look upon such controls as efforts to "keep the patient honest," it is perhaps more appropriate to look upon them as efforts to keep the study honest, since the variables we are attempting to control extend beyond the patient to the clinical milieu itself. There has been a tendency among some clinicians, on the one hand, to denigrate the value of these safeguards, and on the other, to perform them ritualistically as though their use can magically turn a poor, insensitive experiment into a good one. The nature and rationale of the use of these controls in general, and the use of double-blind technique, placebos, and standard medications in particular, has become a matter of some controversy. A critical evaluation of clinical analgetic experimentation requires an understanding of the purposes, uses, and limitations of these experimental procedures and controls.

A. The Double-Blind Technique

The procedure whereby the identity of the factors under test are so disguised that they cannot be distinguished by either the patient or the observer has become known as the double-blind technique. It is a precaution to ensure that the results of any given treatment will not be colored by overt or hidden prejudices that exist before, or may develop during the course of the experiment. Since it is a technique rather than a method of investigation, it does not guarantee the validity or reliability of the results which are dependent on experimental methodology (*34*). It should be emphasized that the observer need not be naive or unaware of the nature of the drugs being investigated, nor is it necessary that the responsible investigator who is not the observer be denied ready access to the code. In terms of ethical consideration alone, "double-blind" should not mean that the patients are to be treated in the dark, nor does the technique rule out intelligent, critical observation or inquiry, as some have implied (*51*). These implications may well have been given impetus by those who feel that confounding the identity of the drugs must be extended to the investigator as well as the observer, and even to the statistician who analyses the results (the so-called "triple-blind" technique) (*52*). These are mere flourishes that contribute little to the basic purpose of the procedure and, indeed, only serve to confuse its intent.

Lasagna (*37*) pointed out that it is not always easy to "deceive" patients or observers as to the identity of the drug. Certainly, there are drugwise subjects and observers who will on occasion be able to identify a drug in terms of properties other than those under test. While this does undoubtedly occur, evidence in the analgetic field would seem to indicate that, in the vast majority of cases, this has not been a major problem. Precaution must be taken, however, to insure that any clues to identity do not carry over as a "halo effect" from one patient to another or from investigator to observer. Asher (*53*) was able to demonstrate that prejudices may occur among observers too, if the medication is presented in different forms or color. Lasagna has mentioned the difficulty of carrying out oral versus parenteral comparisons since it is necessary to give "two kinds of placebos," one oral and one injectable, in order to maintain double-blind conditions (*54*). However, this difficulty has been greatly overrated. The authors have carried out several such comparisons with a high degree of patient acceptance (*10, 44–46*) (Fig. 4). Even if the medications are identical in appearance, double-blind conditions may be broken if a particular medication is constantly associated with a particular code letter or number. This problem is best solved by coding and packaging each dose of medication separately rather than by using multidose containers or vials.

Batterman and Grossman (*36*) have questioned the "double-blindfold" technique as a valid method of distinguishing between the effectiveness of analgetic agents. They have asserted that "the results are confusing and misleading." They attribute this to the high incidence of relief from placebo observed in their studies in outpatients. These investigators have also claimed that the "single-blindfold" technique was not influenced by suggestibility and they present as evidence data indicating that the analgetic effectiveness of placebo did not increase when offered to the patients as a "more potent" drug, although this suggestion did produce a higher incidence of untoward reactions. Since their criteria of satisfactory analgesia was a composite index in which positive values for analgesia and negative values for side effects are combined, it would appear from their data that *both* pain relief and untoward effects were increased by suggestion, although the extent to which this occurred is confounded by the use of global scores. Therefore, despite their claims, the influence of conscious or unconscious suggestion could, in fact, account for the differences between their "single-" and "double-blindfold" results.

Although Keesling and Keats (55) also found a high incidence of pain relief due to placebo, they were able to distinguish between the placebo and active drugs in comparisons utilizing the double-blind technique. They attribute the high placebo effect to the outpatient status of the subjects, since "the investigator cannot control many environmental variables such as social distractions, alcohol, and other therapy," and conclude that to draw conclusions from studies without the safeguards of double-blind evaluations and placebo control would be most hazardous. Indeed, the great weight of evidence indicates that the double-blind technique does not detract from the ability to distinguish between placebos and active drugs in well designed studies (6).

B. Placebo Reaction

1. *What Is a Placebo?*

In the classic sense a placebo provides a "tangible therapeutic symbol" to the patient receiving it (56) and is thus intended to act through some psychological mechanism as an aide to therapeutic suggestion (57).

In the context of an experiment, however, the administration of an inert substance takes on an altogether different meaning—if not to the patient, then at least to the physician. Its two functions, as Gaddum sees them, are to distinguish pharmacological effects from those of suggestion and to obtain an unbiased assessment of experimental results. Since it serves as a counterfeit drug, Gaddum prefers to use the term "dummy" when it is administered under these circumstances (57). Although the inert substance is, indeed, a dummy, its administration to the patient is performed as part of the ritual of therapy even in an experiment, and what we eventually measure has all the connotations of placebo effect. Too many investigators consider only the dummy as a variable, and fail to take into account the circumstances under which it is administered, although the latter is the true determinant of placebo effect and the former merely the instrument for its accomplishment. The term "placebo" is so commonly used to refer to inert medication that it is unlikely that the term "dummy" will ever replace it. To be precise, "placebo" should be used to indicate inert medication only when it serves as an index of placebo effect in the above context.

Some years ago, we conducted a study of the effects of inert medication on the analgetic responses of patients with pain due to cancer to 5 mg doses of

TABLE I

THE ANALGETIC RESPONSES TO ORAL AND PARENTERAL DOSES OF 5 MG OF RACEMORPHAN ADMINISTERED WITH AND WITHOUT AN ORAL OR PARENTERAL DUMMY MEDICATION

Test medications				
Intramuscular injection	Capsule	Drug effect	"Placebo" effect	Analgetic score
(None)	Racemorphan	Oral	"caps"	118
Saline +	Racemorphan	Oral	"caps"+"hypo"	117
Racemorphan	(None)	Intramuscular	"hypo"	211
Racemorphan +	Lactose	Intramuscular	"hypo"+"caps"	207

oral and intramuscular racemorphan (58). This experiment is summarized in Table I. Although the oral and parenteral forms of racemorphan differed in effectiveness, the addition of a dummy corresponding in form to the other administration route did not alter the responses (Fig. 5). Any placebo effect inherent in the act of ministering to these patients was neither enhanced nor diminished by the addition of a lactose capsule or sterile saline injection. These results indicate that placebo reaction must be considered in the context of the total situation of which the dummy is only a part. Ross et al. (59) carried out a related but somewhat differently orientated experiment of the effects of dextroamphetamine on mood in groups of domiciliary subjects. They were able to isolate the placebo effects from those of the drug and concluded that placebo effect is dependent on the expectations of the subjects, and might even act to cancel the pharmacological effects of drugs when they are in opposite directions. We assume that this is not likely to occur in clinical testing of analgetics since the expectations, at least when the patient is administered medication only on demand for relief of pain, are generally in the direction of the drug effect.

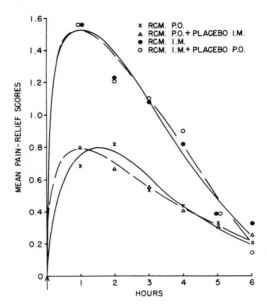

FIG. 5. Time-effect curves for 5 mg of racemorphan administered orally or intramuscularly in the same patients. Changes in pain intensity (ordinate) are plotted against time after drug administration in hours (abscissa). The drug was administered in a random order by either route of administration to 21 patients with pain due to cancer, either alone or together with a dummy corresponding to the other administration route. The study was designed to measure the suggestibility (placebo effect) inherent in the form of administration as it appears to the patient. However, regardless of how it appeared to the patient, the intramuscular form of the drug was significantly more effective than the oral and the inclusion of a lactose capsule or sterile saline injection did not have any appreciable effect at all.

2. Placebo "Reactors" and "Nonreactors"

Several investigators have attempted to characterize populations in terms of their placebo responses. Batterman (36) routinely expects placebo responses of approximately 40% and uses this as a baseline against which to compare test medications. Any placebo response differing significantly from this figure is suspect according to his standards. Beecher (60) in a survey of studies covering a wide variety of clinical situations found the reported incidence of placebo responses to range for 21 to 59% with a mean of 35.2 ±

98

2.2%. This high incidence of placebo response has been a cause of concern to some investigators since it is felt that placebo reaction reduces the sensitivites of drug studies. Attempts have therefore been made to identify so-called "placebo reactors" and to eliminate them from experiments (61). However, the difficulty in identifying them in advance has been pointed out by Lasagna *et al.* (62), and the *ex post facto* elimination of placebo reactors obviously introduces bias. Indeed, there is reason to question even character-

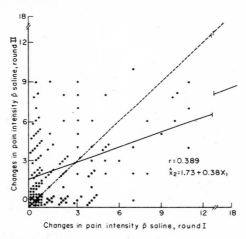

FIG. 6. A correlation of the responses of 150 cancer patients to two random administrations of a placebo medication in the course of analgetic studies. Change in hourly pain intensity scores summed for six hours after the first administration of a sterile saline injection (abscissa) are plotted against similar scores obtained after the subsequent administration (ordinate). The data illustrate the marked variability in placebo responses: 119 patients (80%) reacted to placebo one time or the other; of these, 65 patients (43%) who did not react to one administration of placebo reacted to the other and 54 patients (36%) had varying degrees of response to both administrations. Only 31 patients (20%) consistently failed to react to placebo. The correlation coefficient (r) and the equation for the regression of second dose on first dose are shown in the lower right hand corner of the figure.

izing individuals as placebo reactors. For example, we have found a marked degree of individual variability in the responses of 150 cancer patients to two administrations of a placebo (Fig. 6). Only 20% of the patients in this study could be considered consistent nonreactors. Of those who did react positively, the majority obtained relief from only one of the two placebo administrations, while the remainder had varying degrees of response to both. Rather than to speak of placebo reactors, it seems to us more appropriate to speak of *placebo reaction*, a variable phenomenon; for the individual, his pain and his particular clinical environment are all changing and interacting from time to

99

time. Lasagna *et al.* (*62*) have also attempted to separate reactors and non-reactors in postoperative patients. Using an all-or-none criterion, they found only 14% who consistently failed to obtain pain relief from placebo and this proportion was increased only to 17% by including those who failed to report relief on most occasions, results which agree well with ours. Only

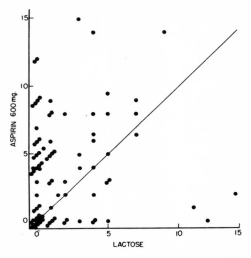

FIG. 7. Scatter diagram of the analgetic responses of 85 cancer patients to 600 mg of aspirin (ordinate) and a lactose placebo medication (abscissa). Each point represents the change in each patient's hourly pain intensity scores summed for six hours after medication. The diagonal represents the equal effect line and separates those who scored higher with aspirin (above) from those who scored better with lactose (below). Fifty-one patients (60%) scored better on aspirin than placebo. Elimination from the study of the 46 "placebo reactors" would result in a loss of 54% of the data and, despite the obvious bias thus introduced, would increase the aspirin superiority to only 67%. The problem of discrimination is one of relative magnitude of response. Since 17 patients obtained more relief from the placebo administration than from aspirin, it must be assumed that an equal number of patients scored higher on aspirin due to chance alone and, therefore, that only 34 of the 51 patients who did better on aspirin can be considered "discriminators." This represents 40% of the total sample and consists of both those who responded and those who failed to react to the placebo medication.

12% of their patients were always relieved by placebo. Psychological tests were carried out in the consistent reactor and nonreactor groups and it was concluded that the reactors were in general more anxious, self-centred, and emotionally labile than the nonreactors. No attempt was made to study the large middle group who responded inconsistently (over 70% of their sample population) as it was assumed that their reponses to the psychological

100

tests would fall between those of the two extremes—however, this remains mere conjecture.

Most investigators consider the so-called "placebo reactors" as nondiscriminators, or at best, poor discriminators of drug effect. Certainly where analgesia is measured as an all-or-none phenomenon (relief or no relief), a positive response to placebo can only imply lack of discrimination *in terms of the scoring system used*. When analgesia is evaluated in terms of a scale of graded effect, however, quite a different picture emerges. For example, Fig. 7 illustrates the responses of 85 cancer patients to lactose and aspirin. Mere inspection of the figure shows that the majority of the patients with positive responses to placebo are still able to discriminate between the pharmacologically active and inactive medications in terms of the *magnitude* of response and, further, that a good proportion of those who failed to respond to the placebo medication also failed to respond to aspirin. Elimination of the "placebo reactors" would result in a loss of over half the data and would increase the proportion of discriminators only from 60 to 67%. Even without considering the introduction of bias, such a procedure would serve to lower rather than raise the efficiency of the experiment. Since the administration of any medication inherently contains a placebo component which may vary in degree or direction, it would seem wise to consider the difference between active drug and placebo effects as one of degree rather than of kind.

3. The "Pharmacology" of Placebos

Placebo medications are known to produce physical as well as psychic effects (*63*), and to mimic active drugs in terms of their onset, peak, and duration of effect to such an extent that the "pharmacology" of placebos has been described (*37*). Of particular relevance to the field of analgetics are studies in which placebo medications and active drugs have been compared, both as to their ability to relieve pain of different severity and their effectiveness under different conditions of "stress." In one study (*64*) Beecher found that the pain relief produced by 10 mg of morphine (as measured by the per cent of the patient population "relieved") was least early in the postoperative period and greater as the postoperative period progressed. The reverse relationship was found for placebo. Since the average severity of pain in a postoperative population tends to decrease as the postoperative period progresses, Beecher concluded that placebo has its greatest effect when the "stress" (pain) was greatest. By the same line of reasoning, it must be concluded that morphine had an opposite effect, being least effective in severe pain and more effective as pain severity decreased. In a subsequent paper (*64a*), Beecher put forth the idea that the efficacy of *both* placebo and morphine is greatest when the pain is most severe, although he presents little

101

in the way of convincing evidence to support this contention which is contrary to that of the study cited above. Lasagna (27) summarized fourteen of his postoperative studies with morphine, and thirty of his postpartum studies with placebo, and demonstrated that effect (peak change in pain intensity) of both morphine and placebo increase with increasing initial pain. However, when using "complete relief" as the criterion of effect in postoperative patients, he found that 92.1% of those with slight pain, 62.3% with moderate pain, 45.7% with severe pain, and only 32.3% with very severe pain experienced relief after morphine. Employing the same criterion with post-partum patients, Lasagna (65) found placebo more frequently produced complete relief in patients who initially had slight to moderate pain than in those with severe to very severe pain. Reichle *et al.* (66), using mean pain relief scores (no relief = 0; pain less than half gone = 1; pain more than half gone = 2; complete relief = 3), also found that both morphine and heroin were more effective in moderate than in severe, and in severe than in very severe pain (patients with slight pain were not used in this study). The interpretations that may be given to these reports hinge upon the meaning given to the term "effectiveness." For example, is complete relief of severe or very severe pain the same or greater effect than complete relief of moder-ate or slight pain? Does a criterion for analgesia, such as "50% relief," imply the same thing early in the postoperative period, when pain is pre-sumably more severe, as it does later in the postoperative course, when the pain has abated? In assays designed to compare drugs, initial pain severity is a randomly distributed variable in the experimental design (if the drugs are randomly assigned to patients) and these questions can be, and usually are, bypassed by the investigator. However, when the experiment is designed to correlate initial pain and effectiveness, and initial pain severity itself becomes the variable under test, these questions of definition become vital to the meaning of the results. Unfortunately, at present they remain merely questions, for no adequate experimental model for evaluating the relation-ship of initial pain intensity and drug effectiveness has been yet designed. "Stress," in this context, is an equally vague term and a catchall for a variety of psychic and physical events. It would seem advisable to avoid use of this word altogether and to speak in terms of the specific events being measured.

4. *What Placebo Response Means*

Although it is generally accepted that the effect of placebo medication is one of suggestion in the direction of the expectation of the patient, some common misconceptions as to the nature of the response exist. A positive placebo response has been variously interpreted as an indication that the pain is purely "psychogenic" (67), that the patient is malingering and actually has no pain at all, or that he is "addicted" and is demanding the medication for purposes other than analgesia. These views are maintained in the face of the great mass of evidence, both experimental and clinical, that pain with a demonstrable physical cause can be influenced by hypnosis and other forms of suggestion, as well as by placebo medication. Although "psychogenic" pain implies "without demonstrable physical cause"—the context in which it is generally employed—it cannot be defined solely in terms of response to suggestion. Furthermore, logic would seem to indicate that the malingerer would be the least likely patient to get relief from anything, including a placebo, and the addict who is presumably more drug wise than the average patient, would be least likely to be fooled by it. The role played by placebo medication in drug assays is commonly misconstrued. Although it has been successfully employed to measure the effect of suggestion, as in the study of Ross *et al.* (*59*), few clinical analgetic trials are designed to ascertain the "no medication" baseline. More frequently, the placebo is a measure of both suggestion and other unpredictable changes in pain occurring in the course of an experiment. It is a means of controlling, but not accurately of measuring, bias due to suggestion.

C. INTERNAL CONTROLS

Standards and controls traditionally serve as a basis of comparison against which the effects of the test medications may be judged; the importance of including standards as a part of the experimental design to control bias in the clinical situation has been alluded to earlier in this chapter. However, in studies of subjective responses, standards and controls serve an additional important purpose. In an evaluation involving a test medication of unknown analgetic value, a real difference between a known analgetic standard and a placebo is a measure of the sensitivity of the method. When a test medication does not differ significantly from placebo, this does not mean very much if no difference can be shown between the standard and the placebo. Thus, a standard and a placebo control serve as an internal measure of the discriminatory ability of the subjects and of the experimental procedure, and allow us to interpret differences (or lack of differences) in the light of the sensitivity of the method we have employed. A significant statistical difference gives us reason to assume that the treatments under test are not alike. However, a failure to establish such a difference need not imply that the treatments are equal. In the latter case, we have merely demonstrated that chance is a *likely* cause, but not a necessary cause, of whatever differences were observed. Real treatment differences may in fact exist, and failure to demonstrate them may be due to inherent limitations in the clinical experiment itself. On the other hand, statistically significant differences do not necessarily imply clinically meaningful differences. This is a judgement based on our system of values rather than on the laws of chance.

Internal controls other than a placebo are often both feasible and desirable. The ability to discriminate between graded doses of a standard medication is in itself an index of sensitivity, and often a more sensitive one than the use of a placebo and a single dose of a standard. Such internal controls can be employed in situations where the use of a placebo is impractical. However, it may be considered worthwhile to include both graded doses of a standard and a placebo control as well, where this is possible, in order to establish a baseline of effect. Graded doses of both the standard and test medication are also advisable in relative potency comparisons in order to establish that one drug is acting essentially as a diluent of the other. Without such assurance, the term relative potency has little meaning.

Where a long-term program of analgetic testing is involved, standards and controls serve the additional purpose of allowing us to compare the small sample population in our study with our over-all patient experience. By this means we are able, within limits, to evaluate whether the particular group we are working with is responding in a manner similar to what we would expect from previous experience or if they differ in a way that would make us cautious about generalizing from our results.

VII. Interpretation of Data

A. Absolute versus Relative Values

It is not uncommon to find analgetic drugs rated in terms of an "optimal," "average," or "minimal effective" dose, or as an "analgetic dose" expressed as an AD_{90} or an AD_{75}. These terms, and results expressed as per cent of population obtaining pain relief, are convenient to use and presumably are easily understood by clinicians. They are also useful in characterizing drug effectiveness in representative samples of particular patient populations. However, their application, even in practical therapeutic terms, is more limited than is generally acknowledged. Individuals vary in response to drugs, and population responses vary as well. Even in well designed clinical analgetic experiments, one is rarely given any assurance that the population sample is indeed representative of the population from which it is drawn. There is even greater chance for error in generalizing from rather limited results in one clinical setting to populations of patients in other institutions or with other types of pain or disease. Furthermore, it should be borne in mind that such statements as "average" or "optimal" doses are derived from arbitrary scales for measuring analgesia or pain, and these scales do vary from one investigator to another. In this context, the fallacies of absolute statements of drug effectiveness, and the danger in comparing drugs in terms of such statements when obtained by different investigators in different settings, become even more apparent.

On the other hand, good evidence exists that well designed experiments can yield information on the *relative* effects of analgetics within a population sample which is reproducible from investigator to investigator and from

TABLE II

RELATIVE POTENCY ESTIMATES OF SEVERAL NARCOTIC ANALGETICS ADAPTED FROM
THE RESULTS OF A NUMBER OF INVESTIGATORS IN DIFFERENT INSTITUTIONS

Drug	Patient Population	Investigator	Potency Relative to Morphine
Oxymorphone	Cancer	Wallenstein and Houde (*68*)	9.8
	Cancer	Eddy and Lee (*69*)	9.9
	Postoperative	DeKornfeld (*70*)	10.0
Phenazocine	Cancer	Houde *et al.* (*71*)	3.2
	Postoperative	DeKornfeld and Lasagna (*72*)	3.3
Dextromoramide	Cancer	Bauer *et al.* (*73*)	2.0
	Postoperative	Keats *et al.* (*74*)	1.9
	Cancer	Houde and Wallenstein (*75*)	1.3
Dipipanone	Cancer	Houde and Wallenstein [a]	0.49
	Cancer	Seed [a]	0.47
	Cancer	Cochin [a]	0.88
Normorphine	Cancer	Houde and Wallenstein (*77*)	0.40
	Postoperative	Lasagna (*39*)	0.25
Dihydrocodeine	Cancer	Seed *et al.* (*16*)	0.15
	Postoperative	Beecher (*16*)	0.17
	Postoperative	Keats *et al.* (*78*)	0.17

[a] Cited in Eddy *et al.* (*76*).

institution to institution. Table II illustrates this point, even though some investigators measured pain intensity and others used all-or-none end points for analgesia. The consistency of these results contrasts with wide variations found in reports of drug effect in absolute terms. Such estimates even vary considerably within the same institution from time to time. Denton and Beecher (*79*) originally reported the AD_{90} of morphine to be 7–9 mg per 150 lb body weight. Later Keats *et al.* (*12*), at that same institution, stated that the mean percentage of patients reporting relief from a dose of 10 mg per 150 lb body weight was 75.5 with a range of from 55 to 94% among subgroups. They point up from this the "dangers of comparing small groups of different patients," a precaution that has unfortunately gone unheeded by too many investigators.

B. GENERALIZING FROM LIMITED EXPERIENCE

The question arises as to the legitimacy of extrapolating an estimate of the comparative effectiveness of analgetics derived in experiments on patients with pain of one cause to all patients. One substantial objection, at least of a theoretical nature, lies in the fact that most investigators feel that the important action of analgetics is in modifying the "reaction component" rather than the "perception component" of the pain experience. Since the reaction component is in large part determined by the significance of the pain to the sufferer, it is not unreasonable, for example, to expect a different reaction to painful stimuli between a group of expectant mothers in labor and a group of patients suffering from terminal cancer. Still another objection stems from the evidence that some analgetics, such as those in the aspirin category, may relieve pain, at least in part, by relieving the cause (7, 80). If some drug specificity exists for certain types of painful conditions, it would naturally lead to contradictory results from various investigations using populations of subjects with pain of different causes and, on the other hand, it could obscure differences in studies in which data from various types of pain were lumped together.

However, there seems to be no good evidence from controlled clinical studies, to date, to indicate that drug specificity for particular types of pain has been a major problem in assaying analgetics (Table II). Both narcotics and the aspirin class of drugs appear to be effective (though in different degrees) in relieving pain in a wide variety of clinical conditions and Beecher (6) feels that, on the basis of comparative results among different investigators, "it seems possible to maintain with considerable assurance that one can generalize cautiously concerning the effectiveness of analgesic agents in treating pain of pathological origin and that neither source (cause) of pain nor type (whether acute or chronic) are important considerations." It must be pointed out though that any such generalization obviously hinges on how one classifies "analgetics." The problem of classification becomes very difficult indeed when one ventures into the realm of nonnarcotic analgetics, particularly those with antiinflammatory or antirheumatic actions. Good correlation of results obtained by different investigators working with different types of patients and disease states has generally been achieved when they have employed drugs drawn from a common class and have reported their results in relative rather than absolute terms.

C. PROPERTIES OF ANALGETIC SCALES

A too rigid interpretation of the subjective scales for analgesia has contributed to confusion in evaluating drug effects. Bross (*81*) has pointed out that a characteristic of subjective scales is that a kind of "slippage" will take place, that is, the borderline between two categories will not coincide for each observer. Since the patient himself makes the measurement in reporting pain or pain relief, we can expect slippage in rating from patient to patient as well as from observer to observer. This would occur whether the scales are graded or quantal.

Different scales will have different properties and must be evaluated in different ways. A quantal scale is simpler and easier to work with than a graded scale, and no assumptions about the distribution of the data need be made. Statistical evaluation can be carried out using chi square or other tests based on the binomial expansion. However, in comparing drugs in analgetic studies, ties are not uncommon and the way to handle them, particularly in terms of crossover data, has been a matter of some controversy. Mosteller (*82*) feels that the chi square test is inappropriate for this type of data and believes that ties should be eliminated from the analysis as they contribute nothing to the evaluation of a drug. He thus evaluates only the responses that are different, using the standard *t*-test. However, Acland (*83*) has pointed out that ties are often obtained as a result of poor discriminatory ability of the subjects and can help to assess the degree of error to which the observations are subject. Throwing them out, he feels, represents a deliberate biasing of the observations in the direction toward which they may tend to run. He presents a method for evaluating paired subjective data which takes into account the number of ties. In an illustration of the effect of increasing numbers of ties on significance levels, he demonstrates that even small increases in the number of ties can rapidly increase the probability that the observed differences are due to chance.[1]

Quantitative or measurement data present other types of problems. Most statistical tests for measurement data rely on the assumption that the data are normally distributed, and subjective data most often are not distributed normally (*81*). Significance levels obtained by using such tests may be subject to some error, although Mainland (*84*) contends "the Gaussian assumption perhaps often does little harm when we are comparing mean values." However, serious doubt about the appropriate test to use can perhaps best be resolved by resorting to nonparametric tests, such as rank-order comparisons.

One of the most useful nonparametric procedures for the handling of subjective data of this type is ridit analysis (*81*). The "ridit" is a probability transformation of the subjective scale in terms of an identified (empirical

[1] See note added in proof on page 122.

rather than theoretical) distribution. Each ridit score is essentially a probability statement, in terms of the reference population, of the chance that an effect up to a given level will be obtained. As a statement of probability, the ridit is distribution free, and since it varies from 0 to 1 (with a mean of 0.5 for the reference group), ridits examining the same effect will tend to be in good numerical agreement even when obtained by different investigators using different scales. It is thus possible, for example, directly to compare the responses of different populations to 10 mg of morphine and a test medication, using the responses to morphine of each population as an identified distribution—even though different scales of analgesia are used by different investigators. This procedure has been successfully used by Paddock and Bellville (*85*) in evaluating results of cooperative analgetic studies carried out in several institutions.

Lasagna (*39*) raised the question of whether or not the steps on the graded scale are actually equal in length. He has investigated this in a variety of ways, using a subjective "pain thermometer" and a ranking scale to evaluate what changes in pain the patients felt were most important. His conclusion was that a drop of pain from severe to moderate was on the average most important to the patient, and from slight to none, least important. There was, however, "amazing variability" in the results, every possible ranking being displayed. Gruber and Baptisti (*20*) have pointed out that both change in pain intensity and estimates of relief are dependent upon initial pain intensity, but tending in opposite directions. They simply added the two scores to balance out the effect of initial pain severity. We have found in our studies that ridit transformations using reference groups with different initial pain severities will most effectively equate the differences in scale (*86*).

The crucial test for any scale is its ability to measure the effect under study. There is no external yardstick for pain and the best possible method of validation is correlation with an independent subjective scale intended to measure the same effect. The extent to which the two measures correlate may serve as an index of the validity of the method. In postpartum patients, Gruber *et al.* (*87*) reported a poor correlation between patients' estimates of change in pain intensity and pain relief. However, they administered their medications by-the-clock regardless of whether the patients had pain. It is conceivable that, under these circumstances, the patients would not relate the drug administration with the intended effect and thus if the patient had no pain either before or after receiving medication, he would not have reported relief. We have found that when drugs are administered on demand to patients with pain due to cancer, there is a remarkably high correlation between the two scales (Fig. 8). A prerequisite of any subjective scale is that a substantially high level of communication exists between the subjects and the observer.

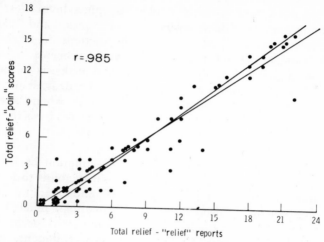

FIG. 8. A correlation between "pain relief" and "pain intensity" as indices of analgesia. Subjective reports of pain intensity based on a four point scale ("none," "slight," "moderate," and "severe" pain) were obtained at hourly intervals. The ordinate represents changes in pain severity summed for a 6 hour period after medication. Relief estimates from a five point subjective scale ("none," "slight," "moderate," "lots," and "complete" relief) were summed for the same period and are plotted on the abscissa. The points represent the responses of 78 patients with pain due to cancer to an intramuscular injection of 8 mg of morphine sulfate. A very high degree of correlation between the two indices was obtained, as shown by the value for the correlation coefficient (r).

VIII. The Analgetic Drugs

In the preceding sections, the discussion was focused chiefly on the problems of measuring pain and analgesia, and of evaluating the analgetic power of drugs, in terms of the design, conduct, and interpretation of clinical experiments. At this point it would be well to consider how these issues relate to the evaluation of particular drugs or classes of drugs, and how successful have been our attempts to develop a sound body of knowledge of the pain relieving properties of the various analgetics. "Success" in this context may be judged by how well different investigators adhering to the same fundamental principles of methodology have been able to come to comparable conclusions on such matters as whether a drug in question is undoubtedly an analgetic in man, its potency relative to other analgetics, its relative effectiveness by different routes of administration, and its efficacy in various types of patients and clinical situations. In order to speak to these questions, it is necessary to reconsider another, that is, how analgetics are generally classified. The most frequently employed schemes, other than merely identifying these drugs with the chemical families to which they belong (e.g., salicylates, *para*-aminophenols, phenylpyrazoles, opiates, opioids), are to categorize them as "potent" or "weak," and "narcotic or "nonnarcotic" analgetics. Although these distinctions do serve a useful purpose, they are not as helpful in evaluating what has been achieved by the pharmacological approach to measuring pain and analgesia in the clinical situation as is a classification based simply on the drug standards with which particular drugs have been compared, for only when there is some such common ground for comparison do we have a solid basis for decision.

A. CHOICE OF STANDARDS

Most clinical analgetic assays are based on the assumption that the "proof" of the soundness and sensitivity of the method lies in its ability to demonstrate significant differences between a known analgetic and a dummy medication in terms of the patients' subjective reports of pain or pain relief. This hypothesis can be tested only by assuming a priori that certain specific drugs are analgetics. For obvious reasons, the drugs most commonly chosen as analgetic standards are morphine and aspirin. Surely, these two drugs have been the most frequently used for the relief of pain, and there are few painful states in which one or the other has not proven effective. Moreover, they are the archetypes of many other effective analgetics in the physician's armamentarium, and they have been the most extensively studied both in the laboratory and in the clinical setting. The selection of two standards rather than one, however, derives from other considerations which are also pertinent to the issues at hand. Morphine is a potent drug in the sense that it is effective in relatively small doses against even the more severe types of pain encountered in medical practice, whereas aspirin is generally considered a "weak" or "mild" analgetic in that, even in relatively large doses, it is much less effective against most types of pain. Morphine is almost always administered by the parenteral route and, because of its more formidable immediate untoward effects, and addiction potential, it is most commonly employed to treat acute pain and used with some reluctance in nonhospitalized patients or in patients with chronic pain. Aspirin, on the other hand, is virtually always administered orally, rarely produces overt side effects, and is much more commonly employed in the management of various types of chronic or low grade pain in both hospitalized patients and outpatients. Thus, on the basis of therapeutic considerations alone, the clinician tends to make a distinction of kind between these two drugs and, depending upon the setting in which he works, the clinical investigator may also find it impractical or inadvisable to use a standard which is inappropriate to common practice in his situation. However, there are other justifications for two standards. First, any putative analgetic which can be shown to be unequivocally better than *either* morphine or aspirin in those conditions in which one or the other is commonly used is a guaranteed "best-seller." Secondly, there are reasons to believe that morphine and aspirin relieve pain by quite different mechanisms of action. Finally, aspirin, being a less potent analgetic and less prone to produce side effects recognizable to an observer, is a more severe test of the sensitivity of a method for assaying analgetics. Morphine, however, has a much wider range of effectiveness in controlling pain of various types and intensities, in a wider range of doses. In graded doses, a linear dose-effect regression can be reliably defined with morphine, whereas there is as yet little information on the properties of aspirin in these terms. Thus the use of parenteral morphine as a standard permits greater flexibility in designing experiments to explore, in the clinical setting, several parameters of analgetic action which are commonly studied in the laboratory.

B. Drugs Compared to Aspirin

Those analgetics which may be considered to fall in this class may be arbitrarily divided into three groups: (i) those which, like aspirin, have antipyretic and/or antirheumatic actions—the salicylates, *para*-aminophenols, phenylpyrazoles, and their derivatives; (ii) the "weak" narcotics and chemically related nonnarcotics—codeine, dextropropoxyphene, ethoheptazine, and prodilidine; and (iii) a variety of chemically unrelated drugs with purported analgetic actions such as phenyramidol, carisoprodol, methopholine, and chlormezanone. These drugs have certain features in common: they are generally administered orally, they are believed to have ceiling effects and thus to be useful only in controlling less than severe pain, and they are frequently employed in combinations, usually with aspirin. In contrast to the widespread use and popularity of these drugs, relatively few well controlled analgetic studies have been conducted and there is still considerable division of opinion on the relative efficacy of several of the drugs in this category.

As mentioned above, aspirin has been employed as a measure of the sensitivity of various clinical analgetic testing methods and, in well controlled experiments, has been demonstrated to be superior to placebo controls in pain due to cancer (*10*), postoperative pain (*61*), headache (*31*), postpartum pain (*65, 88, 89*), pain associated with dental surgery (*90*), acute pain due to trauma and various other causes (*26*), and chronic pain due to arthritis and other diseases (*19, 91, 92*). While most of these studies have been carried out in hospitalized patients, it is evident that similar results can be obtained in well controlled studies in outpatients (*31, 90*).

111

1. *The Antipyretic and Antirheumatic Drugs*

There are few well controlled studies of the comparative analgetic activity of drugs in this group. Of these, virtually all have been carried out using single dose levels of the test drug and standard (usually 600 or 650 mg of aspirin). Although dose-effect data has been reported for graded doses of aspirin (*31, 34*), there have been no reports of relative analgetic potency assays in which graded doses of both the test drug and standard were used; nor has there been any systematic study of comparative ceiling effects of

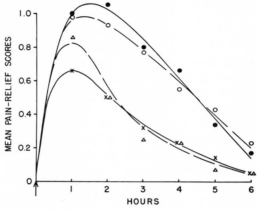

FIG. 9. Time-effect curves for lactose (×) and a fixed dose (600 mg each) of aspirin (●), salicylamide (△), and *N*-acetyl-*p*-aminophenol (○) (APAP, acetaminophen). Changes in pain intensity (ordinate) are plotted against time after drug administration in hours (abscissa). Twenty-seven patients with pain due to cancer received each medication, and 17 of these patients received each medication a second time. The medications were administered in a random order. Both aspirin and APAP were significantly different from either placebo or salicylamide, but not from each other. Although salicylamide was not significantly different from placebo, the relatively high effect obtained in the first hour suggests that the drug may have an early effect which is rapidly dissipated.

these drugs in this context. There is, to be sure, a fairly voluminous literature of uncontrolled analgetic studies and of studies of the antipyretic and antirheumatic or anti-inflammatory action of these drugs, but the information that they provide is subject to the limitations of interpretation discussed above in regard to surveys. A number of studies have also been reported on the blood levels obtained with given doses of various salicylates and other drugs of this group, but there have been no well controlled studies directly correlating analgesia with drug blood levels. The problem may in fact be somewhat more complex than it appears on the surface for both we (*93*) and Lasagna (*94*) have found that, in equimolar doses, aspirin produces significantly more pain relief than sodium salicylate—despite the well known fact that aspirin is rapidly hydrolyzed to salicylic acid and the total salicylate level achieved in the blood is as high or higher after the ingestion of sodium salicylate than after aspirin.

Other than the various formulations of aspirin and APC combinations (88, 92), the only drugs in this group that have been assayed in suitably controlled analgetic studies are salicylamide, acetophenetidin, and aceta-minophen (APAP). An illustration of the results of an experiment which we (95) conducted on salicylamide and acetaminophen is presented in Fig. 9. In this study, as in those conducted by Lasagna (96) on acetophenetidin and acetaminophen, the effects of the test drugs and the aspirin standard were evaluated at only one dose level (identical for all drugs), and compared to placebo. The limitations of such studies are that they provide little inform-ation on relative potency, for the finding that the effects of test medications are not significantly different in equal doses is no proof that they are equi-analgetic. When significant differences in effect are noted (as between salicylamide and aspirin in our study), we have no assurance that a different ratio of doses of the two drugs might not lead to other conclusions. However, the value of plotting time-effect curves of even single dose data can be useful for our results with salicylamide (Fig. 9) suggest that this drug may be rapidly absorbed and eliminated, and studies (97) of the absorption and elimination of this drug in man have shown that this is indeed the case.

2. The "Weak" Narcotics and Related Nonnarcotics

As drugs in this category are apparently most easily detected as potential analgetics by animal screening tests, several have been assayed in man. However, few have been the subjects of published reports and the only drugs of this group on which there is substantial information are codeine, dextropropoxyphene, ethoheptazine, and prodilidine. Codeine is included here in that it is commonly administered orally and has been frequently compared to aspirin. It is, however, a morphine surrogate (98), and a "weak" narcotic only in the sense that its potency relative to morphine is low (see Fig. 3) and its analgetic ceiling is believed to be below that of morphine (99). Dextropropoxyphene, ethoheptazine, and prodilidine are also placed in this category in that they are chemically related to the narcotics, methadone and meperidine, and although more frequently compared to codeine than aspirin, they have been regularly administered orally in studies which more closely resemble the aspirin-standard then the morphine-standard experiments.

There has as yet been no adequately controlled relative potency assay of aspirin and oral codeine based on graded doses of each drug. Thus, at present, there is considerable controversy over what are equi-analgesic doses of these

113

drugs. In our experience, based on the factorial study illustrated in Fig. 1 and other studies in cancer patients (*100*) in which single dose levels of the two drugs were employed, 32 mg of codeine has produced essentially the same analgetic effect as 600 mg of aspirin. However, Beecher *et al.* (*61*) have reported 60 mg of oral codeine to be distinctly inferior to 650 mg of aspirin, while others have found these doses of the two drugs to be approximately equivalent (*14, 101*) or that 30 mg of codeine is superior to 600 mg of aspirin (*91*). Since no two of these studies employed the same criteria or were conducted in the same manner or clinical setting, the differences remain unresolved. This has not deterred investigators in this field from using either aspirin or codeine, or often a combination of the two (sometimes substituting ASA Compound for aspirin) as reference standards in testing other drugs or drug combinations, but it has placed some limitations on conclusions one can make in terms of the relative analgetic effectiveness of drugs in this class. The problems of evaluating the analgetic literature are further compounded by the tendency of many investigators to employ by-the-clock administrations of these drugs and to rely on anamnestic interviews or a variety of observers for the collection of their data. In light of this, and the greater inherent potential variation of responses to orally administered drugs, it is not at all surprising that there is little agreement regarding the analgetic merits of the several drugs which make up this group. Nor can we see any way out of this dilemma until some greater effort is made both to obtain graded dose data based on on-the-spot observations (taken so as to permit the plotting of time-effect curves) and to characterize one's study population in terms of their responses to a given dose of *one* standard drug. The mere use of the double-blind technique and the inclusion of a placebo or active drug control does not compensate for the influences of a number of other variables in either biasing or reducing the sensitivity of analgetic assays.

3. *The Unrelated Miscellaneous Drugs*

This group of drugs presents a greater challenge to the clinical investigator since their spectra of pharmacological actions may be quite different from those of the drugs which we commonly call analgetics. Among these drugs which have been compared to aspirin (or codeine), the majority fall into the category of the so-called "muscle relaxant-analgetics," although some unrelated drugs such as methopholine, indomethacin, and mefenamic acid also belong in this group. The major problem with most of these drugs is to distinguish between the relief of pain produced by an effect on the causal mechanism for pain and that produced by an effect on the central nervous system. However, as mentioned before, this question has also been raised in regard to the mechanism of action of aspirin so that the issue is merely one of classification and, in the final analysis, this will probably be determined by what the drug is predominantly used for in medical practice. Most investigators have carried out their analgetic studies of these agents in mixed populations of patients and have included aspirin as the standard. However, for essentially the same reasons as those mentioned in respect to other categories of drugs in this section, the literature on most of these compounds is difficult to evaluate.

C. Drugs Compared to Morphine

For purposes of this discussion, analgetics falling into this class may also be divided into three groups: (i) the narcotic analgetics—the opiates and the so-called "opioids"; (ii) the narcotic antagonists; and (iii) chemically unrelated drugs with purported analgetic actions. The attributes of these drugs are that they are most frequently administered parenterally, they unquestionably exert their analgetic effects by actions on the central nervous system, and they are employed in the treatment of severe pain of all varieties. In contrast to the drugs compared to aspirin, there is much more uniformity of opinion concerning the analgetic properties and relative analgetic effectiveness of most of these drugs, and there have been a substantial number of well controlled studies of these drugs reported in the literature.

Morphine is commonly used as the standard for these drugs for reasons which have been mentioned before. Its effectiveness in controlling pain of almost all varieties and the fact that graded dose-effect data can be readily obtained with it are obvious advantages for using it in analgetic assays. However it has the following disadvantages: (*a*) it produces side effects which may be recognizable to the observer (and thus compromise a double-blind study which does not make other provisions for controlling this potential source of bias); (*b*) it is not very effective when administered orally; and (*c*) tolerance and physical dependence may develop on its repeated administration. Still another shortcoming is that there is as yet no method sensitive enough for monitoring and correlating with analgesia the blood levels obtained with the usual test doses of morphine.

1. *The Narcotic Analgetics*

These include a large number of drugs which have in common the ability to act in the place of morphine not only in producing analgesia but also in supporting physical dependence. They have thus been designated "morphine surrogates" (*98*) or morphine-mimetic drugs, and include the opiates or morphine congeners, and the "opioids" which, to date, encompass most

115

morphinans, benzomorphans, phenylpiperidines, and methadones, as well as certain diethienylbutenes and substituted benzimidazoles. With the possible exception of codeine, all are commonly spoken of as potent analgetics even though their potencies relative to one another may differ by a factor as great as several hundred.

Although much of the analgetic literature on these drugs can be criticized on the same ground that drugs compared to aspirin were, there have been an encouraging number of reports of well designed and well controlled experiments with these drugs in a variety of clinical settings. This does not imply that analgetic assays are being conducted and analyzed in a completely uniform manner, or even that this is desirable or possible in different clinical settings. However, more laboratories are employing methods of acceptable scientific design and consequently relatively good agreement has been obtained among investigators in rating these drugs as analgetics and in reporting their potencies relative to morphine (see Table II).

There are areas, nonetheless, in which some confusion persists due either to differences in approach or to paucity of experimental data. Among these are the disagreements in regard to the relative oral-parenteral potencies and the ceiling analgetic effects of various drugs. Most of the opinions expressed in the literature concerning the relative oral-parenteral efficacy of the narcotic analgetics have been based on estimates of "average" or "optimal doses" obtained in independent studies in different populations of patients in different institutions. Racemorphan was thus considered to be equally effective by either route of administration (102), whereas in the double-blind study (58) alluded to in Section VI,B,1 (see Table I and Fig. 5) significant differences were observed when the two forms of drug were studied in the same patients. Metopon was similarly considered to be as effective orally as parenterally, but in a relative potency assay carried out double-blind in the same population of patients, Houde and Wallenstein (44) found oral metopon to be less than one-fifth as effective as when it was administered intramuscularly. The question of whether or not the narcotic analgetics differ in their ceiling effects is of interest both for theoretical and practical reasons. On this issue there have been conflicting opinions. We have not found any conclusive evidence from our relative potency studies that the potent narcotic analgetics differ in their ceiling effects. In each instance in which we have attempted to determine whether there is any levelling off of effect with increasing doses of both the test and standard (morphine) medications, we were forced to discontinue before any change occurred in the dose-effect slopes because of the high incidence and severity of untoward effects with both drugs. However, with parenteral codeine, we (103) have observed some change in slope of the codeine dose-effect curve but not that of morphine,

116

when increasing the doses of each medication (to 180 and 360 mg of codeine, and 12 and 24 mg of morphine) in the experiment mentioned in Section V,C (see Fig. 3). Lasagna and Beecher (99) have reported that in post-operative patients, the analgetic effect of parenteral codeine levels off above 60 mg, and that 120 mg fails to equal the performance of 10 mg of morphine. These investigators did not employ any dose above 120 mg and, as in a similar report on dihydrocodeine (104), they have plotted out their dose-effect

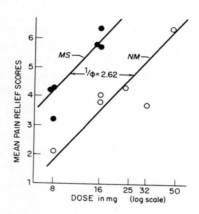

FIG. 10. Dose-effect curves for intramuscular morphine (MS) and normorphine (NM). The change in hourly pain intensity scores summed for 6 hours after medication (ordinate) are plotted against dose on a logarithmic scale (abscissa) for each of three sequential experiments carried out in patients with pain due to cancer. Each experiment consisted of a lower and upper dose of each drug. The common drug slopes for the combined experiments are plotted through the over-all mean effects for each drug. The horizontal line connects the equi-effective doses of the two drugs and indicates that over 2.5 times as much normorphine as morphine was required to produce the same total analgetic effect. In each experiment, 8 and 16 mg of morphine sulfate served as standards. Doses of normorphine hydrochloride in the three sequential series covered a range of from 8 to 50 mg. The analgetic potency of morphine relative to normorphine is represented by the notation $1/\phi$.

curves using an arithmetic scale for dose. Seed et al. (16) have pointed out that a different conclusion would be reached if higher doses of dihydrocodeine were tested and a log dose scale had been employed in plotting the data. As shown in Fig. 10—a relative potency assay of normorphine and morphine—we might have been misled into believing that we had demonstrated a ceiling effect for normorphine (since the effect of the 32 mg dose did not exceed that of the 16 mg dose) had we not persisted in testing still higher doses.

2. The Narcotic Antagonists

That some of the narcotic antagonists are effective and potent analgetics in man has now been firmly established (47, 48, 54). As Lasagna (54) states, "the analgesic powers of nalorphine were discovered by serendipity" since this drug had not been suspected of having analgetic properties on the basis of its preclinical pharmacology. This discovery has subsequently led to the development and analgetic testing of a number of other antagonists of the opiate and opioid class. Since nalorphine and most of the antagonists produce a number of undesirable side effects, these drugs in particular point up the need for measuring analgesia as a distinct phenomenon, since any criterion of "therapeutic" effect which confounds analgesia with side effects would not likely detect these compounds as potentially useful analgetics.

Most clinical analgetic studies of these drugs have been concerned with the effectiveness of narcotic–narcotic antagonist mixtures and the literature on the subject is, at best, confusing. As pointed out in Section V,B (see Fig. 2), the interactions of a narcotic and a narcotic antagonist may be more complex than is commonly appreciated. While there appears to be fairly good agreement between investigators (47, 48, 54) who have carried out analgetic studies of several of the antagonists in postoperative patients, one can predict that conflicting reports of the analgetic effectiveness of these drugs will appear in the literature if care is not taken to exclude patients who are likely to be physically dependent on narcotics, or simply have received a narcotic a few hours prior to being administered the antagonist test drug (105). In this case, crossover studies in which a morphine standard is included may be misleading if care is not taken to examine the first dose data also.

3. Chemically Unrelated Drugs

Putative analgetics of this class present the greatest challenge to the clinical investigator, for while there can be no question that most act primarily on the central nervous system, the pharmacological and purported analgetic effects of some, such as lysergic acid diethylamide and phenycyclidine, are so different from those which we commonly associate with the analgetics as to preclude their being tested by conventional methods. However, whether or not such compounds are to be even considered as analgetics, it is still necessary that they be studied under appropriately controlled conditions and according to established scientific principles. Other drugs which might be included in this group, such as some of the tranquilizers, do have actions which are sufficiently similar to those of the potent narcotics to be tested and evaluated in essentially the same way. While there have been several uncontrolled studies which claim to have shown that promethazine, chlorpromazine, and several other phenothiazines are analgetics or, at least, capable of potentiating narcotics, there have been no reports of well controlled studies substantiating these results. On the other hand, methotrimeprazine was found to be a potent analgetic in postoperative patients by Lasagna and De Kornfeld (*42*), and several other well controlled experiments in patients with labor pain (*106*), postoperative patients (*107*), cancer patients (*108*), and patients with a variety of types of pain (*109*) have confirmed these results.

IX. Conclusions

The clinical evaluation of analgetics and the clinical measurement of pain are just coming of age as scientific disciplines. These areas of investigation have been defined, both through convenience and necessity, in pharmacological terms, for just as the evaluation of analgetics depends on the accurate appraisal of clinical pain, so the measurement of clinical pain itself has come to rely for its validation on the measurable effects of known analgetics. The gaps in our knowledge are large indeed. The mechanisms of action of even the best known centrally acting analgetics are still obscure and the degree to which the salicylates act centrally or in the periphery is still a matter of controversy. The psychological and physical determinants of the pain experience itself remain largely unexplored. There is still much to be learned from the manipulation of psychological variables and from studies correlating analgesia with blood levels or other physical events associated with drug action. Measuring pain and analgesia is deceptively simple, and the complexities have been largely ignored. If the clinic is to be something more than a mere testing ground for putative analgetics and, indeed, if it is even to serve adequately as such a testing ground, basic research in this field must be encouraged and supported.

REFERENCES

1. T. Lewis, "Pain." Macmillan, New York, 1942.
2. H. R. Marshall, "Pain, Pleasure and Aesthetics." Macmillan, London, 1894.
3. C. A. Strong, *Psychol. Rev.* **2**, 329 (1895).
4. J. D. Hardy, H. G. Wolff, and H. Goodell, "Pain Sensations and Reactions." Williams & Wilkins, Baltimore, Maryland, 1952.
5. A. H. Kutscher and H. W. Kutscher, *Intern. Rec. Med.* **170**, 202 (1957).
6. H. K. Beecher, "Measurement of Subjective Responses." Oxford Univ. Press, London and New York, 1959.
7. R. K. S. Lim, F. Guzman, K. Goto, C. Braun, and D. W. Rodgers, *Federation Proc.* **22**, 530 (1963).
8. C. V. Winder, *Nature* **184**, 494 (1959).
9. H. K. Beecher, *Pharmacol. Rev.* **9**, 59 (1957).

119

10. R. W. Houde, S. L. Wallenstein, and Ada Rogers, *Clin. Pharmacol. Therap.* **1**, 163 (1960).
11. J. E. Denton and H. K. Beecher, *J. Am. Med. Assoc.* **141**, 1051 (1949).
12. A. S. Keats, H. K. Beecher, and F. C. Mosteller, *J. Appl. Physiol.* **1**, 35 (1950).
13. S. M. Free, Jr. and F. Peeters, *J. Chronic Diseases* **7**, 379 (1958).
14. R. W. Boyle, C. E. Solomonson, and J. R. Petersen, *Ann. Internal Med.* **52**, 195 (1960).
15. A. J. H. Hewer, C. A. Keele, K. D. Keele, and P. W. Nathan, *Lancet* **256**, 431 (1949).
16. J. C. Seed, S. L. Wallenstein, R. W. Houde, and J. W. Bellville, *Arch. Intern. Pharmacodyn.* **116**, 293 (1958).
17. L. Lasagna, T. J. DeKornfeld, and J. W. Pearson, *J. Pharmacol. Exptl. Therap.* **144**, 12 (1964).
18. C. M. Gruber, Jr., C. L. Miller, J. Finneran, and S. M. Chernish, *J. Pharmacol. Exptl. Therap.* **118**, 280 (1956).
19. L. J. Cass, W. S. Frederik, and A. F. Bartholomay, *J. Am. Med. Assoc.* **166**, 1829 (1958).
20. C. M. Gruber, Jr. and A. Baptisti, Jr., *Clin. Pharmacol. Therap.* **4**, 172 (1963).
21. R. C. Batterman, G. J. Mouratoff, and J. E. Kaufman, *Current Therap. Res.* **4**, 81 (1962).
22. D. Mainland, "Notes from a Laboratory of Medical Statistics," Note 6, p. 3. New York University College of Medicine, New York, 1959.
23. D. Mainland, "Elementary Medical Statistics." Saunders, Philadelphia, Pennsylvania, 1963.
24. T. D. Graff, O. C. Phillips, A. T. Nelson, L. C. Harris, E. T. Fox, and T. M. Frazier, *Southern Med. J.* **54**, 454 (1961).
25. G. L. Jackson and D. A. Smith, *Ann. Internal Med.* **45**, 640 (1956).
26. A. Sunshine, E. Laska, M. Meisner, and S. Morgan, *Clin. Pharmacol. Therap.* (in press).
27. L. Lasagna, *Lancet* **2**, 572 (1962).
28. A. H. B. Masson, *Anaesthesia* **17**, 411 (1962).
29. A. S. Keats and H. K. Beecher, *J. Pharmacol. Exptl. Therap.* **100**, 1 (1950).
30. M. S. Sadove, M. J. Levin, R. F. Rose, L. Schwartz, and F. W. Witt, *J. Am. Med. Assoc.* **155**, 626 (1954).
31. W. J. Murray, *Clin. Pharmacol. Therap.* **5**, 21 (1964).
32. R. W. Houde and S. L. Wallenstein, *Drug Addiction & Narcotics Bull.*, Appendix C, 417 (1953).
33. L. E. Lee, Jr., *J. Pharmacol. Exptl. Therap.* **75**, 161 (1942).
34. W. Modell and R. W. Houde, *J. Am. Med. Assoc.* **167**, 2190 (1958).
35. A. S. Keats, *J. Chronic Diseases* **4**, 72 (1952).
36. R. C. Batterman and A. J. Grossman, *J. Am. Med. Assoc.* **159**, 1619 (1955).
37. L. Lasagna, *Methods Inform. Med.* **1**, 79 (1962).
38. M. Swerdlow, A. Murray, and R. H. Daw, *Acta Anaesthesiol. Scand.* **7**, 1 (1963).
39. L. Lasagna, *Ann. N.Y. Acad. Sci.* **86**, 28 (1960).
40. P. Meier, S. M. Free, Jr., and G. L. Jackson, *Biometrics* **14**, 330 (1958).
41. L. Lasagna and T. J. DeKornfeld, *J. Pharmacol. Exptl. Therap.* **124**, 260 (1958).
42. L. Lasagna and T. J. DeKornfeld, *J. Am. Med. Assoc.* **178**, 887 (1961).
43. A. Sunshine, E. Laska, and M. Meisner, *Drug Addiction & Narcotics Bull.*, Appendix 23, 3955 (1964).
44. R. W. Houde and S. L. Wallenstein, *Federation Proc.* **17**, 379 (1958).
45. S. L. Wallenstein and R. W. Houde, *Federation Proc.* **18**, 456 (1959).

46. R. W. Houde, S. L. Wallenstein, and W. T. Beaver, *Drug Addiction & Narcotics Bull.*, Appendix 22, 3942 (1964).
47. L. Lasagna and H. K. Beecher, *J. Pharmacol. Exptl. Therap.* **112**, 356 (1954).
48. A. S. Keats and J. Telford, *J. Pharmacol. Exptl. Therap.* **117**, 190 (1956).
49. R. W. Houde and S. L. Wallenstein, *Federation Proc.* **15**, 1434 (1956).
50. J. H. Gaddum, *Pharmacol. Rev.* **5**, 87 (1953).
51. A. Hoffer and H. Osmond, *J. Neuropsychiat.* **2**, 221 (1961).
52. L. J. Cass, W. S. Frederik, and J. Teodoro, *Am. J. Med. Sci.* **238**, 529 (1959).
53. R. Asher, *Lancet* **II**, 771 (1948).
54. L. Lasagna, *Pharmacol. Rev.* **16**, 47 (1964).
55. R. Keesling and A. S. Keats, *Oral Surg.* **11**, 736 (1958).
56. L. E. Hollister, *Current Therap. Res.* **2**, 477 (1960).
57, J. H. Gaddum, *Proc. Roy. Soc. Med.* **47**, 195 (1954).
58. R. W. Houde and S. L. Wallenstein, *Federation Proc.* **13**, 367 (1954).
59. S. Ross, A. D. Krugman, S. B. Lyerly, and D. J. Clyde, *Psychol. Rept.* **10**, 383 (1962).
60. H. K. Beecher, *J. Am. Med. Assoc.* **159**, 1602 (1955).
61. H. K. Beecher, A. S. Keats, F. Mosteller, and L. Lasagna, *J. Pharmacol. Exptl. Therap.* **109**, 393 (1953).
62. L. Lasagna, F. Mosteller, J. M. von Felsinger, and H. K. Beecher, *Am. J. Med.* **16**, 770 (1954).
63. S. Wolf, *Pharmacol. Rev.* **11**, 689 (1959).
64. H. K. Beecher, *Am. J. Physiol.* **187**, 163 (1956).
64a. H. K. Beecher, *Science* **132**, 91 (1960).
65. L. Lasagna, V. G. Laites, and J. L. Dohan, *J. Clin. Invest.* **37**, 533 (1958).
66. C. W. Reichle, G. M. Smith, J. S. Gravenstein, S. G. Macris, and H. K. Beecher, *J. Pharmacol. Exptl. Therap.* **136**, 43 (1962).
67. K. D. Keele, *Lancet* **255**, 6 (1948).
68. S. L. Wallenstein and R. W. Houde, *Federation Proc.* **15**, 1611 (1956).
69. N. B. Eddy and L. E. Lee, *J. Pharmacol. Exptl. Therap.* **125**, 116 (1959).
70. T. J. DeKornfeld, *Federation Proc.* **20**, 309 (1961).
71. R. W. Houde, S. L. Wallenstein, J. W. Bellville, A. Rogers, and L. A. Escarraga, *J. Pharmacol. Exptl. Therap.* **144**, 337 (1964).
72. T. J. DeKornfeld and L. Lasagna, *Anesthesiology* **21**, 159 (1960).
73. R. O. Bauer, S. M. Free, Jr., and E. H. Bowen, *J. Pharmacol. Exptl. Therap.* **131**, 373 (1960).
74. A. S. Keats, J. Telford, and Y. Kuroso, *J. Pharmacol. Exptl. Therap.* **130**, 212 (1960).
75. R. W. Houde and S. L. Wallenstein, *Drug Addiction & Narcotics Bull.*, Appendix B, 1934 (1959).
76. N. B. Eddy, H. Halbach, and O. J. Braenden, *Bull. World Health Organ.* **17**, 569 (1957).
77. R. W. Houde and S. L. Wallenstein, *Federation Proc.* **18**, 404 (1959).
78. A. S. Keats, J. Telford, and Y. Kuroso, *J. Pharmacol. Exptl. Therap.* **120**, 354 (1957).
79. J. E. Denton and H. K. Beecher, *J. Am. Med. Assoc.* **141**, 1146 (1949).
80. J. Reid, *Ann. N.Y. Acad. Sci.* **86**, 64 (1960).
81. I. D. J. Bross, *Biometrics* **14**, 18 (1958).
82. F. Mosteller, *Biometrics* **8**, 220 (1952).
83. J. D. Acland, *Clin. Pharmacol. Therap.* **2**, 581 (1961).
84. D. Mainland, *Clin. Pharmacol. Therap.* **1**, 411 (1960).
85. R. B. Paddock and J. W. Bellville, *Drug Addiction & Narcotics Bull.* Appendix 18, 3882 (1964).

86. R. W. Houde, *in* "The Assessment of Pain in Man and Animals" (C. A. Keele and R. Smith, eds.), p. 202. Livingstone, Edinburgh and London, 1962.

87. C. M. Gruber, Jr., J. Doss, A. Baptisti, Jr., and S. M. Chernish, *Clin. Pharmacol. Therap.* **2**, 429 (1961).

88. T. J. DeKornfeld, L. Lasagna, and T. M. Frazier, *J. Am. Med. Assoc.* **182**, 1315 (1962).

89. T. G. Kantor, E. Laska, M. Meisner, and A. Sunshine, *Drug Addiction & Narcotics Bull.* Appendix 20, 3921 (1964).

90. H. S. Brenman, *J. Am. Dental Assoc.* **67**, 23 (1963).

91. L. J. Cass and W. S. Frederik, *Current Therap. Res.* **3**, 97 (1961).

92. L. J. Cass and W. S. Frederik, *Current Therap. Res.* **4**, 583 (1962).

93. R. W. Houde, unpublished data.

94. L. Lasagna, *Am. J. Med. Sci.* **242**, 620 (1961).

95. S. L. Wallenstein and R. W. Houde, *Federation Proc.* **13**, 414 (1954).

96. L. Lasagna and J. W. Pearson, *Drug Addiction & Narcotics Bull.* Appendix 17, 3875 (1964).

97. V. P. Seeberg, D. Hansen, and B. Whitney, *J. Pharmacol. Exptl. Therap.* **101**, 275 (1951).

98. E. Leong Way and T. K. Adler, *Pharmacol. Rev.* **12**, 383 (1960).

99. L. Lasagna and H. K. Beecher, *J. Pharmacol. Exptl. Therap.* **112**, 306 (1954).

100. R. W. Houde, unpublished data.

101. C. M. Gruber, Jr., E. P. King, M. M. Best, J. F. Schieve, F. Elkus, and E. J. Zmolek, *Arch. Intern. Pharmacodyn.* **104**, 156 (1955).

102. C. C. Pfeiffer, *The Modern Hospital* **76**, 100 (1951).

103. R. W. Houde, J. W. Bellville, and S. L. Wallenstein, *Drug Addiction & Narcotics Bull.* Appendix 13, 2533 (1961).

104. J. S. Gravenstein, G. M. Smith, R. D. Sphire, J. P. Isaacs, and H. K. Beecher, *New Engl. J. Med.* **254**, 877 (1956).

105. R. W. Houde, unpublished data.

106. T. J. DeKornfeld, J. W. Pearson, and L. Lasagna, *New Engl. J. Med.* **270**, 391 (1964).

107. A. S. Keats, R. J. Telford, and C. N. Papadopoulos, *Drug Addiction & Narcotics Bull.* Appendix 10, 2816 (1962).

108. R. W. Houde and S. L. Wallenstein, *Drug Addiction & Narcotics Bull.*, Appendix 10, 3264 (1963).

109. E. Montilla, W. S. Frederik, and L. J. Cass, *Arch. Internal Med.* **111**, 725 (1963).

*　　*　　*

Note Added in Proof (see page 107): Since the preparation of this chapter, J. D. Acland has published a retraction of his claim that the proportion of "no preference" decisions or "ties" materially affects the statistical significance of a given difference between the numbers of positive choices for alternative treatments. In this more recent article in *Clin. Pharmacol. Therap.* **5**, 687 (1964), it is pointed out however that the proportion of "ties" is highly relevant to assessing the *quantitative importance* of observed differences of effect in terms of the therapeutic advantage of one treatment (or drug) over another.

CHAPTER IV

Morphine and Its Modifications

EVERETTE L. MAY and LEWIS J. SARGENT

NATIONAL INSTITUTES OF HEALTH,
BETHESDA, MARYLAND

I. The Opium Alkaloids

Opium, the inspissated juice of the unripe seed capsules of the poppy, *Papaver somniferum*, is known to contain some 23 alkaloids, a number of which are very useful clinically. Although records exist of the successful experimental cultivation of the opium poppy (producing opium of satisfactory morphine content) in the temperate zone, as far north as England and Denmark, the bulk of the world supply originates from India, China, Iran, Turkey, the USSR, and southeast Europe. For medicinal purposes, opium, per se, is dried, powdered and standardized to a definite morphine content which ranges between 9.5–10.5%. Pantopon is the proprietary name of one of several widely used opium preparations. The more important alkaloids that occur in opium are as follows: morphine (I, 0.9%), codeine (II, 0.3%); thebaine (III, 0.4%); narcotine (IV, 5%); papaverine (V, 0.8%); cryptopine (0.01%); laudanosine (0.01%); narceine (0.2%) and protopine (0.003%). These are average figures.

Although, at first sight, one may discern two structural types among the opium alkaloids e.g., (a) those related to the 1-benzylisoquinolines, exemplified by norlaudanosoline (VI), and (b) those incorporating the partially hydrogenated phenanthrene system common to morphine (I), codeine (II) and thebaine (III), closer inspection reveals that, logically, all may be considered congeners of the benzylisoquinolines as shown in the accompanying formulas (Fig. 1).

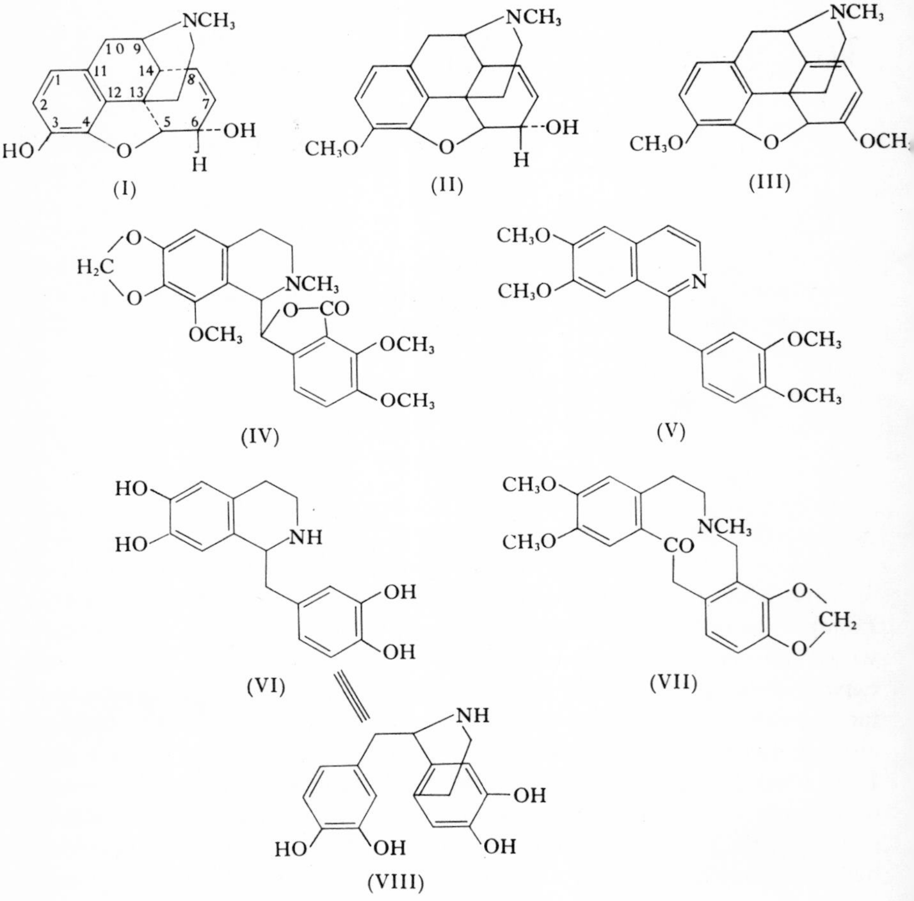

FIG. 1.

As will be noted, papaverine (V) is clearly derivable from (VI), whereas narcotine (IV) requires an additional one-carbon system to account for the carbonyl group of the lactone system. In cryptopine (VII), on the other hand, the new one-carbon unit is incorporated in still another manner to form the novel ring system. In like fashion it is not too difficult to relate the partially

124

hydrogenated phenanthrene system of morphine to that of the benzylisoquinoline redrawn as VIII.

It is of interest to draw attention to the change in pharmacological spectrum that is observed in progressing from papaverine (V), a relatively simple benzylisoquinoline, to the more complicated pentacyclic morphine (I). The former, virtually devoid of central nervous system (CNS) activity, has been utilized as a smooth muscle relaxant while the latter acts principally on the CNS system producing both stimulating and depressing effects as well as contraction of smooth muscle. Morphine, because of its potent analgesic qualities, is by far the most important alkaloid obtained from opium. Opposed, however, to this valuable attribute are certain inherent deficiencies which necessitate circumscribing its medical use. Among these shortcomings are its addiction potential, emetic action, and propensity to cause circulatory and respiratory depression as well as gastrointestinal disturbances. Fortunately it is now possible to counteract the potentially hazardous depressant effects of the drug through the use of certain chemically related antagonists, and this aspect will be considered later on.

II. Morphine, Codeine, Thebaine, and Transformation Products

The possibility of the existence of a relationship between the partially hydrogenated phenanthrene alkaloids (e.g. morphine) and the benzylisoquinoline system led Gulland and Robinson (1) to propose their morphine structure in 1925. It was not until 1952, however, that Gates and Tschudi (2) fully verified this proposal by their elegant synthesis of the alkaloid. Additional synthetic corroboration by Ginsburg (3) and by Barton (4), as well as the elucidation of the stereochemistry (5) and absolute configuration (6) of morphine, have since been reported. In essence, the hydrogens at carbons 5, 6, and 14 are all cis-oriented with respect to the iminoethano system likewise cis-fused to carbons 9 and 13. Mention should be made of an interesting transformation of a morphine derivative to thebaine recently reported by Rapoport (7). Since the reverse alteration has been known for many years, this achievement may be considered a formal chemical synthesis of thebaine.

With the structural picture reasonably complete, attention has recently been directed to the biosynthetic pathways leading to the formation of morphine and its congeners in the opium poppy. The results of several illuminating studies have been admirably summarized by Battersby in his Tilden lecture (8).

The relatively minor structural alteration inherent in proceeding from morphine to codeine results in a marked depression in analgetic potency as well as addiction liability. This knowledge has served as a stimulus, over the years, for the numerous attempts at molecular modification of the morphine molecule with the view to eliminating or, at least, minimizing such deficiencies as addiction potential and respiratory depressant action while retaining the more desirable physiological properties.

The first serious and systematic program which had as its objective the preparation of the ideal morphine substitute was that launched in 1929 under the auspices of the Committee on Drug Addiction of the National Research Council. Competently supervised by Small and Eddy, some 120 morphine derivatives (most of which were synthesized by the former and his colleagues) were carefully evaluated for analgesic as well as other pharmacological properties. The detailed results of these investigations have been summarized in a monograph (9), and the following pertinent general conclusions may be cited. Both the phenolic and alcoholic hydroxyl groups in morphine lend themselves to etherification ($—OCH_3$) or esterification ($—OCOCH_3$). The effect, however, differs and may even be opposite in direction depending on whether the phenolic or the alcoholic group is altered. When the change occurs at the phenolic hydroxyl in morphine or any related compound [heroin (IX) excepted (Fig. 2)] a decrease in morphine-like activity is invariably observed. Similarly, if the alcoholic hydroxyl is transformed or is oxidized to a keto group or replaced by halogen or hydrogen, an increase in morphine-like effect as well as in toxicity generally is elicited. The position of the alcoholic hydroxyl at carbon 6 is of importance; shifting this group to C-8 (e.g., as in pseudocodeine, XXVIII) results in decreased pharmacological activity. On the other hand inverting the hydroxyl at C-6 (α-isomorphine, XXIII, or isocodeine, XXIV) generally enhances potency. Fission of the 4,5-oxygen bridge and substitution in the aromatic ring gives rise to unfavorable activity, while saturation of the 6,7- or 7,8-double bonds may lead to some increase in physiological action, but this is less readily predictable.

Since codeine occurs in opium in relatively small amounts, it is generally prepared commercially by methylation of the more abundant morphine. Codeine is representative of a class of morphine phenolic ethers which are clinically useful for the management of mild to moderate pain and are effective antitussives as well. In view of what has been said regarding the depressed activity that results from muzzling the phenolic hydroxyl, it is interesting to note that acetylation (esterification) of both the phenolic and the alcoholic groups in morphine produces the highly addicting diacetylmorphine (heroin, IX) with about twice the analgetic powers of the parent compound. On balance, then, it appears that O-acetylation of the alcoholic hydroxyl enhances analgetic activity to a degree greater than the weakening effect associated with masking the phenolic hydroxyl. The higher activity of diacetylmorphine probably arises from the greater susceptibility of the 3-acetyl-group to (*in vivo*) hydrolysis thereby implicating 6-acetylmorphine (X) as the active metabolite. Although the latter is known to be about 4 times as effective as morphine, both it, and heroin, are more toxic than the parent alkaloid. Recently described glycyl and *O*-acetyl-L-tyrosyl esters of dihydromorphine (*10*) are reported to exhibit greater solubility and enhanced analgesic effectiveness than morphine.

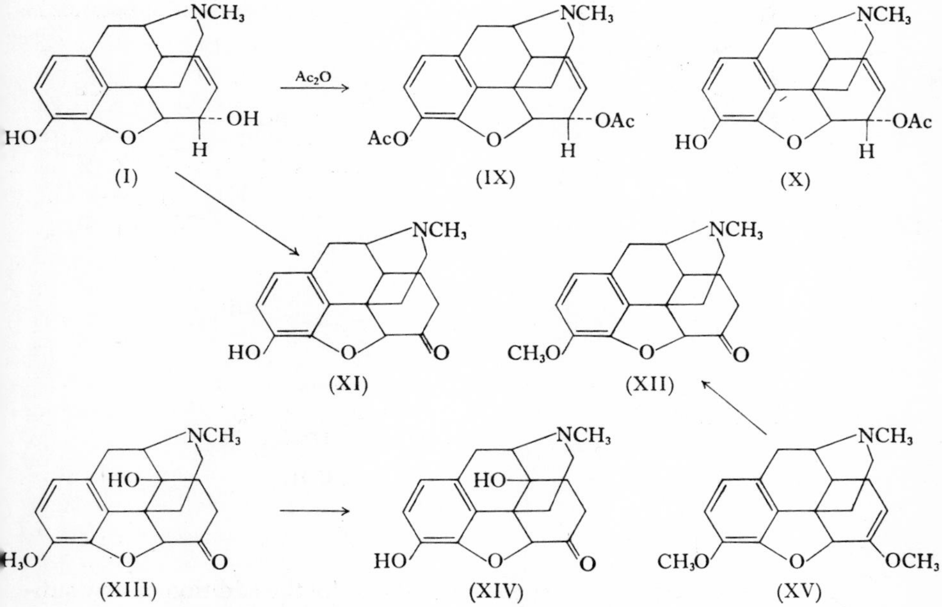

FIG. 2.

Dihydromorphinone (XI) and dihydrocodeinone (Dicodid, XII) exemplify potent analgesics that arise from the catalytic rearrangement of morphine and codeine respectively or, by the hydrolysis of dihydrothebaine (XV). As analgesics, these ketones are about 3–5 times as effective as their hydroxyl counterparts, but fall short because of their relatively higher addiction liability. 14-Hydroxydihydrocodeinone (Eucodal, oxycodone, XIII) of limited clinical utility, is of interest because on controlled demethylation it affords the potent analgesic 14-hydroxydihydromorphinone (Numorphan, XIV) (*11*). Although 6–8 times as effective as morphine, Numorphan is more highly addicting and must be used with caution.

Other modifications at the alcoholic hydroxyl function in morphine have been accomplished with varying effects on analgesic activity. Thus, for example, substitution by chlorine (chloromorphide) enhances activity two to three fold, while replacement by hydrogen leads to dihydrodeoxy-morphine-D (desomorphine, XXII) reputed to be three times as potent as morphine with unusually little emetic or other untoward gastrointestinal effects. 6-Methyl-Δ^6-deoxymorphine (XIX), from the dehydration of 6-methyldihydromorphine (12), is another example where elimination of the alcoholic hydroxyl favorably alters analgetic activity. Although nearly ten times as potent as morphine, duration of action is short and the substance is also highly addicting.

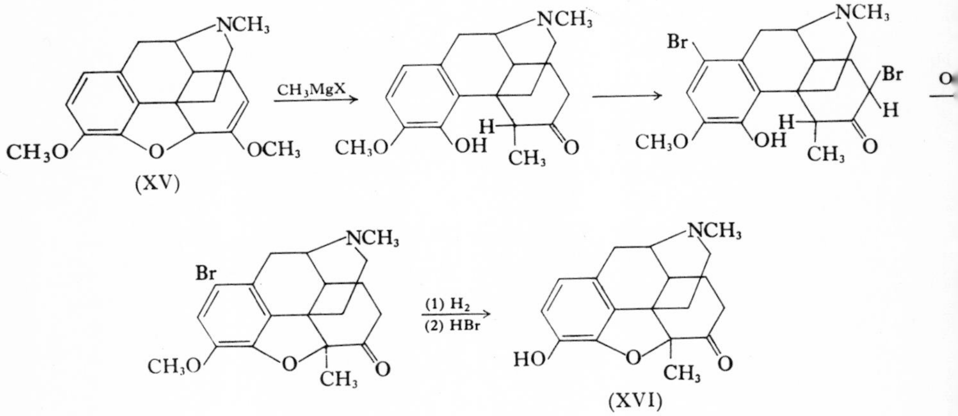

FIG. 3.

As a rule, analgetic effectiveness is depressed by the addition of new substituents to the aromatic or alicyclic rings of the morphine molecule. A notable exception, however, is found in 5-methyldihydromorphinone [metopon, XVI (Fig. 3)] (13), which exhibits about three times the analgesic activity of morphine, and is effective orally. Extensive pharmacological studies (14) have demonstrated that metopon causes little emesis and gives substantial relief in cases of chronic, deep-seated pain. Despite its apparent lower addiction potential the drug has never been promoted for general use —quite possibly because of inherent manufacturing difficulties.

The carbonyl group of the morphine ketones is unusually inert toward the conventional Grignard reagents. Organolithium compounds, on the other hand, readily react to produce 6-substituted tertiary carbinols. Thus when dihydromorphinone (XVII, Eq. 1), was treated with the calculated amount of methyllithium sufficient to compensate for the phenolic hydroxyl, the desired 6-methyldihydromorphine (XVIII) was obtained in good yield (12). Like metopon, the latter derivative not only showed useful analgetic properties but proved to be longer acting than morphine and

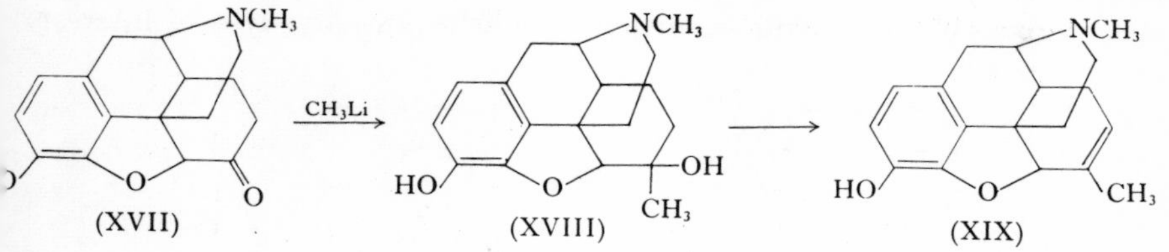

(1)

elicited less intense abstinence phenomena following withdrawal (12). On the basis of these studies, some separation of analgetic effectiveness and physical dependence liability in both metopon and 6-methyldihydromorphine is discernible.

Another variation recently employed to introduce substituents to the alicyclic ring involved treating dihydrocodeinone with triphenylphosphine-methylene reagent to give 6-methylenedihydrodeoxycodeine (15). Controlled catalytic reduction of the latter afforded a good yield of the desired non-phenolic 6-methyldihydrodeoxycodeine along with a quantity of the known phenolic 6-methyltetrahydrodeoxycodeine (Eq. 2). Demethylation

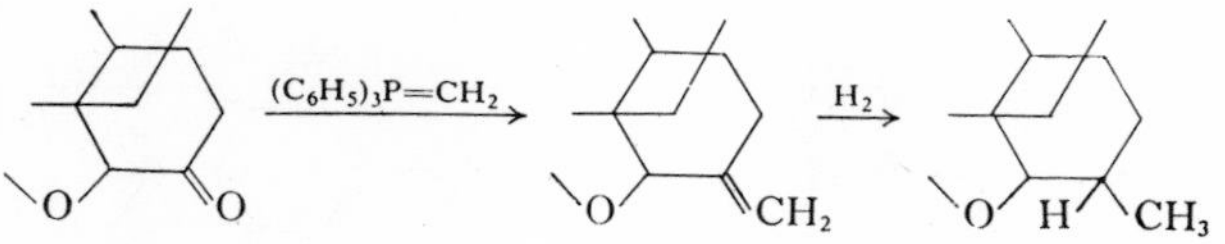

(2)

of the former then led to 6-methyldihydrodeoxymorphine, which showed good analgetic activity.

More recently the medically useless alkaloid thebaine has been transformed via a series of interesting reactions into 14-alkylcodeinones and morphinones whose analgetic activity in rats is reported to be roughly 10,000 times that of morphine (16)—a remarkable value indeed!

In order to test certain postulated mechanisms by which narcotic agents produce analgesia, N-trideuteromethylnormorphine was synthesized and evaluated pharmacologically (17). Briefly stated, deuteration of the N-methyl group was found to depress the analgetic and toxic properties of the alkaloid, while duration of action seemed to be little affected by the isotope substitution.

Whatever other chemical characteristics may be present, a tertiary

129

nitrogen atom constrained in a piperidine-like ring system generally will be found in all potent analgesics derived from morphine. Both the tertiary character of the nitrogen and the heterocyclic ring structure are essential for analgetic action. Fission of the nitrogen ring, as exemplified by the morphimethylmethines, or quaternerization of the nitrogen atom (e.g., methohalides or amine oxides), virtually abolishes activity. It is of interest

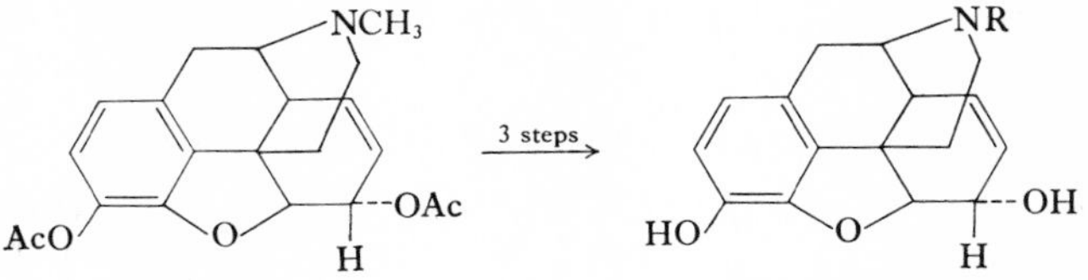

(IX)

3 steps

(XX) R = CH₂CH₂C₆H₅
(XXI) R = CH₂CH=CH₂

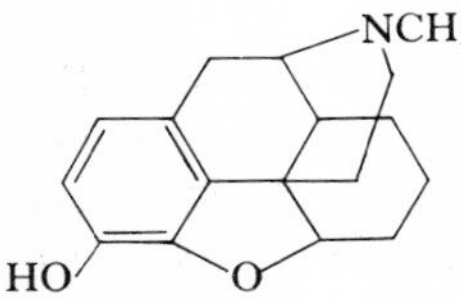

(XXII)

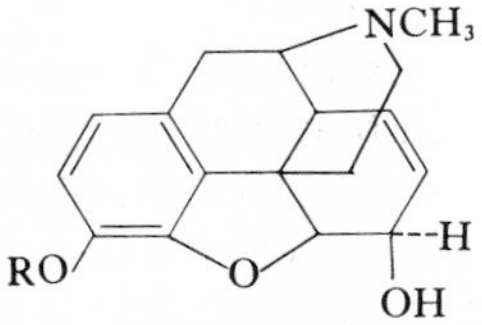

(XXIII) R = H
(XXIV) R = CH₃

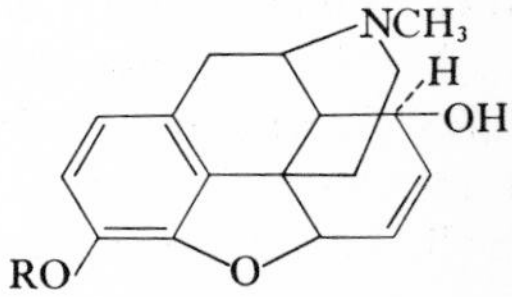

(XXV) R = H
(XXVI) R = CH₃

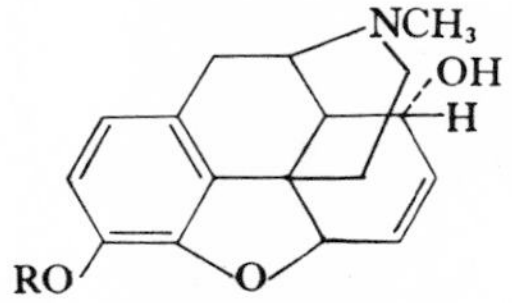

(XXVII) R = H
(XXVIII) R = CH₃

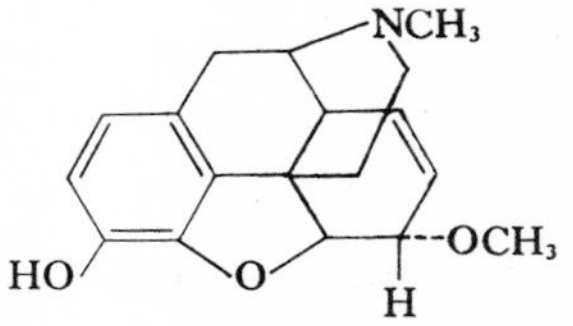

(XXIX)

FIG. 4.

to note, however, that the *N*-oxides of certain morphine congeners, are useful antitussives (*18*).

Novel and interesting pharmacological patterns have recently been uncovered as a result of substituting certain alkyl groups for methyl (on the nitrogen atom). For example, the *N*-(2-phenethyl)nor derivatives (Fig. 4) of morphine (I), desomorphine (XXII), heterocodeine (XXIX), and codeine (II) are far more potent analgetics than the parent alkaloids (*19*). *N*-Allyl-normorphine (nalorphine, XXI) (*20*), on the other hand, is representative of the unusual and unexpected in this area. Not only does it antagonize most of the physiological effects elicited by morphine and other morphine-like analgetics but, in certain cases, may serve effectively in the control of certain types of pain in man. Curiously enough, nalorphine shows little or no analgetic action in animals. Despite significant side-action shortcomings, the drug represents an advance toward the long-sought potent, nonaddicting analgetic.

TABLE I

ACTIVITY OF ANALGESICS IN MICE AND IN MAN

	Analgesic action		
Substance	Mice, ED_{50}, subcutaneously (mg/kg)	Man (equivalence to 10 mg of morphine, mg)	References
Morphine	2.1	10	53
Codeine	14.2	60–120	53, 55
Heroin	0.9	3–5	53
Dihydromorphinone	0.3	2–5	53
Dihydrocodeinone	3.2	15	53
Dihydrodeoxymorphine-D	0.18	1–2	53
Dihydrocodeine	12.4	30	53, 55
Dihydroisocodeine	11.1	30–60	55
Dihydrohydroxymorphinone	0.17	1.5	53
Dihydrohydroxycodeinone	0.6	15	53
Metopon	0.5	3.5	53
6-Methyldihydromorphine	5.4	30	53
Levorphanol	0.5	2–3	53
Meperidine	9.9	50–100	53, 55
Ketobemidone	1.6	5–15	53, 55
($\pm$)-Methadone	1.6	10	53
($-$)-Methadone	0.8	4–6	53
($\pm$)-Isomethadone	2.5	26–30	53
($-$)-Isomethadone	1.2	10	53
($\pm$)-4,4-Diphenyl-6-N-piperidino-3-heptanone	2.0	18	53
($\pm$)-4,4-Diphenyl-6-N-morpholino-3-heptanone	1.1	60	53
($\pm$)-4-Carbethoxy-1-methyl-4-phenylhexamethyleneimine	42.6	50–150	55
Ethylmethylthiambutene	2.4	50	53
Nalorphine	73.0	10	53

TABLE II

PHARMACOLOGICAL EFFECT OF SOME MORPHINE DERIVATIVES (9)

Alkaloidal base	Formula No.	LD$_{50}$[a] (mg/kg)	Analgesia[b] (mg/kg)	Exciting effect[c] (mg/kg)	Emetic action[d] (mg/kg)	General depression[e] (mg/kg)	Respiratory effects[f] (mg/kg)	Convulsant action[g] (mg/kg)
Morphine	I	531	0.75	0.57	0.22	6.75	0.15	531
Codeine	II	241	8.04	8.04	16.0+	36.1	1.3	161
α-Isomorphine	XXIII	890	0.80	0.89	0.13	22.2	0.15	589
Isocodeine	XXIV	589	13.0	13.0		58.9		589
β-Isomorphine	XXV	324	10.1	9.26	4.63	74.0	2.14	324
Allopseudocodeine	XXVI	267	13.3	26.7	13.4+	80.1		178
γ-Isomorphine	XXVII	2000+	7.09	7.09	1.77	133+	2.36	
Pseudocodeine	XXVIII	1780	17.8	22.2	4.45	89.1	48.0	
6-Acetylmorphine	X	293	0.18	0.18	0.18+	0.9		180
Heterocodeine	XXIX	72	0.48	0.32	2.40+	1.40	0.016	65
Dihydromorphinone	XI	84	0.17	0.17	0.08	0.88	0.011	67
Dihydrocodeinone	XII	86	1.28	0.86	2.56+	4.20	0.08	47
Dihydrodeoxymorphine-D	XXII	104	0.08	0.16	Low	0.32	0.012	104
Metopon	XVI	25	0.07	0.10	0.07	3.00	0.012	25
Dihydrohydroxycodeinone	XIII	426	1.34	0.89	0.89+	1.34	0.10	426

[a] LD$_{50}$, subcutaneously in mice.

[b] Analgesia: Minimal dose intramuscularly which caused Eddy pressure test response in at least 80% of cats.

[c] Exciting effect: Minimal dose in cats causing excitement in at least two of five animals.

[d] Emetic action: Minimal dose causing nausea, licking or vomiting in cats.

[e] General depression: Smallest dose preventing immediate righting of at least 15 of 20 rats, 30 minutes after intraperitoneal administration.

[f] Respiratory effect: As defined by Wright and Barbour (114).

[g] Convulsant action: Minimal dose causing convulsions in mice.

III. Partial Structures of Morphine by Total Synthesis

A. MORPHINANS

1. *Chemistry*

Among the early attempts at the total synthesis of morphine were those of the German chemist, Rudolph Grewe. From his investigations have evolved the morphinans (XXX), a class of substances containing the complete carbon-nitrogen skeleton of morphine (I). They are the closest chemical relatives of morphine which have been obtained by total synthesis.

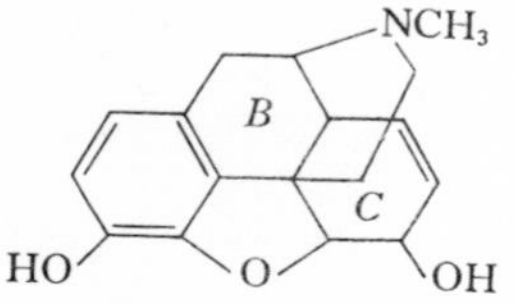

(I) 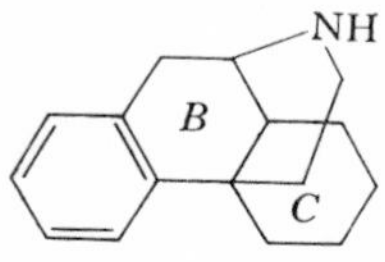   Morphinan (XXX)

The simplest member of the series, *N*-methylmorphinan (XXXIV) showed surprising analgetic activity, nearly one-fifth that of morphine. Furthermore, the 3-hydroxy analog (XXXIX) (numbering the same as in morphine), although lacking the oxygen bridge, the alcoholic hydroxyl, and the alicyclic double bond of morphine, was nevertheless at least four times as potent as morphine with no greater, perhaps less, harmful side effects at optimal doses. Whether or not the high activity shown by these "simplified morphines" was an unexpected by-product of the brilliant researches leading to their synthesis is irrelevant. The fact remains that this discovery provided the stimulus for entirely new areas of research in the narcotics field—investigations that have culminated in the synthesis of strong nonaddicting analgetics of probable clinical utility, as will be indicated later. Furthermore, Grewe's preparation of tetrahydrodeoxycodeine was the first example of the total synthesis of a compound identical with a derivative of morphine and gave further strong support for the Gulland-Robinson (*1*) formula (I).

The first and now basic synthesis of the morphinans devised by Grewe (*21*) was probably modeled after the biogenetic speculations of Robinson (*22*) and Schöpf (*23*) and is shown in Fig. 5. Thus 1-benzyl-2-methyl-1,2,3,4,5, 6,7,8-octahydroisoquinoline (XXXIII), prepared by the reaction of benzyl-magnesium chloride with 2-methyl-5,6,7,8-tetrahydroisoquinolinium iodide (XXXI) and catalytic reduction of the resultant unstable hexahydro base (XXXII) could be cyclized with 85% phosphoric acid to the octahydro-phenanthrene derivative, *N*-methylmorphinan (XXXIV). Hofmann elimination of the methiodide of (XXXIV) and palladium-charcoal aromatization of the methine (XXV) resulting gave phenanthrene (XXVI) and afforded proof of structure. More recently (24), (XXXIV) has been synthesized from 5-hydroxyisoquinoline by the same general method as that developed by Grewe.

It remained for Schnider and his associates in Switzerland to really elaborate the morphinan field. Initially their interest centered on the 3-hydroxy derivative, because of the analogy with morphine, and a practicable synthesis of 5,6,7,8-tetrahydroisoquinoline (XXXVII), which was eventually achieved in six steps from cyclohexanone (25). Schnider and Grüssner effected the

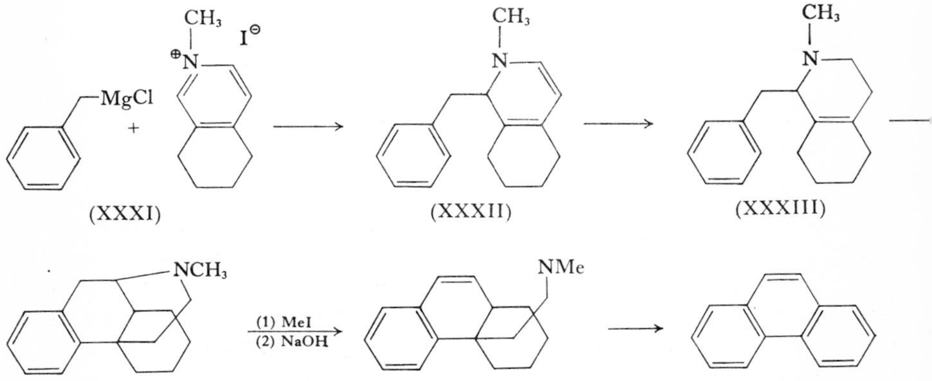

FIG. 5.

synthesis of 3-hydroxy-N-methylmorphinan (XXXIX) (26) utilizing the Grewe method and p-methoxybenzylmagnesium chloride in place of benzylmagnesium chloride (Fig. 6). Almost simultaneously (XXXIX) and tetrahydrodeoxycodeine (XL) were obtained by Grewe (27) by a somewhat different route, although the same XXXVII was used as a starting material (Fig. 7). When 3,4-dimethoxybenzaldehyde was used by Grewe in lieu of anisaldehyde, a small yield of (±)-3-methoxy-4-hydroxy-N-methyl-morphinan (tetrahydrodeoxycodeine, XL) was obtained, a result which established the stereochemical equivalence of the morphinans and morphine (I) at the B:C ring junction and iminoethano system. Several years later a method similar to that of Grewe was developed (28), with 1-chloroiso-quinoline as the key intermediate. This method could also be employed for XXXIV, XXXIX, and XL by using phenylacetonitrile, p-methoxy phenylacetonitrile, or 3,4-dimethoxyphenylacetonitrile, respectively.

3-Hydroxy-N-methylmorphinan (XXXIX) has also been prepared from

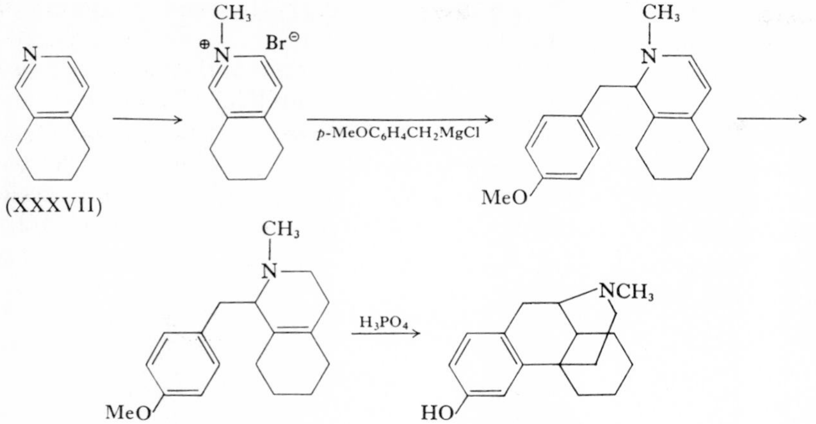

(XXXVII) (XXXVIII) (XXXIX)

FIG. 6.

(XXXIV) by nitration, hydrogenation, and the diazotization reaction (*26*), or by a similar series of reactions on the immediate precursor of XXXIV, the octahydro compound (XXXIII) followed by cyclization (*26*) with phosphoric acid. In the nitration of XXXIV, an isomeric nitromorphinan was

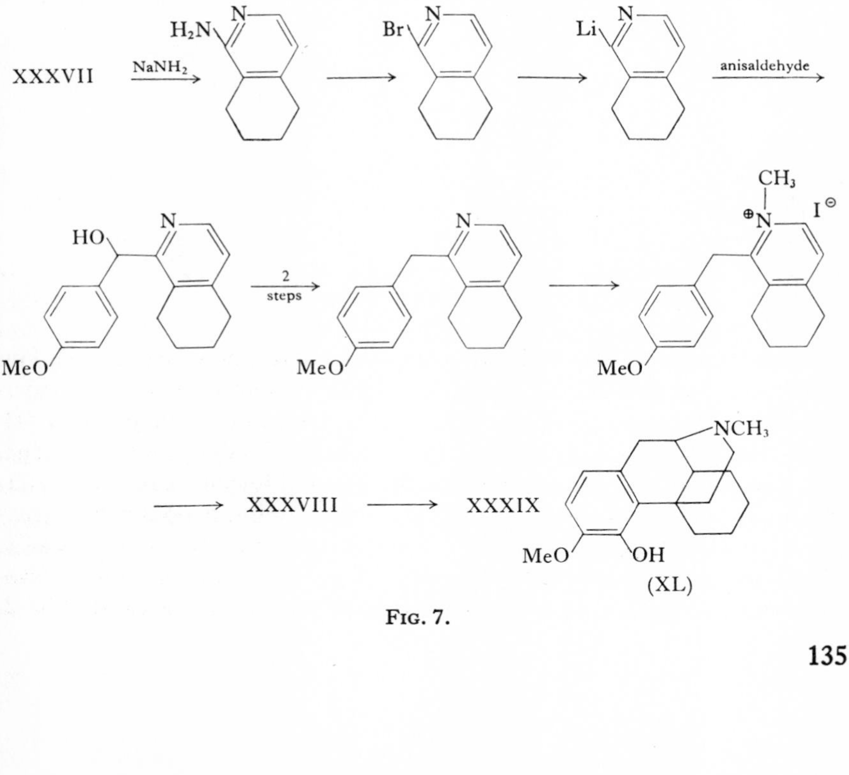

(XL)

FIG. 7.

formed (in low yield) from which the analgetically inert 2-hydroxy-*N*-methylmorphinan could be obtained (*29*).

Perhaps the most practical and versatile synthesis of the morphinans was that developed by Schnider and Hellerbach (*30*) for XXXIX and 3-methoxy-*N*-methylmorphinan (XLV), the *levo*- and *dextro*-isomers, respectively, of which are clinically useful products. In this sequence (Fig. 8) the starting compound, β-cyclohexen-1-ylethylamine (XLI), prepared from cyclohexanone by several methods, is converted to the *p*-methoxyphenylacet-

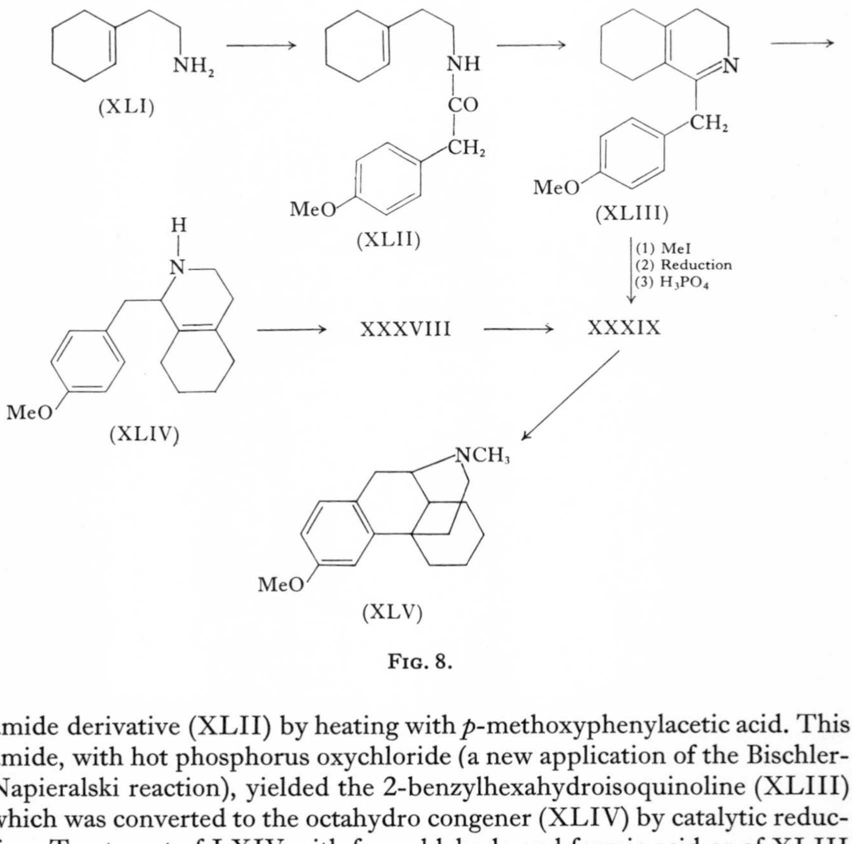

FIG. 8.

amide derivative (XLII) by heating with *p*-methoxyphenylacetic acid. This amide, with hot phosphorus oxychloride (a new application of the Bischler-Napieralski reaction), yielded the 2-benzylhexahydroisoquinoline (XLIII) which was converted to the octahydro congener (XLIV) by catalytic reduction. Treatment of LXIV with formaldehyde and formic acid or of XLIII with methyl iodide followed by reduction of the imminium double bond gave the desired *N*-methyl compound (XXXVIII). In addition to XXXIX, 2-hydroxy- and 2,3-dihydroxy-*N*-methylmorphinan and (±)-tetrahydro-deoxycodeine (XL) have been obtained by this sequence (*29, 30*). The 2-

hydroxy-N-methylmorphinan so obtained was identical with that previously isolated in small yield by nitration, etc. of N-methylmorphinan (26).

Several extensions and modifications of this technically useful synthesis have been made (31–34). All have in common the morphinan precursor, a 1-benzyl-2-methyl-1,2,3,4,5,6,7,8-octahydroisoquinoline such as XXXVIII and appear to offer no particular advantage over the original synthesis (30).

Two other routes to the morphinan nucleus may be mentioned. Ginsburg and Pappo (35) have obtained N-methylmorphinan in low yield starting from 5,10-dioxo-5,6,7,8,9,10,13,14-octahydrophenanthrene, and Barltrop and Saxton (36) have started with β-tetralone, isolating in low yield what is probably N-ethyl-7-oxo-Δ^8-morphinene ethobromide.

2. Resolution and Stereochemistry

Although there are three asymmetric carbons in the morphinan molecule, only two diastereoisomeric (racemic) forms are possible, because the imino-ethano system, attached to positions 9 and 13, is geometrically constrained to a *cis*-(1,3-diaxial)-fusion. These racemates can therefore differ only at the junction of rings B and C—in other words, in the configuration of carbon 14. As stated before, the morphinans have already been shown to be stereochemically equivalent to morphine and congeners (known to possess a *cis* B:C ring fusion (5, 6) at the three common centers of asymmetry. Thus, ($\pm$)-3-hydroxy-N-methylmorphinan may be represented by structural formula XLVI. It was of further interest to compare the optical antipodes of XLVI

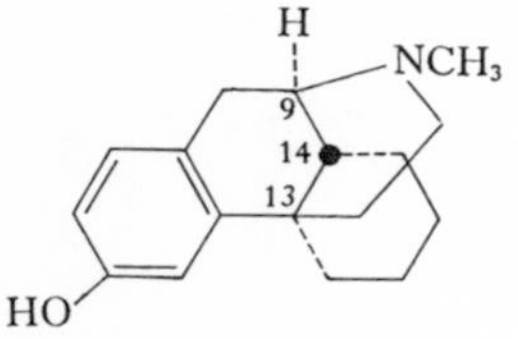

(XLVI) 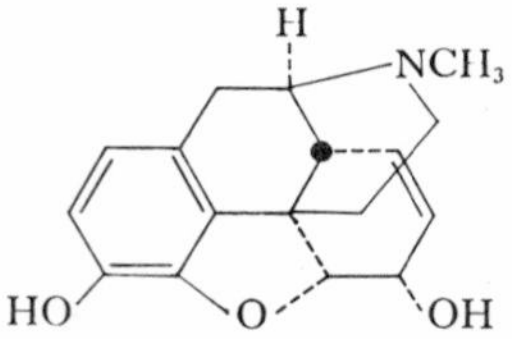   Morphine (I)

with morphine which is levorotatory. There was, of course, the strong suspicion that the bulk of the analgetic activity of XLVI would reside in the *levo*-isomer which, presumably, would have the same absolute configuration as morphine. The resolution of XLVI was effected with L-($+$)-tartaric acid which gave first the pure, ($-$)-isomer (as the tartrate salt). This antipode did indeed contain almost all of the analgetic activity of XLVI and is a clinically useful product (Dromoran®) known generically as levorphanol. To obtain the pure ($+$)-isomer, it was necessary to treat the precursor [($\pm$)-XXXVIII] (Fig. 9) with L-($+$)-tartaric acid which gave [($-$)-XXXVIII] as the less soluble tartrate salt. This enantiomer, on cyclization with phosphoric acid,

137

yielded (+)-3-hydroxy-*N*-methylmorphinan [(+)-XLVI] nearly analgetically inert, the methyl-ether [(+)-XLV, dextromethorphan, Romilar®] of which is an important, nonaddictive antitussive, used extensively in medicine.

Because the commercial demand for dextromethorphan has been much

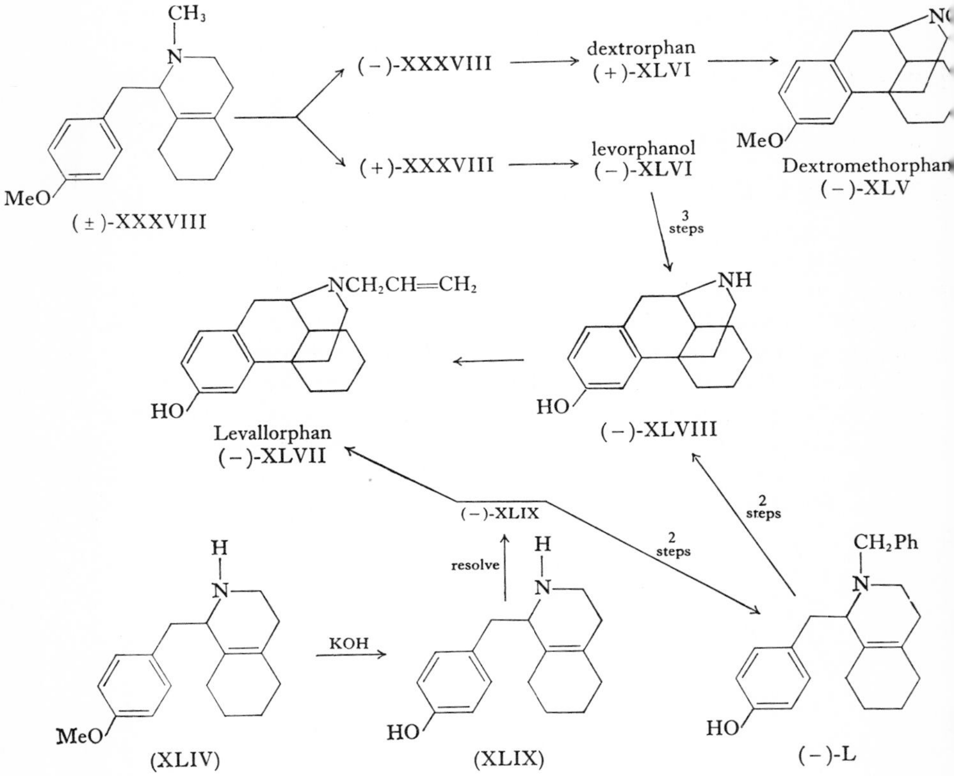

FIG. 9.

greater than that for levorphanol [(−)-XLVI] a procedure for the racemization of (+)-1-(*p*-methoxybenzyl)-1,2,3,4,5,6,7,8-octahydroisoquinoline (XXXVIII) (the cyclization of which gives levorphanol) was developed (*38, 39*). This permits the accumulation of dextromethorphan at the expense of levorphanol (Fig. 9).

Since (−)-3-hydroxy-*N*-methylmorphinan [(−)-XLVI] proved to be the analgetically active antipode, it was logical that variations at the nitrogen

138

would be made primarily with the *levo*-isomer. Consequently (−)-3-hydroxy-*N*-allylmorphinan [levallorphan, (−)-XLVII] was first prepared from the parent *N*-methyl compound (levorphanol) as described in the morphine series (*37*) (Fig. 9), and, like nalorphine (XXI, Fig. 3) found to be

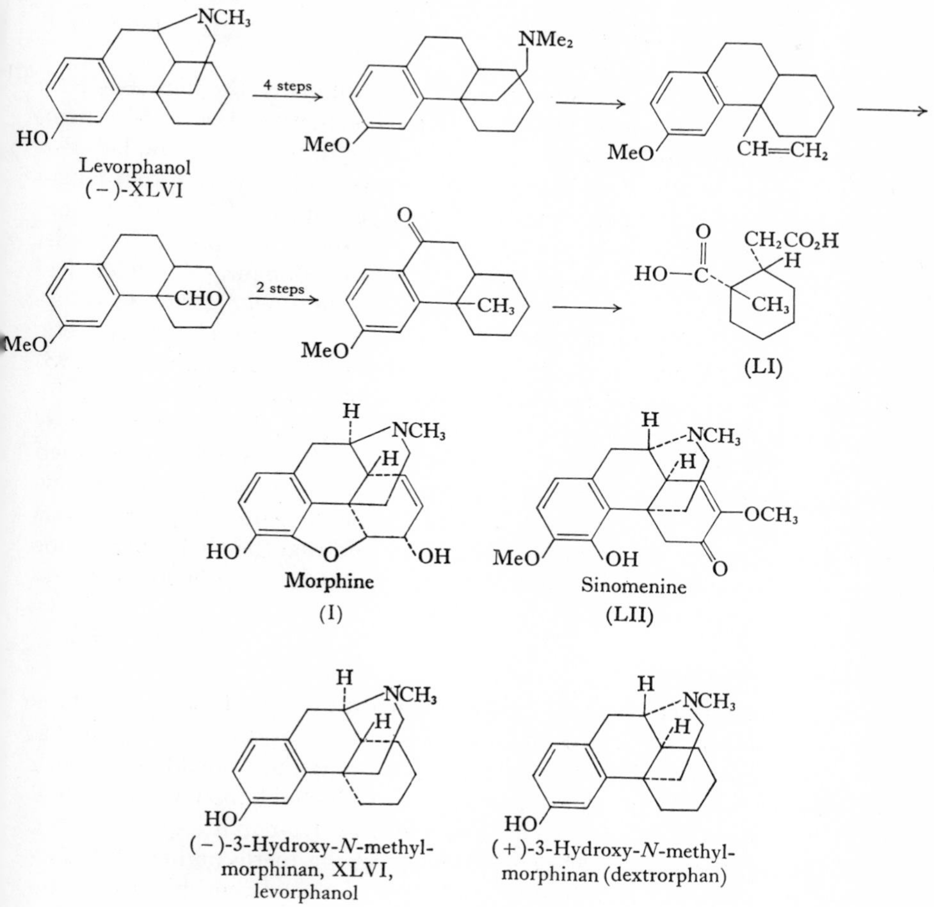

FIG. 10.

a narcotic antagonist, albeit several times as potent as nalorphine. Other N-substituted morphinans may be similarly made.

A more practicable route (Fig. 9) for the preparation of levallorphan consisted in the potassium hydroxide O-demethylation of the octahydro derivative (XLIV), optical resolution of the resulting racemate (XLIX) with tartaric acid, treatment of the (+)-isomer with allyl bromide and subsequent phosphoric acid cyclization to levallorphan. Similarly, benzylation of [(+)-XLIX] gives the (−)-N-benzyl derivative [(−)-L] which can be cyclized and N-debenzylated to give the same (−)-3-hydroxymorphinan (XLVIII) as prepared from levorphanol (40). Many N-substituted derivatives of (−)-XLVIII and its *dextro* enantiomer have been synthesized from these nor compounds.

As for the absolute configuration of the morphinans, the high analgetic activity of the (−)-isomers and the relative inactivity of the (+)-isomers, indicated that the former would be comparable to morphine, the latter to the sinomenine series. Furthermore, Beckett (41) has reported that levorphanol is more strongly adsorbed on silica gel "foot-printed" with morphine than is its enantiomorph, (+)-3-hydroxy-N-methylmorphinan, and is, therefore, probably morphine-like in absolute configuration. Chemical confirmation of this was adduced (Fig. 10) through degradation of levorphanol [(−)-XLVI] to (−)-*cis*-[2-methyl-2-carboxycyclohexyl-(1)] acetic acid (LI) (42) identical to that obtained from thebaine (6) and abietic acid (43) In addition sinomenine (LII) has been transformed into (+)-3-methoxy-N-methylmorphinan (XLV) and dihydrothebaine (XV, Fig. 4) into (−)-3-methoxy-N-methylmorphinan in an elegant series of reactions described by Sawa *et al.* (44). These transformations have provided unambiguous proof that the (−)-morphinans have the same absolute configuration as morphine (I) (5, 6) at carbons 9, 13, and 14, and that the (+)-morphinans have the sinomenine configuration at the three common asymmetric centers. These stereostructures are shown in Fig. 10.

3. *Isomers and Homologs*

The brilliant research which culminated in the total synthesis of morphine has provided another interesting class of compounds, the isomorphinans. The model compound, N-methylisomorphinan, found to be identical with an isomeric (with N-methylmorphinan) by-product obtained in the original Grewe synthesis (21), has been synthesized from 1,2-naphthoquinone (45). A similar synthesis of β-Δ^6-deoxydihydrocodeine methyl ether (46) confirmed the epimeric relationship (at C-14) of the isomorphinans to the morphinans. By the same general method 3-hydroxy-N-methylisomorphinan (LIV) has been prepared and optically resolved (47). The *levo*-isomer containing all of the analgetic activity of LIV is more potent than levorphanol [(−)-XLVI], about nine times as potent as morphine. Appropriately substituted 1,2-naphthoquinones serve as starting materials for the isomorphinans substituted in the aromatic portion. For example, 6-methoxy-1,2-naphthoquinone (LIII, Fig. 11) gives LIV (47).

Many other modifications of the morphinans have been reported. Despite the chemical elegance of these researches (48) none of the compounds resulting have proved to be of especial significance, analgetically, excepting perhaps 3-hydroxy-9-aza-*des*-morphinan (LV, Fig. 11) which appears to be approximately equivalent to morphine (49), although it is more toxic.

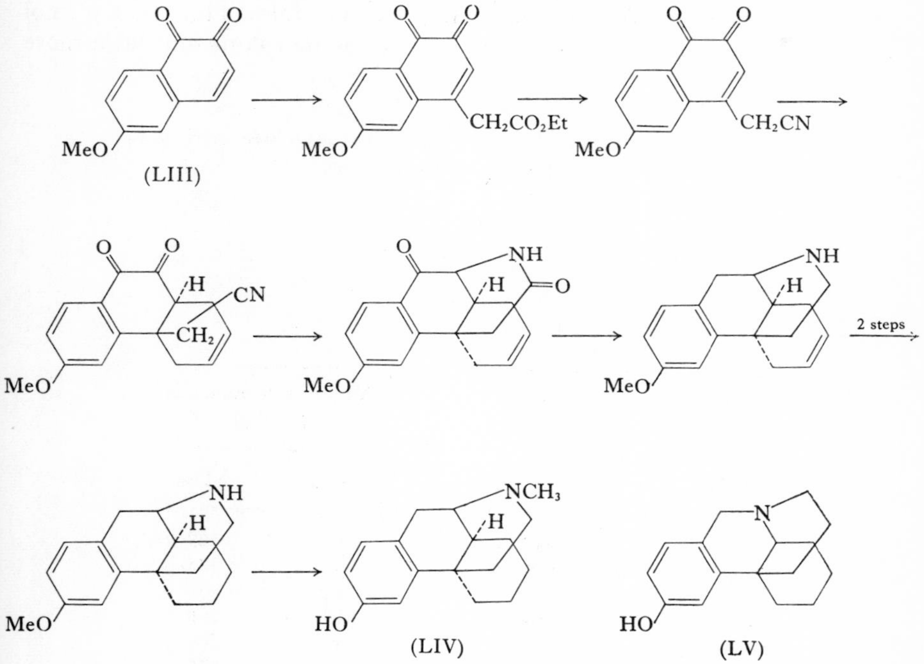

FIG. 11.

4. *Structure-Activity Relationships*

Literally hundreds of morphinans have been evaluated for analgetic activity and acute toxicity, and some for addiction liability and cough suppression. A complete review of these data, not within the scope of this chapter, has been published (50). However, it will be possible to give representative results and indicate trends. All compounds discussed and presented in the following tables have been tested by a standard, reproducible method (51) and the data subjected to probit analysis. Morphine and codeine are given as reference compounds in Table III. As the *dextro* isomers are either substantially inactive or much less active than their *levo* counterparts, only the latter will be treated, with the exception of (±)-*N*-methylmorphinan which has never been resolved.

In Table III are listed *N*-methylmorphinans with alterations in the aromatic portion. The parent compound (XXXIV, H at position 3) as the racemate, is about one-fifth as potent as morphine but more acutely toxic. The introduction of the 3-hydroxyl increases activity twelvefold (based on the racemate) and decreases acute toxicity threefold. Thus levorphanol [(−)-XLVI] is at least four times as potent as morphine and little more

TABLE III

ANALGETIC ACTIVITY OF *N*-METHYLMORPHINANS WITH SUBSTITUENTS IN THE AROMATIC PORTION

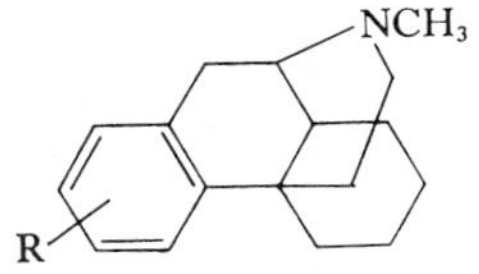

| R | Salt | Mouse, subcutaneous (mg/kg) | |
		ED_{50}	LD_{50}
H[a]	H_3PO_4	11.3	92
3-OH[b]	Tartrate	0.5	365
3-OCOCH$_3$[b]	Tartrate	2.2	—
3-OMe[b]	HBr	3.0	260
3-OH, 2-Me[b]	HCl	Inactive	200
Morphine	HC	2.1	576
Codeine	HC	14.0	270

[a] Racemate.   [b] *Levo* isomer.

toxic. Acetylation of the 3-hydroxyl decreases potency somewhat in contrast to the morphine series, while methylation of the 3-hydroxyl decreases activity to about the same extent, as seen in going from morphine to codeine (Section II). Further substitution in the aromatic moiety of levorphanol or shifting the hydroxyl to position 2 or 4 greatly reduces or abolishes activity. It is worthy of note that 3-hydroxy-*N*-methylisomorphinan (LIV) is about twice as potent as 3-hydroxy-*N*-methylmorphinan (XLVI) while *N*-methylisomorphinan is analgetically inert (*45*).

By far the greatest emphasis has been placed on *l*-3-hydroxy-*N*-substituted morphinans where activity has ranged from zero to about two hundred

TABLE IV

ANALGETIC ACTIVITY OF (−)-3-HYDROXY N-SUBSTITUTED MORPHINANS

N-Substituent	Salt	Mouse, Subcutaneous (mg/kg)	
		ED_{50}	LD_{50}
H	HBr	60.2	222
CH_3	Tartrate	0.5	365
CH_2CH_3	HBr	9.5	243
$CH_2CH_2CH_3$	HBr	Inactive	530
$CH_2(CH_2)_2CH_3$	Tartrate	1.1	—
$CH_2(CH_2)_3CH_3$	HCl	0.4	158
$CH_2(CH_2)_4CH_3$	HCl	0.5	—
$CH_2C_6H_5$	HBr	Inactive	—
$CH_2CH_2C_6H_5$	HBr	0.14	—
$CH_2COC_6H_5$	HCl	0.10	> 400
$CH_2CHOHC_6H_5$	HCl	0.09	225
$CH_2CH_2CH_2C_6H_5$	HBr	25.4	> 400
$CH_2(CH_2)_3C_6H_5$	Tartrate	3.6	> 400
$CH_2CH_2C_6H_{11}$	HCl	2.6	> 750
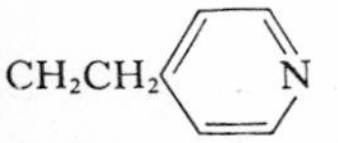 CH_2CH_2-(2-pyridyl)	Tartrate	0.09	500
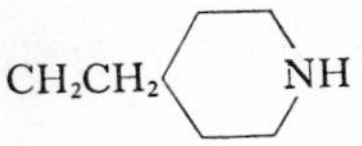 CH_2CH_2-(2-piperidyl, NH)	H_2SO_4	Inactive	—
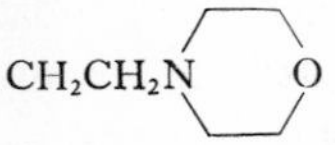 CH_2CH_2N-(morpholino, O)	Salicylate	70.1	> 600
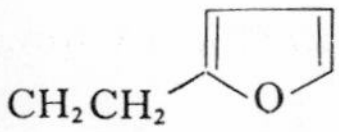 CH_2CH_2-(2-furyl, O)	HCl	0.01	250
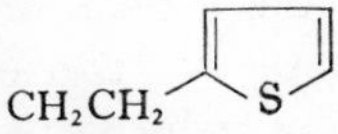 CH_2CH_2-(2-thienyl, S)	HCl	0.02	502
$CH_2CH_2C_6H_4$-p-NH_2	Base	0.02	111
$CH_2CH_2C_6H_4$-m-NH_2	HCl	0.04	176
$CH_2CH_2C_6H_4$-o-NH_2	Base	0.7	665
$CH_2CH_2C_6H_4$-p-OH	HCl	0.2	675
$CH_2CH_2C_6H_4$-p-OCH_3	Tartrate	0.2	> 400
$CH_2CH_2C_6H_4$-p-NO_2	HCl	0.04	> 600
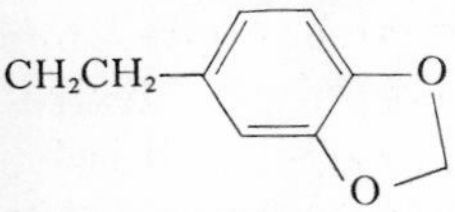 CH_2CH_2-(3,4-methylenedioxyphenyl, O-CH_2-O)	HCl	0.07	> 800
$CH_2CH_2C_6H_4$-p-SCH_3	Base	0.05	> 600

143

times that of morphine, as seen in Table IV. A thorough review of these derivatives is given in Eddy *et al.* (*52*) who treat also the relatively inactive (+)-isomers. It has also been possible to prepare antagonists to morphine-like action in this series more potent than nalorphine. This will be discussed in a later portion of the chapter.

Among groups on the nitrogen conferring highest activity are *p*-substituted phenethyls, phenacyl, 2-furylethyl and 2-thienylethyl. Partial or complete saturation of the aryl group greatly reduces activity as does increasing or decreasing the —CH_2CH_2— chain by one or two carbon atoms. Replacement of methyl on the nitrogen with ethyl also markedly reduces potency, while the substitution of propyl for methyl abolishes activity which begins to return with *N*-butyl and is restored to that of levorphanol with *N*-amyl and *N*-hexyl. Branching the alkyl chain has an unpredictable effect.

In general the toxicity of the *N*-aralkyl derivatives is less than that of the *N*-alkyls. Thus the therapeutic index of the former is much more favorable than that of the latter. There is a fairly good toxicity parallel between the morphinans and similar morphine derivatives.

5. *Clinical Utility of the Morphinans*

Three members of the morphinan series have emerged as medically useful products. They are the strong analgetic, levorphanol [(−)-XLVI] the potent antagonist, levallorphan [(−)-XLVII], and the antitussive agent dextromethorphan [(+)-XLV].

Levorphanol at the recommended dose of 2 mg is comparable in most respects to the optimal dose (10 mg) of morphine. It has at least one advantage over morphine, namely, good activity by the oral route of administration. The addiction liability of levorphanol is also comparable to that of morphine (*50, 53*).

As levorphanol is more potent than morphine as an analgetic, so levallorphan (XLVII) surpasses nalorphine (XXI) in antagonistic potency. Its uses in medicine and research are essentially the same as those of nalorphine: (i) reversal of respiratory depression (especially in overdosage and obstetrics) caused by narcotic analgesics; (ii) as a diagnostic procedure in narcotic addiction; (iii) and as a valuable research tool in assessing the addiction liability of new analgetics. Like nalorphine, levallorphan is not addicting (*50*).

As stated before, the *dextro*-isomers of the morphinan series are relatively inert as analgetics. However, many have proved to be effective suppressants of cough. Most notable is (+)-3-methoxy-*N*-methylmorphinan [dextromethorphan, (+)-XLV], 10–15 mg of which has the same antitussive activity as 15 mg of codeine and is better tolerated (*50*). It is very useful in medicine as an addiction-free (*50, 54*), codeine-like cough remedy and is particularly recommended in pediatrics (*50*).

B. 6,7-BENZOMORPHANS

1. *Chemistry*

The synthesis of (−)-3-hydroxy-*N*-methylmorphinan (levorphanol, XLVI) and the demonstration that this "simplified morphine" can alleviate clinical pain at a much lower dose than morphine (*53*) with no greater harmful side-effects at optimal doses gave hope that the molecule might be still further modified without undue loss in analgetic activity and with possible reduction of deleterious action. Of course it has been recognized for some time that certain of the structural features of morphine and the morphinans should be embodied in any modifications of these molecules obtained by total synthesis. They are : (*a*) the benzene nucleus (*b*) the quaternary carbon (C-13 of compound XLVI) attached to this nucleus ; and (*c*) the tertiary nitrogen two methylene groups removed from the quaternary carbon. The view was also held that the tertiary nitrogen should be in six-membered ring formation and methyl-substituted as in (I) and (XLVI), in which case the phenolic hydroxyl located *meta* to the quaternary carbon attachment should indeed be advantageous (*55*). Finally, optical resolution of any racemate necessarily obtained in ordinary chemical syntheses could be expected to give one analgesically active and one relatively inactive antipode—in effect, a twofold enhancement of activity. These structural considerations are depicted in formula (LVI) and have served as a guide in the syntheses herein described.

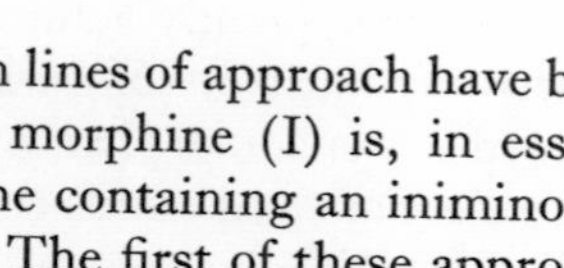

(LVI)

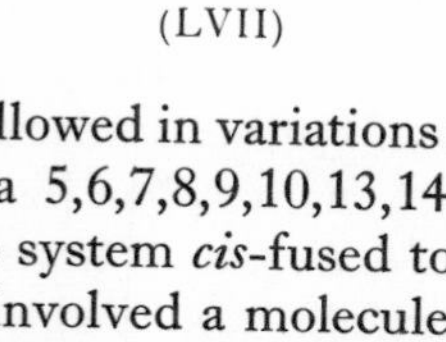

6,7-Benzomorphan

(LVII)

Two main lines of approach have been followed in variations from XLVI which, like morphine (I) is, in essence, a 5,6,7,8,9,10,13,14-octahydro-phenanthrene containing an iniminoethano system *cis*-fused to the 13 and 9-positions. The first of these approaches involved a molecule that would result from elimination of the 9,10-bridge carbons and relocation of nitrogen closure from position 9 to 8. Such a change produces phenylcyclohexane

145

derivatives (LVIII) or phenylmorphans (*56*). In the second line of attack, a series of compounds has evolved, the simplest of which would result from excision of carbons 6, 7, and 8 of ring *C* of XLVI with retention of carbon 5 to preserve the quaternary character of carbon 13. The resultant entity (LVIX) is a hydronaphthalene still containing the *cis*-fused iminoethano system typical of morphine and 3-hydroxy-*N*-methylmorphinan. This entity and its many derivatives are called, briefly, 6,7-benzomorphans (cf. formula LVII). It should be noted that the numbering of the positions in this series is different from that of morphine and morphinan.

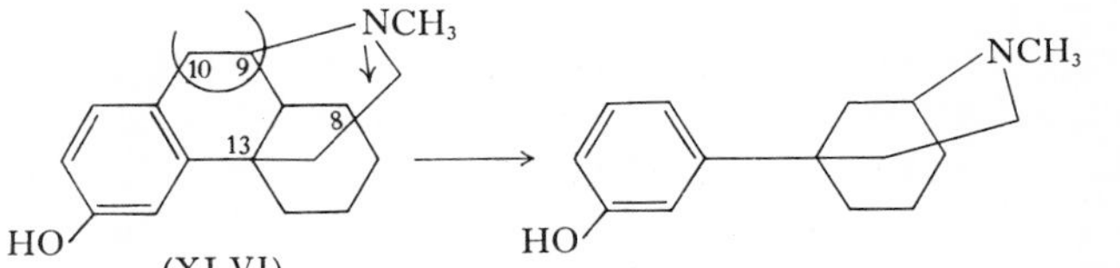

a. 5-Alkyl-2(N)-methyl-6,7-benzomorphans (only hydrogen at position 9). The simplest (model) compound of the benzomorphan series, 2,5-dimethyl-6,7-benzomorphan, (LXI) was synthesized in three different ways. In the first and longest method (*57*), hydratroponitrile (LX) was the starting substance from which both the hydroaromatic and heterocyclic rings of LXI needed to be constructed. Ten relatively straightforward steps were required as shown in Fig. 12. The over-all yield was about 5%. The second route, with a starting compound 3,4-dihydro-1-methyl-2(1*H*)-naphthalenone (LXV) already containing the tetrahydronaphthalene skeleton of LXI initially gave lower yields (*57*) than the longer method. However, significant improvement of the shorter sequence was subsequently achieved (*58, 59*). This method of synthesis was first reported by Barltrop (*60*), who suggested the name 6,7-benzmorphan (later changed to benzomorphan by the editors of the *Journal of Organic Chemistry*) for a class of compounds corresponding to LVII. Barltrop used 2-chloro-*N,N*-diethylethylamine rather than the *N,N*-dimethyl derivative in the alkylation of LXV and did not take his synthesis beyond the stage represented by the quaternary compound (LXIV).

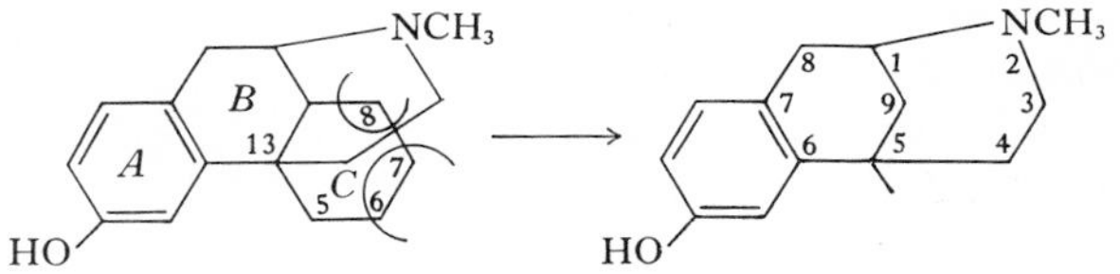

146

Finally, LXI (= LXXId) has been obtained from 1,4-dimethylpyridinium iodide (LXVIa), as shown in Fig. 13. In this instance LXVIa and benzyl-magnesium chloride were brought to reaction (sequence I) in ether to give

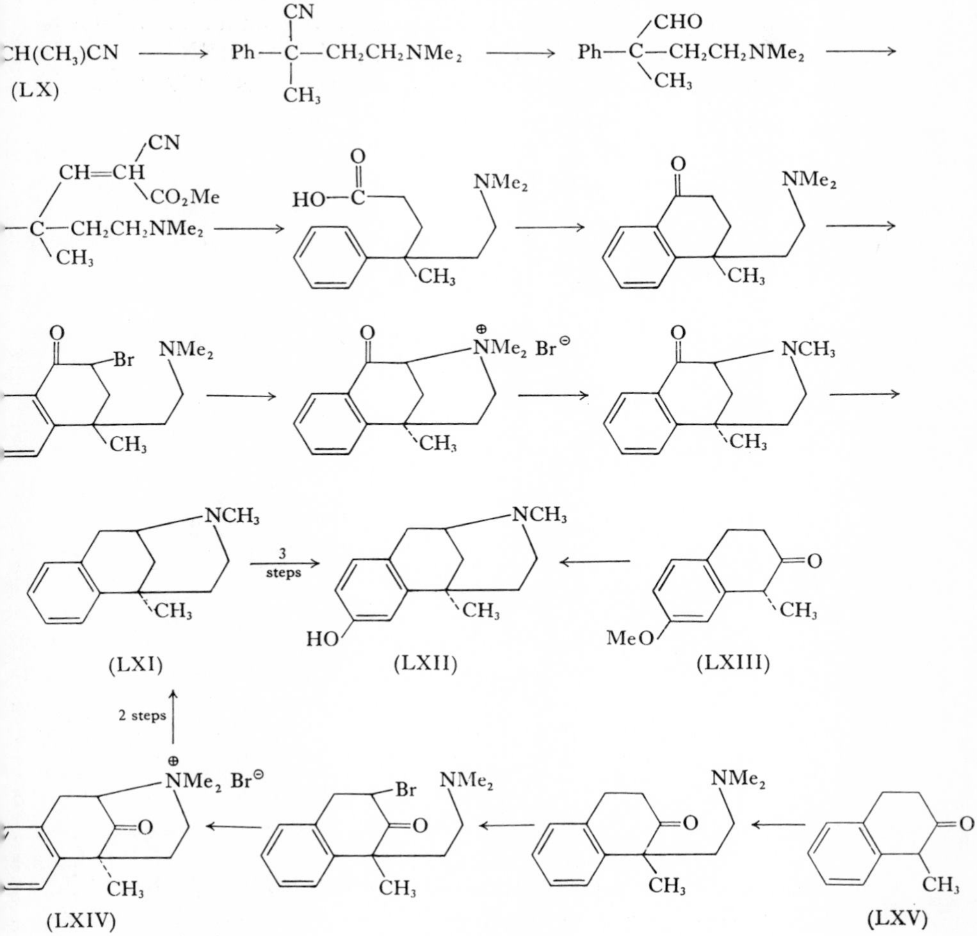

FIG. 12.

the rather unstable dihydro compound LXVIId. This was reduced with palladium-barium sulfate-catalyzed hydrogen (61), or preferably with sodium borohydride, to the tetrahydro derivative (LXVIIId) which could be cyclized with either 48% hydrobromic acid or 85% phosphoric acid. This sequence of reactions will be recognized as an application of the Grewe

147

morphinan synthesis (Section III,A). The fact that LXI could be prepared by the three methods described above is considered to be ample proof of its structure.

The 2′-hydroxy relative (LXII) (*61*) of LXI was first obtained via nitration of LXI, hydrogenation of the resultant 2′-nitro compound and diazotization of the 2′-amino derivative. In addition, LXII (= LXXIf) has been totally synthesized from 3,4-dihydro-7-methoxy-1-methyl-2(1*H*)-naph-

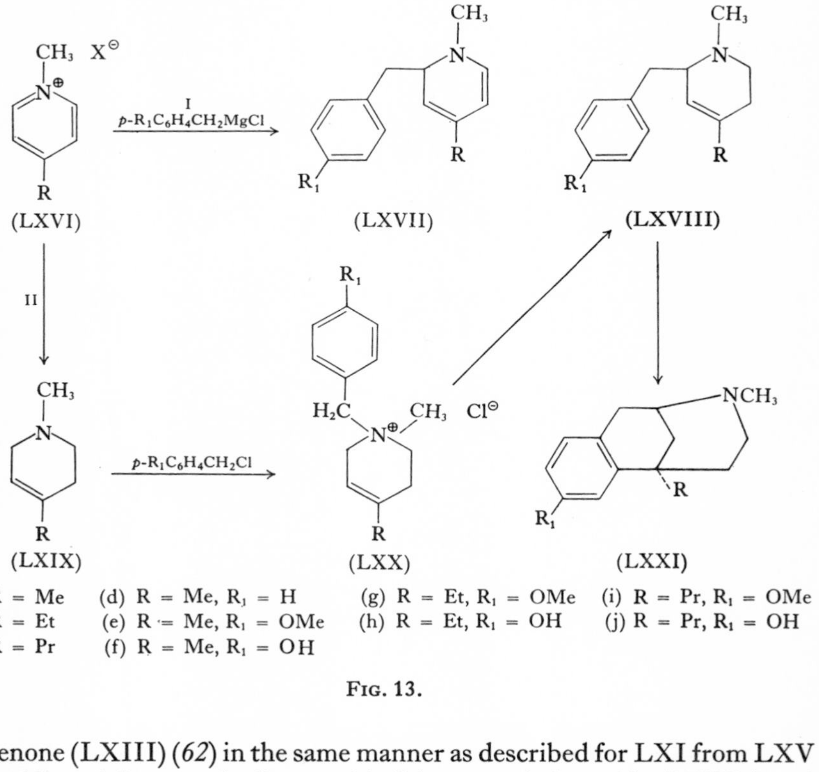

(a) R = Me (b) R = Et (c) R = Pr (d) R = Me, R_1 = H (e) R = Me, R_1 = OMe (f) R = Me, R_1 = OH (g) R = Et, R_1 = OMe (h) R = Et, R_1 = OH (i) R = Pr, R_1 = OMe (j) R = Pr, R_1 = OH

FIG. 13.

thalenone (LXIII) (*62*) in the same manner as described for LXI from LXV (Fig. 12) and from γ-picoline methiodide or methobromide (LXVIa) and *p*-methoxybenzylmagnesium chloride (sequence I, Fig. 13) (*58*, *61*). Alternatively (*63*, *64*) LXVIa was reduced (sequence II) to 1,4-dimethyl-1,2,5,6-tetrahydropyridine (LXIXa) which was quaternized to LXXe with *p*-methoxybenzyl chloride. Treatment of LXXe with ethereal phenyllithium caused rearrangement of the *p*-methoxybenzyl radical from nitrogen to adjacent carbon of the pyridine moiety (Stevens rearrangement) (*63*) giving 2-*p*-methoxybenzyl-1,4-dimethyl-1,2,5,6-tetrahydropyridine

(LXVIIIe) identical with that encountered in sequence I, Fig. 13. Cyclization of (LXVIIIe) afforded LXXIf, O-demethylation occurring simultaneously with ring closure. By sequence II, 5-ethyl- (LXXIh) (*65*) and 5-propyl-(LXXIj) (*64*), 2'-hydroxy-2-methyl-6,7-benzomorphans, have been synthesized from LXVIb and LXVIc in over-all yields of 20–30%.

b. α- and β-5,9-Dialkyl-2(N)-methyl-6,7-benzomorphans. In comparing some of the more intimate structural features of 2'-hydroxy-2,5-dimethyl-6,7-benzomorphans (LXII, LXXIf) with 3-hydroxy-N-methylmorphinan (XLVI), one observes that stereochemically LXII mimics XLVI at assymmetric carbons 5 and 1 (13 and 9 in compound XLVI). The introduction of

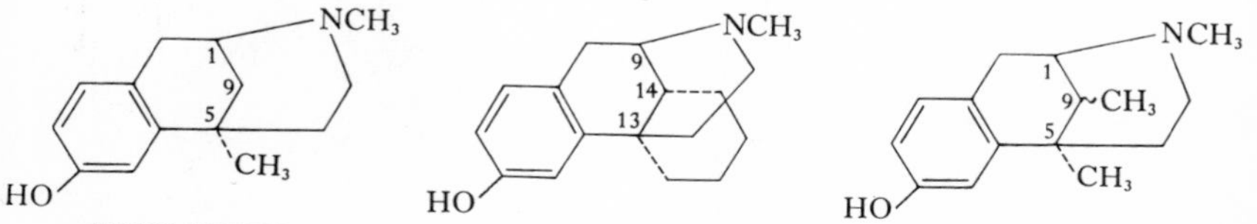

(LXII, LXXIf)   (XLVI)   (LXXII)

a methyl group at position 9 of compound LXII would provide a third assymetric center and would produce the molecule, 2'-hydroxy-2,5,9-trimethyl-6,7-benzomorphan (LXXII), thereby completing the stereochemical approximation of XLVI. Attempts to synthesize such a compound without the phenolic hydroxyl, 2,5,9-trimethyl-6,7-benzomorphan (LXXV)

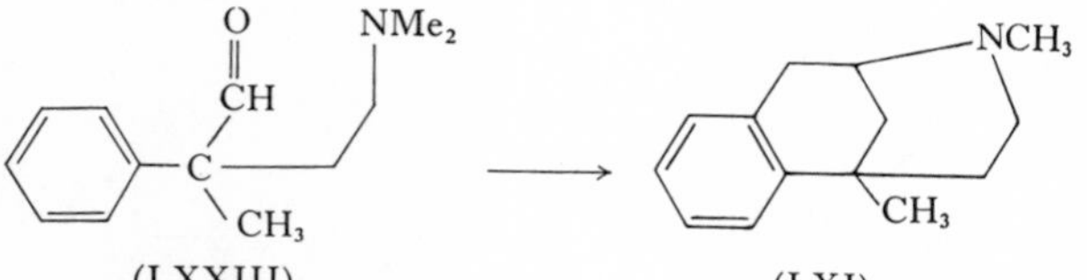

(LXXIII)   (LXI)   (cf. Fig. 12)

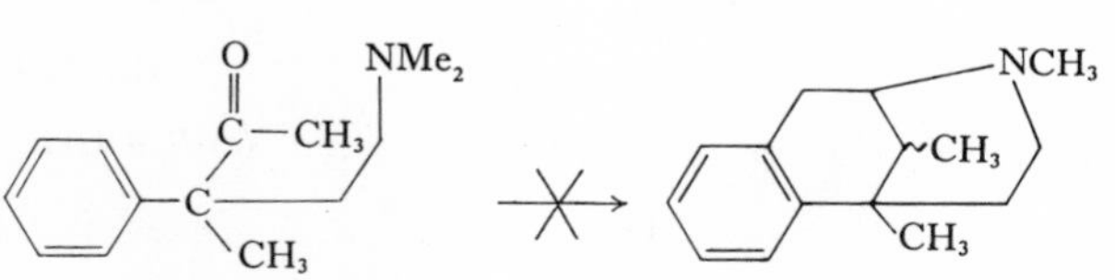

(LXXIV)   (LXXV)

from the methyl ketone (LXXIV) by the method outlined in Fig. 12 were fruitless (*66*).

It was found possible to obtain LXXV and the 2'-hydroxy relative (LXXII) from 1,3,4-trimethylpyridinium bromide or iodide (LXXVI), again by application of the Grewe morphinan synthesis (sequence I, Fig. 14), or by the method based on the Stevens rearrangement (sequence II, Fig. 14) as described previously for 5(mono)-alkyl analogs. The yield of LXXXIa (*67*) was about the same as that of LXXXIc (*67, 68*) (20% based on LXXVI) in sequence I. In sequence II, however, the over-all yield of LXXXIa was

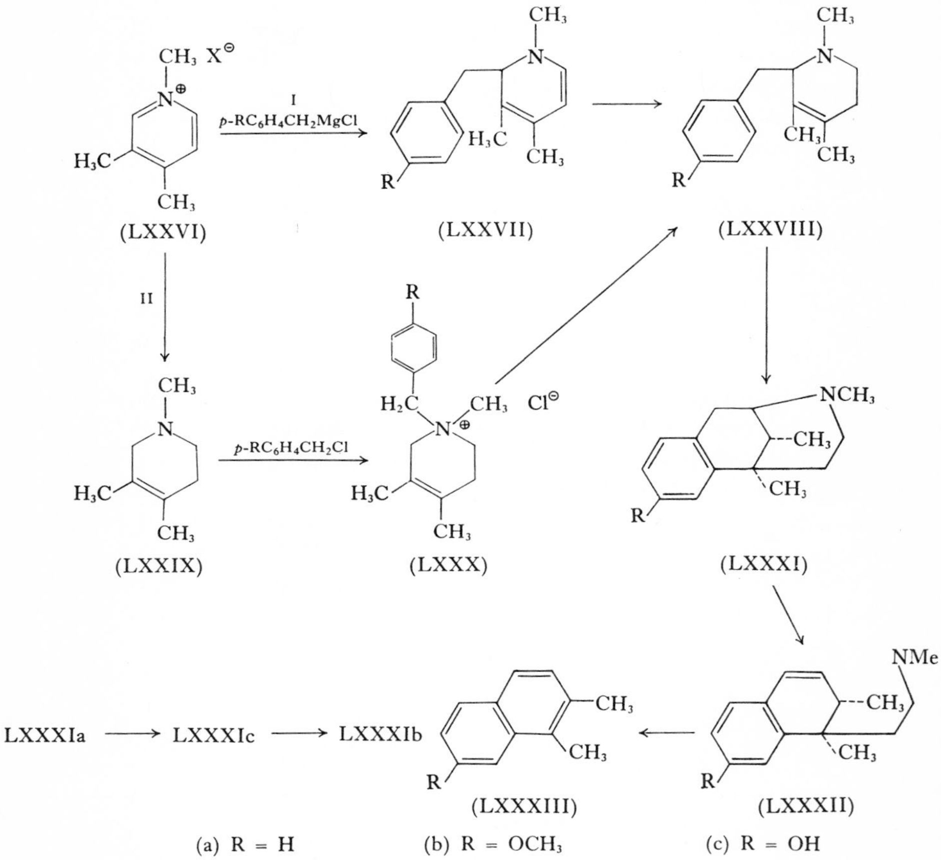

FIG. 14.

markedly lower (only 6.5%), the difference being in the rearrangement step (LXXX→LXXVIII) (*63*). As described before in the 5(mono)-alkyl series (Fig. 13), compound LXXXIa could be converted in three steps to LXXXIc. Nuclear magnetic resonance spectra served to establish the position of the double bond in the borohydride reduction products (LXXIX and LXIX) (*63*).

150

For confirmation of the fundamental skeleton of LXXXI, 2,5,9-trimethyl-6,7-benzomorphan LXXXIa was degraded (67) to 1,2-dimethylnaphthalene (LXXXIIIa) (indistinguishable from authentic material) by exhaustive methylation and palladium-charcoal aromatization of the resulting methine (LXXXIIa) or its dihydro derivative. Similarly (LXXXIb), prepared from LXXXIc by methylation with ethereal diazomethane gave 7-methoxy-1,2-dimethylnaphthalene (LXXXIIIb) (68).

Utilizing the two methods outlined in Fig. 14, the following 3,4-dialkyl-1-methylpyridinium bromides and/or iodides (LXXXIV) have been converted (cf. Fig. 15) to 5,9-dialkyl-2'-hydroxy-6,7-benzomorphans: 3,4-dimethyl (63, 68); 3,4-diethyl (63, 69); 3,4-dipropyl (64); 3-ethyl-4-methyl (70); 3-methyl-4-ethyl (70); and 3-methyl-4-propyl (71). The predominant product (65–75% yields and arbitrarily designated α) obtained in the acid cyclization of LXXXV has been shown (*vide infra*) to conform to the structure and streochemistry represented by LXXXVI. In all instances a small yield (5–8%) of an isomeric product was isolated. The latter (designated β) proved to be diastereoisomeric (at C-9) with the α-isomers by degradation of two representatives (LXXXVIIa and LXXXVIIb) to 1,2-dimethyl- and 1,2-diethyl-7-methoxynaphthalenes (LXXXVIIIa and LXXXVIIIb) respectively (68, 70), identical with those obtained from the corresponding LXXXVIa and LXXXVIb.

That the stereochemistry of the predominant (α) products and the lesser diastereomers (β) is accurately represented by LXXXVI and LXXXVII respectively, in addition to having been predicted by theory (67), has been demonstrated by methiodide-reaction-rate data (72). Quaternization of the α-compounds with methyl iodide occurred from five to ten times as rapidly as the β-counterparts. This could only mean that in the α-compounds the 9-alkyl substituent is oriented away from the nitrogen (axial for the hydroaromatic ring) of the iminoethano system of LXXXVI geometrically constrained to a *cis* (diaxial) fusion as in morphine (I) and the morphinans (XLVI). The slower reacting β-compounds must therefore be assigned structure LXXXVII in which the 9-alkyl substituent, equatorially oriented for the hydroaromatic ring, is close enough to the nitrogen to cause steric hindrance. It was noted in the rate studies (72) that, as the size of R_1 increased in the β series, reaction with methyl iodide became slower. This, then, related the α-compounds (LXXXVI), with their *cis* juxtaposed (for the hydroaromatic ring) 5,9-dialkyl groups, to morphine, and the morphinans whose *cis*-fusion of rings B and C is a certainty (cf. Sections I and III,A,2).

Further confirmation of these configurational assignments was observed in nuclear magnetic resonance spectra of the 5,9-dimethyl compounds

151

(LXXXVIa and LXXXVIIa) (72). Thus the 9-methyl frequencies (doublet) of the α-isomer are at higher field (about 25 c.p.s.) than those of the β-isomer attributable to aromatic ring current effects. This is possible in structure LXXXVIa, not LXXXVIIa.

c. α- and β-9-Hydroxy-2(N)-methyl-6,7-benzomorphans. The substitution of a hydroxyl group at position 14 of morphin-like structures generally has

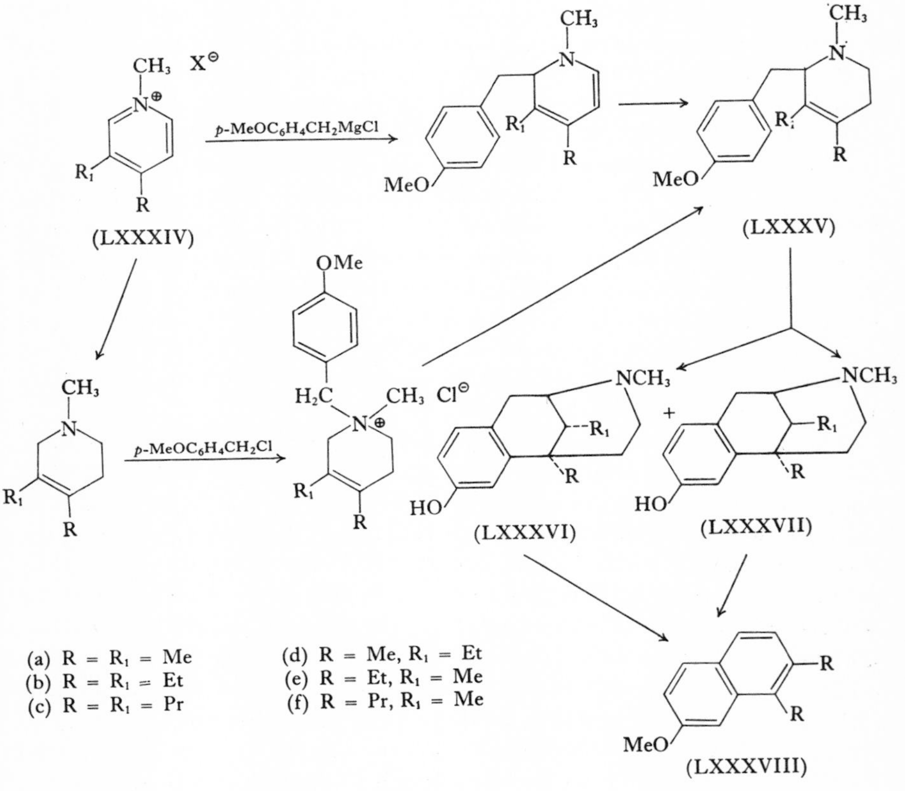

Fig. 15.

an enhancing effect on analgetic activity. For example, 14-hydroxydihydro-codeinone (oxycodone, XIII) and 14-hydroxydihydromorphinone (oxymorphone, XIV), are from two to four times as potent as dihydrocodeinone (hydrocodone, XII) and dihydromorphinone (hydromorphone, XI), respectively (14c). A similar modification of the basic benzomorphan structures LXI, LXII, and derivatives is represented by LXXXIX.

Appropriate starting materials for the synthesis of compounds of structure

152

LXXXIX were 2,5-dimethyl-9-oxo-6,7-benzomorphan methobromide [(XCa) (*57*) and the 2′-methoxy relative (XCb) (*62*). When each (Fig. 16) was brought to reaction with ethereal methylmagnesium iodide, 9-methyl carbinols of the structure and configuration shown in (XCIIe) (*73*) and (XCIIh)

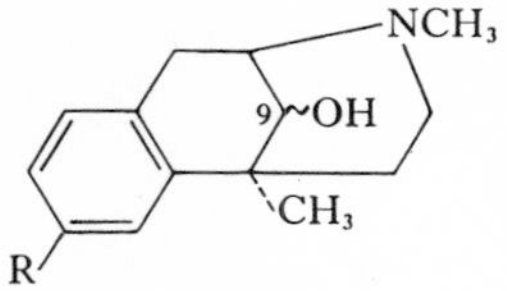

(a) R = OMe

(b) R = OH

(c) R = H

(LXXXIX)

(*74*) were obtained in 75% yield after pyrolytic extrusion of methyl bromide or iodide from the intermediates (XCIe and XCIg), respectively. On the other hand, addition of methylmagnesium iodide or methyllithium to the bases XCIVa and XCIVb occurred in the reverse manner to give the methyl carbinols XCVe (*73*) and XCVg (*74*). The assignment of an equatorial (for the hydroaromatic ring) conformation to the 9-hydroxyl substituent of XCIIe and XCIIg (designated α for convenience) and an axial arrangement for XCVe and XCVg (called β-isomers) was based principally on infrared spectral measurements. With the α-isomers was noted a maximum (at 3450 cm^{-1}) indicative of strong OH...N bonding, to be expected when the hydroxyl is oriented toward the nitrogen of the *cis*, diaxial fused iminoethano system as in XCIIe and XCIIg. The β-isomers, however, gave spectra clearly indicating OH...π bonding, compatible with structures XCVe and XCVg. Furthermore, double Hormann degradation (followed by hydrogenation) (*75*) of XCIIe (*73*) and XCIIg (*74*) produced nitrogen-free products of the structures XCIIIe and XCIIIg, respectively (*cis*-fusion of hydrofurano and hydroaromatic rings) as determined by spectral data and an alternative, relatively unambiguous synthesis (*76*) of XCIIIe. Compound XCVe and XCVg gave nitrogen-free products having spectral characteristics which are accomodated by structures XCVIe and XCVIg (*trans*-fusion of the two hydrogenated rings.) Thus structures XCII conform to the oxymorphone (XIV) (*11*) and oxycodone (XIII) stereochemistry (*11*, *77*).

This same stereochemical pattern of addition was followed by platinum oxide-catalyzed hydrogen. Thus, XCa and XCb yielded (through XCId and XCIf), XCIId (*73*) and XCIIf (*78*), respectively, while XCIVa and XCIVb gave XCVd (*73*) and XCVf (*78*). Furthermore, changing R$_1$ to ethyl made no difference in the stereochemistry of the products (although the additions were markedly slower due to steric effects) and XCc led ultimately to XCIIj and XCIIk, whereas XCIVc yielded XCVj and XCVk (*79*). Finally, neither

153

ethyl- nor propylmagnesium iodide or bromide could be induced to add to the carbonyl group of XCb although a small yield of hydrogenation product XCIIf could be isolated in each instance (79). However, the less hindered

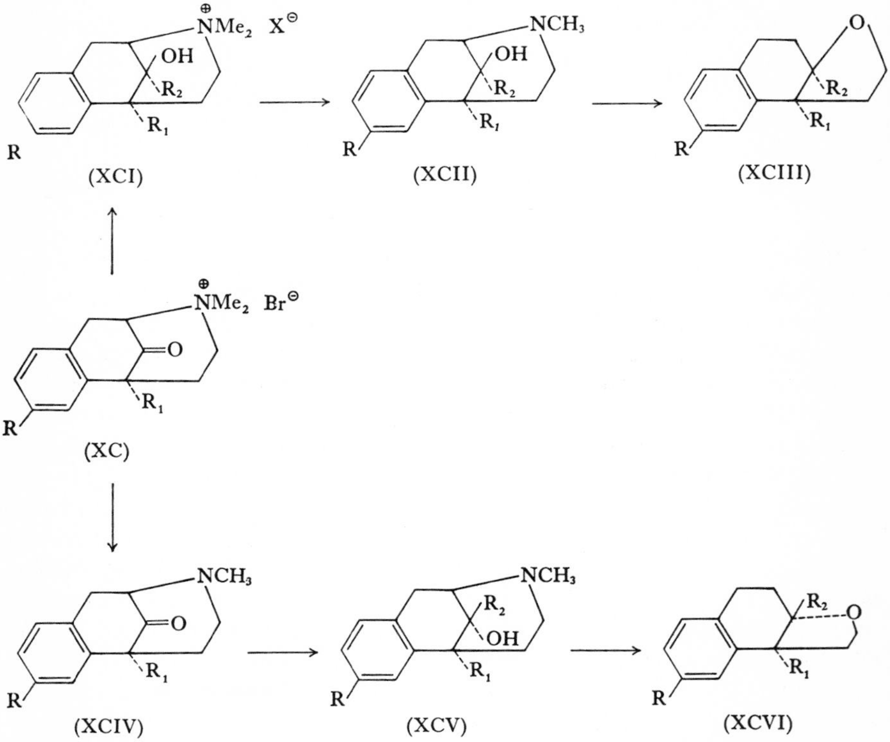

(a) R = H, R$_1$ = Me
(b) R = MeO, R$_1$ = Me
(c) R = MeO, R$_2$ = Et
(d) R = H, R$_1$ = Me, R$_2$ = H
(e) R = H, R$_1$ = R$_2$ = Me
(f) R = MeO, R$_1$ = Me, R$_2$ = H
(g) R = MeO, R$_1$ = R$_2$ = Me

(h) R = HO, R$_1$ = Me, R$_2$ = H
(i) R = HO, R$_1$ = R$_2$ = Me
(j) R = MeO, R$_1$ = Et, R$_2$ = H
(k) R = MeO, R$_1$ = Et, R$_2$ = Me
(l) R = HO, R$_1$ = Et, R$_2$ = H
(m) R = HO, R$_1$ = Et, R$_2$ = Me
(n) R = MeO, R$_1$ = Me, R$_2$ = Et

FIG. 16.

carbonyl group of XCIVb received ethylmagnesium bromide to give the β-carbinol (XCVn) (79).

The direction of addition to the carbonyl function of the above 9-oxo-benzomorphans appears, therefore, to depend principally upon the electrical environment of the neighboring nitrogen. When the nitrogen is cationic

154

as in XC, carbinols are formed with hydroxyl oriented toward it. With negative nitrogen (XCIV) the additions are reversed in stereochemistry. Within the narrow limits of the study, increased steric hindrance has retarded or voided reaction, but has not essentially altered stereochemistry.

Phenolic compounds XCIIh, XCIIi, XCIII, XCIIm, XCVh, XCVi, XCVl, and XCVm were obtained by treatment of the corresponding methyl ethers with boiling 48% hydrobromic acid (74, 78, 79). There was no inversion of the hydroxyl or skeletal rearrangement as shown by diazomethane conversion of the phenols to the original methyl ethers.

Stereoselectivity of addition of platinum oxide-catalyzed hydrogen has been observed also with 2'-methoxy-2,5-dimethyl-9-methylene-6,7-benzo-morphan (XCVII) obtained from the methyl carbinol (XCIIg) and thionyl

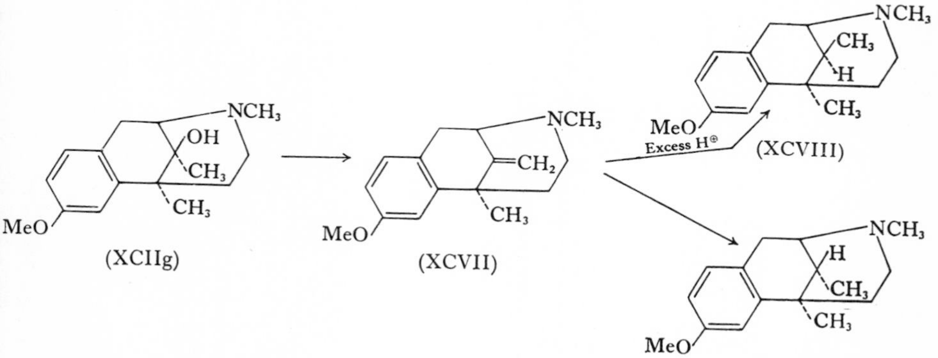

chloride. As the free base or hydrochloride salt in alcohol, this 9-methylene compound received hydrogen from the top side of the molecule giving α-2'-methoxy-2,5,9-trimethyl-6,7-benzomorphan (XCIX) in good yield. In the presence of excess hydrochloric or perchloric acid (presumably to keep the nitrogen positive), on the other hand, the direction of addition was reversed and β-2'-methoxy-2,5,9-trimethyl-6,7-benzomorphan (XCVIII) was obtained in 70% yield. O-Demethylation of XCIX and XCVIII to LXXVIa and LXXXVIIa, respectively, proved their identity (80).

d. N-Substituted 6,7-benzomorphans. As implied earlier, it has been the feeling that substitution of any group for the N-methyl of morphine and similar entities would have a detrimental effect on analgetic activity. However, in 1956 it was reported that replacement of methyl by phenethyl in the morphine molecule resulted in an eight-fold increase in potency (19c). A short time later this and similar modifications were reported for the morphinans (52, 81). In many instances the increase in potency was dramatic.

155

Consequently, a fairly representative group of N-substituted 6,7-benzomorphans has been synthesized. The most interesting of this group have proved to be N-phenethyl derivatives initially synthesized from parent N-methyl compounds, as shown in Fig. 17 for α-2′-hydroxy-5,9-dimethyl-2-phenethyl-6,7-benzomorphan (phenazocine, CIVc) (*82*). In this route, α-2′-acetoxy- or methoxy-2,5,9-trimethyl-6,7-benzomorphan (Ca) or (Cb) was converted to the secondary amine (CIc) or (CIb) in two steps (cyanogen bromide followed by acid hydrolysis) (*82, 83*). Phenylacetylation of CI with phenylacetyl chloride in the presence of aqueous methanolic potassium carbonate produced the amide (CIII) which can be reduced to CIVb or CIVc with ethereal lithium aluminum hydride. Conversion of CIVb to CIVc was effected with boiling 48% hydrobromic acid (*82*).

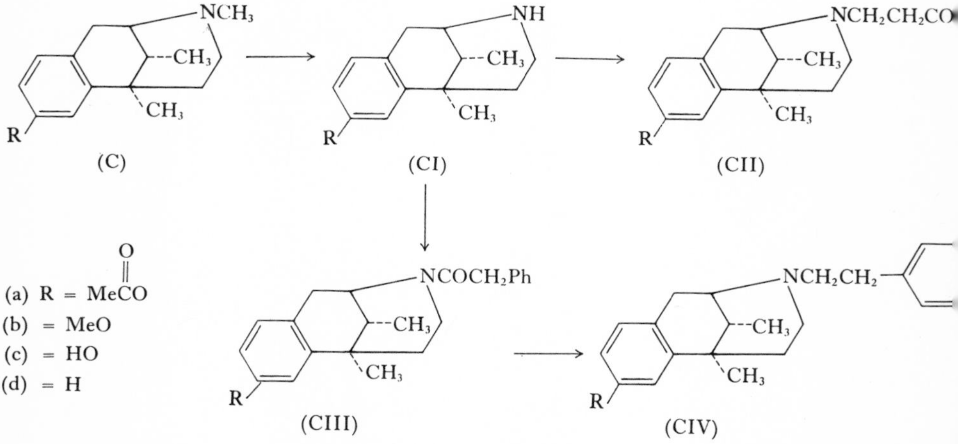

(a) R = MeCO
(b) = MeO
(c) = HO
(d) = H

Fig. 17.

Similarly, the following 6,7-benzomorphans have been prepared: 5-methyl-2-phenethyl (*83*); 2′-hydroxy-5-methyl-2-phenethyl (*62*); 5-ethyl-2′-hydroxy-2-phenethyl (*65*); α-2′,9-dihydroxy-5,9-dimethyl-2-phenethyl (*74*); α-5,9-diethyl-2′-hydroxy-2-phenethyl (*69*); α-2-ethyl-2′-hydroxy-5,9-dimethyl (*84*); α-2′-hydroxy-5,9-dimethyl-2-propyl (*84*); α-2-butyl-2′-hydroxy-5,9-dimethyl (*84*); and α-2-amyl-2′-hydroxy-5,9-dimethyl (*84*). Alternatively, 2′-hydroxy-5-methyl-2-phenethyl-6,7-benzomorphan (*58, 62*), 5-ethyl-2′-hydroxy-2-phenethyl-6,7-benzomorphan (*65*) and (CIVc) (*58, 83*) have been prepared from appropriate 1-phenethylpyridinium bromides or iodides by the general methods outlined in Figs. 13, 14, and 15. Finally, 5,9-dimethyl-2-(3-phenyl-3-oxopropyl)-6,7-benzomorphan (CIId) and the 2′-hydroxy congener (CIIc) were obtained from CId and CIc, respectively, via the Mannich reaction using formaldehyde and aceto-phenone (*85*). Many other *N*-substituted 6,7-benzomorphans have been synthesized in other laboratories (*86, 87*). Some are tabulated in the pharma-cological section.

   e. Optically active 5,9-dialkyl-6,7-benzomorphans: absolute configuration. It has been stated in Section III,A,2 that 3-hydroxy-*N*-methylmorphinan has three asymmetric carbon atoms (at 9, 13, and 14). However, since the iminoethano system is geometrically constrained to a *cis*-fusion, only two (racemic) diastereoisomers are possible. Of these, (±)-3-hydroxy-*N*-methylmorphinan has been shown to conform to structure XLVI (*cis*-fusion

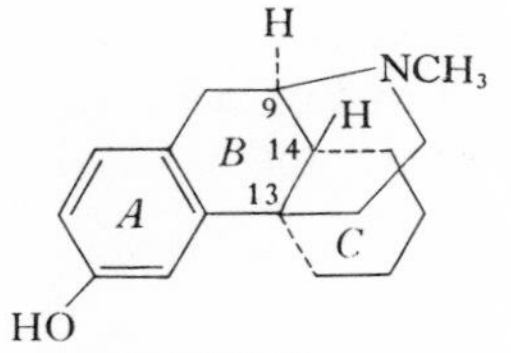

(XLVI)

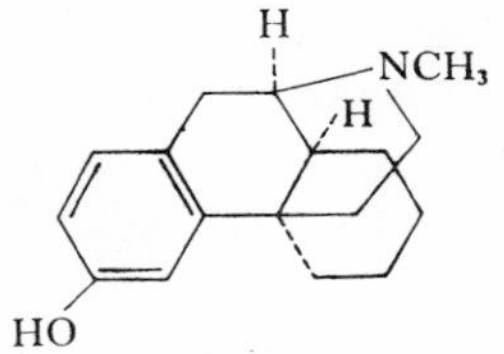

(CV)

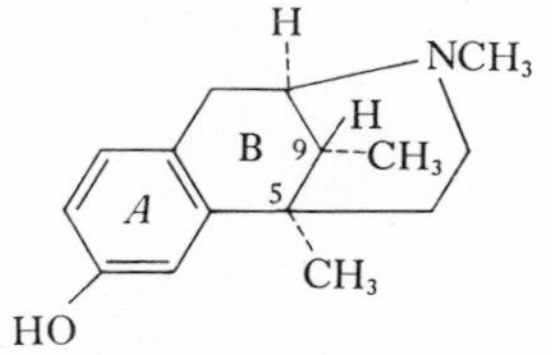

(CVI)

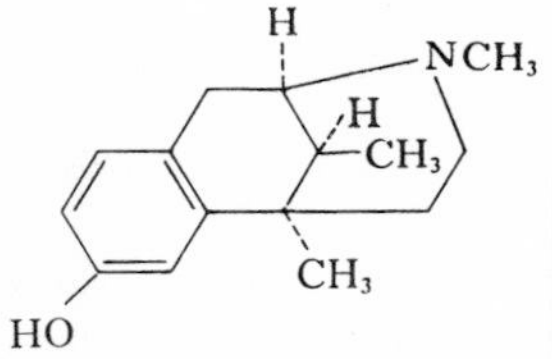

(CVII)

of rings *B* and *C*), while the second racemate may be represented by stereo-structure CV, (±)-3-hydroxy-*N*-methylisomorphinan with a *trans*-fusion of rings *B* and *C* (*47*). Similar considerations apply to the 5,9-dialkyl-6,7-benzomorphans in which it is has been shown that the 5,9-dialkyl groups (attached to ring *B*) may be in either *cis* (predominant, α-isomers, CVI) or *trans* (lesser, β-isomers, CVII) juxtaposition for the hydroaromatic ring *B*. Thus CVI corresponds to XLVI and CVII to CV. It is also well known (Section III,A) that nearly all of the analgetic activity of XLVI and CV is due in each instance to the *levo*-antipode which in the case of XLVI con-forms to the absolute configuration of (*levo*) morphine at the three common asymmetric centers. Optical resolution of the α- and β-2′-hydroxy-2,5,9-trimethyl-6,7-benzomorphans (CVI, CVII), the 5,9-dimethyl groups repre-

157

senting vestiges of ring C of the morphinans, has revealed an analogous relationship. The *dextro*-isomers of CVI and CVII were not only substantially inactive but were also more toxic than the *levo*-counterparts.

Resolution was effected with (+)-3-bromo-8-camphorsulfonic acid (*82*); the resultant diastereoisomeric salts could be easily separated in aqueous

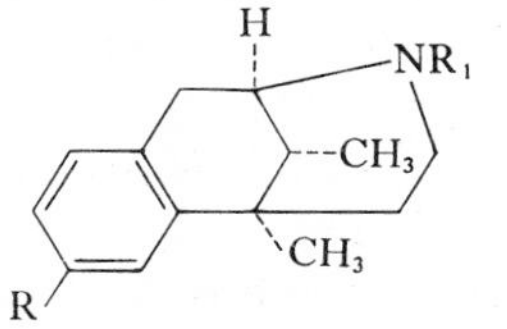

(a) R = MeO, R_1 = Me

(b) R = MeO, R_1 = CH_2CH_2Ph

(c) R = HO, R_1 = CH_2CH_2Ph

(CVIII)

medium. The antipodes of the α-series (CVI) were then converted to the *N*-phenethyl derivatives (CVIIIc) as outlined in Fig. 6 for the racemates. In addition, antipodes corresponding to CVIIIa and CVIIIb have been prepared and characterized (*88*).

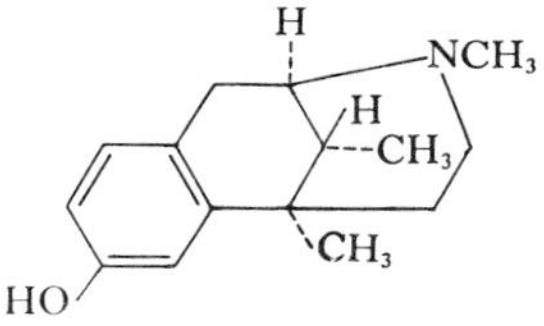

(CIX) (−)

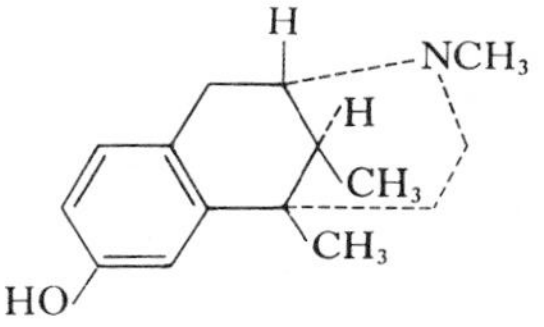

(CX) (+)

In view of the fact that the analgesic activity of CVI does reside in the *levo*-isomer, and as it has been shown by the method of stereoselective adsorbents (*41*) that (−)-CVI is configurationally related to (−)-3-hydroxy-

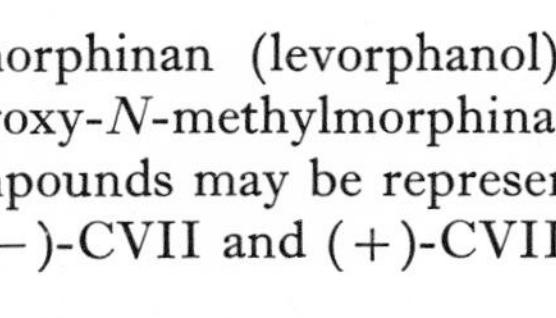

(CXI)

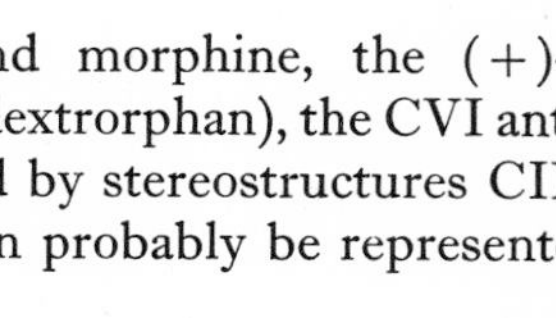

(CXII)

N-methylmorphinan (levorphanol) and morphine, the (+)-isomer to (+)-3-hydroxy-*N*-methylmorphinan (dextrorphan), the CVI antipodes and related compounds may be represented by stereostructures CIX and CX. Similarly (−)-CVII and (+)-CVII can probably be represented by CXI and CXII.

158

f. 5-Carbethoxy-2-methyl-6,7-benzomorphan and derivatives. If one replaces the 5-methyl substituent of 2,5-dimethyl-6,7-benzomorphan (LXI) with a carbethoxy group, a structure (CXV) is obtained which is in essence a hybrid of this benzomorphan and the well-known analgetic, meperidine (4-carbethoxy-1-methyl-4-phenylpiperidine, CXVIII). Compound CXV

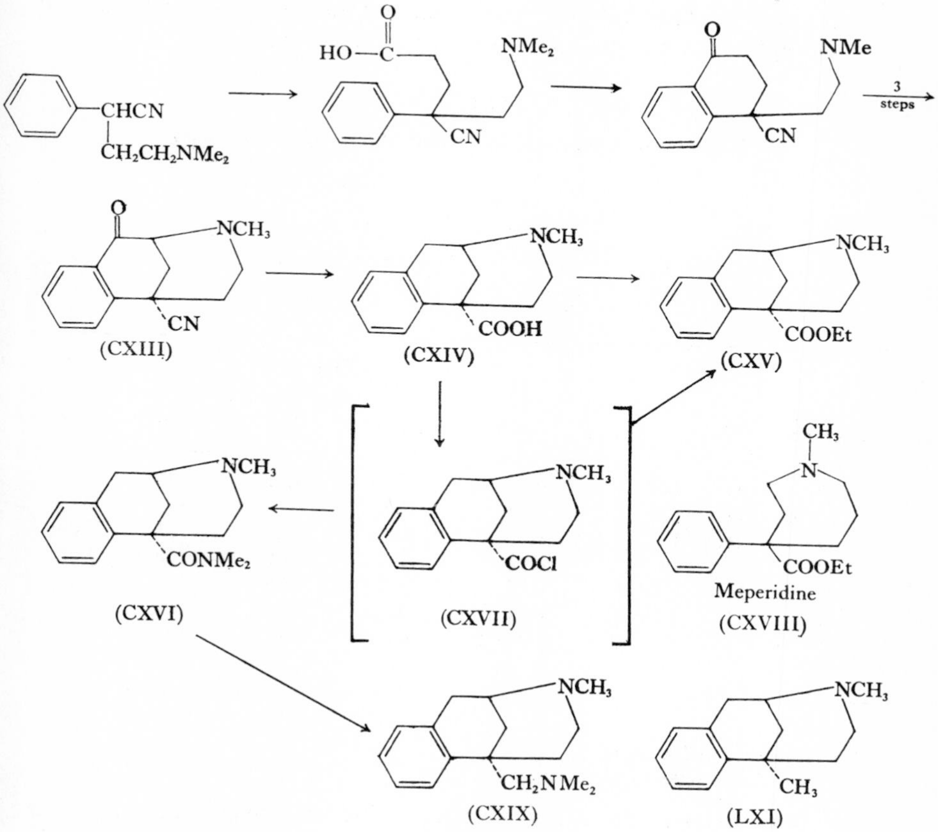

FIG. 18.

was synthesized from phenylacetonitrile by a method closely approximating that used for LXI (Fig. 12) as outlined in Fig. 18 (*89*). The reactions were all relatively straightforward and good yields were obtained. Wolff-Kishner conditions (Huang-Minlon modification) for cyanoketone (CXIII) effected both hydrogenolysis of the oxo group and hydrolysis of the cyano group. The resultant CXIV could be esterified directly with ethanolic hydrogen

159

chloride or indirectly via the acid chloride (CXVII). The latter with dimethylamine yielded amide CXVI which was reduced with lithium aluminum hydride to the aminomethyl compound CXIX.

2. Pharmacology

A thorough review of the analgetic activity, addiction liability, and opiate-antagonistic effects of 6,7-benzomorphans has just been written (90). Only the highlights will be presented in the present chapter.

TABLE V

5-ALKYL-(OR CARBOXYL)-2(N)-METHYL-6,7-BENZOMORPHANS

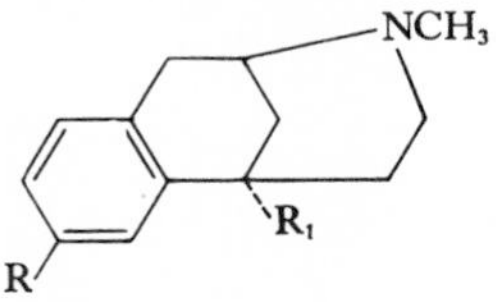

Reference	R	R_1	Salt	ED$_{50}$ Subcut.	ED$_{50}$ Oral	LD$_{50}$ Subcut.[a]	PDC
57	H	Me	HCl	22.1	42.1	148	—
62, 63	HO	Me	HCl	10.4	—	175	None
65	HO	Et	HCl	2.3	11.2	171	Low
64	HO	Pr	HCl	2.1	14.8	130	Low
89	H	CO$_2$Et	HCl	10.1	43.8	141	None
89	H	CONMe$_2$	HCl	18.3	33.8	[1]	—
89	H	CH$_2$NMe$_2$	Di-HBr	None to 100	—	[2]	—

[a] Notes:
[1] None died at 100 mg/kg.
[2] None died at 400 mg/kg.

a. Analgetic and toxic effects in animals. The same techniques have been employed for the study of nearly all compounds which were first tested by the subcutaneous route of administration in mice (51, 90). Most of the more active ones were tested by the oral route as well. If sufficient material was available the subcutaneous acute toxicities of the compounds were determined and an LD$_{50}$ calculated by probit analysis. In most instances the generally very water-soluble hydrochloride or hydrobromide salts were used. If necessary, propylene glycol-water not in excess of 25% aqueous solution could be used for the less soluble aralkyl compounds. The ED$_{50}$'s and LD_{50}'s are in milligrams of salt/kilogram of mouse. When salts were not available, the bases were dissolved in the stoichiometric amount of $1N$ hydrochloric acid and the solution diluted to the desired volume. Unless otherwise specified the racemates have been used.

In Tables V–XII are presented analgetic and toxicity data for most of the

TABLE VI

5,9-DIALKYL-2(N)-METHYL-6,7-BENZOMORPHANS

(a) α-SERIES

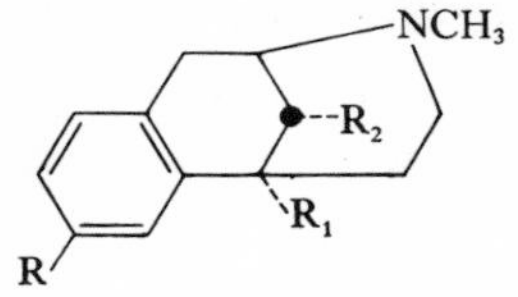

| | | | | | ED$_{50}$ | | LD$_{50}$ | |
| | | | | | --- | --- | --- | |
Reference	R	R$_1$	R$_2$	Salt	Subcut.	Oral	Subcut.[a]	PDC
62	H	Me	Me	HCl	27.3	—	155	—
91	H	Et	Et	HCl	5.0	36.7	83	None
64	HO	Me	Me	HCl	3.0	23.9	175	Low
68	MeO	Me	Me	HBr	9.8	21.7	—	Low
72	AcO	Me	Me	HCl	1.17	3.3	[1]	Intermediate
64, 70	HO	Et	Me	HCl	4.9	31.7	309	Low
64, 70	HO	Me	Et	HCl	1.5	14.8	134	None
69	HO	Et	Et	HCl	4.2	Inactive	423	None
58	AcO	Et	Et	HCl	3.0	28.9	252	None
64	HO	Pr	Me	HBr	2.9	72.1	[2]	—
64	HO	Pr	Pr	HCl	71.2	—	[3]	—

[a] *Notes*:
[1] Ten of 20 died at 200; three of 9 died at 300 mg/kg; $LD_{50} > 300$.
[2] One of 10 died at 200; three of 9 died at 300 mg/kg; $LD_{50} > 300$.
[3] One of 10 died at 400 mg/kg.

benzomorphans (excepting the antagonists, to be discussed in a later section) synthesized to date. The range in subcutaneous activity for the 5-alkyl and 5,9-dialkyl-2-methyl-6,7-benzomorphans (not substituted at 2′) is from about one-half to one-fifteenth that of morphine (ED_{50} 4.2 to 27.3, cf. Tables V–VII). Replacement of the 5-methyl substituent (R_1, TableV) with carbethoxy or carbodimethylamino has little effect. The introduction of a 2′-hydroxyl substituent ($R = OH$) in general markedly increases activity

161

especially in the β-5,9-dialkyl series (Table VII). The most potent of the 2'-hydroxy compounds is β-($\pm$)-5-ethyl-2,9-dimethyl-2'-hydroxy-6,7-benzomorphan (Table VII, R = OH, R_1 = Et, R_2 = Me) about thirty times (ED_{50} 0.07) as potent as (*levo*) morphine (ED_{50}) 2.0). In the 5,9-dialkyl series (Tables VI and VII), maximum activity is shown when the total number of saturated carbons in the 5- and 9- positions is three. There is a very marked drop in activity when going from 5,9-diethyl to 5,9-dipropyl. The β-isomers are from five to seventy times more potent than their α

TABLE VII

5,9-DIALKYL-2(N)-METHYL-6,7-BENZOMORPHANS

(*b*) β-SERIES

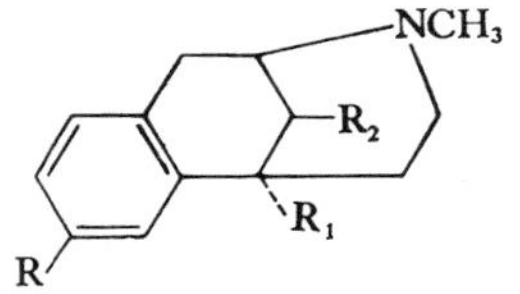

| Reference | R | R_1 | R_2 | Salt | ED_{50} | | LD_{50} | |
					Subcut.	Oral	Subcut.	PDC
92	H	Me	Me	HBr	8.9	37.1	178	—
91	H	Et	Et	HBr	4.2	38.6	~80	Very low
64, 68	HO	Me	Me	HCl	0.44	8.2	67	Low
64, 70	HO	Et	Me	HCl	0.07	1.1	60.15	Intermediate
64, 70	HO	Me	Et	HCl	0.47	17.2	85.0	—
69	HO	Et	Et	HCl	0.28	6.5	116	None
64	HO	Pr	Pr	HCl	0.87	—	62	—

counterparts. Data not yet ready for publication indicate that in the 5(mono)-alkyl series (Table V) also activity reaches a maximum with three carbons (5-propyl) then begins to recede. Methylation of the phenolic hydroxyl lowers activity (cf. Tables V, VI, CIII, IX, and X) while acetylation has a slight, enhancing effect. Substitution of a hydroxyl for hydrogen at position 9 (Tables VIII and IX) in contrast to the morphine series (Section II), has a deleterious effect on activity unless the hydroxyls are protected with acetyl (Table X). These changes also vastly increase toxicity.

Replacement of the 2(N)-methyl substituent by ethyl, propyl, or butyl in 2'-hydroxy-2,5,9-trimethyl-6,7-benzomorphan abolishes activity which is completely restored with N-amyl (Table XI). Phenethyl p-substituted phenethyl, or 2-thienylethyl, when substituted for methyl on the nitrogen, increases the activity of 2'-hydroxy compounds many times in most instances (Table XI; compare compounds of Tables VI and VII). Little effect is seen in replacing 2-methyl with phenacyl or 3-phenyl-3-oxypropyl. Also phenethyl has little effect if there is no 2'-hydroxy substituent in the molecule.

TABLE VIII

9-HYDROXY-2(N)-METHYL-6,7-BENZOMORPHANS

(a) α-SERIES

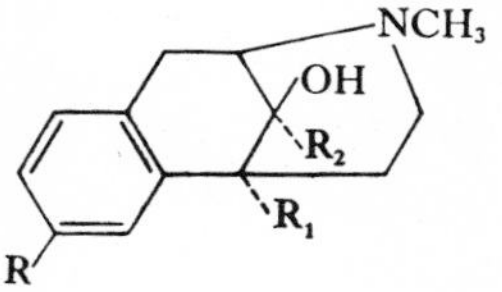

Reference	R	R_1	R_2	Salt	ED$_{50}$ Subcut.	ED$_{50}$ Oral	LD$_{50}$ Subcut.[a]	PDC
73	H	Me	H	HBr	63.8	—	[1]	—
73	H	Me	Me	HBr	43.7	—	[1]	—
73	HO	Me	H	HBr	79.9	—	—	—
73	HO	Me	Me	HBr	6.9	—	—	—
73	MeO	Me	H	HBr	>100	—	[2]	—
73	MeO	Me	Me	HCl	19.7	13.5	373	Very low
79	HO	Et	H	HCl	Inactive	—	[3]	—
79	MeO	Et	H	HCl	67.4	—	[4]	—
79	HO	Et	Me	Base	6.7	55.3	[5]	—
79	MeO	Et	Me	HCl	13.8	43.0	—	—

[a] Notes:
[1] Two of 10 died at 400 mg/kg.
[2] None died at 200 mg/kg.
[3] Three of 10 died at 400, none at 200 mg/kg.
[4] Eight of 10 died at 400, none at 200 mg/kg; LD$_{50}$ ca. 400 mg/kg.
[5] None of 10 died at 300 mg/kg.

As is true in the morphinan series (Section III,A,3), the analgetic activity of the *racemic*-benzomorphans is due principally to the *levo*-isomers (Table XII). Two *dextro*-isomers, α-(+)-2'-hydroxy-5,9-dimethyl-2-phenethyl-6,7-benzomorphan (ED$_{50}$ 6.6) and β-(+)-2'-hydroxy-2,5,9-trimethyl-6,7-benzomorphan (ED$_{50}$ 15.8), do, however, have significant activity, although

163

only about one-fiftieth that of their *levo*-counterparts. In the case of α-(±)-2′-hydroxy2,5,9-trimethyl-6,7-benzomorphan toxicity is definitely favorably influenced by resolution.

Oral analgetic effectiveness was determined for about half of the compounds listed in Tables V–XII. With only one exception (cf. Table VIII)

TABLE IX

9-Hydroxy-2(N)-methyl-6,7-benzomorphans

(*b*) β-Series

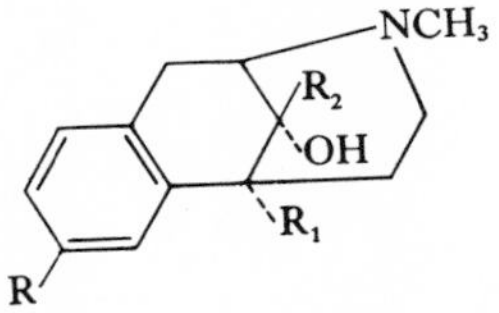

					ED$_{50}$		LD$_{50}$
Reference	R	R$_1$	R$_2$	Salt	Subcut.	Oral	Subcut.[b]
73	H	Me	Me	HCl	112.1	—	—
73	HO	Me	H	HBr	[I][a]	—	[1]
73	MeO	Me	H	HBr	47.3	—	[2]
73	HO	Me	Me	HBr	6.0	—	55
73	MeO	Me	Me	HBr	[I at 20]	—	63
79	HO	Et	H	HCl	12.2	—	[3]
79	HO	Et	Me	HBr	1.7	—	74
79	MeO	Me	Et	HCl	8.4	—	[4]

[a] [I] = Inactive.
[b] *Notes:*
[1] One of 10 died at 200 mg/kg.
[2] Four of 10 died at 100 mg/kg.
[3] Three of 10 died at 400, none at 200 mg/kg.
[4] Three of 16 died at 50 mg/kg while resting for analgesia.

the oral dose was two or more times the parenteral. When the subcutaneous ED$_{50}$ was less than 1.0 mg/kg the oral ED$_{50}$ was 8–100 times greater (average 41). When the subcutaneous ED$_{50}$ was 2.0 mg/kg or more the oral ED$_{50}$ was rarely more than eight times greater. There is, however, no indication of a structural relationship in these ratios.

Regarding acute toxicity, the LD$_{50}$'s of all compounds are reasonably high excepting a few having a hydroxyl group in position 9 (β-series,

Table IX). The 5(mono)-alkyl compounds (Table V) are comparable to the α-5,9-dialkyls (Table VI). Toxicity in the β-series (Table VII) is somewhat greater, although not parallel with the increase in analgetic potency. Thus the therapeutic indexes in the β series are more favorable than those of the α or 5(mono)-alkyl compounds.

TABLE X

9-Acetoxy-2(N)-methyl-6,7-benzomorphans

(a) α-Series

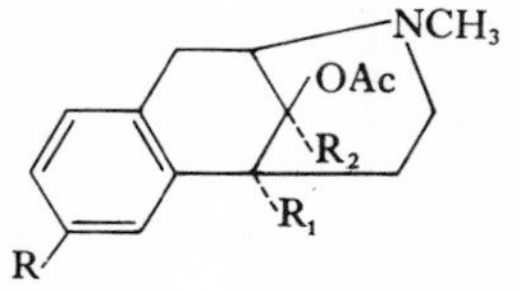

Reference	R	R_1	R_2	Salt	ED$_{50}$ Subcut.	ED$_{50}$ Oral	LD$_{50}$ Subcut.[a]	PDC
73	H	Me	H	HBr	29.0	—	367	—
73	AcO	Me	H	HBr	0.5	40.5	[1]	High (48.0)[b]
73	AcO	Me	Me	HBr	1.1	22.5	—	Low
79	MeO	Et	H	HCl	22.6	—	197	—
79	AcO	Et	H	HCl	2.2	10.6	262	—
79	HO	Et	Me	HCl	1.13	Inactive	[2]	—
79	MeO	Et	Me	HCl	14.8	—	[3]	—
79	AcO	Et	Me	HCl	1.15	72.3	[3]	—

[a] *Notes*:
[1] One of 10 died at 200 mg/kg.
[2] Five of 10 died at 400, one of 10 at 200 mg/kg; LD$_{50}$ ca. 400 mg/kg.
[3] Three of 10 died at 400 mg/kg; none at lower doses; LD$_{50}$ > 400 mg/kg.
[b] Equivalence to 3 mg of morphine.

b. *Addiction liability in monkeys.* About a third of the benzomorphans included in the tables have been studied for addiction liability in the monkey. The selection of compounds for study has not been wholly systematic, because of a limited supply in many instances. Enough data have been accumulated, however, to warrant some discussion. We are indebted to Drs. M. Seevers and G. A. Deneau of the Department of Pharmacology, University of Michigan, for permission to quote their results, most of which have been reported (93).

TABLE XI

N-Substituted (Other than Methyl)-6,7-benzomorphans

(a) 5-Alkyl and α-5,9-Dialkyl-2(N)-alkyl or Aralkyl-6,7-benzomorphans

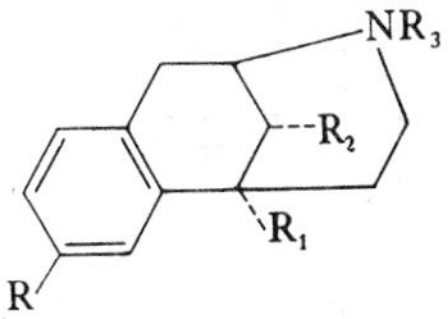

Reference	R	R_1	R_2	R_3	Salt	ED50 Subcut.	ED50 Oral[a]	LD50 Subcut.[b]	PDC
83	H	Me	H	CH₂CH₂Ph	HCl	35.9	—	>400	—
62	HO	Me	H	CH₂CH₂Ph	HBr	0.48	7.9	55	None
65	HO	Et	H	CH₂CH₂Ph	HCl	0.16	6.0	88	Intermediate
82	HO	Me	Me	CH₂CH₂Ph	HBr	0.25	6.4	332	High (17.0)
82	MeO	Me	Me	CH₂CH₂Ph	HBr	6.5	10.6	—	Very low
86	AcO	Me	Me	CH₂CH₂Ph	HBr	0.19	6.1	169	Low
69	HO	Et	Et	CH₂CH₂Ph	HBr	2.1	[1]	292	—
71	HO	Pr	Me	CH₂CH₂Ph	HCl	0.92	38.1	[1]	—
85	H	Me	Me	CH₂CH₂COPh	HCl	8.7	[1]	[2]	—
85	HO	Me	Me	CH₂CH₂COPh	Base	2.3	30.2	83	None
85	MeO	Me	Me	CH₂COPh	HCl	42.9	—	[3]	—
86	HO	Me	Me	CH₂CH₂CH₂Ph	Base	13.6	83.9	—	None
86	HO	Me	Me	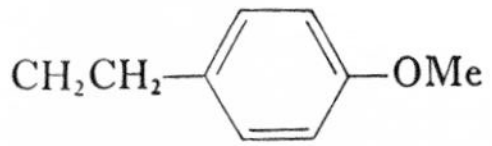 CH₂CH₂—〈OMe〉	Base	0.11	10.7	125	Intermediate
86	HO	Me	Me	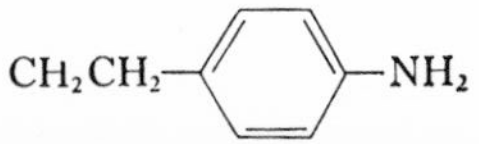 CH₂CH₂—〈NH₂〉	HBr	0.32	18.9	[4]	Low

No.	3-Position			R	Salt				
86	HO	Me	Me	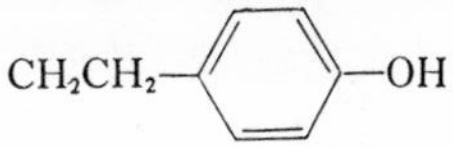 $CH_2CH_2C_6H_4OH$	HBr	0.2 (rat)	—	—	—
86	HO	Me	Me	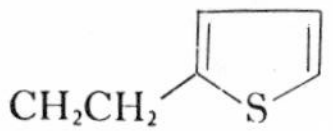 CH_2CH_2(2-thienyl)	Base	0.055	5.8	88	Low
84, 86	HO	Me	Me	H	HCl	[I]	—	84	—
61, 67	HO	Me	Me	Me	HCl	3.0	23.9	175	—
84	HO	Me	Me	Et	HBr	[I]	—	[5]	—
84	HO	Me	Me	Pr	HCl	[I]	—	137	—
84	HO	Me	Me	Bu	HBr	[I]	—	341	—
84	HO	Me	Me	Am	HCl	2.2	88.7	[6]	Low
86	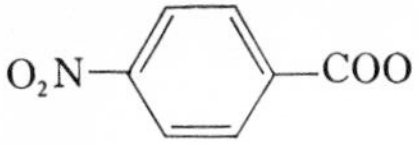 O_2N–C_6H_4–COO	Me	Me	CH_2CH_2Ph	HCl	0.41	14.6	—	None
86, 87	HO	Me	Me	$CH_2CH=CH_2$	HCl	[I]	—	—	None
87	HO	Me	Me	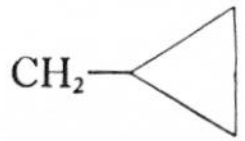 CH_2–(cyclopropyl)	Base	23.1	—	[8]	None
87	HO	Me	Me	$CH_2CH=CMe_2$	Base	[I]	—	[9]	None
87	HO	Et	Me	$CH_2CH=CMe_2$	Base	15.9	—	[10]	—

a [I] = Inactive.

b Notes:

[1] None of 10 died at 400 mg/kg.
[2] One of 10 died at 400 mg/kg.
[3] None of 10 died at 400 mg/kg.
[4] Three of 10 died at 450 mg/kg.
[5] Two of 10 died at 100 mg/kg during analgesic testing.
[6] Ten of 10 died at 400, none of 10 at 200 mg/kg; LD$_{50}$ = 400 mg/kg or less.
[7] Four of 8 died at 50 mg/kg; LD$_{50}$ = ca. 50 mg/kg.
[8] One of 10 died at 300 mg/kg.
[9] Eight of 10 died at 400 mg/kg; LD$_{50}$ ca. 400 mg/kg.
[10] Two of ten died at 300 mg/kg.

TABLE XII

OPTICALLY ACTIVE 5,9-DIMETHYL-6,7-BENZOMORPHANS

(a) α-SERIES

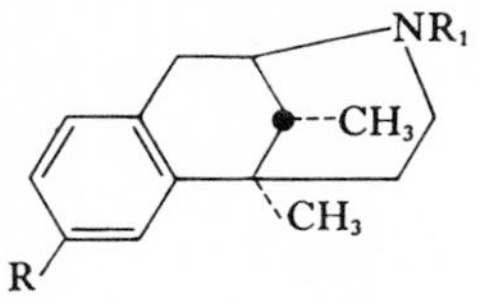

Reference	Isomer	R	R_1	Salt	ED_{50} Subcut.[a]	Oral	LD_{50} Subcut.[b]	PDC
82	levo	HO	Me	HBr	1.69	14.1	[1]	Very low
82	dextro	HO	Me	HBr	[I]	—	[2]	—
88	levo	MeO	Me	HBr	8.7	17.9	175	—
88	dextro	MeO	Me	HBr	[I]	—	176	—
82	levo	HO	CH_2CH_2Ph	HBr	0.11	3.9	147	High (9.0)
82	dextro	HO	CH_2CH_2Ph	HBr	6.6	12.9	201	None
88	levo	MeO	CH_2CH_2Ph	HBr	1.83	—	[3]	None
88	dextro	MeO	CH_2CH_2Ph	HBr	[I]	—	—	—

(b) SERIES-β

| 72 | levo | — | — | HBr | 0.39 | 6.6 | 118 | Low |
| 72 | dextro | — | — | HBr | 15.75 | — | — | — |

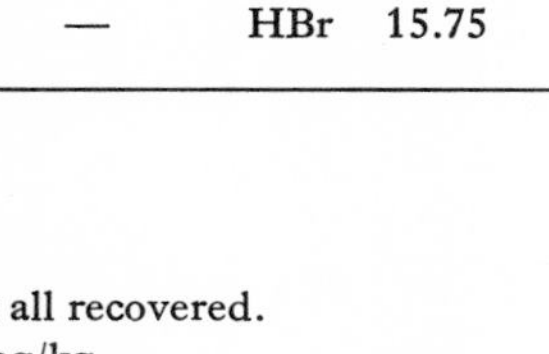

[a] I = Inactive.
[b] *Notes*:
[1] None died at 400 mg/kg.
[2] Convulsant at 20 mg/kg.; all recovered.
[3] Three of 10 died at 500 mg/kg.

The procedure for the preliminary assessment of addiction liability (physical dependence capacity, PDC) has been described in detail *(93, 94)*. The primary objective is to determine whether or not a test drug will suppress all of the abstinence signs in a morphine-dependent monkey stabilized on

3 mg/kg of morphine sulfate every 6 hours without interruption for a minimum of 60 days. This is based on the principle, demonstrated in animals and man, that any chemical substance capable of complete suppression of all the specific signs of morphine abstinence is also capable of creating physical dependence (perhaps the most important component of addiction) during chronic administration. For testing, regular morphine injections are withheld for 12–14 hours until abstinence signs of intermediate intensity are present. If left untreated the abstinence signs increase during the next several hours, but the administration of morphine or any drug with morphine-like physical dependence capacity results in a partial or complete suppression of abstinence symptoms. A test drug is therefore characterized *High*, *Intermediate*, or *Low* in physical dependence capacity depending upon the degree of suppression of abstinence signs. The physical dependence potency of a drug is a measure of the amount (relative to 3 mg/kg of morphine) of drug required to completely suppress all abstinence signs, if indeed it is capable of such suppression. The preselected quantity of test drug is based on its analgesic potency in mice.

The physical dependence capacity (PDC) ratings for those benzomorphans studied are given in the last column of Tables V–XII. Whenever a compound showed high PDC, its morphine equivalent is given in parentheses beside the rating.

It is immediately apparent that the benzomorphans as a class have low physical dependence capacity, especially so relative to their analgesic effectiveness. The standard abstinence-suppressing dose of morphine is only a little above its analgesic ED_{50}, 3.0 verus 2.1 mg/kg. On the other hand, 19 of the benzomorphans had an ED_{50} for analgesia less than that for morphine, but only one had a morphine equivalence dose less than 3.0 mg.; only three were rated high and only three others intermediate in PDC. There is a rough parallelism between analgesic activity and PDC in this group, but there are some notable exceptions. Most of the compounds which were weaker than morphine with respect to analgesia are in the group which had no physical dependence capacity, but in this same group there are three which had a greater analgesic effect than morphine. Also in the group rated low in PDC seven were more effective than morphine as analgesics and among these is the most potent analgesic yet encountered in the benzomorphan series.

The over-all addictiveness of α-($\pm$)-2'-hydroxy-5,9-dimethyl-2-phenethyl-6,7-benzomorphan (phenazocine) (Table XI) will be discussed later since it is one benzomorphan which has been studied extensively in man and is presently marketed. It and its *levo*-isomer (Table XII) were rated high in PDC but whereas their ED_{50}'s were 0.25 and 0.11 mg/kg, their morphine

169

equivalent doses for abstinence suppression were 17.0 and 9.0 mg/kg, respectively. Phenazocine was also administered chronically to monkeys. Animals which had not previously received drug were given phenazocine subcutaneously every 6 hours without interruption, 2 mg/kg the first week, 4 mg/kg the second week, 8 mg/kg the third week 16 mg/kg, the fourth and fifth weeks. The animals were challenged with nalorphine, 2 mg/kg on the 28th day and abruptly withdrawn on the 35th day. The degree of abstinence precipitated by nalorphine and observed on withdrawal was of only inter-mediate intensity, definitely less than would be expected with similar ad-ministration and increase in dosage of morphine. Furthermore, α-($\pm$)-2'-hydroxy-5,9-diethyl-2-methyl-6,7-benzomorphan (Table VI), showing no PDC from doses of 4–60 mg/kg, was also chronically administered to monkeys for a total of 31 days, the dose finally reaching 20 mg/kg. Both the nalorphine-induced and abrupt withdrawls were attended by a very mild degree of abstinence phenomena. This drug is therefore rated *low* in physical dependence capacity on chronic administration.

c. Clinical application. Initial animal studies of the analgesic potency of α-($\pm$)-2'-hydroxy-5,9-dimethyl-2-phenethyl-6,7-benzomorphan (generic name, phenazocine; trade names, Prinadol, Narphen, CIVc) indicated an increase in effect of about tenfold over morphine (Table XI). However, a dose of 17.0 mg/kg of phenazocine was required to equal the effect of 3.0 mg/kg of morphine. As low abstinence-suppressant potency was believed to be indicative of reduced ability to cause addiction, the first such indication in so potent an analgetic, extensive studies in man have been made. A thorough review of these studies has been published (*90*). In short, phena-zocine has proved to be an effective analgetic in almost all types of severe pain at a parenteral dose of 1–3 mg (compared with 5–10 mg of morphine). Its effect on respiration is comparable to that of morphine, but it causes much less circulatory depression than does morphine and is generally attended with fewer undesirable side-effects in the management of clinical pain. Phenazocine is also effective by the oral route of administration, especially in chronic pain (*90*) at 2–5 mg, another, advantage over morphine, The onset of action is, of course, slower than when administration is parenteral. The development of tolerance is definitely slower (*95*) and the over-all addiction liability certainly less than with morphine.

Two other benzomorphan analgetics which have been studied in man are α-($-$)-2'-hydroxy-2,5,9-trimethyl-6,7-benzomorphan (CIX) and α-($\pm$)-2'-hydroxy-5,9-diethyl-2-methyl-6,7-benzomorphan (LXXXVIb). Com-pound CIX was slightly more potent than morphine in mice [ED_{50} 1.7 mg/kg (Table XII) as compared with 2.0 for morphine], and in the monkey physical dependence capacity was very low. It produced no significant toxic effects on chronic administration to rats (*90*). When tested in man (*90*) for postoperative pain at parenteral doses of 3–15 mg, no untoward effects were seen; it was concluded that a dose of 15 mg was as good as or somewhat better than 10 mg of morphine in pain-relieving power. The addictiveness of this drug in man is somewhat less than that of morphine (*90*). As a substitute for morphine in an established addiction it proved to be only one-eighth as potent as morphine, little better than a placebo. Tolerance development was slower and physical dependence less severe on chronic administration of CIX to post-addicts. Compound LXXXVIb [ED_{50} 4.2 mg/kg subcutaneously in mice (Table V)], administered subcutaneously to postoperative patients was inferior to 10 mg of morphine at a dose of 10 mg but definitely superior in peak effect at 20 mg through four hours of observation. Its onset and duration of action were comparable to those of morphine and there were no untoward side actions. It will be recalled that this benzomorphan is practically devoid of addiction liability in the monkey (Section III,B,2*b*).

IV. Narcotic Antagonists of the Morphine, Morphinan, and Benzomorphan Series as Analgetics

The capacity of *N*-allylnormorphine (XXI) to antagonize most of the pharmacologic effects of narcotic analgetics was first demonstrated in 1943 (*96*), although this property was recognized for *N*-allylnorcodeine in 1914 (*97*). Clark *et al.* (*19a*) reported that *n*-propyl, methallyl, and isobutyl substituted for the *N*-methyl group of morphine and close relatives also conferred antagonistic properties on the molecule, albeit to a lesser degree than allyl. Similar findings have been reported for the morphinan series. In fact (−)-3-hydroxy-*N*-allylmorphinan (levallorphan, XLVII) is more than twice as potent an antagonist (*87*) as nalorphine as is the benzomorphan counterpart, α-(±)-2-allyl-5,9-dimethyl-2′-hydroxy-6,7-benzomorphan (*87*, *98*). These antagonists, especially nalorphine (*55*), have proved useful in various ways in clinical practice and research (Section III,A,5).

All three of the *N*-allyl derivatives just mentioned appear to have little analgetic action in animals. However, nalorphine, without addiction liability (*99*), is now known to be comparable to morphine in analgetic potency in man (*100*). Although the high incidence of side-effects, particularly of a psychotomimetic nature precludes its use as a substitute for morphine, the fact that it did prove to be a nonaddicting, strong analgetic in man has stimulated further work along these lines. For example, Gates and Montzka have replaced the methyl group with cyclopropylmethyl (chosen because of its similarity to allyl) (*101*) in various morphine and morphinan congeners. Not only were the resulting compounds more powerful antagonists

171

than nalorphine or levallorphan, but at least one, (−)-3-hydroxy-N-cyclo-propylmethylmorphinan is a potent analgetic in man.

A broader effort (87) was undertaken in the 6,7-benzomorphan (cf. Section II,B,2) series in which some dissociation of analgetic activity and addiction liability had already been shown (64, 90). Archer and associates synthesized over twenty N-substituted derivatives of α-(±)-5,9-dimethyl-2′-hydroxy-6,7-benzomorphan and α-(±)-5-ethyl-9-methyl-2′-hydroxy-6,7-benzo-morphan (87). These were tested for antagonistic action to meperidine, morphine, and phenazocine and for other pharmacologic properties. The range in antagonistic activity was from about one-hundredth that of nalor-phine (N-cyclohexylmethyl derivative) to six times that of nalorphine (N-cyclopropylmethyl, -cis-3-chloroallyl, and -propyl derivatives). Most of these substances showed little or no analgetic activity in the usual animal tests (51, 87). Three of the negative compounds were, however, selected for clinical trial on the basis of their interesting pharmacological and favor-able toxicological properties. Of these, at least one [α-(±)-5,9-dimethyl-2-(3,3-dimethylallyl)-2′-hydroxy-6,7-benzomorphan, pentazocine], appears to be a clinically acceptable, strong analgetic of insignificant addiction liabil-ity (102). Pentazocine (also a weak antagonist), at a dose of 20–30 mg appears to be comparable to 10 mg of morphine in controlling postoperative pain (87, 103). Another, the very strong antagonist, α-(±)-2-cyclopropyl-methyl-5,9-dimethyl-2′-hydroxy-6,7-benzomorphan (cyclazocine), has about forty times the potency of morphine in postoperative patients (104). If, indeed, either pentazocine or cyclazocine does prove to be acceptable in medical practice, then many problems of the physician in controlling pain (especially chronic pain) would be greatly ameliorated.

V. Metabolism of Morphine, Codeine, and Levorphanol

The metabolic fate of narcotic analgesics in both animals and man has been the subject of numerous investigations which have been greatly facilitated by the advent of isotopic tracer methodology and thin-layer chromato-graphy (105). An elegant review of this subject which considers in detail the absorption, distribution, biotransformation, elimination and estimation of morphine and congeners as well as the more important synthetic analogs, has been written by Way and Adler (106).

In general, absorption of morphine and congeners (including synthetic analogs) is relatively rapid after parenteral administration and erratic after oral medication. Pharmacological or clinical effects can be noted within a few minutes after injection but peak effects may not occur for an hour or more.

The predominant metabolic changes for morphine, codeine, and levorphanol are N-demethylation, O-demethylation, and conjugation with glucuronic acid (at the 3-hydroxyl position for morphine and levorphanol and at the 6-hydroxyl for codeine). Experiments (*107*) with either O-methyl or N-methyl C^{14}-labeled codeine have shown that rapid disposal occurs in man and that 24 hours after injection, the maximum of morphine (4–13%), norcodeine (8%), bound codeine (35–40%), and unchanged codeine (5–12%) is present in the urine; negligible amounts are found in the feces and only part of the detached O-methyl and N-methyl radicals can be recovered as expired carbon dioxide. Similar studies with N-methyl C^{14}-labeled morphine (*108*) revealed a somewhat parallel pattern. Although in this instance 7–10% of morphine was found in the feces, urinary excretion of bound (conjugated) morphine accounted for most of the recovered activity. The pulmonary excretion of $C^{14}O_2$ amounted to 3.5–6% of the injected dose, yet neither normorphine nor its conjugate have ever been detected in the urine (*106*).

The absorption of levorphanol and analogs is rapid after administration by the usual routes in all species studied. It is likely that the marked superiority of levorphanol to morphine as an oral analgetic is due largely to its more rapid absorption (than morphine) after oral administration. The biologic half-life of N-methyl C^{14}-labeled levorphanol (*106, 109*) in the plasma was 75 to 90 minutes for free levorphanol and 3 hours for conjugated levorphanol when injected subcutaneously in the monkey and the dog. About 2.5% of the dose administered to the monkey appeared in the urine as free levorphanol; 35%, as conjugated. In dogs the percentages were 4.4 and 42%, respectively. Less than 0.1% appeared in the feces of either species. The monkey eliminates about 20% of the radioactivity of administered levorphanol as $C^{14}O_2$; the rat, 5%; the dog, very little. In spite of this 3-hydroxymorphinan (norlevorphanol) has not been detected in the urine or feces, again a parallel to morphine.

The results just presented are in fairly good agreement with those obtained by other investigators and are representative of the morphine and morphinan series. There are, of course, species differences, particularly between man and lower animals and in respect to variations related to sex. However, these differences are generally of a quantitative nature and are usually not so pronounced as to invalidate a qualitative prediction of the behavior of a morphine-like analgetic in transferring from animal to man. It is also the consensus that altered distribution or fate of narcotic drugs, in a gross sense, is not associated with or responsible for the development of tolerance or physical dependence (*106*). Fundamental studies at the cellular level (*110*) may yet reveal initimate differences which will ultimately prove significant.

As for the possible role of N-dealkylation (the metabolic pathway most common to morphine and surrogates) in the mediation of analgesia, it is concluded (*111*) that the main pharmacological actions of these narcotic analgesics cannot be explained through an action of N-demethylated products. Although morphine, codeine, and relatives become localized only to a minor extent in the central nervous system, peak levels of the unchanged drugs in the central nervous system are correlative with pharmacological activity (*112*) as measured by the pain-reaction time method.

Counter to this view, however, is the hypothesis advanced by Beckett (*113*) that "oxidative dealkylation to produce *nor*-compounds is presumed to be the first step in the reaction sequence leading to analgesia."

REFERENCES

1. J. M. Gulland and R. Robinson, *Mem. Proc. Manchester Lit. Phil. Soc.* **69**, 79 (1925).
2. M. Gates and G. Tschudi, *J. Am. Chem. Soc.* **74**, 1109 (1952); **78**, 1380 (1956).
3. D. Elad and D. Ginsburg, *J. Chem. Soc.* p. 3052 (1954).
4. D. H. R. Barton, G. W. Kirby, W. Steglich, and G. M. Thomas, *Proc. Chem. Soc.* p. 203 (1963).
5. H. Rapoport and J. B. Lavigne, *J. Am. Chem. Soc.* **75**, 5329 (1953); K. W. Bentley and H. M. E. Cardwell, *J. Chem. Soc.* 3252 (1955); G. Stork and F. H. Clarke, *J. Am. Chem. Soc.* **78**, 4619 (1956).
6. J. Kalvoda, P. Buchschacher, and O. Jeger, *Helv. Chim. Acta* **38**, 1847 (1955).
7. H. Rapoport, H. N. Reist, and C. H. Lovell, *J. Am. Chem. Soc.* **78**, 5128 (1956).
8. A. R. Battersby, *Proc. Chem. Soc.*, p. 189 (1963).
9. L. F. Small, N. B. Eddy, E. Mosettig, and C. K. Himmelsbach, "Studies on Drug Addiction," Suppl. No. 138 to the Public Health Repts. U.S. Govt. Printing Office, Washington, D.C. 1938.
10. P. Karrer and H. Heynemann, *Helv. Chim. Acta* **31**, 398 (1948).
11. U. Weiss, *J. Am. Chem. Soc.* **77**, 5891 (1955).
12. L. F. Small and H. Rapoport, *J. Org. Chem.* **12**, 284 (1947); H. Isbell and H. F. Fraser, *Pharmacol Rev.* **2**, 355 (1950).
13. L. F. Small, H. M. Fitch, and W. E. Smith, *J. Am. Chem. Soc.* **58**, 1457 (1936); *cf.* also M. Gates and M. S. Shepard, *J. Am. Chem. Soc.* **84**, 4125 (1962).
14. (a) N. B. Eddy, *Ann. N.Y. Acad. Sci.* **51**, 51 (1948); (b) R. W. Houde, L. H. Rasmussen, and J. S. LaDue, *Ann. N.Y. Acad. Sci.* **51**, 161 (1948); (c) N. B. Eddy, H. Halbach, and O. J. Braenden, *Bull. World Health Organ.* **14**, 353 (1956).
15. M. S. Chadha and H. Rapoport, *J. Am. Chem. Soc.* **79**, 5730 (1957).
16. K. W. Bentley and D. G. Hardy, *Proc. Chem. Soc.* **220** (1963).
17. C. Elison, H. W. Elliot, M. Look, and H. Rapoport, *J. Med. Chem.* **6**, 237 (1963).
18. B. Kelentei, E. Stenszky, F. Czollner, L. Szlavik, and Z. Meszaros, *Arzneimittel-Forsch.* **7**, 594 (1957; *Chem. Abstr.* **52**, 3163 (1958); K. Takagi and H. Fukuda, *Yakugaku Zasshi* **80**, 1499 (1960); *Chem. Abstr.* **55**, 8648 (1961).
19. (a) R. L. Clark, A. A. Pessolano, J. Weijlard, and K. Pfister, 3rd, *J. Am. Chem. Soc.* **75**, 4963 (1953); (b) N. B. Eddy, L. F. Small, and E. L. May, *J. Org. Chem.* **23**, 1387 (1958); (c) J. Weijlard, P. D. Orahovats, A. P. Sullivan, Jr., G. Purdue, F. K. Heath, and K. Pfister, 3rd, *J. Am. Chem. Soc.* **78**, 2342 (1956).

20. (a) J. Weijlard and A. E. Erickson, *J. Am. Chem. Soc.* **64**, 869 (1942); (b) L. Lasagna and H. K. Beecher, *J. Pharmacol. Exptl. Therap.* **112**, 306 (1954); (c) A. S. Keats and J. Telford, *J. Pharmacol. Exptl. Therap.* **117**, 190 (1956).

21. R. Grewe and A. Mondon, *Ber. Deut. Chem. Ges.* **81**, 279 (1948); R. Grewe, *Angew Chem.* **59**, 194 (1947); R. Grewe, *Naturwissenschaften* **33**, 333 (1946).

22. R. Robinson, "The Structural Relations of Natural Products." Oxford Univ. Press (Clarendon), London and New York 1955.

23. C. Schöpf and K. Thierfelder, *Ann. Chem.* **537**, 143 (1939).

24. C. F. Koelsch and N. F. Albertson, *J. Am. Chem. Soc.* **75**, 2095 (1953).

25. O. Schnider, Swiss Pat. 252,755 (1946).

26. O. Schnider and A. Grüssner, *Helv. Chim. Acta* **32**, 821 (1949).

27. R. Grewe, A. Mondon, and E. Nolte, *Ann. Chem.* **564**, 161 (1949).

28. E. Ochiai and M. Ikehara, *Pharm. Bull. (Tokyo)* **3**, 291 (1955).

29. O. Schnider and J. Hellerbach, unpublished results.

30. O. Schnider and J. Hellerbach, *Helv. Chim. Acta* **33**, 1437 (1950).

31. R. Grewe, R. Hamann, G. Jacobsen, E. Nolte, and K. Riecke, *Ann. Chem.* **581**, 85 (1953).

32. H. Henecka, *Ann. Chem.* **583**, 110 (1953); H. Henecka and W. Wirth, *Med. Chem. (Verlag Chemie GmbH "Bayer" Leverkusen)* **5**, 321 (1956).

33. M. Sasamoto, *Pharm. Bull. Nippon Univ.* **8**, 324, 329, 980 (1960).

34. S. Sugasawa and R. Tachikawa, *J. Org. Chem.* **24**, 2043 (1959).

35. D. Ginsburg and R. Pappo, *J. Chem. Soc.* p. 938 (1951).

36. J. A. Barltrop and J. E. Saxton, *J. Chem. Soc.* p. 1038 (1952).

37. (a) O Schnider and A. Grüssner, *Helv. Chim. Acta* **34**, 2211 (1951); (b) O. Schnider, A. Brossi, and K. Vogler, *Helv. Chim. Acta* **37**, 710 (1954).

38. C. W. Den Hollander, U.S. Pats. 2,819,272 (1958); 2,915,479, (1959); A. Brossi and O. Schnider, *Helv. Chim. Acta* **39**, 1376 (1956).

39. N. C. Handley, Brit. Pat. 832,025 (1960).

40. J. Hellerbach, A. Grüssner, and O. Schnider, *Helv. Chim. Acta* **39**, 429 (1956).

41. A. H. Beckett and P. Anderson, *J. Pharm. Pharmacol.* **12**, 228T (1960).

42. H. Corrodi, J. Hellerbach, A. Zust, E. Hardegger, and O. Schnider, *Helv. Chim. Acta* **42**, 212 (1959).

43. D. Arigoni, J. Kalvoda, H. Heusser, O. Jeger, and L. Ruzicka, *Helv. Chim. Acta* **38**, 1857 (1955).

44. Y. K. Sawa, N. Tsuizi, and S. Maeda, *Tetrahedron* **15**, 144, 154 (1961).

45. M. Gates, R. B. Woodward, W. F. Newhall, and R. Künzli, *J. Am. Chem. Soc.* **72**, 1141 (1950).

46. M. Gates and G. Tschudi, *J. Am. Chem. Soc.* **72**, 4839 (1950).

47. M. Gates and W. G. Webb, *J. Am. Chem. Soc.* **80**, 1186 (1958).

48. S. Sugasawa and S. Saito, *Pharm. Bull (Tokyo)* **4**, 237 (1956); M. S. Newman and B. J. Magerlein, *J. Am. Chem. Soc.* **69**, 942 (1947); S. Saito, *Pharm. Bull. (Tokyo)* **4**, 438 (1956); M. Protiva, V. Mychajlyszyn, and J. O. Jilek, *Chem. Listy* **49**, 1045 (1955); E. L. May and J. G. Murphy, *J. Org. Chem.* **19**, 618 (1954); N. Sugimoto, *J. Pharm. Soc. (Japan)* **75**, 183 (1955); N. Sugimoto and S. Ohshiro, *Pharm. Bull. (Tokyo)* **4**, 353, 357 (1956); K. Harasawa, *J. Pharm. Soc. (Japan)* **77**, 168, 172, 794 (1957); N. Sugimoto, S. Ohshiro, H. Kugita, and S. Saito, *Pharm. Bull. (Tokyo)* **5**, 62 (1957); N. Sugimoto and S. Ohshiro, *Pharm. Bull. (Tokyo)* **5**, 316 (1957); N. Sugimoto and H. Kugita, *Pharm. Bull. (Tokyo)* **5**, 67 (1957); **6**, 429 (1958); N. Sugimoto and S. Ohshiro, *Tetrahedron* **8**, 296 304 (1960); H. Kugita, *Pharm. Bull. (Tokyo)* **4**, 29 189 (1956).

49. N. Sugimoto and H. Kugita, *Pharm. Bull.* (*Tokyo*) **3**, 11 (1955); **5**, 378 (1957).

50. J. Hellerbach, O. Schnider, H. Besendorf, and B. Pellmont, *In* "Synthetic Analgesics," Part II-A; Morphinans. Pergamon Press, London 1965.

51. N. B. Eddy and D. Leimbach, *J. Pharmacol. Exptl. Therap.* **107**, 385 (1953).

52. N. B. Eddy, H. Besendorf, and B. Pellmont, *Bull. Narcotics* **10**, 23 (1958).

53. N. B. Eddy, H. Halbach, and O. J. Braenden, *Bull. World Health Organ.* **17**, 569 (1957).

54. H. Isbell and H. F. Fraser, *J. Pharmacol. Exptl. Therap.* **107**, 524 (1953).

55. E. L. May, *in* "Medicinal Chemistry" (A. Burger, ed.), p. 311. Wiley (Interscience), New York, 1960.

56. E. L. May and J. G. Murphy, *J. Org. Chem.* **20**, 1197 (1955); E. L. May, *J. Org. Chem.* **23**, 947 (1958).

57. E. L. May, and J. G. Murphy, *J. Org. Chem.* **20**, 257 (1955).

58. E. M. Fry, J. H. Ager, and E. L. May, Nat. Inst. of Health, unpublished results.

59. E. L. May, H. Kugita, and J. H. Ager, *J. Org. Chem.* **26**, 1621 (1961).

60. J. A. Barltrop, *J. Chem. Soc.* p. 399 (1947).

61. N. B. Eddy, J. G. Murphy, and E. L. May, *J. Org. Chem.* **22**, 1370 (1957).

62. J. G. Murphy, J. H. Ager, and E. L. May, *J. Org. Chem.* **25**, 1386 (1960).

63. E. M. Fry and E. L. May, *J. Org. Chem.* **26**, 2592 (1961).

64. J. H. Ager, S. E. Fullerton, and E. L. May, *J. Med. Chem.* **6**, 322 (1963).

65. S. Saito and E. L. May, *J. Org. Chem.* **27**, 948 (1962).

66. E. L. May, *J. Org. Chem.* **22**, 593 (1957).

67. E. L. May and E. M. Fry, *J. Org. Chem.* **22**, 1366 (1957).

68. E. L. May and J. H. Ager, *J. Org. Chem.* **24**, 1432 (1959).

69. J. H. Ager and E. L. May, *J. Org. Chem.* **27**, 245 (1962).

70. S. E. Fullerton, J. H. Ager, and E. L. May, *J. Org. Chem.* **27**, 2554 (1962).

71. J. H. Ager, Nat. Inst. of Health, unpublished results.

72. S. E. Fullerton, E. L. May, and E. D. Becker, *J. Org. Chem.* **27**, 2144 (1962).

73. E. L. May, H. Kugita, and J. H. Ager, *J. Org. Chem.* **26**, 1621 (1961).

74. E. L. May and H. Kugita, *J. Org. Chem.* **26**, 188 (1961).

75. C. Schöpf and F. Borkowsky, *Ann. Chem.* **452**, 249 (1927).

76. E. M. Fry, *J. Org. Chem.* **22**, 1710 (1957).

77. T. B. Zalucky and G. Hite, *J. Med. Pharm. Chem.* **3**, 615 (1961).

78. H. Kugita and E. L. May, *J. Org. Chem.* **26**, 1954 (1961).

79. S. Saito and E. L. May, *J. Org. Chem.* **26**, 4356 (1961).

80. S. Saito and E. L. May, *J. Org. Chem.* **27**, 1087 (1962).

81. A. Grüssner, J. Hellerbach, and O. Schnider, *Helv. Chim. Acta*, **40**, 1232 (1957).

82. E. L. May and N. B. Eddy, *J. Org. Chem.* **24**, 1435 (1959).

83. E. L. May, *J. Org. Chem.* **21**, 899 (1956).

84. J. H. Ager and E. L. May, *J. Org. Chem.* **25**, 984 (1960).

85. E. M. Fry and E. L. May, *J. Org. Chem.* **24**, 116 (1959).

86. M. Gordon, J. J. Lafferty, D. H. Tedeschi, B. M. Sutton, N. B. Eddy, and E. L. May, *J. Med. Pharm. Chem.* **5**, 633 (1962).

87. S. Archer, N. F. Albertson, L. S. Harris, A. K. Pierson, and J. G. Bird, *J. Med. Chem.* **7**, 123 (1964).

88. E. L. May, Nat. Inst. of Health, unpublished results.

89. H. Kugita, S. Saito, and E. L. May, *J. Med. Pharm. Chem.* **5**, 357 (1962).

90. N. B. Eddy and E. L. May, *in* "Synthetic Analgesics," (J. Rolfe, Ed.), Part-II-B, 6.7-Benzomorphans. Pergamon Press, London 1965.

91. A. E. Jacobsen and E. L. May, *J. Med. Chem.* **7**, 409 (1964).
92. J. H. Ager, S. E. Fullerton, E. M. Fry, and E. L. May, *J. Org. Chem.* **28**, 2470 (1963).
93. M. H. Seevers and G. A. Deneau, Addenda to the Minutes of the Committee on Drug Addiction and Narcotics. Nat. Acad. Sci. Nat. Res. Council, Washington, D.C., 1958–1962.
94. H. Halbach and N. B. Eddy, *Bull. World Health Organ.* **28**, 139 (1963).
95. H. F. Fraser and H. Isbell, *Bull. Narcotics* **12**, 15 (1960).
96. K. Unna, *J. Pharmacol. Exptl. Therap.* **79**, 27 (1943).
97. J. Pohl, *Z. Exptl. Pathol. Therap.* **17**, 370 (1914).
98. M. Gordon, J. J. Lafferty, D. H. Tedeschi, N. B. Eddy, and E. L. May, *Nature* **192**, 1089 (1961).
99. H. Isbell, *Federation Proc.* **15**, 442 (1956).
100. L. Lasagna and H. K. Beecher, *J. Pharmacol. Exptl. Therap.* **112**, 356 (1954); A. S. Keats and J. Telford, *J. Pharmacol. Exptl. Therap.* **117**, 190 (1956).
101. M. Gates and T. A. Montzka, *J. Med. Chem.* **7**, 127 (1964).
102. H. F. Fraser, D. E. Rosenberg, and H. Isbell, *J. Pharmacol. Exptl. Therap.* in press.
103. A. S. Keats and J. Telford, *J. Pharmacol. Exptl. Therap.* in press.
104. L. Lasagna and T. DeKornfeld, *Federation Proc.* **22**, 248 (1963).
105. J. Cochin and J. W. Daly, *Experientia* **18**, 294 (1962).
106. E. L. Way and T. K. Adler, *in* "The Biological Disposition of Morphine and Its Surrogates." World Health Organ., Geneva, Switzerland, 1962; *cf.* also *Bull. World Health Organ.* **25**, 227 (1961); **26**, 51, 261 (1962); **27**, 359 (1962).
107. T. K. Adler, J. M. Fugimoto, E. L. Way, and E. M. Baker, *J. Pharmacol. Exptl. Therap.* **114**, 251 (1955).
108. H. W. Elliot, B. M. Tolbert, T. K. Adler, and H. H. Anderson, *Proc. Soc. Exptl. Biol. Med.* **85**, 77 (1954).
109. L. A. Woods, L. B. Mellett, and K. S. Anderson, *J. Pharmacol. Exptl. Therap.* **124**, 1 (1958).
110. J. Axelrod, *Science* **124**, 263 (1956).
111. J. W. Miller and H. H. Anderson, *J. Pharmacol. Exptl. Therap.* **112**, 191 (1954).
112. J. W. Miller and H. W. Elliot, *J. Pharmacol. Exptl. Therap.* **113**, 283 (1955).
113. A. H. Beckett, A. F. Casy, and N. J. Harper, *J. Pharm. Pharmacol.* **8**, 874 (1956).
114. C. I. Wright and F. A. Barbour, *J. Pharmacol. Exptl. Therap.* **61**, 422 (1937).

CHAPTER V

Synthetic Analgetics with Morphine-like Actions

ROBERT A. HARDY, Jr.

and M. GERTRUDE HOWELL

LEDERLE LABORATORIES,

A DIVISION OF AMERICAN CYANAMID CO.,

PEARL RIVER, NEW YORK

I. Introduction

The synthetic morphine-like compounds discussed in this chapter are distinguished from morphine and the related compounds described in Chapter IV by increased stereochemical flexibility. These compounds are generally moderately to highly potent, narcotic-type analgetics which tend to exhibit a spectrum of pharmacological and clinical actions qualitatively similar to that of morphine. These include pain-killing capacity, development of tolerance, physical dependence capacity, addiction liability, respiratory depression, and antagonism by nalorphine and related compounds.

Extensive studies of structure versus morphine-like actions have provided highly specific hypotheses concerning the structural requirements for this type of analgetic. These hypotheses have been elegantly summarized by Beckett and Casy (1) and Braenden et al. (2), among others. The structural features generally found in all the families of compounds discussed in this chapter (and in morphine and the modifications covered in Chapter IV, as well) can be summarized, in part, as follows.

$$\overset{R}{\underset{|}{\text{Am}—C_nH_{2n}—X—Ar}}$$

A basic amine function (Am), usually tertiary, is connected through a hydrocarbon chain, generally of two carbon atoms, to a highly substituted central atom (X). This central atom is usually a quaternary carbon atom, but may also be a tertiary nitrogen, and is attached to a flat, aromatic ring (Ar) such as benzene or a 5- or 6-membered heteroaromatic ring. The structure of the remaining group(s) (R) attached to the central atom is less critical and frequently has an oxygen function in the vicinity of the central atom. In morphine (I) the stereochemical arrangement of the basic amine, the alkylene chain, the central carbon atom, and the flat, aromatic ring is essentially rigid. However, the structures of the synthetic morphine-like analgetics covered in this chapter usually allow considerable rotational or conformational freedom. Thus, these compounds are generally capable of forming a morphine-like configuration (II) even though it may not be a preferred

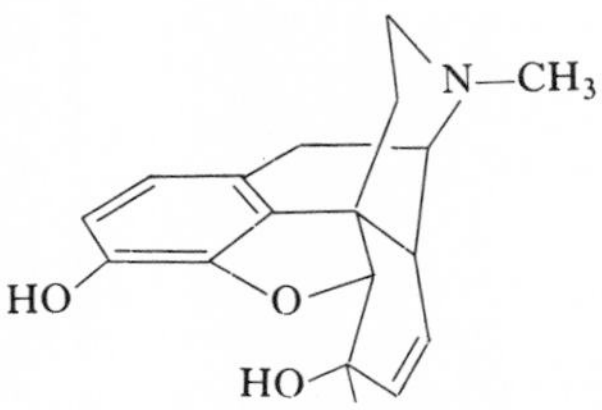

(I) 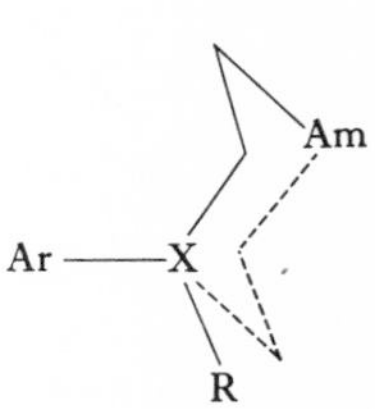   (II)

conformation. These structural features provide the background for understanding the analgetic properties of the widely diversified chemical types covered in this chapter.

The study of synthetic morphine-like analgetics dates from the development in 1939 of meperidine, 4-carbethoxy-1-methyl-4-phenylpiperidine (3). Since then, synthetic analgetic research has expanded exponentially. Few other fields of pharmaceutical research have attracted such a continuing and expanding volume of work over a period of 25 years. This chapter can not cover this field in every detail; rather it is designed to review highlights of the more significant work during the past few years. An over-all picture of the present general state of knowledge of synthetic morphine-like compounds and their activity is presented, with emphasis on recent results which are contributing to the direction of current research.

The synthetic morphine-like analgetics have been the subject of a number of excellent reviews. Bergel and Morrison (4) have surveyed work in this field before 1948. A series of reviews sponsored by the World Health Organization present a detailed picture of progress to about 1956. Braenden and Wolff (5) covered aspects of chemical synthesis. The relationship between chemical structure and analgetic action was surveyed by Braenden and co-workers (2). Eddy et al. (6) reviewed the relationship between analgetic action and addiction liability with a discussion of chemical structure. The same authors (7) have also covered clinical aspects of the morphine-like analgetics. More recently, May (8) and Beckett and Casy (9) have reviewed the chemistry of morphine-like compounds to about 1960–1961. Additionally, brief reviews have been presented by Eddy (10), by Janssen (11a,b), and by Pfeifer (12). Mellett and Woods (13) have surveyed analgesia and addiction with a detailed comparative compilation of mouse analgesia data, addiction liability in man, and physical dependence in the monkey for many of the compounds covered in this chapter.

II. 4-Phenylpiperidine Derivatives

The 4-phenylpiperidine class of synthetic morphine-like analgetic agent is historically the oldest (since 1939) synthetic group. It has probably attracted the greatest amount of research toward related compounds of any of the synthetics. This research continues to expand even today. However, the first drug in this series, meperidine, is still the most widely accepted substitute for morphine (and codeine) for moderate to severe pain. This class of compounds may be summarized by the general formula:

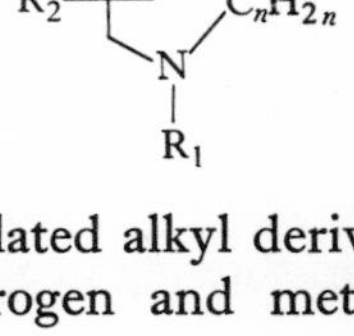

R_1 includes methyl and related alkyl derivatives, particularly including phenalkyl types; R_2 is hydrogen and methyl, etc. (principally in the

181

3-position); Ar is a phenyl group with a variety of substituents or related heteroaromatic groups such as furyl; R_3 is principally an oxygen function including carbalkoxy, acyloxy, alkyl ketone, alkyl ether groups, and related chemical or isosteric functions; n is 1, 2, or 3 for 5-, 6-, and 7-membered analogs.

A. 4-CARBALKOXY TYPES (MEPERIDINE FAMILY)

4-Carbethoxy-1-methyl-4-phenylpiperidine (III), or 1-methyl-4-phenyl-isonipecotic acid ethyl ester, was synthesized in Germany and investigated as an antispasmodic agent. However, clinical trials demonstrated powerful analgetic action (3). This drug is now widely known as meperidine or pethidine (Europe) and also a variety of other names (14).

1. Stereochemical Considerations

A conformational structure of meperidine showing the aliphatic amino group, the ethylene chain, the central quaternary carbon atom, and the flat, aromatic moiety in a morphine-like configuration is illustrated (IV; compare with I).

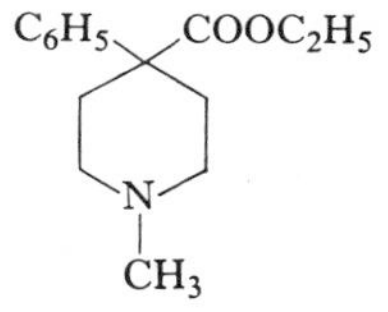

(III) 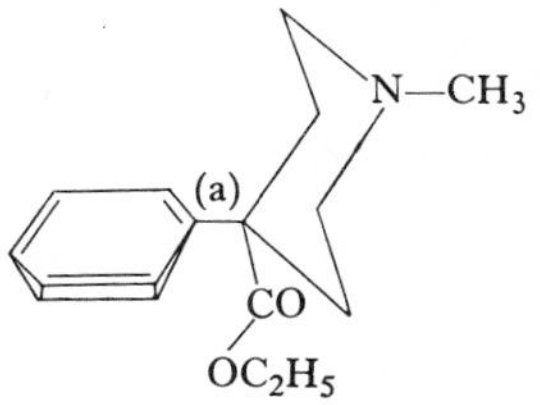   (IV)

Although the axial 4-phenyl group may not be the preferred conformation (by analogy with the detailed stereochemistry know in the prodine series—see Section II,A), it illustrates that meperidine can apparently fit the same biological receptor as morphine. Structural analogies between meperidine and morphine were observed only after the morphine-like actions of the synthetic derivative became known.

The importance of a specific stereochemical fit between a "morphine receptor" and the analgetic drug was gradually recognized, and was best outlined by Beckett and Casy (1, 15) in 1954. This concept has now been accepted, with some modification, by virtually all analgetic researchers and has been an important factor in studying many of the compounds described in this chapter. Important features of the Beckett and Casy stereospecific receptor include sites for specific binding with the analgetic agent. An area for binding with the aromatic ring of the analgetic agent, perhaps by van der Waals forces or chelation with the π-electrons, and an anionic center for binding with the cationic amine hydrochloride group (at physiological pH) are primary sites. These are stereospecifically oriented on a receptor (enzyme) surface with a suitable cavity such that (+) and (−) enantiomers (where possible) may show different degrees of drug-receptor fit. This results in different degrees of analgetic potency. Secondary binding sites involving others parts of the analgetic molecule such as the oxygen function(s) may also be important. Many compounds studied as analgetics appear to have all the structural and stereochemical requirements of the "morphine receptor," but are completely devoid of morphine-like actions. Factors such as absorption, distribution, penetration into the central nervous system, metabolism, etc. may prevent satisfactory transport of the analgetic-like compound to the receptor. It is also noteworthy that these structural analogs which are not active as analgetics at times have other useful central nervous system activity (e.g., as tranquilizers, antiemetics, etc.).

2. Synthesis

The first synthesis of meperidine was reported by Eisleb in 1941 (16). Modifications have been described by Eisleb and others and reviewed by Braenden and Wolff (5) and by Bergel and Morrison (4). New methods have not been introduced in recent years. Scheme 1 shows the principal routes to the meperidine family of compounds (VIII).

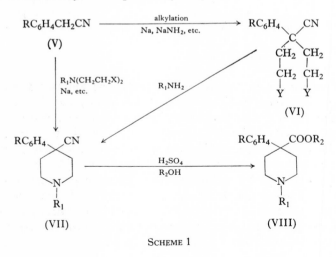

SCHEME 1

183

Basic intermediates for this series are phenylacetonitrile and its ring substituted derivatives (V). One of the original syntheses used the nitrogen mustard, bis(2-chloroethyl)methylamine. The 4-cyano-4-phenylpiperidine (VII) was thereby obtained and converted to the 4-carbalkoxy compound (VIII). Other reactive groups, such as the p-toluenesulfonyloxy group, have been used in place of halogen to avoid the toxic properties of the 2-halo-ethylamines. The piperidine ring may also be formed by the reaction of an amine with a dialkylated phenylacetontrile derivative (VI). The phenyl-acetonitrile is first treated with a compound of the type XCH_2H_2Y in which the nature of the Y grouping does not permit it to react during the initial alkylation. The Y function is then converted to a reactive moiety prior to cyclization with the amine. The acid-labile vinyloxy function is such a group and is replaced by a halogen or arylsulfonyloxy moiety prior to ring closure.

If R_1 is a benzyl or benzenesulfonyl group it may be removed by hydro-genolysis or hydrolysis. The resulting 1-H (or nor) compound can then be converted to a wide variety of N-substituted derivatives. The synthesis of the 3-methyl derivatives (XII) by a variation of the general scheme is illustrated here (17).

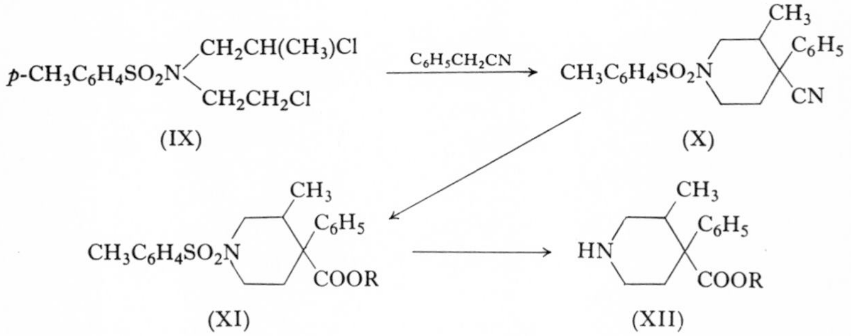

The 3-substituent confers asymmetry to the ring, and two diastereomeric racemates are formed (X). The α and β forms are separated by their differ-ential solubility in methanol. Alkaline hydrolysis of the nitrile gives the acid which is converted, via the acid chloride, to the methyl, ethyl, and isopropyl esters (XI). Removal of the tosyl moiety with a mixture of phenol–acetic acid–HBr, produces the α and β forms of the nor compounds (XII) which can then be used for a variety of 1-substituted 3-methylnormeperidine derivatives.

Virtually all recent work on the meperidine series has been directed towards the synthesis of new, N-1 substituted derivatives. Most of the common methods for alkylating amines have been employed; typical methods are illustrated in Scheme 2.

184

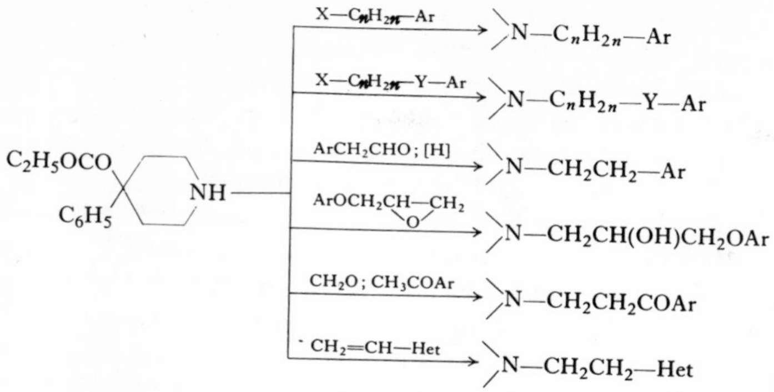

$$C_2H_5OCO, \quad C_6H_5 \bigotimes NH$$

Reagent	Product
$X-C_nH_{2n}-Ar$	$\rangle N-C_nH_{2n}-Ar$
$X-C_nH_{2n}-Y-Ar$	$\rangle N-C_nH_{2n}-Y-Ar$
$ArCH_2CHO; [H]$	$\rangle N-CH_2CH_2-Ar$
$ArOCH_2CH-CH_2 \; (O)$	$\rangle N-CH_2CH(OH)CH_2OAr$
$CH_2O; CH_3COAr$	$\rangle N-CH_2CH_2COAr$
$CH_2=CH-Het$	$\rangle N-CH_2CH_2-Het$

SCHEME 2

3. Structure-Activity Relationships

The excellent clinical acceptance of meperidine and the accessability of this type of compound has prompted the synthesis of inumerable related substances. Structure-activity correlations rapidly became apparent and, by about 1955 the following generalizations were well accepted (6, 9).

(a) Substitution on the 4-phenyl ring generally reduced activity except for a few special cases. For example, the m-hydroxy (bemidone; 1.5 × meperidine) and o-methyl derivatives were somewhat more potent than the parent compounds.

(b) The carbethoxy function proved to be more active than the methyl and higher alkyl esters. Replacement of the ester by other groups generally diminished activity. However, high potency can be obtained by reversal of the ester function (see Section II,B).

(c) Shifting the phenyl and (or) carbethoxy groups from the 4-position reduced or eliminated activity.

(d) The N-1 methyl appeared to be the optimal group at this position. Hydrogen and other lower alkyl groups were less potent.

However, in 1956 Perrine and Eddy (18) reported that the 1-phenethyl and 1-(2-hydroxy-2-phenylethyl) derivatives were 2–3 times more potent than meperidine. That phenethyl substitution on the nitrogen atom of the rigid analgetics (19) (morphine and related compounds, the morphinans and the benzomorphans; see Chapter IV) markedly increased activity had been previously recognized. About that time Millar and Stephenson (20) found that 1-(2-morpholinoethyl)normeperidine was more potent than the parent drug, and its toxicity was not correspondingly increased. The high activity of the phenalkyl and heteroalkyl derivatives was rapidly confirmed by other laboratories (21, 22) and provided new impetus for intensified research on 1-substituted 4-phenylpiperidine analgetics. The same compounds were occasionally synthesized and evaluated simultaneously and independently by different laboratories. Impressive increases in potency have been achieved (to more than $3000 \times$ meperidine in animal assays). However, the side effects, including addiction liability potential have, generally, also increased with the analgetic potency.

Meperidine is intermediate in analgetic potency between codeine and morphine. By the Eddy hot-plate procedure using mice (23), it is approximately one-fifth as potent as morphine. Throughout this chapter the mouse hot-plate results of Eddy, as compiled by Mellett and Woods (13), are used for potency comparisons based on animal data whenever possible. This procedure as carried out in Dr. Eddy's laboratory over a number of years has assayed virtually all of the important analgetic agents known today, and provides a uniform basis for comparison. Other animal testing procedures are well known and a considerable range of relative potency values is obtained depending on the species, the method of pain stimulus, and the route of administration. However, the order of ranking by relative potency (e.g., codeine < meperidine < morphine) is generally consistent despite different animal procedures and clinical results.

A cross-section of 1-substituted normeperidine derivatives reported since 1956 is given in Table I. The 1-substituents illustrate those moieties which have generally increased the potency of the parent molecule, sometimes to levels many times morphine. Invariably, the most potent derivatives also show high physical dependence capacity in monkeys (13). The normeperidine derivatives which have been used clinically as analgetic drugs have also shown addiction liability in man, and are controlled as narcotics. It is noteworthy that the changes in the meperidine molecule which so markedly increase the potency are somewhat removed from the basic skeleton of the hypothetical potent analgetic (i.e., the basic nitrogen, the alkylene chain, the central atom, and the aromatic ring). The side chain might be expected to have a relatively minor influence on the stereospecific drug-receptor interaction. The results indicate the shape and configuration of the chain on the basic nitrogen may be very important factors, however.

Many derivatives structurally related to the compounds listed in Table I have been synthesized. However, their analgetic activity is generally not pronounced or has been unreported. Several 3β-methyl derivatives of meperidine (Table I, No. 1) have been described recently (55). They have 1-alkyl substituents ranging from methyl to heptyl. These derivatives are noteworthy due to the asymmetry conferred on the molecule by the 3-substituent. When diastereomeric isomers are isolated, they usually exhibit significantly different analgetic potencies. Detailed studies of the stereochemistry and

TABLE I

1-SUBSTITUTED NORMEPERIDINE DERIVATIVES

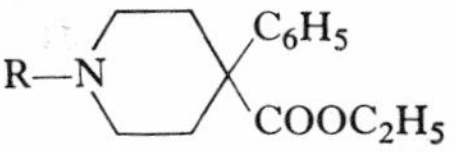

$$R-N \diagdown \begin{array}{l} C_6H_5 \\ COOC_2H_5 \end{array}$$

No.	R	Activity[a]	References
1.	CH_3 (meperidine)[b]	1.0	16
2.	H (normeperidine)	0.3	24
3.	$CH_2=CHCH_2$	0.7[24]	24
4.	$C_6H_5CH_2CH_2$(pheneridine)	2–3	18, 25, 26
5.	$C_6H_5CH(OH)CH_2$	3.3	18, 27
6.	$C_6H_5(CH_2)_3$	13[22]	22, 27, 28
7.	$C_6H_5(CH_2)_4$ (4-m-HOC_6H_4)	0.9	33
8.	p-$NH_2C_6H_4CH_2CH_2$(anileridine)	3	21, 22, 28, 29a, b
9.	$C_6H_5NHCH_2CH_2$ (Win 13,797)	60	30
10.	$C_6H_5NH(CH_2)_3$ (piminodine)	9	30
11.	$C_6H_5NHCOCH_2CH_2$	5[31]	31
12.	$C_6H_5CH=CHCH_2$	29[22]	22, 27
13.	p-$NH_2C_6H_4CH=CHCH_2$	12[22]	22, 28, 32
14.	p-$CH_3OC_6H_4CH=CHCH_2$ (4-m-HOC_6H_4)	11	33
15.	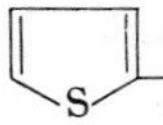 [thiophene]$-CH=CHCH_2(3-\beta-CH_3)$	> 100[34]	34
16.	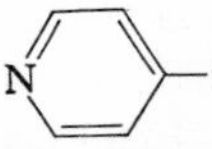 [pyridine]$-CH_2CH_2$	5[22]	22, 35, 36
17.	$C_6H_5COCH_2CH_2$ (R-951)	100	37–40
18.	$C_6H_5CH(OH)CH_2CH_2$ (phenoperidine)	150	27, 40, 41
19.	$CH_3(CH_2)_5$	7[42]	42, 43
20.	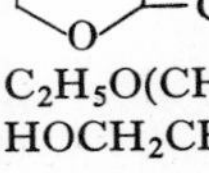 O[morpholine]NCH_2CH_2	2.5	44
21.	$C_6H_5OCH_2CH_2$	9	45
22.	$C_6H_5OCH_2CH(OH)CH_2$	12[47]	46, 47
23.	$C_6H_5CH_2OCH_2CH_2$ (benzethidine)	8	48, 49
24.	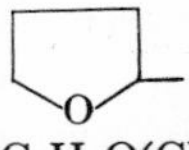 [tetrahydrofuran]$-CH_2OCH_2CH_2$	80	49, 50
25.	$C_2H_5O(CH_2)_4$	20	51, 52
26.	$HOCH_2CH_2OCH_2CH_2$ (etoxeridine)	5[54]	53, 54

[a] Unless otherwise noted by superscript citation of the appropriate reference, the analgetic activity, compared to meperidine, is taken from the Eddy hot-plate data in mice (13,56a,b,c).

[b] The generic names or code numbers in parentheses, except for normeperidine, generally indicate these compounds have shown clinical utility in man.

187

activity of 3-substituted compounds have been carried out with the prodine series (see Section II,B), but the corresponding meperidine analogs have not received as much attention.

Normeperidine (Table I, No. 2) is considerably less active than meperidine and shows no physical dependence capacity in monkeys (56b). 1-Allyl-normeperidine (No. 3) has attracted renewed interest following the increasing importance of N-alkenyl type derivatives of the rigid analgetics (morphine, etc.; see Chapter IV) as antagonists with non-narcotic analgetic activity. The carbomethoxy and carbopropoxy analogs of No. 3 and its quaternary allobromide (57) do not appear to be either analgetics or antagonists (56b). However, the 1-(4-phenylbutyl)derivative (No. 7) exhibited both types of activity in animals (56c).

In the simple N-phenylalkyl series (Table I, Nos. 4 and 6) the 3-phenylpropyl compound proved to be 6–7 times more active than the corresponding phenethyl and 4-phenylbutyl derivatives (27). Recently, the N-(2-cyclohexyl-2-phenylethyl) analog of No. 4 was reported to be as active as meperidine (58). Substitution of the phenethyl side chain with a β-hydroxyl group did not affect the activity markedly but acetylation lowered it somewhat.

The p-aminophenethyl derivative (anileridine; Table I, No. 8) was among the first of the phenalkyl derivatives to be studied in man, and has been introduced for general clinical use. In rats (radiant heat method), anileridine is 11 times more potent than meperidine (22), while in clinical use it is about $2\frac{1}{2}$ times more active. In the p-$NH_2C_6H_4(CH_2)_n$ series, peak activity was obtained with $n = 2$. A variety of compounds with substituents on the phenethyl aromatic ring have been synthesized (27, 29a, b). The 3,4-di-CH_3O, 2-NH_2, 4-NO_2, 4-CH_3CONH and 4-C_2H_5NH compounds exhibited potencies between meperidine and anileridine. Other substituents had activity in the meperidine range.

The isomeric anilinoalkyl derivatives (Table I, Nos. 9 and 10) are somewhat more active than anileridine. Piminodine (No. 10) has also been introduced for general clinical use. Its clinical potency is in the morphine range. Substitution of the aniline ring generally lowered the activity (30) of piminodine. The related $C_6H_5NHCOCH_2CH_2$ derivative (No. 11) was the best of a series of 1-$ArNHCOC_nH_{2n}$ and 1-$ArNHCH_2CH(OH)CH_2$ compounds (31).

1-Cinnamylnormeperidines (Table I, Nos. 12–15) have also exhibited very high activity. Several 3-β-methyl derivatives (Me, Et, iso-Pr esters) of the parent compound (No. 12) have also been synthesized (59).

The $ArCOCH_2CH_2$ compounds (Table I, No. 17) are Mannich bases derived from normeperidine. These and the reduced derivatives, $ArCH(OH)CH_2CH_2$ (No. 18), show the highest potency of all the 4-phenyl-

188

4-carbalkoxy compounds. Janssen *et al.* (*37*) synthesized forty-four $RC_6H_4COCH_2CH_2$ derivatives (of No. 17) with a variety of aromatic substituents. With the exception of the *m*-fluoro derivative, all were significantly less active than the parent compound in which $R = H$. Recently, several alkyl 1-(2-benzoylethyl)-3β-methyl-4-phenylpiperidine-4-carboxylates have also been prepared (*60*). The secondary alcohols (e.g., No. 18) have been acetylated (*40*, *61*) and have also been dehydrated to the cinnamyl compounds (*32*). Phenoperidine ($R = C_6H_5CH(OH)CH_2CH_2$, No. 18) has been resolved (*41*). The (−)-enantiomer is almost twice as potent as the racemate, while the (+)-isomer is about one-half as active as the *dl*-compound. The (−)-isomer has been related to (−)-(*S*)-ethylphenylcarbinol. Thus, the configuration of the side chain can play an important role, perhaps by influencing a stereospecific drug-receptor interaction. Phenacyl (or acetophenone) analogs, $ArCOCH_2$, have been obtained and reduced to the secondary alcohols, $ArCH(OH)CH_2$, converted to esters and ethers (*58*, *62*, *63*). This series is markedly less active than the corresponding propiophenone derivatives (*27*). The butyrophenone compounds, $ArCO(CH_2)_3$, also exhibit reduced activity when compared to the propiophenones (*27*, *39*).

The 1-*n*-hexyl derivative (Table I, No. 19) exhibited the best activity of a group of higher alkyl substituents. The homologs with 3-heptyl, nonyl, 1-heptyl, octyl, and 2-hexyl side chains, showed increasing activity from 2 to 6 times the potency of meperidine (*42*). The decyl compound was inactive.

The 2-morpholinoethyl derivative (Table I, No. 20) was the most active of a series of morpholinoalkyl and thiamorpholinoalkyl compounds (*44*). This led to the synthesis of a variety of oxyalkyl compounds (Nos. 21–26). In general, the highest activity was found in compounds with 2–4 carbon atoms between the basic nitrogen and the ether function. Substitution of the aromatic ring, $ArOCH_2CH_2$ (No. 21), reduced activity. The tetrahydropyranylmethoxy analogs of the very active tetrahydrofurfuryl compound (No. 24) were about 10 times more active than meperidine (*50*).

Except for the 1-(higher alkyl) series (Table I, No. 19), all of the normeperidine derivatives with increased activity have groups with high electron density about 2–4 carbon atoms removed from the nitrogen atom. These observations were used to suggest (*64*) an extension of the analgetic receptor surface described by Beckett and Casy (*1*). On this extended surface there is a sterically oriented grouping which can interact with the high electron density moieties of the N-1 chain. This additional binding site might increase the stability (or rigidity) of the drug-receptor complex and explain the enhanced analgetic potency of the normeperidine derivatives in Table I. This is an interesting postulate. However, the wide latitude of structural

189

changes in the 1-substituent which markedly improve the potency of meperidine suggests that the steric requirements of this portion of the drug-receptor complex may be much less specific than those of the remainder of the molecule. Also, other factors such as absorption, distribution, metabolism, etc. can not be ignored in the over-all explanation of drug action. The difficulty in obtaining significant data for these parameters on a large number of compounds is apparent. However, as more information becomes available, structure-activity correlations can be expected to encompass these factors in addition to the concept of the specific receptor for morphine-like activity.

An interesting meperidine analog is the 3-α-phenyltropane-3-β-carboxylic ester (XIV) synthesized by Bell and Archer (65). It was obtained from 3-α-phenyl-3-β-tropanyl phenyl ketone (XIII) via the oxime and Beckmann rearrangement to the 3-β-carboxylic acid. The conformational

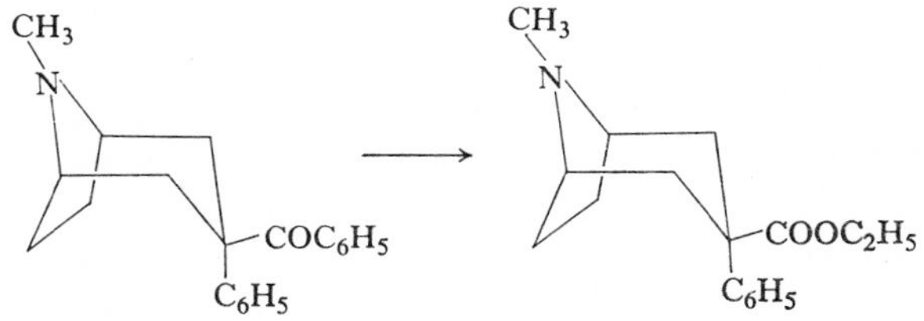

(XIII)   (XIV)

freedom of the piperidine ring is restricted by the 2,6-ethylene bridge and the phenyl group is held in the axial position (like morphine). This compound was slightly more active than meperidine. The norester related to XIV was synthesized by a similar route and groups which led to enhancement of activity in the meperidine series were introduced. However, any change from the N-methyl substituent led to a considerable decrease in activity. The 3-β-phenyl-3-α-tropanyl phenyl ketone isomeric with XIII was obtained in low yield, but the 3-β-phenyl (equatorial) isomer of XIV apparently has not been prepared.

Some meperidine derivatives are of interest because they are poor analgetics but nonetheless show significant physical dependence capacity or addiction liability. Diphenoxylate (XV), developed by Janssen (11 a, b, 66) showed an unusual dissociation of morphine-like effects. It seemed to have no analgetic action in animals or man, but retained to a high degree a morphine-like action on intestinal motility. It was a very effective antidiarrheal agent and also showed antitussive properties. Signs of physical dependence capacity in monkeys and opiate-like effects in man with a definite but mild abstinence syndrome were observed (10). Structurally, this compound is related to both the meperidine and methadone families (see Section III,A). The carbobutoxy analog also showed high physical dependence capacity in monkeys with a very long duration of action (56b).

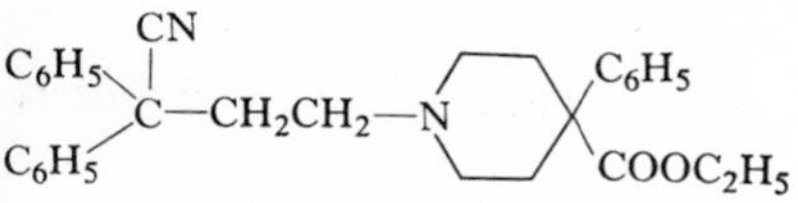

(XV)

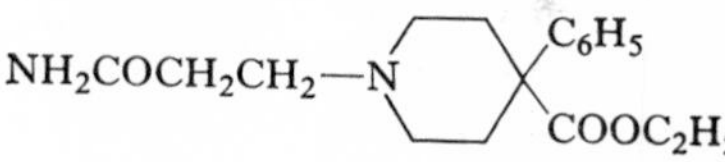

(XVI)

Another compound with the unusual combination of little or no analgetic activity in mice and high physical dependence capacity in monkeys (13) is the 1-(2-carbamylethyl) derivative (XVI). A variety of substituted amides have also been synthesized (67).

The increasing scope and complexity of the groups introduced on the nitrogen of normeperidine is illustrated with XVII and XVIII. The pheno-thiazine derivative (XVII) combines the elements of meperidine with structures known for their tranquilizing activity (68). Anti-hypertensive activity is reported for XVII.

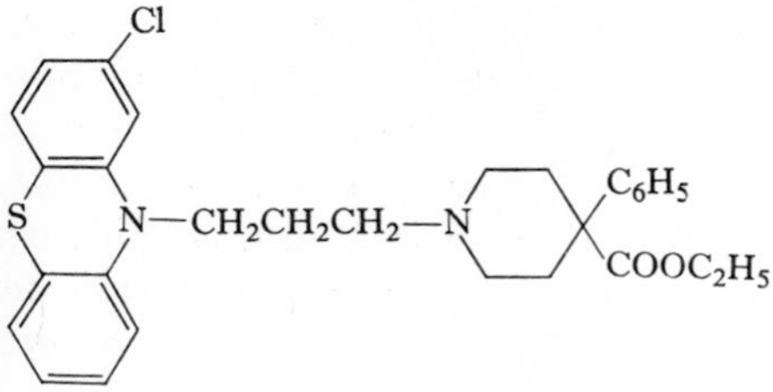

(XVII)

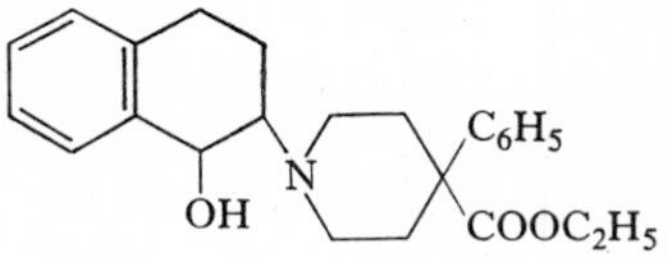

(XVIII)

Tetralin derivatives including XVIII and related compounds from 2-bromoindanes have been obtained by alkylation of normeperidine (69).

4. Distribution and Metabolic Fate

An enormous amount of work has been carried out on biological disposition of the morphine-like analgetics. This area was capably surveyed by Way and Adler (70a, b, c) in 1962. Meperidine has been the subject of several such investigations on biological disposition, but none of the 1-substituted-nor-meperidine derivatives (Table I) except for anileridine, have received similar attention.

The absorption of meperidine and anileridine (and other morphine-like analgetics) is rapid by all routes of administration in animals and man. Peak plasma levels of meperidine are obtained 1–2 hours after oral administration in man. High levels of anileridine are found in rat brain 15 minutes after sub-cutaneous administration. These drugs are widely distributed in various tissues. The liver, kidneys, and lungs are invariably organs in which high concentrations are observed in all species. Concentration in the brain was also found in rats and dogs.

The known metabolic transformations of meperidine (XIX) and anileri-dine (XXV) are summarized in Scheme 3.

Meperidine and the five transformation products shown in Scheme 3(a) have been identified by countercurrent distribution studies on urines of persons receiving the drug. The percentage figures represent that part of the administered dose excreted in human urines during the first 24 hours after administration. They indicate that both meperidine and anileridine are extensively metabolized and relatively small amounts are excreted un-changed. It is of interest that the immediate precursor of the normeperidinic acid (XXIII) is apparently nomeperidine itself (XXII) rather than meperi-dinic acid (XX). The structures of the conjugated forms, XXI and XXIV, have not been established. Anileridine (Scheme 3, *b*) undergoes similar hydrolysis to the 4-piperidinecarboxylic acid (XXVI), but can also undergo acetylation on the aromatic amine function (XXVII). Subsequent acetylation or hydrolysis produces acetylanileridinic acid (XXVIII). It is not evident which route predominates. An additional metabolite of anileridine is an unidentified diazotizable substance which might be acetylamino-phenylacetic acid. The source of this fragment was not established, but it has been suggested that simple N-dealkylation of anileridine to give nor-meperidine may be possible. This would represent an important common route that could be involved in the metabolic fate of most of the potent 1-substituted normeperidine derivatives (Table I).

The metabolic changes indicated in Scheme 3 take place chiefly in the liver. N-Demethylation (or N-dealkylation) may be a particularly significant step in the biological disposition of meperidine and related compounds. This might be accomplished by oxidation of the tertiary amine to the amine oxide, followed by rearrangement to a carbinol, and subsequent hydrolysis giving the nor compound and formaldehyde. Alternately, the N-dealkylation process might involve direct replacement of an alkyl hydrogen by a hydroxyl. Some interesting questions pertaining to the importance of metabolic dealkylation have been raised. N-Demethylation has been viewed as an activation process for analgetic effects and has also been implicated in the development of tolerance on chronic administration.

Beckett *et al.* (*71*), in 1956, postulated that formation of a drug-receptor complex by itself does not produce an analgetic effect, but oxidative dealkyla-tion must first occur on the receptor surface. Release of the N-dealkylated

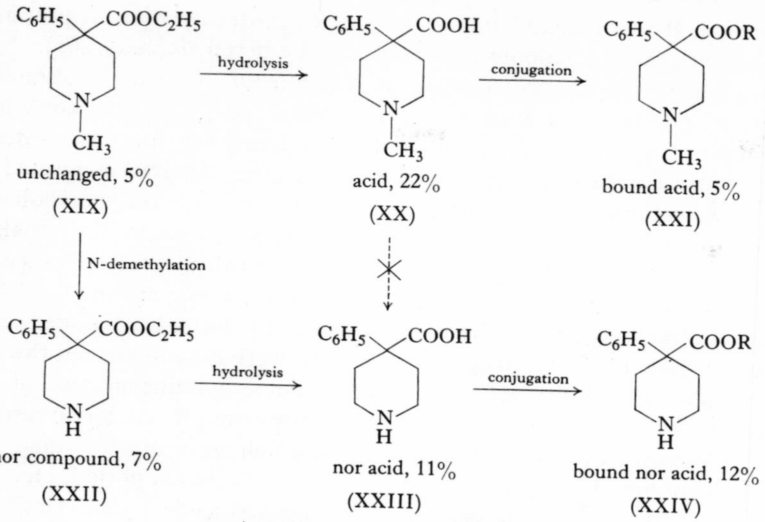
hydrolysis
conjugation
unchanged, 5%
(XIX)
acid, 22%
(XX)
bound acid, 5%
(XXI)
N-demethylation
hydrolysis
conjugation
nor compound, 7%
(XXII)
nor acid, 11%
(XXIII)
bound nor acid, 12%
(XXIV)

(*a*) Metabolic Pathways of Meperidine

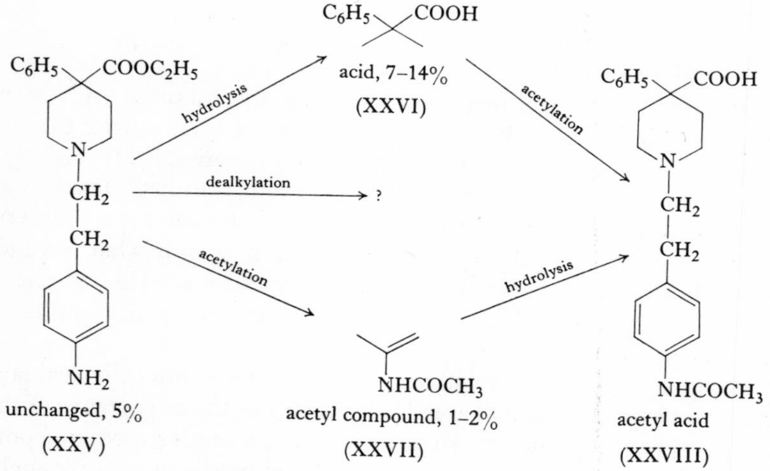
acid, 7–14%
(XXVI)
hydrolysis
acetylation
dealkylation
?
acetylation
hydrolysis
unchanged, 5%
(XXV)
acetyl compound, 1–2%
(XXVII)
acetyl acid
(XXVIII)

(*b*) Metabolic Pathways of Anileridine

Scheme 3

derivative on the receptor surface then produces the analgetic response. This interesting hypothesis only partially explains the wide range of activity observed with 1-substituted-normeperidines and other morphine-type analgetics. It was concluded that the role of N-dealkylation in promoting or limiting analgetic responses remained to be better defined (70b).

Another interesting correlation of the role of N-demethylation with biological effects is the suggestion of Axelrod (72a, b, c) that continuous interaction of the narcotic drugs with demethylating enzymes inactivates the enzyme and leads to the development of tolerance. Axelrod suggested that liver microsomes, which are principally responsible for the metabolism of meperidine and related compounds, could serve as a model for the "analgetic receptor" in the central nervous system. In chronically narcotized rats which had developed tolerance to the analgetic effects of meperidine (and other morphine-like analgetics), the liver microsomes showed a reduced ability to demethylate analgetic drugs. Correlations were noted between the analgetic response and the activity of the N-demethylating system of liver microsomes under a variety of conditions. For example, analgetic response and N-demethylation ability showed parallel changes during antagonism with nalorphine, during recovery in the post-withdrawal period, etc. After considering the variety of evidence relating reduced N-dealkylation by liver microsomes to the development of tolerance, Way and Adler (70b,) concluded the many exceptions cast doubt upon the validity of this correlation.

5. Clinical Utility

As the clinical utility of meperidine was rapidly and universally accepted throughout the world, it became an important reference drug for clinical comparison with all succeeding morphine-like analgetics. Eddy et al. (7) have surveyed the clinical literature on meperidine in complete detail to about 1957. A detailed bibliography of more recent clinical papers describing meperidine is not included in this chapter as it is somewhat beyond the scope of the present survey of synthesis and structure-activity relationships. Generally, recent clinical papers have used meperidine as a standard for judging newer drugs.

A survey of meperidine relatives which have been clinically evaluated in recent years is presented in Table II. It illustrates the importance of the N-phenalkyl substituent that was so prominent in promoting increased potency in animal assays (Table I). In general, the clinical potency parallels the animal potency but may be somewhat reduced in magnitude. For example, phenoperidine $(R = C_6H_5CH(OH)CH_2CH_2)$ is about 150 times as potent as meperidine in the mouse hot plate test (Table I, No. 18) whereas clinically it is perhaps 25–50 times as potent. Clinical potency on a milligram scale is one of the least important properties of the ideal analgetic drug. Whether 1 or 10 or 100 mg of a new drug is required for a satisfactory pain-killing effect is a secondary consideration to the side effects which may be evident at analgetic dose levels. The recognition of worthwhile new drugs, therefore, rests on an improved spectrum of activity versus side effects. This must ultimately be done in man as predictions from animal data do not always carry over without significant changes. The compounds listed in

TABLE II

CLINICAL UTILITY OF 4-CARBALKOXY-4-PHENYLPIPERIDINE ANALGETICS

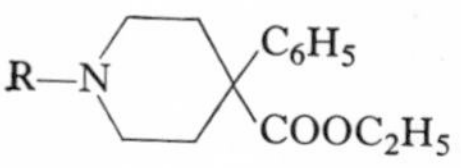

$$R-N \diagup \diagdown \quad \diagup C_6H_5 \diagdown COOC_2H_5$$

Name	Structure (R)	Human Dose, mg.	Remarks	Year	References
Meperidine	CH_3	50–100	Analgetic, sedative, and spasmolytic	1939	7
Properidine	$CH_3[4\text{-}COOCH(CH_3)_2]$	5–10	For pain from muscle spasm	1944	7
Anileridine	$p\text{-}NH_2C_6H_4CH_2CH_2$	10–50	Similar duration as meperidine	1957	7, 73–77
Piminodine	$C_6H_5NH(CH_2)_3$	10–40	Like morphine with less drowsiness	1959	77–89
Pheneridine	$C_6H_5CH_2CH_2$	10–50	Similar duration as meperidine	1961	11a, b
Win-13,741	$3,4\text{-}(CH_3O)_2C_6H_3CH_2CH_2$	20–30	Short acting	1961	85
R-951	$C_6H_5COCH_2CH_2$	0.5–3	Short acting	1961	11a, b
Phenoperidine	$C_6H_5CH(OH)CH_2CH_2$	0.3–2	Short acting	1961	11a, b, 90–92
Etoexeridine	$HOCH_2CH_2OCH_2CH_2$	75	Like meperidine	1961	11a, b
Win-16,516	$(CH_3)_2NCOCH_2CH_2$	10–15	High respiratory depression	1961	85

Table II represent attempts to accomplish these aims. However, they have not provided any particularly significant separation of the potent analgetic action of meperidine from its side effects, including addiction liability, respiratory depression, etc. Anileridine and piminodine are the principal newer compounds from this group which have been introduced for general medical use (in the United States). They are controlled as narcotic analgetics in the same manner as meperidine.

B. 4-ACYLOXY TYPES (PRODINE FAMILY)

The 4-phenyl-4-acyloxypiperidines are "reversed ester" analogs of the meperidine series. This type of compound was first described, in 1943, by Jensen and Ziering (*93*) who found that reversal of the ester function increased analgetic activity. Extensive study of this series of 4-phenylpiperidines by Lee and co-workers (*94*) led to the synthesis of the isomeric derivatives, alphaprodine (XXIX) and betaprodine (XXX). Alphaprodine has been accepted as an effective analgetic drug in general medical use. Many related compounds have been investigated for analgetic action and several have been tried clinically. Alpha- and betaprodine are two diasteroisomeric racemates;

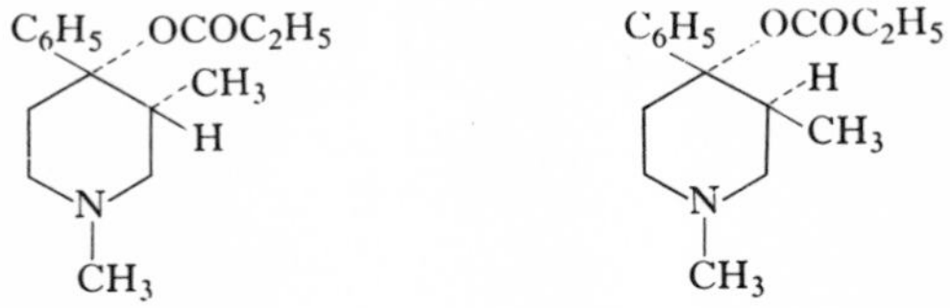

$$\text{(XXIX)} \qquad \text{(XXX)}$$

the α-isomer is the more abundant synthetic product. Alphaprodine is approximately equal to morphine in analgetic potency, and betaprodine is about 3 times more active than morphine.

1. *Synthesis*

The principal synthetic route to the prodine family involves the addition of a phenyllithium derivative (or its equivalent) to a 4-piperidone (XXXI), followed by acylation of the resulting 4-aryl-4-piperidinol (*5, 94, 95*).

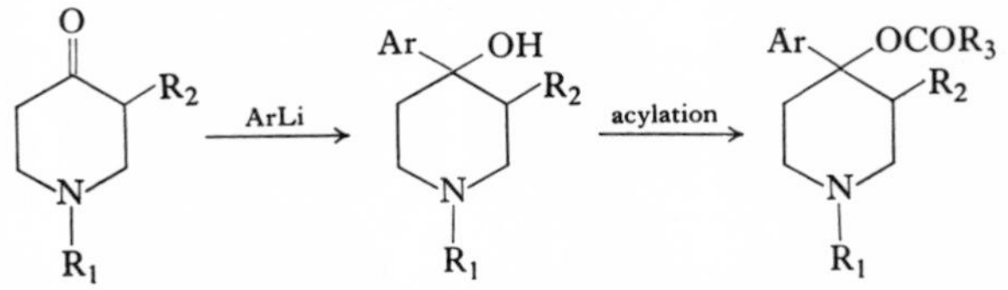

$$\text{(XXXI)} \qquad \text{(XXXII)} \qquad \text{(XXXIII)}$$

Addition of the lithium aryls can produce diasteromeric alcohols if the piperidone (XXXI) has an asymmetric center ($R_2 \neq H$). These α- and β-piperidinols (XXXII) differ in the *cis-trans* relationship of the R_2 (usually alkyl) and Ar groups. The isomers are sometimes separated before acylation, but frequently the mixture is acylated and studied for analgetic activity before the individual compounds are isolated. In some cases, particularly

196

with RArLi intermediates carrying bulky *ortho*-substituents, only one isomer is produced (*95*).

The 4-piperidone (and 4-piperidinol) precursors are obtained by several methods illustrated in Scheme 4. The most common route (*a*) involves a Dieckmann cyclization of an iminodiester (XXXIV) followed by hydrolysis and decarboxylation. This method is versatile, and has been used for piperidones (XXXV) with a variety of R_1 and R_2 groups. A variation (*b*) of this

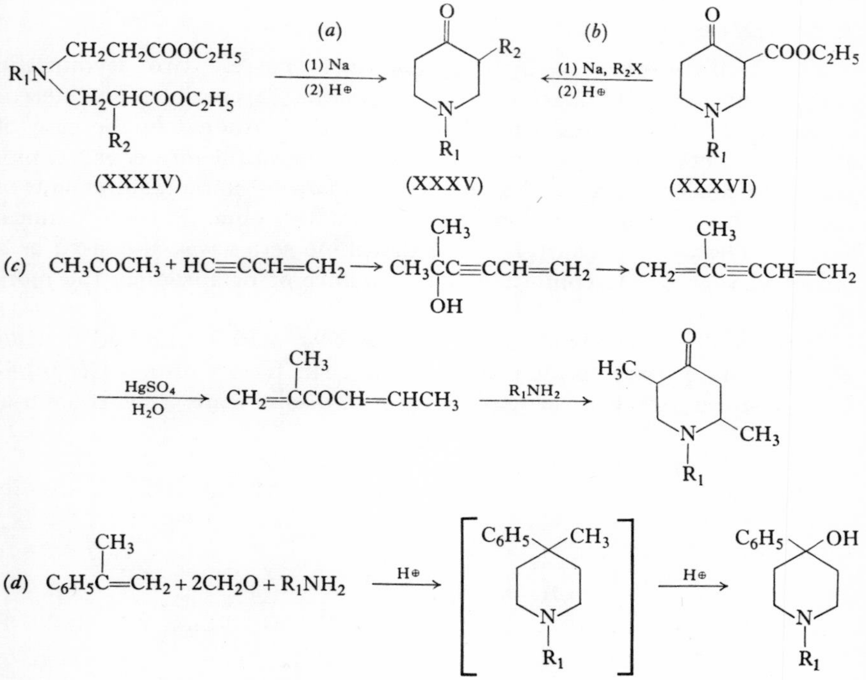

SCHEME 4

route which produces 3-substituent derivatives consists of alkylation of the 3-carbalkoxy-4-piperidone (XXXVI) followed by hydrolysis of the β-keto ester (*96*). Sometimes the 4-piperidone is obtained as the ketal and is liberated by further acid hydrolysis. Sequence (*c*) illustrates another method of forming the piperidone ring and involves the reaction of an amine with a divinylketone (*97a, b, c*). Several variations of this method have also been employed (*97a, b, c*). The 4-phenyl-4-piperidinol synthesis (*d*) of Schmidle and Mansfield (*98*) has been used for prodine intermediates which do not have ring substituents.

197

As was the case in the meperidine series, synthetic efforts on the prodine class in recent years have largely been directed towards the preparation of a variety of N-substituted derivatives. The choice of the R_1 group is frequently determined by the choice of the amine used to prepare the iminodiester intermediates by successive Michael additions to acrylate esters. In other cases, the appropriate R_1 substituent may be obtained by amine substitution reaction on the 1-*H*-4-phenyl-4-piperidinols.

2. *Stereochemistry*

The 3-alkyl-4-phenyl-4-hydroxypiperidines possess two asymmetric centers and thus two diastereomeric racemates are possible. The stereochemistry of these isomers has been extensively studied in the case of alpha- and betaprodine because of the importance of the former as a clinically useful analgetic drug and to further elucidate the steric requirements of the biological receptor site. Conflicting results were obtained from chemical studies. The stereochemistry of the morphine series was also used as a model to suggest the conformational structure of betaprodine, the more potent isomer.

In 1959, X-ray crystallographic studies (*99a, b, c*) established that *dl*-alphaprodine hydrochloride existed in the chair form with a 3-CH$_3$(e)/4-C$_6$H$_5$(e)-*trans*-arrangement (XXXVII) in the solid state. This equatorial

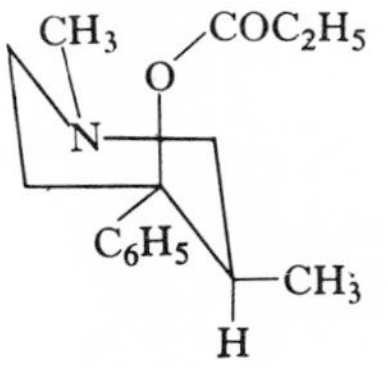

(XXXVII) 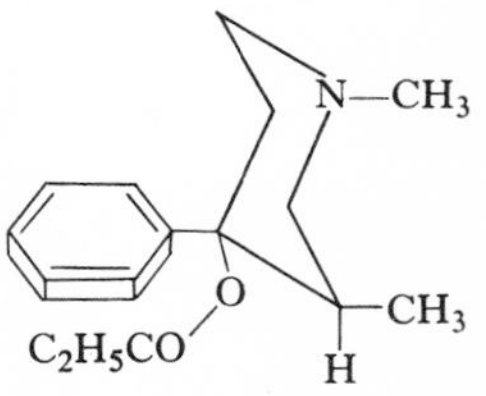   (XXXVIII)

4-phenyl conformation would not appear to satisfy the stereochemical requirements of the postulated morphine receptor. However, the conformational isomer with an axial 4-phenyl group (XXXVIII), obtained by inversion through a boat form, shows considerable similarity to the stereochemical structure of morphine (I). It is well established that the polar, asymmetric environment of an *in vivo* biochemical system can influence the manner in which a substrate (or drug) presents itself to an enzyme surface (or receptor) (*100*). In such an environment the preferred conformation of alphaprodine in solution, or, more specifically, the difference in energy between the conformational isomers, is unknown. However, for a highly substituted molecule like alphaprodine the energy difference between the two conformations may be relatively small.

The X-ray crystallographic study of *dl*-betaprodine hydrobromide, published in 1962 (*101*), established that the solid exists in the chair form with a 3-CH$_3$(a)/4-C$_6$H$_5$(e)-*cis* configuration (XXXIX). Again, the 4-phenyl group assumed the equatorial conformation in the crystal lattice. The

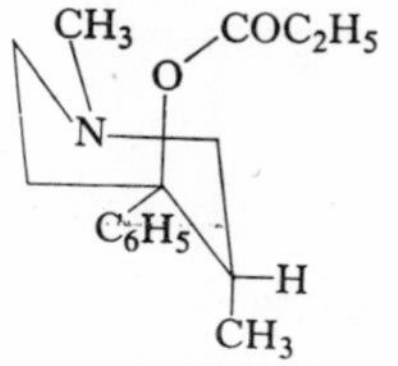

(XXXIX) 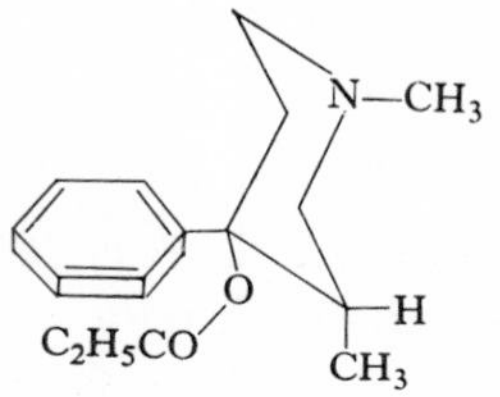   (XL)

opposite conformational isomer of betaprodine which illustrates its similarity with morphine is shown by XL. Comparison of XL with XXXVIII indicates betaprodine is a slightly better configurational replicate of morphine than α-prodine and thus might be expected to be somewhat more active. This relative activity of the α- and β-isomers does not hold for other substituents in the 3-position, however. The 3-ethyl analogs showed little difference in potency between the α- and β-isomers, and in the 3-allyl series the α-compound was considerably more active than its β-isomer (*102*). Thus, correlations of the activity of isomers in the prodine series are not always consistent. However, the configurations of the 3-ethyl, and 3-allyl derivatives have not been established with the certainty of the steric forms of alpha- and betaprodine.

The chemical data concerning the stereochemistry of alpha- and betaprodines was generally consistent with the structures determined by the X-ray studies. Archer (*103*) suggested identical structures after reviewing the chemical evidence. Beckett and co-workers have conducted the most extensive synthetic research in this area. Their work was summarized in 1959 (*104*). They analyzed the stereochemistry of ArLi additions to a 3(e)-CH$_3$-4-piperidone (XLII) and concluded that α-piperidinol (XLIII), formed in larger amount, should result from attack on the 4-ketone from the less hindered side, and the minor product XLI, or β-isomer, by attack from the more hindered side. This led to formulation of the *trans* (CH$_3$/C$_6$H$_5$) configuration for alphaprodine, identical with the X-ray conclusions. However, attack on the ketone from the more hindered side would produce

199

the axial phenyl conformation (XLI) resulting in a *cis* (CH_3/C_6H_5) configuration, and this structure was postulated for betaprodine. When a bulky ArLi intermediate (2,6-dimethylphenyl) was used, only the *trans* configuration was possible according to models, and only one isomer was obtained, in

(XLI)   (XLII)   (XLIII)

almost quantitative yield (*95, 105*). Kinetic studies showed the β-esters hydrolyzed more rapidly than the α-esters. Beckett *et al.* interpreted these results in favor of an equatorial propionoxy group for betaprodine (*104*), in contrast with the axial conformation shown by X-ray studies. Furthermore, reaction of α-prodine alcohol with thionyl chloride was entirely analogous to the facile dehydration of N-methyl-4-phenyl-4-piperidinol by *trans* elimination involving an axial hydroxyl (XLIII). Betaprodine alcohol with thionyl chloride gave a chloro compound in high yield indicating steric hindrance in the dehydration reaction, i.e., the *cis* (4-OH/3-H) configuration (XLI) was less suitable for facile dehydration.

Ziering *et al.* (*102*) had earlier interpreted the infrared spectra of the prodine alcohols to suggest the reverse configurations for alpha- and betaprodine. Beckett and co-workers also found significant differences in the infrared spectra of the two series (*104*). Beckett *et al.* (*95, 105*) have extended the stereochemical studies of the prodine family to compounds with N-phenethyl groups in place of *N*-methyl, and to the compounds with 3-ethyl and 3-propyl groups. They also investigated derivatives in which the 4-phenyl group carried substituents in the *o-*, *m-* and *p-*positions. Ziering *et al.* (*102*) studied the stereochemistry of the 3-ethyl, 3-allyl, and 3-crotyl analogs of alpha- and betaprodine. The results are consistent with the stereochemical considerations just described. Recent studies of prodine type compounds with more than one asymmetric center have generally not included detailed analyses of the stereochemistry.

3. *Structure-Activity Relationships*

Structure-activity correlations for the prodine series are quite similar to the relationships outlined for the meperidine family. For example, propionoxy esters are generally more active than the acetoxy or butyryloxy analogs

200

and substitution on the 4-phenyl ring usually reduces activity. Until the importance of the 1-phenalkyl and 1-heteroalkyl types became known in the meperidine series, the 1-methyl group of alphaprodine was thought to confer optimal activity. Generally, the reversed ester isomers (4-OCOR) were more active than the corresponding meperidine analogs (4-COOR). Introduction of a 3-alkyl group increases the stereochemical complexity of the molecule, and sometimes increases the analgetic potency. Recently, attention has been directed to the synthesis of 1-phenalkyl derivatives both with and without 3-alkyl substituents. In Table III there is presented a representative selection of the more interesting prodine derivatives, generally arranged to emphasize comparison with similar compounds in the meperidine series (Table I).

The influence of 3-substituents on activity is illustrated with compounds 2–6 (Table III). Correlation of the analgetic activity with the α- and β-stereoisomers has already been discussed, noting the lack of consistency between the relative activity of the α- and β-isomers with varied groups in the 3-position. The 3-ethyl derivatives (Nos. 4 and 5) even show markedly different potency ratios when studied in different laboratories. The 3-allyl compound (No. 6) represents the approximate upper limit of the size of 3-alkyl groups with good activity. The 3-crotyl derivative was much less active (102). Patchett and Giarrusso (116) thoroughly investigated the 3-phenyl derivatives related to α- and β-prodine. These compounds may also be considered cyclic analogs of propoxyphene (see Section V). Synthesis of the 3-phenyl-4-acetoxy and 3-phenyl-4-propionoxy derivatives yielded predominantly the α-isomers (7:1) which were separated by chromatography. All of these compounds were inactive as analgetics.

The 1-allyl derivative (Table III, No. 7) demonstrates that substitution of the more flexible analgetics with an N-allyl group does not produce antagonists. Quite the contrary, the compound shows increased analgetic potency and high physical dependence capacity in monkeys (13). A 1-isobutyl-3-H-norprodine derivative was intermediate in activity between meperidine and alphaprodine (13). Compound No. 8 is the best of a group of dimethylpiperidino compounds (2,5-, 2,3-, and 3,5-) studied in Russia. It is known as trimeperidine and has been used clinically. This compound was obtained as a mixture of four geometric isomers among which the α-form was the most active.

Studies of the 1-phenethylnorprodines (Table III, Nos. 9 and 10) have paralleled those of 1-phenalkylnormeperidines (Table I). The stereochemistry and relative activity of Nos. 9 and 10 are similar to that of α- and β-prodine. However, the 1-phenethyl derivatives are more active than the 1-methyl analogs. Compound No. 11 is unusual in that the 4-acetoxy group

TABLE III

1-SUBSTITUTED-4-ACYLOXY-4-PHENYLPIPERIDINES

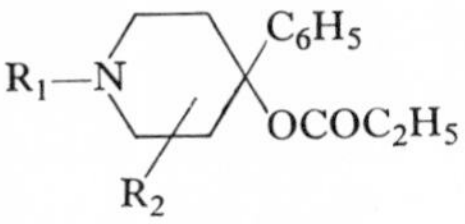

No.	R_1	R_2	Activity[a]	References
	Meperidine		1	
1.	CH_3	H	5–10[93]	93, 106
2.	CH_3	3-CH_3(α-prodine)	5	5, 94
3.	CH_3	3-CH_3(β-prodine)	14	5, 94
4.	CH_3	3-C_2H_5(α-meprodine)	8(5.5[102])	102
5.	CH_3	3-C_2H_5(β-meprodine)	1(6.3[102])	102
6.	CH_3	3-CH_2=$CHCH_2$	12	102
7.	CH_2=$CHCH_2$	3-CH_2=$CHCH_2$	52	13
8.	CH_3	2,5-di-CH_3(α-trimeperidine)	40–50[97]	97a, b, c
9.	$C_6H_5CH_2CH_2$	3-CH_3(α)	23[95]	95, 107
10.	$C_6H_5CH_2CH_2$	3-(CH_3(β)	110[95]	95, 107
11.	$C_6H_5CH_2CH_2$	3-CH_3(4-acetoxy-4-o-tolyl)	65[95]	95
12.	$C_6H_5NHCH_2CH_2$	H	1300[108]	108
13.	$C_6H_5N(CH_3)CH_2CH_2$	3-CH_3	20	107, 109
14.	$C_6H_5CH(OH)CH_2CH_2$	H	3200[108]	108
15.	$C_6H_5CH(OCOC_2H_5)CH_2CH_2$	H	1000(3000[27])	27, 110, 111
16.	O⟩NCH_2CH_2	H	active[112]	112
17.	$F(CH_2)_7$	H	2200[113]	113a, b
18.	$(CH_3)_2N$	H	inactive[114]	114
19.	CH_3O	3-CH_3(β)	1[115]	115

[a] Unless otherwise noted by superscript citation of the appropriate reference, the analgetic activity, compared to meperidine, is taken from the Eddy hot-plate data in mice (13, 56b).

is better than the corresponding 4-propionoxy group and the o-tolyl derivative is more active than the unsubstituted phenyl. Other substituents on the phenyl ring reduced activity (95).

The 2-anilinoethyl derivative (Table III, No. 12) is a direct analog of piminodine (meperidine series, Table I, No. 10) and shows remarkable potency. Since 1-(2-anilinoethyl)-4-phenyl-4-piperidinol has two groups

(O and N) which can be acylated, a special synthesis was developed when selective deacylation proved unsuccessful:

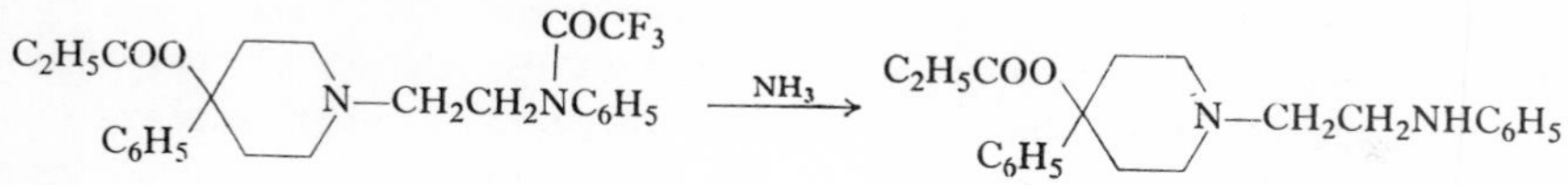

Selective hydrolysis of the trifluoroacetyl group was confirmed by infrared spectra. The propionanilide derivative, $R_1 = C_6H_5N(COC_2H_5)CH_2CH_2$, related to No. 12 (Table III), was about 3 times more active than meperidine (117). This compound may also be considered to be a basic anilide type (see Section VI). The tertiary N-methylanilinoethyl derivative (Table III, No. 13) was prepared by the conventional Dieckmann cyclization with the R_1 group introduced at the beginning of the sequence. The corresponding N-ethylanilinoethyl compound was intermediate in potency between No. 13 and meperidine. Other analogs of the 1-anilinoethylnor-prodines include the $1-C_6H_5SCH_2CH_2$ and $1-C_6H_5SCH_2CH_2$ compounds which were about 3 and 40 times more active than meperidine, respectively (108).

Analogous to the meperidine series, the 1-(3-phenyl-3-propanol) derivatives (Table III, Nos. 14 and 15) are the most potent of the prodine family. The precursor to No. 14, $R_1 = C_6H_5COCH_2CH_2$, had about 1300 times the activity of meperidine (27). The 1-(3-acetoxy-3-phenylpropyl)-4-acetoxy analog of No. 15 was 120 times meperidine (27). These compounds are the most potent of the 4-phenylpiperidine analgetics and are among the most active of all the morphine-like agents.

The fluoroheptyl side chain of compound No. 17 (Table III) represents an interesting variation of the higher alkyl substituents which enhanced potency in the meperidine series. This compound is also very active. Other related compounds with activity claimed in the range of 250 to 1500 times morphine are the 1-(6-nitrohexyl)-, 1-(6-chlorohexyl), 1-(7-fluoroheptyl)-3-methyl-, and 1-(8-fluorooctyl)-4-acetoxy analogs (113a, b).

The 1-dimethylaminonorprodine compound (Table III, No. 18) is an example of a rather extensive group of hydrazine analogs of the 4-phenyl-piperidine analgetics. The carbon isostere of No. 18 is more active than morphine. Since the 1-isopropyl group is about the same size as the 1-dimethylamino function, the inactivity of the hydrazine analogs was attributed to their lowered basicity (ca 3 to 4 pK_a units). The necessity of a cationic amine function in the analgetic molecule at physiological pH which could bind with a specific anionic site on the receptor surface was, thus, further emphasized. The study of hydrazine analogs was extended to include both the α- and β-isomers of 1-dimethylamino-3-methyl-4-phenyl-4-acyloxypiperidines, and to compounds with 2-thienyl, $2,6\text{-}(CH_3)_2C_6H_3$, and $C_6H_5C{\equiv}C$ groups in place of the 4-phenyl group (*114*). None of these compounds was active. A number of 1-alkoxy derivatives have also been studied. Only the 1-methoxy (No. 19) and 1-ethoxy analogs of betaprodine showed activity somewhat equivalent to meperidine when administered orally (rats). They were inactive by the subcutaneous route (*115*). Some difficulty was encountered in the acylation of the 4-piperidinol precursors to compounds Nos. 18 and 19. This was resolved by treating the 4-piperidinols with phenyllithium (or MeLi or MeMgBr) followed by an acyl chloride or anhydride. The stereochemistry of No. 19 was established by relating the α-form of the 4-piperidinol precursor to α-prodine alcohol in a series of synthetic transformations.

The 4-phenyl-4-piperidinols, which are the immediate precursors of the 4-acyloxy compounds illustrated in Table III, have generally been studied as analgetics, and are frequently less active than their acylated derivatives. However, two interesting compounds in this area have widely divergent types of activity. The butyrophenone derivative (XLIV), haloperidol (*118*), is not an analgetic and does not show physical dependence capacity in monkeys (*56c*), but it is a powerful tranquilizer which has found clinical

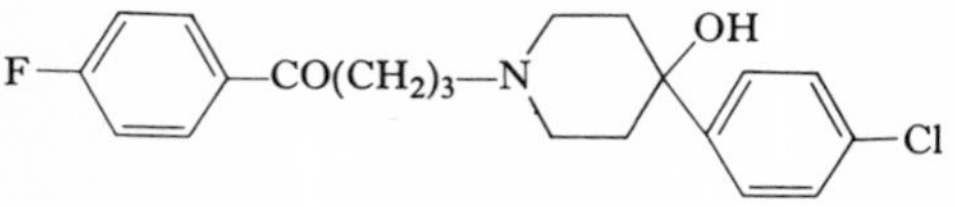

(XLIV) 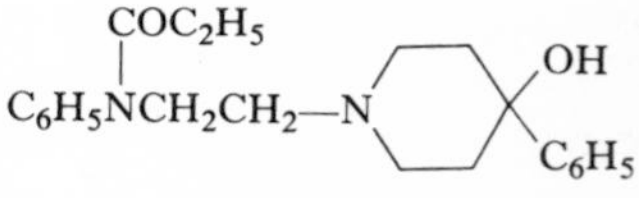   (XLV)

utility. This compound appears to meet the steric requirements of the postulated analgetic receptor, but has potent central nervous system action markedly different from that of the opiates. In contrast, the propionanilide-piperidinol (XLV) has narcotic type analgetic properties [$50 \times$ meperidine (*117*)]. This compound may also be considered a basic anilide type analgetic (see Section VI). It was obtained during an attempted preferential O-acylation to give the anilinoethylnorprodine derivative (Table III, No. 12). Several related derivatives (acetanilide, butyranilide and 3-methyl analogs) also showed good analgetic activity ($5\text{-}30 \times$ meperidine).

4. *Pharmacological and Clinical Evaluation*

The detailed pharmacological evaluation of 4-acyloxy-4-phenylpiperidines of the prodine series has generally paralleled the analogous investigations in the meperidine family. However, relatively few 4-acyloxy derivatives have

204

been selected for extensive study and clinical trial. Randall and Lehmann (*119*) described the pharmacology of alpha- and betaprodines in 1948 and clinical reports on the analgetic activity of alphaprodine appeared about the same time (*7*). Comparative analgetic activity, toxicity, spasmolytic effects, and respiratory effects were reported for a number of related compounds including *dl*-alpha- and *dl*-betaprodine, and the enantiomers of betaprodine (*119*). Virtually all of these compounds show intermediate to high physical dependence capacity in the monkey (*13*). Apparently, quantitative studies on the metabolic disposition of alphaprodine have not been carried out in

TABLE IV

<small>CLINICAL UTILITY OF 4-ACYLOXY-4-PHENYLPIPERIDINE ANALGETICS</small>

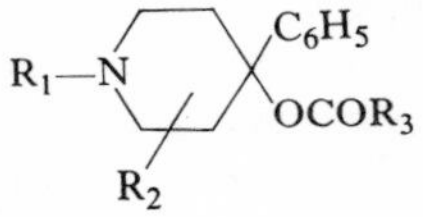

$$R_1-N \diagup \diagdown \diagup \diagdown \begin{smallmatrix} C_6H_5 \\ OCOR_3 \end{smallmatrix}$$

$$R_2$$

Name	Structure (R_1, R_2, R_3)	Human dose (mg.)	Remarks	Year	References
Meperidine		50–100			
Morphine		10			
Alphaprodine	1,3-dimethyl-4-pro-pionoxy-	40–60	Short duration	1948	*7, 120*
Trimeperidine (Promedol)	1,2,5-trimethyl-4-propionoxy-	10–20	Longer duration than meperidine; hypotensive	1955	*7, 9*
Wy-2247	1-phenethyl-3-methyl-4-acetoxy-4-*o*-tolyl-	3–4	Severe respiratory depression	1960	*121*

a manner similar to the detailed studies on meperidine (*70a, b, c*). N-Demethylation and hydrolysis of the 4-propionoxy group would be expected as the principal primary metabolic transformations, by analogy to the metabolism of meperidine.

Relatively few compounds of the prodine class have been investigated in man, and current clinical interest in new derivatives of this family appears to be low. Table IV summarizes several 4-acyloxypiperidines which have been studied clinically. Alphaprodine has been studied extensively and the clinical literature to about 1957 is covered in detail by Eddy *et al.* (*7*). This compound is available for general medical use as a rapid-onset, short-duration analgetic drug. It is, therefore, used for special purposes such as

205

preparation for local anesthesia, for endoscopies, obstetrical analgesia, etc. Its milligram potency in humans is significantly less than that of morphine, but it is approximately equipotent in animals. Alphaprodine is an addicting agent of the same order as meperidine.

The 2,5-dimethyl derivative, trimeperidine (or promedol), was developed in the U.S.S.R. and a stereoisomer, isopromedol, has also been used clinically (7). 1-Phenethyl-3-methyl-4-acetoxy-4-o-tolylpiperidine (or Wy-2247), although unacceptable as a clinical analgetic because it produced severe respiratory depression at analgetic doses, was of interest since it demonstrated a remarkable dissociation of the usual side actions expected of a morphine-like drug. It produced more respiratory depression, but less nausea and vomiting than morphine. These results encouraged Keats and co-workers (121) to reaffirm their opinion that further study of newer chemical types could produce a potent analgetic agent with a more favorable clinical separation of analgetic activity and side actions. This is the aim of all current clinical investigations of new analgetic agents and further emphasizes the importance of quantitative clinical evaluation of side effects which may be difficult or impossible to predict from animal data.

C. HEXAMETHYLENEIMINE TYPES (ETHOHEPTAZINE FAMILY)

With the vigorous development of the meperidine and prodine families of morphine-like analgetics, it was natural that attention was directed to the 7- and 8- membered analogs. In 1953 and 1954, synthesis of the hexamethyleneimine analog of meperidine was described independently by two different laboratories (122, 123). One group found this compound was about one-half as potent as meperidine in mice (124a, b), and its clinical utility in man was reported in 1955 (125a, b); this drug is known as ethoheptazine (XLVI).

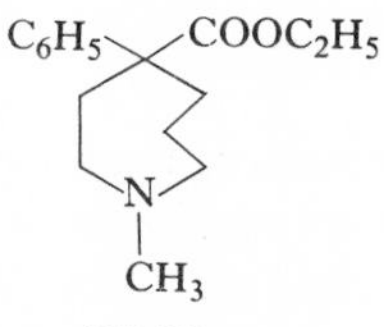

C_6H_5 $COOC_2H_5$

N

CH_3

(XLVI)

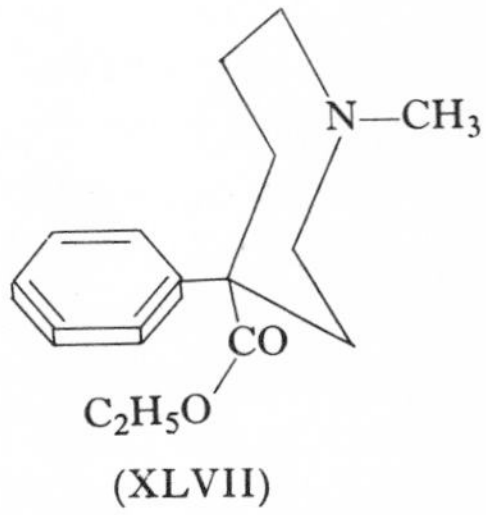

N—CH_3

CO

C_2H_5O

(XLVII)

A conformational representation of ethoheptazine (XLVII) shows that it is another somewhat flexible molecule which can assume a morphine-like configuration and thus interact with a stereospecific "analgetic-receptor."

Ethoheptazine shows activity in the range of codeine or somewhat weaker and is marketed in combination with aspirin (in the United States).

1. Synthesis

Hexamethyleneimine analogs (including ethoheptazine) have been synthesized by methods which are generally analogous to those used for the meperidine and prodine families. Several variations, including methods applicable to the synthesis of 2-, 3-, and 5-methyl derivatives, are outlined in Scheme 5. The principal synthesis (*122, 123, 126*) involves alkylation of 4-dimethylamino-2-phenylbutyronitrile (XLIX) with a trimethylene dihalide followed by ring closure of the resulting 1-dimethylamino-3-phenyl-3-cyano-6-chlorohexane (L). The intermediate, cyclized quaternary salt need not be isolated. The resulting 4-cyano-4-phenylhexamethyleneimine (LI) is converted to the acid by hydrolysis and then esterified to give ethoheptazine and its homologous esters (LII). Treatment of the same 4-methylamino-2-phenylbutyronitrile (XLIX) with crotonaldehyde gave a hexanal derivative (LIII) which was reduced, chlorinated with thionyl chloride, and cyclized to the 5-methyl derivative (LIV). Similar sequences with methacrolein and methyl vinyl ketone gave the 6- and 7-methyl derivatives, respectively (*127*). The 2- and 3-methyl isomers were obtained by a sequence (*b*) commencing with the treatment of phenylacetonitrile with sodium amide and β-dimethylaminoisopropyl chloride (*128a,b*). The mixture of isomeric aminobutyronitriles (LV and LVI), formed by isomerization of the β-dimethylaminoisopropyl chloride through a cyclic immonium chloride, was not separated but treated with $NaNH_2$ and trimethylene chlorobromide as in the synthesis of the demethyl compound (L). Separation of the isomers followed by cyclization gave the 2 (and 3) -methyl-4-cyano-4-phenylhexamethyleneimines (LVII and LVIII). However, detailed proof of structure for these intermediates was not given (*128a, b*). Dieckmann cyclization of the iminodiester derived from LIX, followed by hydrolysis and decarboxylation, gave a 3-methyl-4-ketohexamethyleneimine which was converted to the seven-membered analog (LX) of alphaprodine (*129, 130*). Only one diastereoisomer was formed and was designated the α-derivative. The stereochemistry of other 2-, 3-, 5-, 6-, and 7-methyl derivatives was not investigated. Derivatives with substituents on the aromatic ring were prepared by using substituted phenylacetonitriles (*123*).

2. Structure-Activity Relationships

The study of analgetic activity in the hexamethyleneimine series has been considerably more limited than with the corresponding piperidines (meperidine and prodine families). This is undoubtedly due to the lower activity of

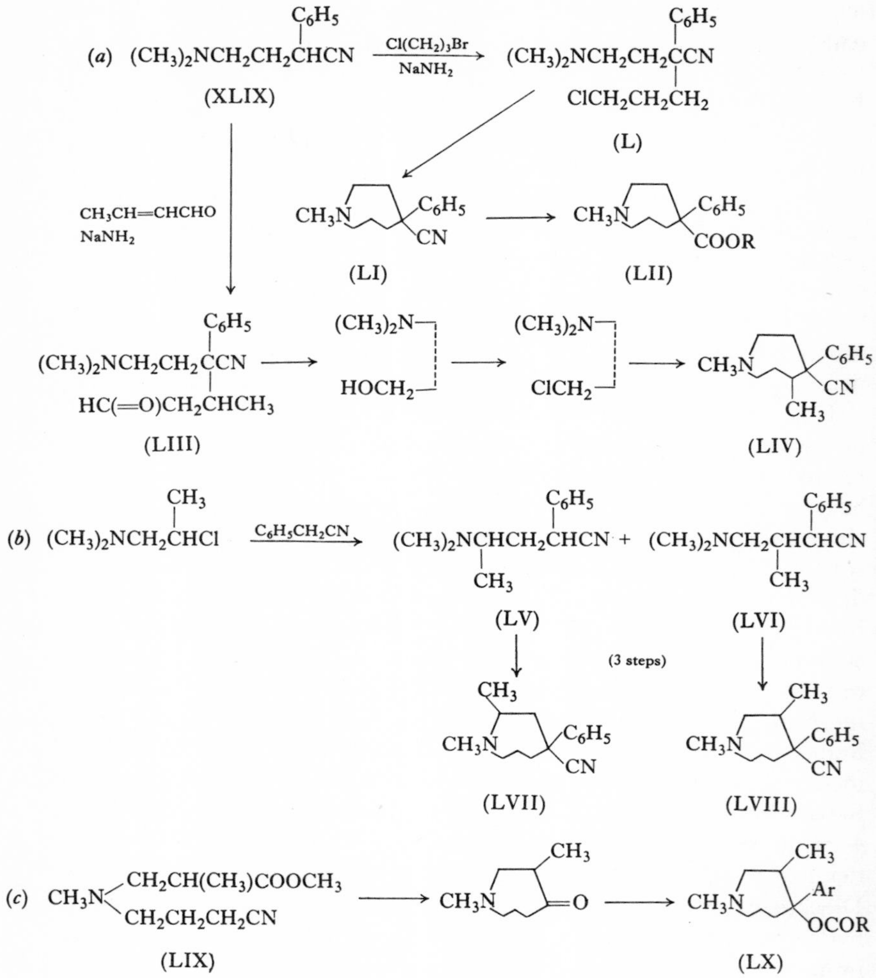

(a) $(CH_3)_2NCH_2CH_2\overset{\underset{\displaystyle C_6H_5}{|}}{C}HCN$ $\xrightarrow[\text{NaNH}_2]{\text{Cl(CH}_2)_3\text{Br}}$ $(CH_3)_2NCH_2CH_2\overset{\underset{\displaystyle ClCH_2CH_2CH_2}{|}}{\overset{\underset{\displaystyle C_6H_5}{|}}{C}}CN$

(XLIX)   (L)

$CH_3CH{=}CHCHO$
$NaNH_2$

(LI)   (LII)

$(CH_3)_2NCH_2CH_2\overset{\underset{\displaystyle HC(=O)CH_2\overset{\underset{\displaystyle CH_3}{|}}{C}H}{|}}{\overset{\underset{\displaystyle }{|}}{\overset{\displaystyle C_6H_5}{C}}}CN \longrightarrow$

(LIII)

(b) $(CH_3)_2NCH_2\overset{\underset{\displaystyle CH_3}{|}}{C}HCl$ $\xrightarrow{C_6H_5CH_2CN}$ $(CH_3)_2NCH\overset{\underset{\displaystyle CH_3}{|}}{C}H_2\overset{\underset{\displaystyle }{|}}{\overset{\displaystyle C_6H_5}{C}}HCN$ + $(CH_3)_2NCH_2\overset{\underset{\displaystyle CH_3}{|}}{C}H\overset{\underset{\displaystyle }{|}}{\overset{\displaystyle C_6H_5}{C}}HCN$

(LV)   (3 steps)   (LVI)

(LVII)   (LVIII)

(c) $CH_3N{<}^{CH_2CH(CH_3)COOCH_3}_{CH_2CH_2CH_2CN}$ $\longrightarrow$ $\longrightarrow$

(LIX)   (LX)

SCHEME 5

the hexamethyleneimines compared to that of their piperidine counterparts. Table V lists several hexamethyleneimine derivatives which have received special attention. Ethoheptazine (Table V, No. 1) is less active than meperidine and codeine by the Eddy hot-plate method in mice (13), and does not show evidence of addiction liability (126). It was found to be more potent but less toxic than codeine in clinical trials (126). On the other hand, Blicke and Tsao (122), who first described ethoheptazine, reported that its analgetic

208

activity in animals was uninteresting because it would be observed only at large, toxic doses.

The 2- and 3-methyl derivatives (Table V, Nos. 2 and 3) were slightly more potent then ethoheptazine in the mouse hot-plate method (*13*). This is

TABLE V

HEXAMETHYLENEIMINE AND PYRROLIDINE ANALOGS

No.	R_1	R_2 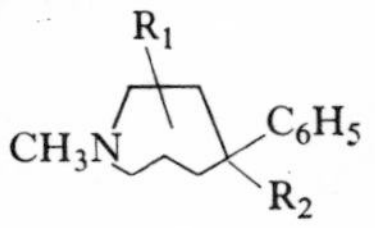	Activity[a]	References

	meperidine		1	
	codeine		0.8	
1.	H (ethoheptazine)	$COOC_2H_5$	0.25	*122, 123, 126*
2.	3-CH_3	$COOC_2H_5$	0.5	*128a, b*
3.	2-CH_3	$COOC_2H_5$	0.4	*128a, b*
4.	3α-CH_3 (proheptazine)	$OCOC_2H_5$ 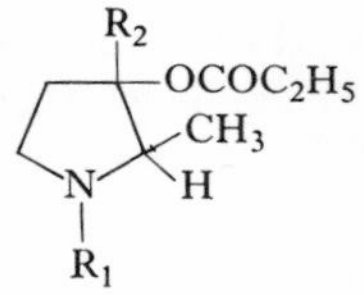	10	*129, 130*

5.	CH_3 (prodilidene)	C_6H_5	0.6	*143, 148a, b, 149, 150*
6.	$CH_2=CHCH_2$	C_6H_5	0.5[143]	*143*
7.	$C_6H_5CH_2CH_2$	C_6H_5	0.3[151]	*151*
8.	p-$NH_2C_6H_4CH_2CH_2$	C_6H_5	1[151]	*151*
9.	$C_6H_5CH(OH)CH_2CH_2$	C_6H_5	0.6[151]	*151*
10.	CH_3	o-$CH_3C_6H_4$	0.2[151]	*151*
11.	CH_3	m-$CH_3OC_6H_4$	none[151]	*151*

[a] Unless otherwise noted by superscript citation of the appropriate reference, the analgetic activity, compared to meperidine, is taken from the Eddy hot-plate data in mice (*13*).

consistent with the improved activity observed upon introduction of the 3-methyl substituent in the prodine series. The 3-methyl derivative of ethoheptazine (No. 2) has been extensively evaluated in animals (*131–133*). It had analgetic activity in rats and monkeys greater than that of codeine or meperidine with few of the side effects of the narcotic analgetics (*132*). The reversed ester derivative, proheptazine (No. 4), showed markedly improved analgetic potency (like the prodine series) compared to the 4-carbethoxy derivatives, and produced high physical dependence in monkeys at high doses (*13*). This indicates that high analgetic potency is possible in the hexamethyleneimine series, but that concomitant addiction liability is also probable. The 4-acetoxy analog of proheptazine has been studied, and it, too, shows high physical dependence capacity (*56a*).

Azacyclooctane analogs of ethoheptazine and proheptazine were synthesized (*134, 135*) but were less interesting as analgetics. 4-Acyl analogs of ethophetazine have also been prepared (*136*). These are derivatives which have a 4-ketone moiety (i.e., propionyl) in place of the 4-carbethoxy group. They are obtained by Grignard addition to the 4-cyano intermediate.

3. *Pharmacological and Clinical Evaluation*

In the hexamethyleneimine series, ethoheptazine is the only compound which has undergone extensive evaluation including clinical investigation. Pharmacological properties were reported by Seifter *et al.* (*124a, b*), in 1954 and the first clinical reports appeared in 1955 (*7*). The absorption and metabolism of ethoheptazine was studied by Walkenstein *et al.* (*137*), and is generally similar to that of the related 4-phenylpiperidine analgetics (*70a, b, c*). This drug is rapidly absorbed, with liver and kidney showing the highest levels of radioactivity 30 minutes after administration of C^{14}-labeled compound. Ethoheptazine is metabolized by at least three routes. Hydrolysis to the corresponding acid (7–8% in dogs and rats) was established by paper chromatography, electrophoresis, and infrared studies. This parallels one of the established pathways for meperidine. Oxidative hydroxylation of the hexamethyleneimine ring (9% in dogs) was demonstrated by isolation of a monohydroxy derivative which was characterized by its elemental analysis and infrared spectrum, but the location of the hydroxyl group was not established. Metabolic hydroxylation on an alicyclic carbon atom has, apparently, not been reported with the 4-phenylpiperidine analgetics. N-Demethylation of ethoheptazine was also suggested, based on a color test for a secondary amine on a paper chromatogram. Very little of the drug was excreted unchanged (2–4% in dogs and rats).

In humans, ethoheptazine is orally effective against moderate pain in doses of 50–100 mg (*7*). The lower dose was preferable for ambulatory patients since prolonged repeated administration of doses averaging 100 mg resulted in cumulative toxicity manifested as central nervous system stimulation. A double-blind study of the clinical effectiveness of ethoheptazine, aspirin, codeine, and various combinations with aspirin indicated ethoheptazine alone or aspirin alone was more effective than placebo. However, addition of aspirin to ethoheptazine or to codeine increased the analgetic effectiveness, and ethoheptazine plus aspirin was as effective as codeine plus aspirin. A combination of 75 mg of ethoheptazine citrate and 325 mg of aspirin has been made available for general clinical use as an orally effective drug for moderate pain. It has given satisfactory results for postpartum pain (*138*). Ethoheptazine (75 mg given three or four times daily) has also been effective in conditions with an inflammatory component (*139*). This drug has shown no physical dependence inducing or sustaining properties in doses up to those which produce toxic reactions. Therapeutic doses for a period of three months followed by withdrawal did not produce symptoms suggestive of physical dependence (*140*). Ethoheptazine is not subjected to narcotics regulations.

The 1,2-dimethyl- and 1,3-dimethyl-4-phenyl-4-carbethoxyhexamethyl-imines (Table V, Nos. 2 and 3) were briefly studied in man and were approximately as active as ethoheptazine (*125a, b*).

D. Pyrrolidine Types (Prodilidene Family)

A pyrrolidine analog (LXI) of meperidine was first described in 1944 but was inactive in analgetic testing (*141*). Other related pyrrolidine derivatives were also inactive (*142*), and research in this field became quiescent for a number of years, in contrast to the extensive exploitation of the 6- (and 7-) membered ring series. However, within a few months during 1961 chemical, pharmacological, and clinical publications (*143–146*) indicated two laboratories were independently evaluating the same pyrrolidine derivative (LXII). This compound is named prodilidine, and is a pyrrolidine analog of alpha-prodine. Clinical evaluation is continuing.

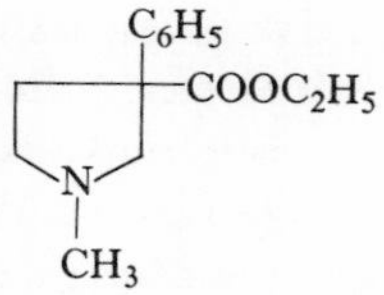

(LXI) 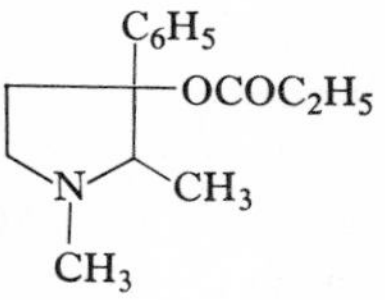   (LXII) 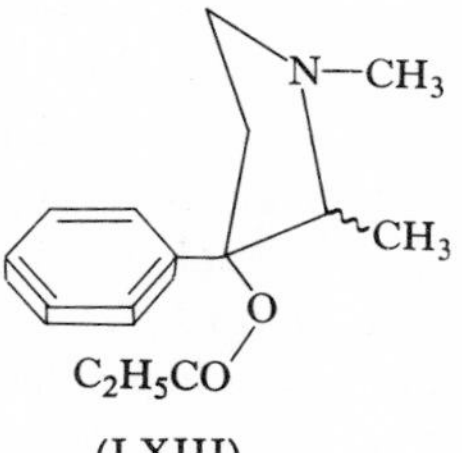   (LXIII)

A conformational representation LXIII shows a certain similarity to the rigid morphine configuration (I) and perhaps some degree of "fit" on a morphine receptor. The preferred conformation of this 1,2,3,3-tetra-substituted pyrrolidine derivative has not been determined and would be difficult to predict. However, a half-chair form has been suggested as the predominant form for pyrrolidine rings (*147*).

1. *Synthesis*

Prodilidine and its relatives have been synthesized by two similar routes (Scheme 6). One of these (*a*) consists of the Dieckmann cyclization of the appropriate iminodicarboxylate diester to a 3-pyrrolidone, followed by addition of an aryl lithium derivative and acylation of the resulting 3-pyrrolidinol (*143*). This route is entirely analogous to the synthesis of alpha- and betaprodine. The iminodicarboxylate diesters were generally obtained from β-aminopropionic esters or nitriles and a substituted α-bromoacetic ester.

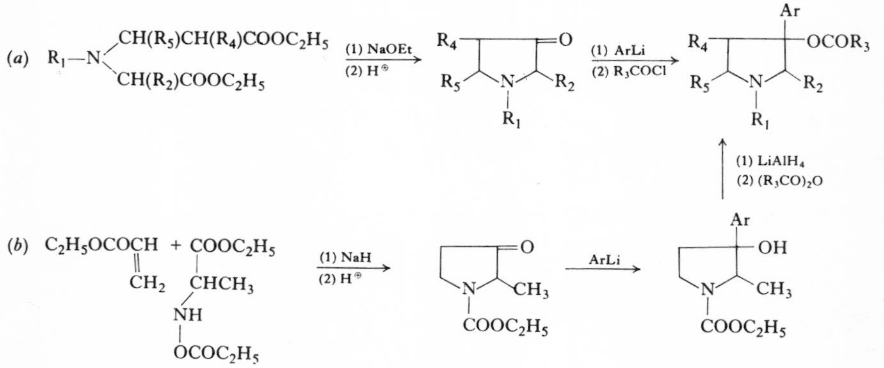

SCHEME 6

Wu and co-workers (*148a, b*) adopted a slightly different approach since early workers had reported that 3-pyrrolidones, produced by Dieckmann cyclization, were unstable. The alternate cyclization sequence (*b*) consists of the reaction between an α,β-unsaturated ester and an *N*-carbethoxy-α-amino acid ester. The resulting 1-carbethoxy-3-pyrrolidone is converted to the corresponding 1-carbethoxy-3-anyl-3-pyrrolidinol and reduced to the *N*-methyl derivative with LiAlH₄ before acylation of the 3-hydroxyl function. Using an *N*-acetyl-α-amino acid ester, a 1-acetyl-3-pyrrolidone was obtained and LiAlH₄ reduction gave the 1-ethylpyrrolidine derivative. When the N-substituent (R_1) is benzyl in the Dieckmann cyclization sequence (*a*), the product could be reductively hydrogenolyzed, and the norprodilidine derivative was available for introduction of a variety of *N*-phenalkyl type substituents (similar to the 1-substituted normeperidines, Table I).

Resolution of prodilidene was effected smoothly by fractional crystallization of the tartrates of the corresponding alcohol (*143*). Investigation of additional stereoisomers of prodilidene, which can potentially exist as two diastereomeric racemates, has not been reported in detail. However, addition of phenylmagnesium bromide to 1,2-dimethyl-3-pyrrolidone yielded 41% of a mixture of hydroxy compounds, from which 3-hydroxy-3-phenyl-1,1,2-

trimethylpyrrolidinium iodide was obtained. In contrast, phenyllithium yielded 76% of the desired prodilidene precursor, 1,2-dimethyl-3-phenyl-3-pyrrolidinol (melting point 83–84°C). With acetone and methyl iodide, this tertiary base gave the identical quaternary salt obtained previously.

2. Structure-Activity Relationships

The recent synthesis and analgetic screening of derivatives in the pyrrolidine series has generally paralleled that of the related meperidine and prodine families. A few of the more interesting pyrrolidine analogs are listed in Table V. Prodilidene (Table V, No. 5) is the principal compound in this series, which has received extensive evaluation in animals and in man. This compound is somewhat less potent than meperidine and codeine using the Eddy hot-plate procedure in mice, and its physical dependence in monkeys is low (13). When the enantiomers of prodilidene are resolved, the (+)-isomer is about 1.4 times the potency of the racemate, while the (−)-isomer is 0.6 as active (146). Derivatives with methyl and ethyl groups in the 2-, 4-, and 5-positions have been studied in some detail (143, 148a, b). The 2-methyl substituent (prodilidene) clearly produces optimal activity, although the 4-methyl and 4-ethyl derivatives are about one-half as active. A 2-phenyl derivative is about one-half as potent as prodilidene. Other analogs are markedly less active or inactive. Variation of the 4-acyloxy function indicates that the propionyloxy group is the best of a homologous series, although the isobutyryloxy derivative is nearly as active as prodilidene. Quaternary methiodides are inactive.

The influence of N-substituents upon activity is illustrated with N-allyl-norprodilidene (Table V, No. 6) and the phenalkyl types (Nos. 7–9.) Relatively comparable activity is maintained with methyl, ethyl, propyl, and allyl groups on the nitrogen. The 1-H derivative, norprodilidene, shows similar potency, but is several times more toxic than the N-methyl compound. A variety of phenalkyl, heteroalkyl, and oxyalkyl substituents have been introduced in the 1-position similar to those used in the meperidine family (Table I) but these changes generally do not improve the activity of prodilidene. The p-aminophenethyl compound (No. 8) is the only derivative with significantly improved activity over the parent compound. The aryl substituted compounds (Nos. 10 and 11) illustrate the general findings that substituents on the 3-phenyl moiety, or its replacement by a 2-pyridyl group, reduce or abolish analgetic activity.

3. Pharmacological and Clinical Evaluation

Prodilidene is the only compound in this series which has received extensive evaluation and clinical investigation. Winder et al. (146) and Kissel and co-workers (*144, 152, 153*) have reported their detailed pharmacological investigations. The action of prodilidene hydrochloride in rodents is fairly prompt and unusually well sustained (like morphine). Its analgetic potency is generally similar to that of codeine sulfate when given orally, but is significantly less potent than codeine when administered by parenteral routes. Prodilidene differs from the aspirin-like agents in exhibiting greater analgetic potency but lacking antipyretic and anti-inflammatory effects. On the other hand, prodilidene differs from other morphine-like drugs in lacking antitussive action, a constipating action, respiratory depression, or significant cardiovascular effects except at high dosage. Its acute toxicity is in the range of codeine. The effects of prodilidene are not antagonized by nalorphine, and this drug does not support morphine physical dependence in monkeys. Hence, it has been assumed that significant capacity for addiction ability in man may be lacking.

When the enantiomers are separated, one isomer (+) is more active than the racemate by the intraperitoneal route while the other is less active, as is true with most optically active analgetic structures. When the enantiomers of prodilidene are administered orally, however, there is a marked reduction in the difference between the (+)- and (−)-isomers. In fact, it appears that the racemate is less potent as an analgetic than either optical isomer administered alone. This is unusual for analgetic enantiomers and racemates and it is difficult to interpret these results in the light of the current concepts of a stereospecific receptor. Winder *et al.* (*146*) suggest a mutual interference between the enantiomers by the gastric route. Another noteworthy point concerning the analgetic potency of enantiomers is the general finding that when a lower potency racemate, such as prodilidene, is resolved, the difference in activity of the enantiomers is much less than that achieved by the resolution of a high potency racemate. Among analgetic compounds with the potency of morphine or greater the activity of the racemate is largely due to the more potent enantiomer.

The absorption and metabolism of prodilidene has been studied by Weikel and La Budde (*154*) and shows certain similarities to the metabolic transformations of other analgetic agents such as meperidine, ethoheptazine, etc. Prodilidene is well absorbed from the gastrointestinal tract, is extensively metabolized and, thus, achieves only relatively low blood levels. It appears to be either more extensively transformed than other agents or the pathways are different. Prior knowledge of the metabolism of related compounds suggests prodilidene could undergo N-demethylation to LXIV, ester hydrolysis, to LXV and ring hydroxylation. These possibilities are illustrated in Scheme 7. However, none of these suspected metabolites (LXIV, LXV, or LXVI) were found in rat urines following oral administration of prodilidene, and only traces of the unchanged drug were detected. A small amount of an unidentified metabolite which could have been a secondary amine was also observed. N-Demethylation of prodilidene to norprodilidene (LXIV) was demonstrated by an *in vitro* drug-metabolizing system composed of the microsomes plus soluble fraction of liver. A comparative study with prodilidene, meperidine, and propoxyphene (see Section V) indicates that all three drugs are demethylated *in vitro* at approximately equal rates. The ($-$)-isomer is demethylated by rat liver microsomes to a greater extent than the ($+$)-isomer which is analgetically more active.

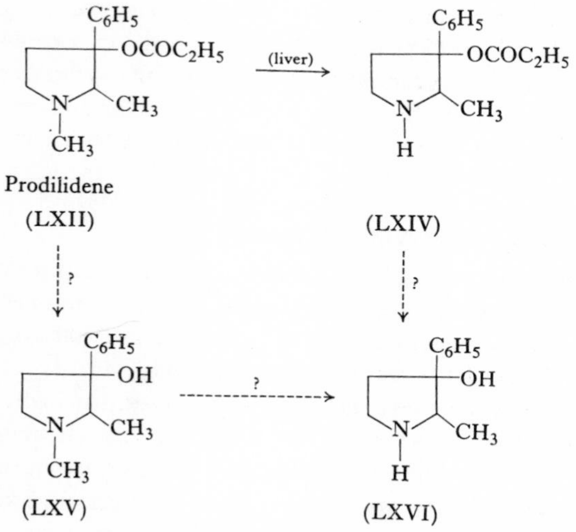

Prodilidene
(LXII)

(LXIV)

(LXV)

(LXVI)

SCHEME 7

Several independent clinical trials have reported that prodilidene is a safe, moderately potent analgetic drug. Cass and Frederik (*145*) reported that 50 mg of prodilidene hydrochloride was better than a placebo and equivalent to 600 mg of aspirin, while 100 mg of prodilidene hydrochloride approached the activity of 30 mg of codeine sulfate. These trials were carried out by a triple blind crossover technique with hospitalized patients suffering from chronic pain caused by miscellaneous diseases. In a later, similar trial by the same investigators (*155*), 100 mg of prodilidene hydrochloride was superior to a placebo but less effective than 600 mg of aspirin, a finding in disagreement with the initial trial. In the second trial, prodilidene was found to be less than half as potent as codeine, milligram for milligram. Splitter (*156*) found that 50–100 mg of prodilidene hydrochloride every 4 hours was about 90% effective in 100 ambulatory patients seen in private practice. Batterman *et al.*

(157) have also reported on the effectiveness of prodilidene hydrochloride, d-propoxyphene hydrochloride and placebo administered orally to more than 200 ambulatory patients with musculoskeletal disorders. Fifty milligrams of prodilidene was 69% effective without eliciting an unusual incidence of side effects. With 75 mg of prodilidene, an increased incidence of side effects decreased the over-all patient acceptance of the drug so that satisfactory pain relief was obtained in only 61% of the patients. Placebo medication was 36% effective under identical conditions. d-Propoxyphene was intermediate in activity between the placebo and prodilidene.

Although the limited clinical experience with prodilidene has not shown any suggestion of physical dependence, the propensity of prodilidene to produce drug addiction is not yet adequately answered. It is apparent, however, that moderate to lower potency morphine-like analgetic (less potent than codeine) drugs generally have significantly less addiction liability than meperidine and morphine or their derivatives with increased analgetic potency.

E. Miscellaneous 4-Phenylpiperidine Types

The high analgetic activity associated with the 4-carbalkoxy- (meperidine series) and 4-acyloxy-4-phenylpiperidines (prodine series) inevitably prompted the synthesis and study of compounds with other groups in the 4-position. These have included ketone, acid, amide, ether, and alkyl analogs, etc. For the synthesis of these derivatives, the same intermediates were generally utilized which were required for the meperidine and prodine series. For example, the 4-cyano-4-phenylpiperidines, key intermediates in the meperidine series, have been converted to keto analogs via the Grignard reaction or have been hydrolyzed to the corresponding acids prior to amide formation. The 4-hydroxy- and 4-acyloxy-4-phenylpiperidines of the prodine series have served as precursors for the corresponding 4-ether analogs.

1. Structure-Activity Relationships

The synthesis and analgetic testing of the miscellaneous 4-substituted 4-phenylpiperidines again parallels that of the meperidine and prodine series. A number of the more interesting compounds are listed in Table VI. The 4-keto analogs have received the most attention and the m-hydroxy-4-propionyl derivative, ketobemidone (Table VI, No. 1), has undergone clinical investigation. It is more active than meperidine and approximately equipotent with alphaprodine and morphine by the Eddy hot-plate procedure. It shows high physical dependence capacity in monkeys (13), and is at least as addicting as morphine in man (7). This compound was first described by Eisleb in 1942, and the initial clinical report appeared in 1946. Since then, a number of clinical papers have appeared (7) and this drug has been used commercially, principally in Europe. The human dose of keto-bemidone is 5 to 10 mg. Thus, its potency is somewhat greater than that of

TABLE VI

MISCELLANEOUS 4-PHENYLPIPERIDINES

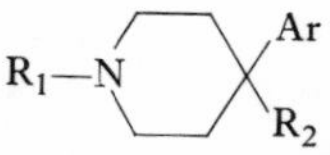

$$R_1-N \diagup \diagdown \begin{array}{c} Ar \\ R_2 \end{array}$$

No.	R_1	R_2	Ar	Activity[a]	References
	Meperidine			1	
4-Ketones					
1.	CH_3(ketobemidone)	COC_2H_5	m-HOC_6H_4	6	5, 158
2.	$C_6H_5(CH_2)_3$	COC_2H_5	m-HOC_6H_4	1	56c
3.	$C_6H_5NHCH_2CH_2$	COC_3H_7	C_6H_5	9[159]	159, 160
4.	$C_6H_5NH(CH_2)_3$	COC_2H_5	C_6H_5	6[159]	159, 160
5.	$C_6H_5CH{=}CHCH_2$	COC_2H_5	m-HOC_6H_4	0.9	56b
6.	$C_6H_5OCH_2CH(OH)CH_2$	COC_3H_7	C_6H_5	1.4	161a, b
4-Amides					
7.	$C_6H_5CO(CH_2)_3$	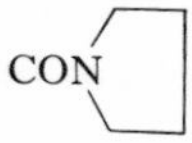 $CON\diagdown$	p-$CH_3C_6H_4$	anti-emetic	165a, b
4-Ethers					
8.	$C_6H_5CH_2CH_2$	OC_2H_5	2-furyl	inactive[167]	166–169
9.	$C_6H_5CH_2CH_2$	$OC_2H_5(3{-}CH_3)$	2-furyl	18	166–169
10.	$C_6H_5CO(CH_2)_3$	OC_2H_5	2-furyl	2[167]	166–169
4-Alkyls					
11.	CH_3	C_3H_7	m-HOC_6H_4	8	171, 172a,b
12.	$C_2H_5OCH_2CH_2$	CH_2OH	C_6H_5	<0.1	173
13.	$C_6H_5CH(C_6H_{13})CH_2$	CH_2OH	C_6H_5	1[58]	58

[a] Unless otherwise noted by superscript citation of the appropriate reference, the analgetic activity, compared to meperidine, is taken from the Eddy hot-plate data in mice (13, 56a,b,c)

morphine and its duration of action is at least as long. Quantitative studies on the disposition of ketobemidone have not been reported (70a, b, c), but it appears to be N-demethylated to the corresponding nor derivative on the basis of paper chromatographic studies on urine.

217

1-Phenalkyl-substituted derivatives have been studied in the ketobemidone series (Table VI, Nos. 2–6) only relatively recently. The *N*-(3-phenylpropyl) analog (No. 2) of ketobemidone is about equal to meperidine in potency (Eddy hot-plate procedure) but has no physical dependence capacity (monkeys) and is not an antagonist (*56c*). This degree of potency combined with the lack of physical dependence capacity is unusual if this compound is truly morphine-like in its action. The N-(anilinoalkyl) derivatives (Nos. 3 and 4) are the best of a series which parallel the 1-(anilinoalkyl)normeperidines which include piminodine (Table I, No. 10). In this series the *N*-anilinoalkyl derivatives with 4-propionyl and 4-butyryl substituents are somewhat more active than the *N*-methyl congeners, but the increased potency is not as marked as that produced by the introduction of this type of substituent in the meperidine series (Table I). The *N*-cinnamyl analog (No. 5) shows reduced activity compared to the parent compound, ketobemidone, just the opposite of the markedly improved activity of *N*-cinnamyl analogs in the meperidine series. *N*-Cinnamylnorketobemidone is about equal to meperidine in potency (Eddy hot-plate), does not support physical dependence in monkeys, and is not an antagonist. This is another example of an unusual combination of good analgetic properties without serious side effects, if this compound is truly a potent analgetic rather than a general central nervous system depressant. The corresponding *N*-cinnamyl-4-(*m*-fluorophenyl) derivative has been studied recently and is one-third to one-half as potent as meperidine and is not an antagonist (*56c*). Elpern has described the analog of No. 5 which lacks the *m*-hydroxyl function (ca. 4 × meperidine) and a number of derivatives with substituents on the aromatic ring of the cinnamyl moiety (*159, 162*).

A variety of *N*-oxyalkyl derivatives related to ketobemidone have also been synthesized. These include the 2-hydroxy-3-phenoxypropyl derivative (Table VI, No. 6), which is somewhat more active than meperidine, but also has high physical dependence capacity (*56a*). This compound is equal to codeine as a cough suppressant. A number of related 2-hydroxy-3-(substituted phenoxy)propyl derivatives have also been synthesized (*161*). The related *N*-(2-phenoxyethyl) derivative (*163*) also has antitussive properties. *N*-(2-Morpholinoethyl)- (*163*) and *N*-tetrahydrofurfuryl- (*163, 164*) derivatives have also been synthesized.

The 4-amide derivative (Table VI, No. 7) is one example of an extensive series developed by Janssen (*165a, b*) and claimed to be antiemetic agents. A variety of substituents on both phenyl rings are included. The amide functions are generally those derived from pyrrolidine and dimethylamine.

The 4-ethers (Table VI, Nos. 8–10) indicate that a piperidine derivative with a 4-ethoxy group in place of the 4-carbethoxy or 4-propionoxy groups and with a 2-furyl group replacing the 4-phenyl ring can exhibit excellent morphine-like activity. Comparison of Nos. 8 and 9 demonstrates that the 3-methyl substituent is necessary for the activity of the latter derivative. These compounds were obtained by an alkyl-oxygen heterolysis of the acetoxy or propionoxy esters of the 4-piperidinol:

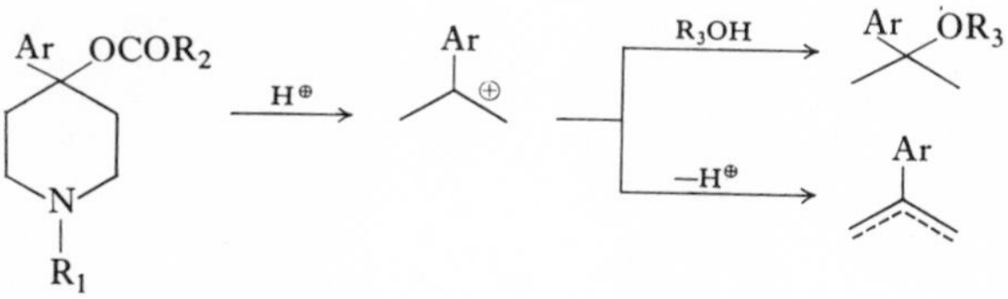

This reaction was considered to proceed via a carbonium ion which could react with an alcohol forming an ether or, by loss of a proton, giving a 3,4 (or 4,5)-olefin (*168*). A variety of alcohols (methanol, ethanol, isopropanol, etc.) were reacted with a number of 4-arylpiperidinol (phenyl, thienyl, pyridyl, etc.) derivatives (*168, 170*). Several N-aroylalkyl derivatives related to the butyrophenone compound No. 10 exhibited about the same analgesic activity as No. 10. These include the propiophenone analog and its derived secondary alcohol, and the 3-methyl derivative of No. 10. The ethyl ethers are superior to the methyl and propyl homologs. It has been suggested that the 4-alkoxy-4-phenylpiperidines may not be as susceptible to metabolic deactivation as the 4-carbethoxy derivatives (meperidine, anileridine, and ethoheptazine) which are hydrolyzed *in vivo* (*166*).

Studies on a series of 4-alkyl-4-phenylpiperidines synthesized by McElvain and Clemens (*171*) indicate that substitution of a nonpolar hydrocarbon residue of the appropriate size (C_3) for the polar, oxygenated function usually found in the 4-position still maintains good morphine-like activity in selected cases. The 4-*m*-hydroxyphenyl-4-propyl compound (Table VI, No. 11) was the best of a series of related derivatives, but exhibited high physical dependence capacity (*13*) along with its high analgetic potency. The *m*-methoxy derivative was less active, just as codeine is less active than morphine, and the 4-phenyl analog exhibited even lower activity. The *m*-hydroxyl was the best of a series of *o*-, *m*-, and *p*-isomers. These compounds were synthesized from ethyl (1-arylalkylidene)cyanoacetates by the sequence overleaf.

The 4-(hydroxyphenyl)piperidines were obtained by demethylation of the corresponding methoxyphenyl compounds with hydrobromic acid.

Compound No. 12 (Table VI) is representative of a group of recently described 4-(1'-hydroxyalkyl)-1-oxyalkyl-4-phenylpiperidines. It is virtually inactive as an analgetic and has no capacity for inducing physical

219

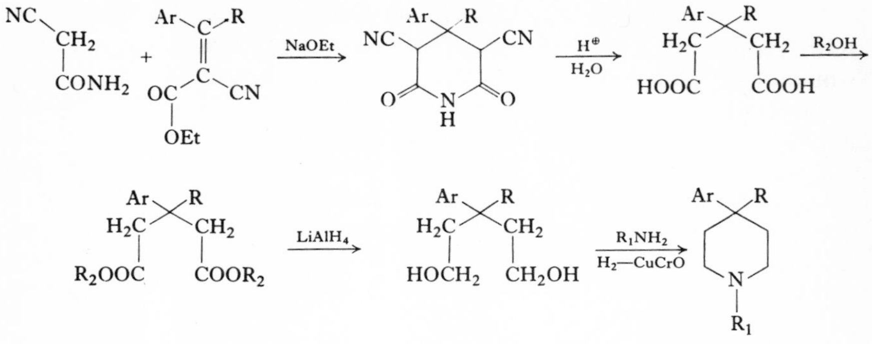

dependence in monkeys. Compound No. 13 is another recently reported 4-hydroxymethyl-4-phenylpiperidine derivative.

Structures LXVII and LXVIII represent compounds in which an additional methylene group has been inserted in a 4-phenylpiperidine structure.

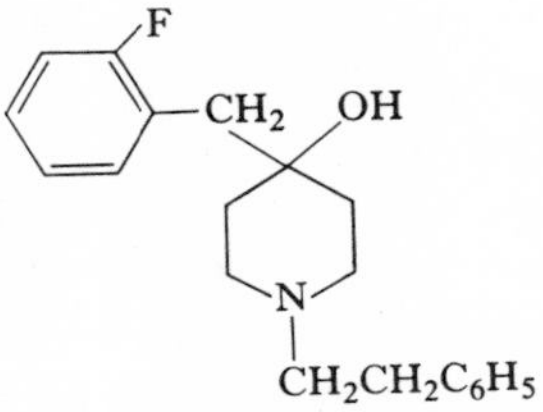

(LXVII)

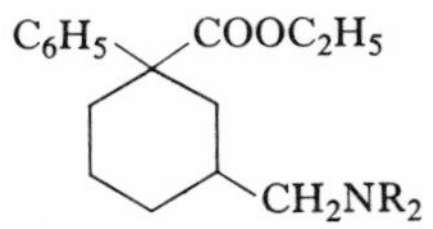

(LXVIII)

The 4-(m-fluorobenzyl)piperidine derivative (LXVII) is the most interesting pharmacological agent in an extensive series of N-substituted 4-fluoro-benzyl-4-piperidinols and their acyl esters synthesized by Harper and Simmonds (174). This compound appears to have analgetic activity by the mouse hot-plate method, but other related testing procedures indicate that the compound is a general central nervous system depressant rather than a true morphine-like analgetic. Thus, a hydrocarbon residue inserted between the central atom and the aromatic ring in the generalized structure postulated for potent morphine-like activity may sufficiently alter the steric fit of the drug with the analgetic receptor to markedly change its pharmacological actions. The aminomethylcyclohexane compound (LXVIII) is one group of a series claimed as antitussive agents (175). This alteration of the tertiary amine function and the alkylene chain might also be expected to affect the fit of the drug and the morphine-like receptor with a resulting modification of the spectrum of activity.

Harper and Fullerton (*176*) studied a series of ethynyl, phenylethynyl, and styryl compounds of the prodine type to determine whether the aromatic ring could be replaced by other groups which were not aromatic, but which also possessed a π-cloud of electrons. Only the 4-phenylethynyl derivative (LXIX) showed pronounced pharmacological activity which was judged to be of a general central nervous depressant type rather than morphine-like activity. The acetyl and propionyl esters of LXIX were uninteresting, and reduction to the *cis*-and *trans*-styryl analogs resulted in a loss of the central nervous effects. These compounds were also reduced to the fully saturated 4-phenethyl derivatives which showed general central nervous system activity, but not morphine-like actions.

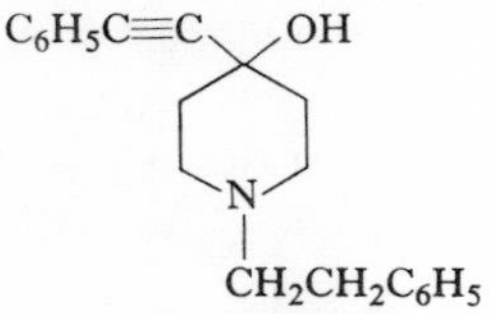

$C_6H_5C{\equiv}C$ OH

$CH_2CH_2C_6H_5$

(LXIX)

$HC{\equiv}CCH_2$ $OCOC_2H_5$

$CH_2CH_2C_6H_5$

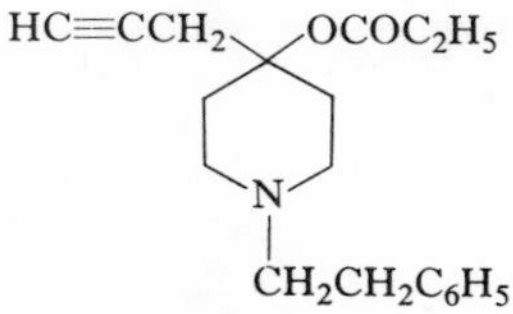

(LXX)

Another compound (LXX) related to the Harper and Fullerton series has recently been evaluated independently by Deltour *et al.* (*177, 178*), as an antitussive (ca. 3 × codeine) agent, and has been assigned the generic name propinetidine. These studies also indicate that LXX does not have true morphine-like actions. From this evidence, it is apparent that the 4-phenyl substituent is necessary for its bonding capacity with the morphine-like analgetic receptor, and can not be replaced by a nonaromatic group which has a π-electron cloud. Nor can the phenyl group be separated from the 4-position by an ethylene, a vinyl, or a ethynyl connective moiety with retention of morphine-like activity.

Other closely related 4-phenylpiperidine derivatives which should be capable of a relatively good steric fit with an analgetic receptor are the meperidine intermediates, LXXI and LXXII. However, these compounds did not exhibit significant analgetic activity by the Eddy hot-plate method,

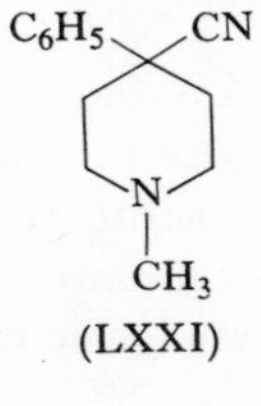

C_6H_5 CN

CH_3

(LXXI)

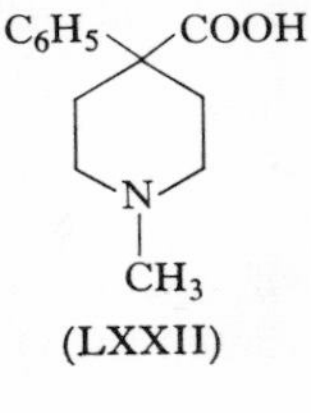

C_6H_5 COOH

CH_3

(LXXII)

C_6H_5 R

CH_3

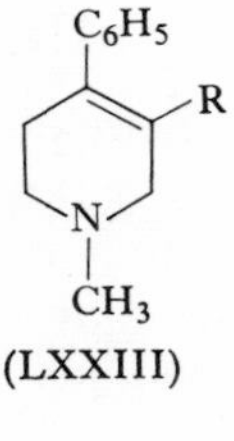

(LXXIII)

221

and showed no physical dependence capacity in monkeys (*13*). The unsaturated compounds (LXXIII), where R is H and methyl, obtained by dehydration of the corresponding prodines, similarly did not possess analgetic activity or physical dependence capacity (*13*). The steric position occupied by a 4-phenyl group attached to the 3,4 double bond is apparently sufficiently altered in these compounds (compared to a saturated 4-phenylpiperidine structure) that a satisfactory drug-receptor complex for morphine-like activity may not be obtained.

Two types of sulfur analogs of the 4-phenylpiperidines should also be mentioned. These include the 4-alkylsulfonyl derivatives (LXXIV) and a meperidine analog in which the basic nitrogen function is replaced by sulfur (LXXV). They were synthesized by methods entirely analogous to those used for the meperidine series (see Section II,A,2). Several of the 4-alkyl-

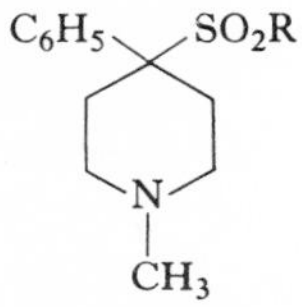

(LXXIV) 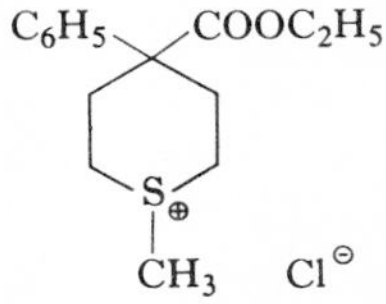   (LXXV)

sulfonyl-4-phenylpiperidines (*179, 180*) showed meperidine-like activity in mice, but the sulfonium analog (*181*) was inactive.

Extensive investigation of the broad class of 4-phenylpiperidines and their congeners has thus yielded an enormous number of compounds for analgetic testing, some impressive increases in analgetic potency, a few clinically accepted drugs, and a great deal of information supporting the concept of a stereospecific drug-receptor complex required for morphine-like analgetic activity. However, the idealized goal of a highly potent, nonaddicting drug without series side effects (such as addiction liability, respiratory depression, etc.) has not been attained, even though significant progress in this direction has been achieved.

III. Diphenylpropylamine Derivatives

The diphenylpropylamine class of synthetic morphine-like analgetics followed the 4-phenylpiperidines as the second major group of synthetic analgetics. Reports from Germany (about 1945) concerning the highly potent morphine-like actions of 6-dimethylamino-4,4-diphenyl-3-heptanone (methadone, LXXVI), initiated the synthesis and analgesic testing of hundreds of related diphenylpropylamine compounds. This general class may be summarized by the formula:

$$\text{Am}-\text{C}_n\text{H}_{2n}-\underset{\underset{\text{Aryl}}{|}}{\overset{\overset{\text{Aryl}}{|}}{\text{C}}}-\text{Z}$$

where Am represents an aliphatic amine moiety, which is usually tertiary, attached to an acyclic alkylene chain, $-\text{C}_n\text{H}_{2n}-$, which is connected to the central quaternary carbon atom. Two aryl groups, principally unsubstituted phenyl, are attached to the central carbon atom, and the fourth substituent, Z, includes a variety of groups such as ketones, alcohols, amides, esters, sulfones, and nitriles. All of the general requirements for morphine-like analgetics may be recognized in this structure with the additional feature that two aryl groups are attached to the central atom instead of one. In all probability, only one of the aryl groups in these diphenylpropylamine derivatives is necessary for the postulated stereospecific complex between the active drug and a morphine-like receptor. However, the second aryl group may provide bulk and electronic effects which allow the remainder of the molecule to more readily assume a morphine-like configuration. Or it simply may provide optimum solubility and other properties for absorption and distribution. The acyclic nature of the diphenylpropylamine analgetics compared to the 4-phenylpiperidines makes for markedly increased conformational flexibility. That a highly flexible aliphatic chain with its associated groups may assume a morphine-like configuration, forming a satisfactory drug-receptor complex leading to potent analgetic activity is attested by the fact that a number of diphenylpropylamine derivatives mimic morphine in many pharmacological actions (allowing for quantitative differences). These include pain-killing power, tolerance, physical dependence and addiction, reduced intestinal motility, and antagonism by nalorphine, etc. The number of structural variations in the diphenylpropylamine class which retain morphine-like actions is sharply limited, compared to the 4-phenylpiperidine class. This is particularly true with respect to substituents on the basic nitrogen atom.

General reviews which include the diphenylpropylamine class as well as other morphine-like synthetic analgetics have been described in Section I. In addition, two reviews specifically restricted to the diphenylpropylamines should be mentioned. Carney (182) has covered the literature through 1952, particularly summarizing the chemistry of methadone and related compounds. New synthetic methods have generally not been introduced since then. Janssen (183) has compiled a massive summary of almost six hundred

223

diphenylpropylamines (to mid-1958), and has tabulated their synthesis and physical properties together with detailed analgetic testing results (including method, animal, route of administration, etc.).

A. Ketone Types (Methadone-Isomethadone Family)

The initial investigations which established the diphenylpropylamine class of synthetic analgetics were conducted in Germany during World War II by Bockmühl, Ehrhart, and Schaumann. These were research activities of I. G. Farbenindustrie in the field of medicinal chemistry, and resulted in the discovery that 6-dimethylamino-4,4-diphenyl-3-heptanone (LXXVI) was a powerful analgetic, 5 to 10 times more potent than meperidine.

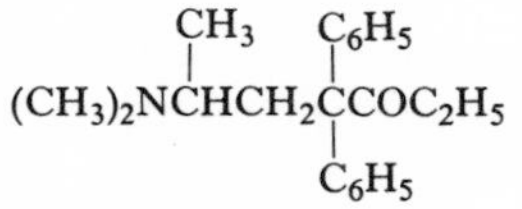

$$(CH_3)_2NCHCH_2CCOC_2H_5$$

$$\overset{\displaystyle CH_3 \quad C_6H_5}{\underset{\displaystyle C_6H_5}{|}}$$

(LXXVI)

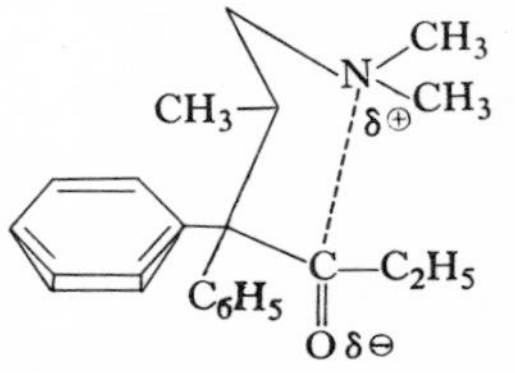

(LXXVII)

This compound, known as methadone (or amidone), has become a clinically accepted narcotic analgetic which is slightly more potent that morphine, and with similar side effects. The report of Kleiderer *et al.* (*184*) of research activities in Germany during the war, describing the synthesis of methadone, led to immediate investigations of related 3-dialkylamino-1,1-diphenylpropyl alkyl ketones in a number of laboratories around the world.

It was some years later that the suggestion was made that methadone could fit the same stereospecific analgetic receptor as morphine (*1*). A conformational representation of methadone is shown by LXXVII, and illustrates one way in which the flexible methadone molecule may approximate the morphine configuration and thereby facilitate its association with the proposed analgetic receptor. Beckett (*185*) suggested that a mutual interaction between the unprotonated amino nitrogen and the carbonyl carbon atom assists in the formation of a favorable conformation. Infrared data, dissociation constants, and chemical data were used to support this type of nitrogen-carbonyl interaction illustrated in LXXVII. Beckett also considered the possibility that intramolecular hydrogen bonding between the protonated amine (at physiological pH) and the carbonyl oxygen function could assist formation of an analgetically favorable conformation, but preferred the fomer type of interaction. It is noteworthy that an intramolecular association between the basic group and an oxygen containing function (or its equivalent)

224

is possible in all of the potent, morphine-like diphenylpropylamine derivatives, which include ketones, ketimines, alcohols, and amides.

1. *Synthesis*

The initial synthesis of methadone is outlined by sequence (*a*) in Scheme 8. It is an equivocal method with respect to the position of the branched methyl group on the alkylene chain (*186*). Treatment of diphenylacetonitrile with sodium amide and 2-chloro-*N*,*N*-dimethylpropylamine, which isomerizes through a cyclic immonium chloride, gave a mixture of isomeric aminonitriles (LXXVIII and LXXIX) in nearly equal amounts. These

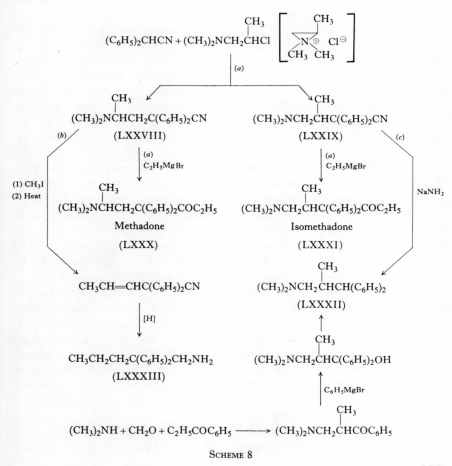

SCHEME 8

225

nitriles were separated by solubility differences and converted to methadone (LXXX) and isomethadone (LXXXI), respectively, by Grignard addition of ethylmagnesium bromide followed by hydrolysis of the resulting ketimines. These structures were established both by degradation and independent synthesis using a variety of methods. Isomethadone, with the branched methyl group adjacent to the central quaternary carbon atom, was only slightly less potent than methadone in animals and in clinical trials (in 1948). Thus, the importance of isomeric forms of the alkylene chain was quickly established, and has been an important factor in subsequent studies of the diphenylpropylamines and other acyclic analgetic compounds.

Two general degradation schemes were used to prove the structure of each of the isomeric nitriles which gave methadone and isomethadone. Sequence (b) in Scheme 8 illustrates degradation of the tertiary amino function of methadonenitrile (LXXVIII) by exhaustive methylation (187). The unsaturated compound was hydrogenated, and the product (LXXXIII) was identical with the amine obtained by hydrogenation of diphenyl-n-propyl-acetonitrile. A similar series of reactions from isomethadonenitrile (LXXIX) gave the amine obtained by hydrogenation of diphenylisopropylacetonitrile. Bockmühl and Ehrhart (186) degraded the nitriles by heating them with sodium amide, replacing the cyano group with hydrogen. This method, for isomethadonenitrile (LXXIX), is illustrated by sequence (c) in Scheme 8. The 2-methyl-3,3-diphenylpropylamine derivative (LXXXII) obtained from isomethadonenitrile was identical with material synthesized independently. Dimethylamine, formaldehyde, and propiophenone gave the Mannich ketone which was converted to the diphenyl tertiary carbinol by a Grignard reaction. Reduction of the corresponding tertiary chloro derivative then gave the authentic propylamine derivative (LXXXII) for comparison. The corresponding degradative removal of the nitrile group from methadonenitrile gave a propylamine derivative which was synthesized by the reductive amination of benzhydrylacetone with dimethylamine.

The hindered nature of the nitrile group in isomethadone-type isomers is evident by the relative stability of the ketimines formed by reaction with ethylmagnesium bromide (188–190). The ketimine precursor to isomethadone is much more resistant to hydrolysis than the isomeric methadone ketimine. Furthermore, isomethadonenitrile (LXXIX) is more resistant both to hydrolysis and to the action of sodamide. The lower reactivity of isomethadone-type nitriles has also been used to suggest the structures of methadone-isomethadone-type isomers before they have been established by degradation or unequivocal synthesis (191).

A variety of related compounds have been obtained by analogous procedures. Alkylation of diphenylacetonitrile with 2-haloethylamines (in place of 2-halopropylamines or 2-haloisopropylamines) produced 4-amino-2,2-diphenylbutyronitrile derivatives which lack the branched-chain methyl groups of methadone and isomethadone, and thus avoid the problem of mixtures of isomers. The variety of amino functions have principally included dimethylamino, morpholino, and piperidino groups, etc. Diphenylacetonitrile derivatives with substituents on the aromatic rings have also been employed. Variations in the alkyl ketone portion of methadone and isomethadone have been obtained by using a variety of alkyl Grignard reagents.

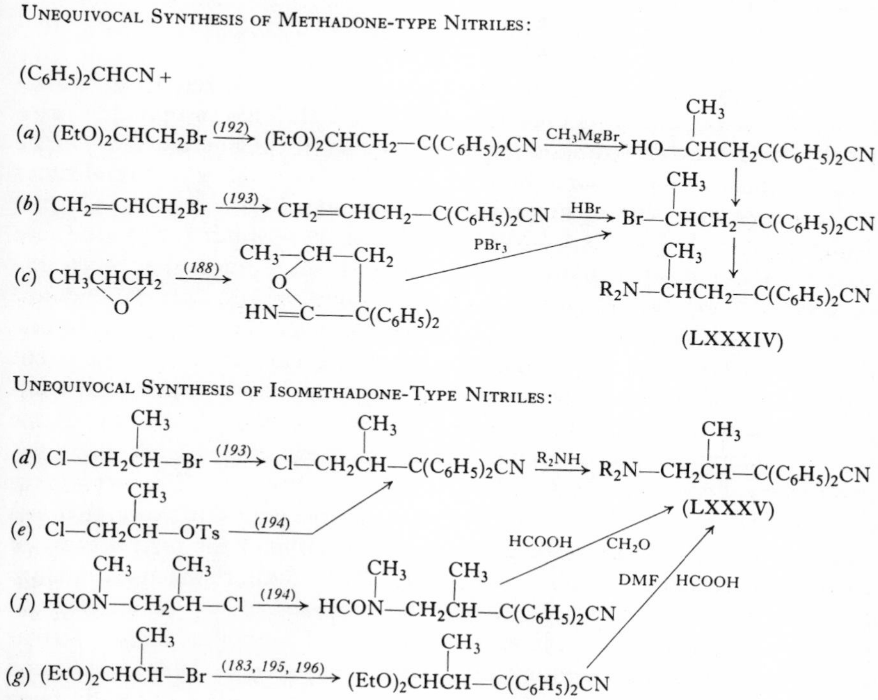

UNEQUIVOCAL SYNTHESIS OF METHADONE-TYPE NITRILES:

$(C_6H_5)_2CHCN +$

(a) $(EtO)_2CHCH_2Br \xrightarrow{(192)} (EtO)_2CHCH_2—C(C_6H_5)_2CN \xrightarrow{CH_3MgBr} HO—\overset{\overset{\displaystyle CH_3}{|}}{C}HCH_2C(C_6H_5)_2CN$

(b) $CH_2=CHCH_2Br \xrightarrow{(193)} CH_2=CHCH_2—C(C_6H_5)_2CN \xrightarrow{HBr} Br—\overset{\overset{\displaystyle CH_3}{|}}{C}HCH_2—C(C_6H_5)_2CN$

(c) $CH_3\overset{\overset{\displaystyle}{}}{C}HCH_2 \underset{O}{\overset{(188)}{\longrightarrow}}$ $\begin{array}{c} CH_3—CH—CH_2 \\ O \quad | \\ HN=C——C(C_6H_5)_2 \end{array} \xrightarrow{PBr_3}$ $R_2N—\overset{\overset{\displaystyle CH_3}{|}}{C}HCH_2—C(C_6H_5)_2CN$

(LXXXIV)

UNEQUIVOCAL SYNTHESIS OF ISOMETHADONE-TYPE NITRILES:

(d) $Cl—CH_2\overset{\overset{\displaystyle CH_3}{|}}{C}H—Br \xrightarrow{(193)} Cl—CH_2\overset{\overset{\displaystyle CH_3}{|}}{C}H—C(C_6H_5)_2CN \xrightarrow{R_2NH} R_2N—CH_2\overset{\overset{\displaystyle CH_3}{|}}{C}H—C(C_6H_5)_2CN$

(LXXXV)

(e) $Cl—CH_2\overset{\overset{\displaystyle CH_3}{|}}{C}H—OTs \xrightarrow{(194)}$

(f) $HCO\overset{\overset{\displaystyle CH_3}{|}}{N}—CH_2\overset{\overset{\displaystyle CH_3}{|}}{C}H—Cl \xrightarrow{(194)} HCO\overset{\overset{\displaystyle CH_3}{|}}{N}—CH_2\overset{\overset{\displaystyle CH_3}{|}}{C}H—C(C_6H_5)_2CN$

(g) $(EtO)_2CH\overset{\overset{\displaystyle CH_3}{|}}{C}H—Br \xrightarrow{(183, 195, 196)} (EtO)_2CH\overset{\overset{\displaystyle CH_3}{|}}{C}H—C(C_6H_5)_2CN$

$\xrightarrow[HCOOH]{CH_2O}$ / $\xrightarrow[HCOOH]{DMF}$

SCHEME 9

A number of unequivocal syntheses of methadone and isomethadone have been developed. Scheme 9 summarizes the synthesis of methadone-type nitriles (LXXXIV) and isomethadone-type nitriles (LXXXV) by methods which do not produce isomers. These nitriles are then converted, by the Grignard reaction, to ketone derivatives corresponding to methadone and isomethadone, respectively. In each case, alkylation of diphenylacetonitrile with a 2-halopropylamine derivative (which can isomerize via a cyclic immonium quaternary salt) is avoided, and the basic amino function is formed as the last step in the synthesis of the appropriate nitrile. In addition, methadonenitrile has been synthesized from 2-methyl-4-cyano-4,4-diphenylbutyric acid by a procedure in which the carboxyl group is transformed to a dimethylamino group by Curtius degradation of the azide to the isocyanate followed by reaction with formaldehyde and formic acid (*197*). This method appears to be less desirable, since it is a multistep procedure from a relatively unusual cyanobutyric acid derivative that itself requires several preparative steps.

2. *Structure-Activity Relationships*

A summary of the more interesting ketone derivatives related to methadone and isomethadone is presented in Table VII. This compilation principally describes those compounds which have shown analgetic activity in the range of methadone or isomethadone. This level of activity is several times more potent than that of meperidine, the standard for comparison in the 4-phenylpiperidine series. *dl*-Methadone (No. 1) is about 5–6 times more potent than meperidine in animals, and is slightly more potent than morphine in these procedures. It produces definite signs of physical dependence capacity in monkeys (*13*), and is addicting in man (*7*). About six ketone derivatives related to methadone have been used clinically. As was evident with the 4-phenylpiperidines, and is equally true in this series, high analgetic potency is paralleled by the usual morphine-like side effects. These include tolerance, intermediate to high physical dependence capacity, respiratory depression, reduced intestinal motility, etc. The structure-activity relationships presented in Table VII represent information that was developed relatively promptly following publication of the high activity of methadone and isomethadone in the late 1940's. Other structural analogs generally show markedly reduced activity compared to methadone and isomethadone, or are inactive. Janssen (*183*) lists 115 individual ketone derivatives (exclusive of salts and optical isomers) prepared by 1958. Continued synthesis of new examples of methadone-like ketones has generally been reported only occasionally in the past 5 to 7 years, in contrast with the vigorous activity in the investigation of new N-substituted 4-phenylpiperidine types.

Methadone and isomethadone were the first synthetic analgetics which possess only one asymmetric center, and separation of the optical isomers was accomplished without difficulty. Analgetic testing of the enantiomers indicated that the morphine-like actions of methadone reside principally in one isomer. The (−)-isomer, or *l*-methadone (Table VII, No. 2), is approximately twice as potent as the racemate and shows intermediate physical

TABLE VII

DIPHENYLPROPYLAMINE DERIVATIVES; KETONES

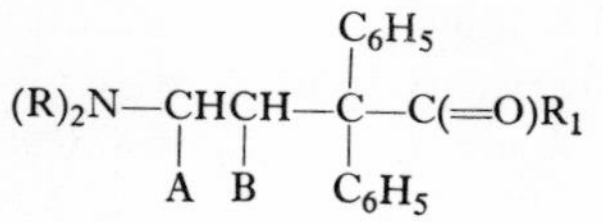

$$(R)_2N-CHCH-\underset{\underset{C_6H_5}{|}}{\overset{\overset{C_6H_5}{|}}{C}}-C(=O)R_1$$
$$\underset{A}{|}\ \underset{B}{|}$$

No.	$(R)_2N$	A	B	$C(=O)R_1$	Activity[a]	References
	Morphine				0.8	
	Meperidine				0.17	
1.	$(CH_3)_2N$	CH_3	H	COC_2H_5 (dl-methadone)	1.0	186–189
2.	$(CH_3)_2N$	CH_3	H	COC_2H_5 (−)	2.0	189, 198–200
3.	$(CH_3)_2N$	CH_3	H	COC_2H_5 (+)	0.07	189, 198–200,
4.	$(CH_3)_2N(O)$	CH_3	H	COC_2H_5 (dl-N-oxide)	0.05	206a, b
5.	$(CH_3)_2N$	H	CH_3	COC_2H_5 (dl-isomethadone)	0.7	186–189, 200
6.	$(CH_3)_2N$	H	H	COC_2H_5 (normethadone)	0.7 (0.4[183])	186, 207, 210
7.	$(C_2H_5)_2N$	CH_3	H	COC_2H_5	0.7[183]	208
8.	$C_5H_{10}N^b$	CH_3	H	COC_2H_5 (dipipanone)	0.9 (1.8[183])	208
9.	$C_5H_{10}N^b$	H	H	COC_2H_5 (Hexalgon)	0.7	186, 207, 210, 211
10.	$C_5H_{10}N^b$	H	H	$COCH(CH_3)_2$	0.2[183]	186
11.	$C_5H_{10}N^b$	H	H	CHO	0.3[183]	186
12.	$OC_4H_8N^c$	CH_3	H	COC_2H_5 (phenadoxone)	1.6 (2.1[183])	186, 193, 211
13.	$OC_4H_8N^c$	H	H	COC_2H_5	0.8[183]	186, 210, 211
14.	$C_4H_8N^d$	CH_3	H	COC_2H_5	0.8[183]	212
15.	$C_9H_{12}N^e$	H	H	$COCH_2CH_2CH_3$	<0.05[183]	183
16.	$OC_4H_8N^c$	H	CH_3	$(C=NCOCH_3)C_2H_5$	0.7[183]	211
17.	$OC_4H_8N^c$	H	CH_3	$C(=NH)C_2H_5$	0.3[183]	193, 211

[a] Unless otherwise noted by superscript citation of the appropriate reference, the analgetic activity, compared to methadone, is taken from the Eddy hot-plate data in mice (13, 56a).

[b] $C_5H_{10}N$ = piperidino.

[c] OC_4H_8N = morpholino.

[d] C_4H_8N = pyrrolidino.

[e] $C_9H_{12}N$ = $C_6H_5CH_2CH_2N(CH_3)$—.

dependence capacity in monkeys (13). The (+)-isomer (No. 3) is virtually inactive and, furthermore, does not suppress the morphine abstinence syndrome in man (13) indicating the addiction liability properties are also associated with the analgetically more active enantiomer. These findings were important factors contributing to the suggestions concerning the stereospecific drug-receptor complex for morphine-like activity proposed by Beckett and Casy in 1954 (1). They also led to the study of the optical isomers of virtually all the important racemic, synthetic analgetics which followed methadone and isomethadone. Resolutions of dl-methadone, dl-isomethadone, and/or dl-methadonenitrile with (+)-tartaric acid (189, 198, 199), ammonium (+)-α-bromocamphor-π-sulfonate (200), and p-nitrobenzoyl-L-glutamic acid (200) were reported in 1947–1949. Optical isomers of the piperidino, pyrrolidino, and morpholino analogs obtained with D-tartaric acid have also been described (201). Janssen (183) has compiled optical rotation data on the enantiomers obtained by the resolution of approximately twenty-five diphenylpropylamine derivatives of all types (to 1958). Additional details concerning the resolution of isomethadonenitrile with (+)-tartaric acid were described in 1959 (202), and differential evaluation of the pharmacodynamic effects of methadone enantiomers has continued in 1963 (203). These results indicated the toxicity of (−)-methadone was 1.3–1.5 times that of the racemate. This was somewhat less than the two-fold increase in analgetic potency.

Beckett and co-workers have related the absolute configuration of (−)-methadone to that of D-(−)-alanine (204, 205). D-Alanine was converted to N-formylalanine and reduction with lithium aluminium hydride afforded the alcohol (LXXXVI). This was formylated and converted to the chloride

$$\underset{\text{HCONHCHCOOH}}{\overset{\overset{\displaystyle CH_3}{|}}{}} \quad \longrightarrow \quad \underset{\text{(LXXXVI)}}{\underset{\text{CH}_3\text{NHCHCH}_2\text{OH}}{\overset{\overset{\displaystyle CH_3}{|}}{}}} \quad \xrightarrow{\text{2 steps}} \quad \underset{\text{(LXXXVII)}}{\underset{\overset{\displaystyle \backslash CH_3}{}}{\overset{\overset{\displaystyle CH_3}{|}}{\text{HCONCHCH}_2\text{Cl}}}}$$

(LXXXVII). Alkylation of diphenylacetonitrile with LXXXVII and transformation to D-(−)-methadonenitrile, the precursor of (−)-methadone, was analogous to the method used by Sletzinger et al. (194) for the preparation of isomethadonenitrile [Scheme 9(f)]. This series of reactions does not involve the asymmetric center. Previous work had also related (−)-methadone (and the (−)-ethyl sulfone analog) to D-alanine, but required the Wolff rearrangement of a diazoketone in which the asymmetric group migrated with complete retention of configuration. The key reaction was the conversion of D-alanine to β-aminobutyric acid without inversion or racemization. This was confirmed by the later work.

Methadone N-oxide (Table VII, No. 4) was much less active than its parent and showed low physical dependence capacity in monkeys (13). Apparently, the dipolar N-oxide moiety inhibits formation of a good drug-receptor complex for morphine-like actions. The importance of isomethadone (No. 5) has already been emphasized in discussing synthetic methods. This compound showed high physical dependence capacity in monkeys, and sustained addiction in man at a somewhat higher dose than morphine (*13*). The derivative without the branched chain methyl group (normethadone, No. 6) was somewhat less active than methadone or isomethadone, particularly by methods other than the hot-plate procedure using mice. This represents approximately the limit of permissible variations in the alkylene chain portion of the molecule for good analgetic activity. The alkylene chain structures of methadone, isomethadone, and normethadone, therefore, represent variations which have been studied in many related compounds, and the analgetic activity generally follows a similar pattern. Optimum activity is frequently found in the methadone-type isomer, and the straight-chain analogs are usually less active (or inactive).

Several variations in the amino function also retain significant analgetic activity. The diethylamino analog (Table VII, No. 7) is somewhat less potent than methadone, and other dialkylamino derivatives are usually markedly less potent. Saturated heterocyclic moieties such as piperidino, morpholino, and pyrrolidino groups have good activity in selected cases. The piperidino analog of methadone (No. 8), known as dipipanone, is one of the few ketone derivatives which is somewhat more potent than methadone, although its relative potency varies with the testing procedure. Variations of the ethyl ketone portion of methadone with higher and lower homologs usually reduces analgetic activity, as illustrated by Nos. 10 and 11. The aldehyde derivative (No. 11) did not support physical dependence in monkeys (*56a*), but appeared to have analgetic potency in animals equivalent to meperidine. Phenadoxone (No. 12) is the morpholino analog of methadone, and is another methadone-like ketone with improved activity (1.5–2.0 times) over the parent compound in several test procedures. The (−)-enantiomer of phenadoxone possessed nearly all of the analgetic activity of the racemate, and has been related to the absolute configuration of (−)-methadone (and hence D-alanine) by a study of molecular rotations in various solvents. (*209*). The pyrrolidino compound (No. 14) also has activity comparable to methadone and isomethadone. Thus, the dimethylamino, diethylamino, piperidino, morpholino, and pyrrolidino moieties represent the limits of variation of the basic group which permit retention of potent, methadone-like activity. Other variations, such as the hexamethyleneimino group, are less active (*183*). A derivative with an *N*-methylphenethylamine basic moiety (No. 15) was inactive. This type of substituent on the 4-phenylpiperidine ring markedly improved the potency of the meperidine and prodine families, and stimulated renewed interest in 4-phenylpiperidines. This, apparently, is not the case in the diphenylpropylamine series.

The ketimine derivatives (Table VII, Nos. 16 and 17) illustrate the

231

findings that a moiety isosteric with the ketone function can provide compounds with meperidine-to-methadone-like potency in a few carefully selected examples. This type of methadone derivative has generally not been evaluated further.

Beckett and co-workers (185, 213) have carried out a detailed study of the dissociation constants of methadone-type compounds, and have discussed the correlation of ionization and other physical properties with analgetic activity. No relation could be shown to exist between analgetic activity and pK_a's which ranged from 6.8 to 9.2 for the more potent compounds. However, minor modifications of the basic group vary the analgetic activity rather markedly at times, and steric factors such as effective width of the basic group were correlated with analgetic activity. It was concluded that the anionic site on the morphine-like receptor had certain dimensions (ca. 6.5×8 Å), and, if the cationic or basic amine portion of the analgetic drug exceeded these, a weaker drug-receptor complex was formed with concomitant reduction in analgetic activity. These conclusions appear to be valid for the several diphenylpropylamine types of analgetic agent, but would appear to require some modification upon consideration of the variety of N-phenethyl and related substituents which markedly improve the analgetic potency of the 4-phenylpiperidines.

Mellett and Woods (13) have discussed additional factors concerning the influence of ionization (pK_a) on analgetic activity. They point out that anionic sites on the analgetic receptor which potentially bind the protonated amino function of the analgetic agent could be carboxyl, sulfhydryl, or phosphoric acid groups ($pK_a \leq 4$). Another factor pertaining to ionization constants and analgetic activity (or many other drug actions) is the rate of penetration of the drug into the brain or across a cell barrier. It is generally recognized that drugs are transported across a cell membrane more readily when in the neutral or un-ionized form (214). Thus, these analgetic compounds as free bases would be favored for transport across one or more cell membranes to the receptor site. The pK_a's then determine that fraction of the drug in a given system (such as blood plasma) which is available in both the protonated or free base forms. Thus, the individual lipid solubility of the un-ionized forms of an analgetic drug is another factor which could affect the facility with which the drug molecules reach the morphine-like receptor. The importance of acid-base equilibria and relative lipid solubilities are obviously not problems unique to the field of analgetic drugs, or even to the methadone-like ketones as a narrow class of morphine-like agents.

Other pH-dependent phenomena have been studied by Mellett and co-workers (215, 216). The binding of various analgetics (not necessarily diphenylpropylamines) to plasma proteins and to brain fractions were

232

measured at a variety of pH's. There was an increase in binding of the individual drugs both to plasma proteins and brain fractions as the pH was increased from 5.5 to about 9.0. With further increases in the pH, the binding remained at 95–100%, except for drugs possessing a free phenolic group which showed decreased binding. These data were interpreted as suggesting the analgetic drugs are preferentially bound in the un-ionized or free base form. The decreased binding of the phenolic compounds at high pH then paralleled the ionization of the phenolic group (pK_a's 9–11). If these systems are useful models for the morphine-like receptor, these data would suggest that the amine function in the analgetic agent may be bound to the complimentary site on the receptor surface as the free base rather than as the protonated form suggested by Beckett and Casy (1). This would represent a relatively minor modification of the structure-activity hypotheses which apply to the morphine-like analgetics covered in this chapter.

Three additional methadone-isomethadone analogs should be mentioned to illustrate the direction of more recent investigations in this field. The pyrrolidine analog (LXXXVIII) was less active than methadone, and the corresponding N-phenethyl compound was inactive (217). These were obtained from the N-substituted 3-pyrrolidinols by conversion to the 3-chloro derivatives and condensation with diphenylacetonitrile, followed by Grignard synthesis of the ketones.

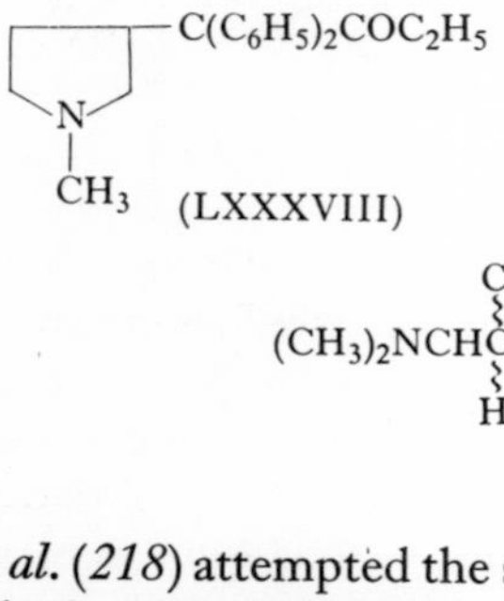

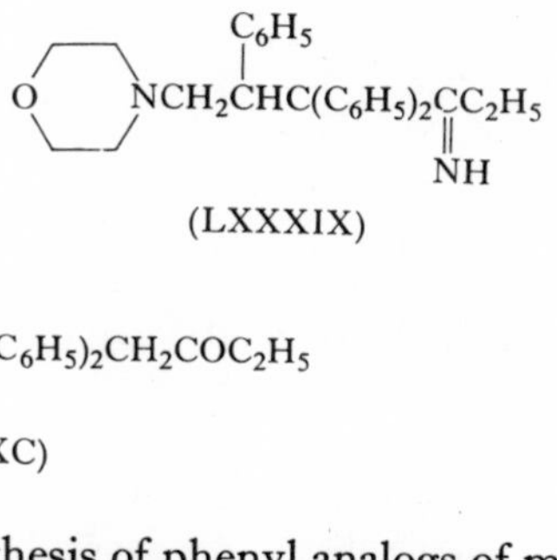

Shapiro et al. (218) attempted the synthesis of phenyl analogs of methadone (or isomethadone) in which the branched-chain methyl group was replaced by an aromatic group. The ketimine derivative (LXXXIX) was the closest these authors came to their goal, as this ketimine was unusually resistant to hydrolysis. This compound was approximately one-fifth as potent as methadone. The position of the branched-chain phenyl group, as related to the isomethadone series, was assigned on the basis of mechanistic analogy rather than degradation or unequivocal synthesis. Patchett and Giarrusso (219) synthesized several homologous methadone derivatives including

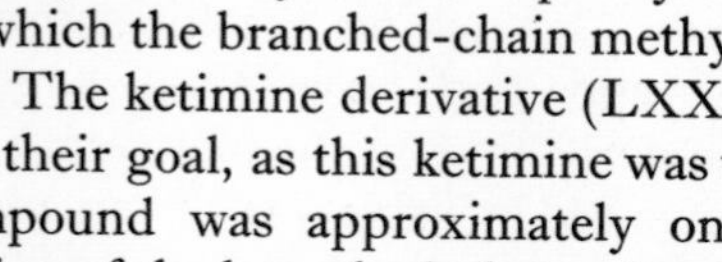

233

(XC). All of the compounds in this series were inactive in the rat tail-flick test. They were obtained by alkylation of 1,1-diphenyl-3-pentanone ethylene ketal with 2-chloro-N,N-dimethylisopropylamine. No attempt was made to identify the methyl isomer isolated.

3. *Pharmacological and Clinical Evaluation*

The detailed pharmacology of methadone, in addition to its analgetic activity, has been intensively studied (*220, 221*) as both the racemate and the optical isomers. More recently, a comparison of toxicities and anesthetic and antiacetylcholine activities of the piperidyl methadone isomers (dipipanone) has been described (*222*).

The biological disposition of methadone has shown similarities with the disposition of other morphine-like analgetics (*70a, b, c*). Absorption of methadone is rapid in the rat with a prompt onset of analgetic action. It is firmly bound to tissue, and organs with high concentrations include the lungs, liver, kidneys, spleen, and adrenal and thyroid glands. Both *in vivo* as well as *in vitro* evidence indicates methadone is rapidly metabolized in man and the rat. N-Demethylation appears to be an important pathway, but unequivocal proof is complicated by the facile conversion of N-demethylmethadone (XCI) to the cyclic compound (XCII). Evidence for both XCI

$$\underset{\text{CH}_3}{\overset{\text{CH}_3}{|}}$$

$$(\text{CH}_3)_2\text{NCHCH}_2\text{C}(\text{C}_6\text{H}_5)_2\text{COC}_2\text{H}_5 \rightarrow \text{CH}_3\text{NHCHCH}_2\text{C}(\text{C}_6\text{H}_5)_2\text{COC}_2\text{H}_5 \rightarrow$$

$$\text{(XCI)}$$

$$\text{(XCII)}$$

and XCII have been obtained in biochemical studies (*70a, b, c*). N-Demethylation represents the principal metabolic pathway which is common to many of the varied types of morphine-like analgetics including the diphenylpropylamines. Less than 10% of methadone is excreted unchanged. Most of the drug is accounted for in the urine and feces as unknown metabolic products. The rate of metabolism and excretion appears to be quite similar for both optical isomers. Detailed studies on the biological disposition of other methadone-like ketones apparently have not been reported.

A number of ketone derivatives in the methadone series have been used clinically. These are reviewed in Table VIII. Methadone was introduced for general clinical use in 1946, and remains the principal ketone derivative of the diphenylpropylamines which is used in man, both as an analgetic drug and an antitussive agent. Its analgetic potency is slightly superior to that of morphine, and is sedative effect is somewhat less. Methadone shows a slower onset of action compared to morphine. Addiction to methadone is of the same order as that to morphine. The analgetic activity and the addiction liability are possessed by the $(-)$-isomer. The $(+)$-isomer is relatively less effective (*223*).

The clinical activity of the additional methadone-like ketones which have been used in man has generally paralleled the animal activity (Table VII),

TABLE VIII

CLINICAL UTILITY OF DIPHENYLPROPYLAMINES; KETONE DERIVATIVES

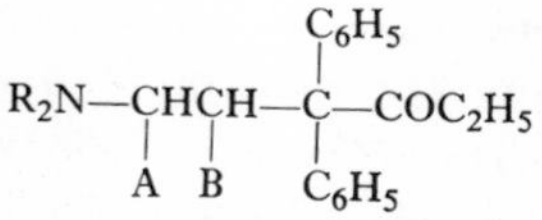

$$R_2N-CHCH-\underset{\underset{C_6H_5}{|}}{\overset{\overset{C_6H_5}{|}}{C}}-COC_2H_5$$

$$\underset{A}{|}\ \underset{B}{|}$$

Name	R_2N	A	B	Human dose (mg)	Remarks	Year	References
Meperidine				50–100			
Morphine				10			
Methadone	$(CH_3)_2N$	CH_3	H	5–15	Slow onset; power-ful antitussive	1946	7
$(-)$-Isomethadone	$(CH_3)_2N$	H	CH_3	10	Like morphine	1948	7
Normethadone	$(CH_3)_2N$	H	H	7.5–50	Antitussive at low doses	1948	7
Phenadoxone	$OC_4H_8N^a$	CH_3	H	10–60	Shorter duration than morphine	1948	7
Dipipanone	$C_5H_{10}N^b$	CH_3	H	20–25	For moderate pain	1956	7, *224, 225*
Orfenso (Hexalgon)	$C_5H_{10}N^b$	H	H	6	Combined with non-narcotics	1962	*183, 226, 227*

[a] OC_4H_8N = morpholino.　　[b] $C_5H_{10}N$ = piperidino.

although dipipanone is less active in man than in animals when compared to methadone. Clinical trials of isomethadone were carried out mainly with the $(-)$-isomer, which possessed practically all of the analgetic activity and was approximately equipotent with *dl*-methadone. Normethadone was less active, and produced frequent side effects at the 50 mg dose required for an analgetic effect in man. It has been used principally as an antitussive agent in the form of a mixture with a sympathomimetic agent (7.5 mg of normethadone orally in solution). Phenadoxone produced a wide divergence in the dose equivalent to 16 mg of morphine in different trials, with more frequent side effects at the higher dose. Dipipanone, or piperidyl methadone, was

235

studied clinically somewhat later than the initial group of methadone-like ketones, and is more effective against moderate pain than against severe pain. More recently, a low dose of the piperidyl analog of normethadone has been studied in a combination with p-hydroxyacetanilide, a pyrazolone, caffeine, and an antispasmodic for oral administration (Orfenso). Thus, methadone remains the principal ketone analog from this family which has gained acceptance as a clinically useful drug.

B. ALCOHOL TYPES (METHADOL FAMILY)

With the rapid development of a variety of diphenylpropylamine analgetics containing the ketone function, it was natural that transformations of this moiety followed promptly. Reduction of methadone gave the secondary alcohol, methadol (XCIII), and subsequent acetylation gave acetylmethadol (XCIV), the prototypes of the diphenylpropylamine alcohol derivatives. The reduction introduces a second asymmetric center, and a study of the analgetic activity of all four optical isomers from two diastereomeric racemates has been an important feature in the investigation of this series. The acetylmethadols are somewhat more potent in animal tests than the parent ketone, methadone, and in part this activity has carried over to human trials. Therefore, a number of the active ketone derivatives in Table VII have been reduced to the corresponding alcohols and converted to acylated derivatives.

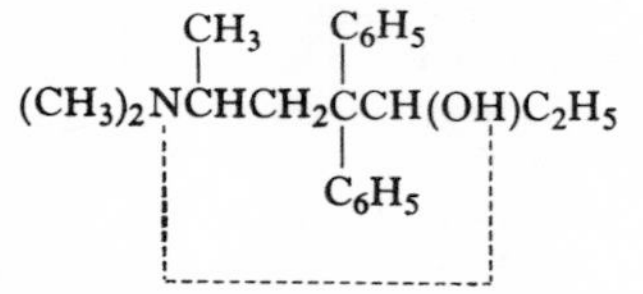

$$(CH_3)_2NCHCH_2CCH(OH)C_2H_5 \qquad (CH_3)_2NCHCH_2CCH(OCOCH_3)C_2H_5$$

with CH_3 and C_6H_5 groups on the central chain and C_6H_5 below

(XCIII) 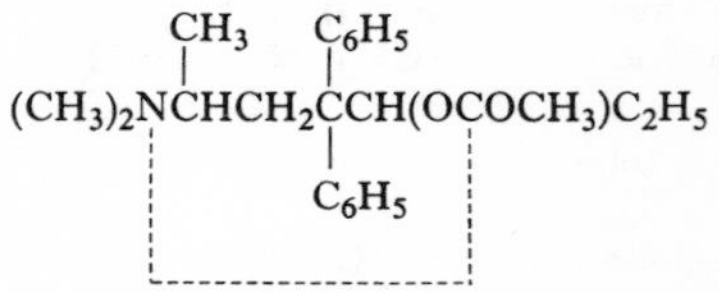   (XCIV)

The dotted lines in structures XCIII and XCIV illustrate potential mutual interactions between the basic group and the oxygen-containing functions which may contribute to the formation of an analgetically favorable conformation approximating the morphine configuration. Thus, the methadols are, apparently, capable of forming the stereospecific morphine-like drug-receptor complex postulated for potent narcotic actions. Intramolecular hydrogen bonding in the alcohols or nitrogen-carbonyl interactions in the esters may provide a cyclic conformation in the same manner as discussed in detail by Beckett (185) for the ketone derivatives.

1. Synthesis

Synthesis of the methadols and their acylated derivatives has been generally straight forward from the preparative viewpoint, but complicated by the isolation, under the appropriate conditions, of all four possible optical isomers from two racemates. This detailed investigation of optical isomers has been carried out only on alcohols and acetyl derivatives derived from methadone and isomethadone.

The facility with which the ketone function is reduced is directly related to the nature of substituents on the alkylene chain. Compounds with the ethylene chain without a branched methyl group, as in normethadone (Table VII) are reduced with relative ease. The methadone-type ketones, with the branched methyl group adjacent to the basic nitrogen, are somewhat resistant to reduction. The isomethadone types, with the branched methyl group adjacent to the central quaternary carbon, are more resistant. This behavior parallels the relative reactivity of methadonenitrile and isomethadonenitrile, and the resistance to hydrolysis of the ketimine precursor to isomethadone.

The reductions of normethadone, methadone, and isomethadone are summarized in part in Scheme 10. The unbranched ketone, normethadone, was readily reduced in ethanol with hydrogen and a nickel catalyst, but this procedure failed to reduce the branched ketones, methadone or isomethadone (186). Aluminium isopropoxide in boiling toluene, also reduced nor-

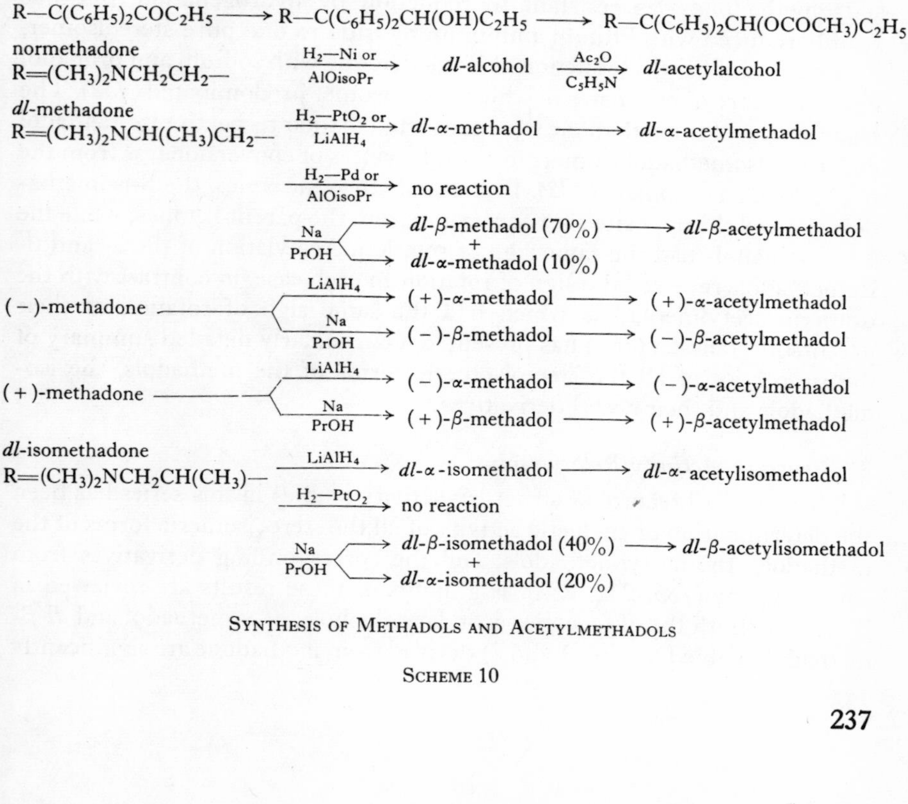

$$R—C(C_6H_5)_2COC_2H_5 \longrightarrow R—C(C_6H_5)_2CH(OH)C_2H_5 \longrightarrow R—C(C_6H_5)_2CH(OCOCH_3)C_2H_5$$

normethadone
$R = (CH_3)_2NCH_2CH_2—$ $\xrightarrow[\text{AlOisoPr}]{\text{H}_2\text{—Ni or}}$ dl-alcohol $\xrightarrow[\text{C}_5\text{H}_5\text{N}]{\text{Ac}_2\text{O}}$ dl-acetylalcohol

dl-methadone
$R = (CH_3)_2NCH(CH_3)CH_2—$ $\xrightarrow[\text{LiAlH}_4]{\text{H}_2\text{—PtO}_2 \text{ or}}$ dl-α-methadol $\longrightarrow$ dl-α-acetylmethadol

$\xrightarrow[\text{AlOisoPr}]{\text{H}_2\text{—Pd or}}$ no reaction

$\xrightarrow[\text{PrOH}]{\text{Na}}$ dl-β-methadol (70%) $\longrightarrow$ dl-β-acetylmethadol
+
dl-α-methadol (10%)

(−)-methadone $\xrightarrow{\text{LiAlH}_4}$ (+)-α-methadol $\longrightarrow$ (+)-α-acetylmethadol

$\xrightarrow[\text{PrOH}]{\text{Na}}$ (−)-β-methadol $\longrightarrow$ (−)-β-acetylmethadol

(+)-methadone $\xrightarrow{\text{LiAlH}_4}$ (−)-α-methadol $\longrightarrow$ (−)-α-acetylmethadol

$\xrightarrow[\text{PrOH}]{\text{Na}}$ (+)-β-methadol $\longrightarrow$ (+)-β-acetylmethadol

dl-isomethadone
$R = (CH_3)_2NCH_2CH(CH_3)—$ $\xrightarrow{\text{LiAlH}_4}$ dl-α-isomethadol $\longrightarrow$ dl-α-acetylisomethadol

$\xrightarrow{\text{H}_2\text{—PtO}_2}$ no reaction

$\xrightarrow[\text{PrOH}]{\text{Na}}$ dl-β-isomethadol (40%) $\longrightarrow$ dl-β-acetylisomethadol
+
dl-α-isomethadol (20%)

Synthesis of Methadols and Acetylmethadols

Scheme 10

methadone (*228*), and did not affect methadone (*229*). Methadone was more resistant to reduction, but was readily converted to methadol by the use of hydrogen and Adams platinum oxide (*211, 229*). A palladium catalyst was unsuccessful. Only one isomer of methadol was obtained by catalytic reduction. It is the same isomer as obtained, in virtually quantitative yield, by reduction with lithium aluminium hydride (*211, 230*). This isomer has been designated as the α-racemate, and this convention has been followed with other methadol analogs. Branched ketone derivatives reduced with lithium aluminium hydride gave only the stereoisomer, designated as the α-form. In order to obtain the β-isomers of methadol, reduction of *dl*-methadone with sodium and propanol was carried out, and the predominant product was the β-methadol racemate (65–70%) together with a minor amount of the α-racemate (*186, 231*). Subsequently, the predominant isomer from sodium and alcohol reductions of related ketone derivatives has similarly been designated as the β-isomer.

The conversion of the enantiomers of methadone to the appropriate methadol and acetylmethadol isomers is also outlined in Scheme 10. The α-methadols and α-acetylmethadols showed the opposite rotation from the parent ketones, while the β-series showed the same sign of rotation.

Isomethadone was resistant to reduction by hydrogenation, but was readily reduced with lithium aluminum hydride to one pure stereoisomer, α-isomethadol (*229*). Reduction of isomethadone with sodium and propanol gave a mixture of racemates in which the β-isomer predominated (*232*). The enantiomers of isomethadone were converted to their respective isomethadol and acetylisomethadol isomers in a similar series of conversions, as from the methadone enantiomers (*232*). In the isomethadone series, the β-isomethadols showed the opposite sign of rotation from the parent ketones, while the α-isomethadols had the same sign of rotation. Acetylation of the α- and β-isomethadols reversed the sign of rotation in each case, in contrast with the isomeric acetylmethadols which had the same sign of rotation as their precursors. Janssen (*183*) has presented a particularly detailed summary of the properties of all the stereoisomeric forms of the methadols, the isomethadols and their acetyl derivatives.

2. *Structure-Activity Relationships*

The principal feature of structure-activity studies in this series has been the determination of analgetic activity of all the stereoisomeric forms of the methadols, the acetylmethadols, and the corresponding derivatives from isomethadone (*183, 231, 232*). Highlights of these results are reviewed in Table IX. Both the of racemic secondary alcohols, *dl*-α-methadol and *dl*-β-methadol (Table IX, Nos. 1 and 2) derived from methadone are significantly

TABLE

DIPHENYLPROPYLAMINES; ALCOHOLS AND AMIDES

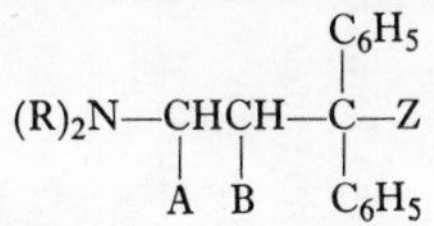

$$\text{(R)}_2\text{N}-\underset{\text{A}}{\text{CH}}\underset{\text{B}}{\text{CH}}-\overset{\text{C}_6\text{H}_5}{\underset{\text{C}_6\text{H}_5}{\text{C}}}-\text{Z}$$

No.	$\text{(R)}_2\text{N}$	A	B	Z	Activity[a]	References
	Methadone				1.0	
	Alcohols (and derived esters); $Z = CH(OH)C_2H_5$ and $CH(OCOR_1)C_2H_5$					
1.	$(CH_3)_2N$	CH_3	H	$CH(OH)C_2H_5$ (dl-α-methadol)	0.08	183, 231
2.	$(CH_3)_2N$	CH_3	H	$CH(OH)C_2H_5$ (dl-β-methadol)	0.2	183, 231
3.	$(CH_3)_2N$	CH_3	H	$CH(OCOCH_3)C_2H_5$ (dl-α-acetylmethadol)	1.5	183, 231
4.	$(CH_3)_2N$	CH_3	H	$CH(OCOCH_3)C_2H_5$ [(+)-α-]	5.0	183, 231
5.	$(CH_3)_2N$	CH_3	H	$CH(OCOCH_3)C_2H_5$ [(−)-α-]	0.9	183, 231
6.	$(CH_3)_2N$	CH_3	H	$CH(OCOCH_3)C_2H_5$ (dl-β-acetylmethadol)	2.3	183, 231
7.	$(CH_3)_2N$	H	CH_3	$CH(OCOCH_3)C_2H_5$ (dl-α-acetylisomethadol)	0.3	183, 232
8.	$(CH_3)_2N$	CH_3	H	$CH(OCOC_2H_5)C_2H_5$	0.3^{183}	183, 211, 229
9.	$(CH_3)_2N$	CH_3	H	$CH(OCOCH_2Cl)C_2H_5$	17^{230}	183, 230
10.	$OC_4H_8N^b$	CH_3	H	$CH(OCOCH_3)C_2H_5$	6^{211}	183, 211
11.	CH_3NH	CH_3	H	$CH(OH)C_2H_5$ (dl-α-)	1.6	233
12.	CH_3NH	CH_3	H	$CH(OCOCH_3)C_2H_5$ (dl-α-; noracimethadol)	3.0	233, 234
	Amides; $Z = CON(R_1)_2$					
13.	$(CH_3)_2N$	H	CH_3	$CONH_2$ (aminopentamide)	0^e	183
14.	$OC_4H_8N^b$	H	CH_3	$CONHC_2H_5$	0.15^{183}	183, 238, 239
15.	$OC_4H_8N^b$	H	CH_3	$CON(CH_3)_2$	3.8^{183}	183, 238, 239
16.	$C_5H_{10}N^c$	H	CH_3	$CON(CH_3)_2$	0.5^{183}	183, 238, 239
17.	$OC_4H_8N^b$	H	CH_3	$CONC_4H_8{}^d$ (dl; racemoramide)	3.6^{183}	183, 238, 239
18.	$OC_4H_8N^b$	H	CH_3	$CONC_4H_8{}^d$ [(+); dextromoramide]	$13(7^{183})$	183, 238, 239

[a] Unless otherwise noted by superscript citation of the appropriate reference, the analgetic activity, compared to methadone, is taken from the Eddy hot-plate data in mice (13, 56a,).

[b] OC_4H_8N = morpholino.   [c] $C_5H_{10}N$ = piperidino.   [d] C_4H_8N = pyrrolidino.

[e] Possesses clinically useful anticholinergic activity.

239

less active than the parent ketone, but potent analgetic activity is reinstated upon acetylation. The *dl*-α-acetylmethadol and *dl*-β-acetylmethadol racemates (Nos. 3 and 6) are somewhat more active than the parent ketone. Analgetic testing of the various enantiomers has generally shown that one isomer from a given racemate is more active than the racemate, and the opposite isomer is less active. However, the relative potencies of the pairs of enantiomers have not always been consistent with the concept that the more active enantiomer may be expected to be up to twice as active as the racemic mixture while the other isomer is proportionately less active. For example, (+)-α-acetylmethadol (No. 4) is apparently more than twice as active as the corresponding racemate (No. 3) On the other hand, the opposite enantiomer (−)-α-acetylmethadol (No. 5) is surprisingly potent for an "inactive" isomer; it is derived from (+)-methadone (which is virtually inactive), and is therefore related to the absolute configuration of L-alanine with respect to the branched methyl asymmetric center. These findings are contrasted with the configurations of the methadone-like ketones (and sulfones) where the potent optical isomers have identical absolute configurations related to D-(−)-alanine.

The isomethadols and acetylisomethadols derived from isomethadone are generally less active than the corresponding derivatives from methadone. *dl*-α-Acetylisomethadol (Table IX, No. 7) is the most active of this group of derivatives. The optical isomers in this series have also been studied for analgetic activity (*232*).

All of the active secondary alcohols and secondary esters in this series are derived from ethyl ketones. Examples derived from methyl and propyl ketone derivatives were inactive. The acetyl group appeared to provide optimal activity for the ester portion of the molecule. Formyl and propionyl (Table IX, No. 8) esters were less active, but chloroacetylmethadols (No. 9) and isomethadols were somewhat more active than the acetyl esters. Acetyl-mandelic esters of α- and β-methadols have recently been described as strong analgetics (*235*). Nearly all of the methadol and isomethadol types studied for analgetic activity have the dimethylamino basic group. However, a few morpholino derivatives (such as No. 10) also have high activity. The recently studied monomethylamino derivatives (Nos. 11 and 12) are exceptional examples in which the secondary amines are more potent than the corresponding tertiary amino derivatives. The reverse is the usual pattern (4-phenylpiperidines, methadone-like ketones, etc.). These compounds were prepared from intermediates containing the benzylmethylamino group, and the benzyl group was removed by hydrogenolysis as the final step. Both the α- and β-forms were obtained by reduction of the ketone derivative with lithium aluminium hydride and sodium in alcohol, respectively.

A group of recently described diphenylcyclopropane derivatives (*236*) bear some resemblance to the methadols and have been claimed as analgetics. Compound (XCV) is illustrative of this series. The usual structural elements of the morphine-like analgetics appear to be present in this series, but it is difficult to predict how well such a molecule could fit a morphine-

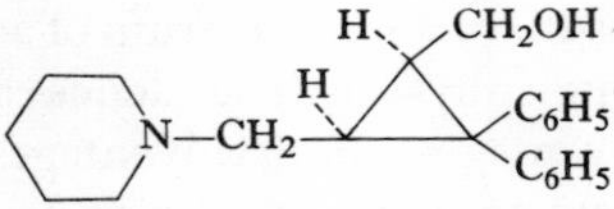

$$
\text{H} \diagdown \quad \diagup \text{CH}_2\text{OH}
$$

(XCV)

like receptor. Acetoxy derivatives have also been made and dimethylamino and morpholino groups have been included in variations of the basic function.

3. *Clinical Evaluation*

The number of secondary alcohol derivatives of the methadol family which have been tried in man is rather limited. Earlier trials (1952) studied the α-acetylmethadols (Table IX, Nos. 3–5) as the racemate and as both optical isomers (*7*). More recently (1963), the monomethylamino derivative, noracimethadol (Table IX, No. 12), has been studied (*237*).

Pharmacological evaluation of the α-acetylmethadols indicated they were at least as potent as the parent ketones, and that their relative toxicity was slightly decreased. Furthermore, they showed comparatively high activity by the oral route of administration. *dl*-α-Acetylmethadol was effective against chronic pain in human trials at an oral dose of 5 or 10 mg, several times a day. These doses were sometimes accompanied by morphine-like side effects. The less active isomer, ($-$)-α-acetylmethadol, was effective in relieving postoperative pain when administered subcutaneously only at doses greater than 40 mg. The dose equivalent to 10 mg of morphine was estimated as 50 mg. However, repeated administration of the ($-$)-α-isomer in the 20–40 mg dose range sometimes produced a dangerous comatose state like that of morphine poisoning. Relatively little investigation of the more potent isomer, ($+$)-α-acetylmethadol, was carried out. A subcutaneous dose of 2.5 mg was somewhat less effective than 10 mg of morphine in the same patients. The racemate and both optical isomers are addicting in man (*7*).

The secondary amine, noracimethadol, was suggested for human trials on the basis of its relatively high activity by the oral route, slower development of tolerance than morphine, and longer duration than morphine or

241

methadone. Single oral doses of 20–30 mg of noracimethadol were approximately equivalent to 60–90 mg doses of morphine given orally to postpartum patients (237). Noracimethadol was approximately 3.25 times as potent as morphine in producing a satisfactory analgetic effect compared to placebo controls and had fewer undesirable effects than morphine at equally effective doses. While this drug appears to have some advantages over morphine under these conditions, it still has the general spectrum of activity of the morphine-like analgetics. It showed high physical dependence capacity in monkeys (13). Therefore, its relative advantages, or disadvantages, over the established morphine-like drugs remain to be more fully proven.

C. Amide Types (Dextromoramide Family)

Diphenylpropylamine derivatives with a tertiary amide moiety in place of the alkyl ketone group found in the methadone family represent another closely related type of highly potent, morphine-like analgetic agent. Although several 4-amino-2,2-diphenylbutyramide derivatives were known as early as 1943, and additional derivatives were studied as analgetics (186, 207) following the introduction of methadone (1946), it was not until 1956 that Janssen and co-workers (183, 238, 239) established that this type of derivative could possess potent analgetic activity. The early derivatives were inactive as analgetics. Furthermore, a number of primary amide derivatives related to the methadone structure were found to have antispasmodic actions (186, 240, 241), apparently diverting interest from the analgetic field. The (+)-isomer of N-(2,2-diphenyl-3-methyl-4-morpholinobutyryl)-pyrrolidine (XCVI), or dextromoramide, is the principal tertiary amide derivative which has been extensively evaluated as an analgetic agent.

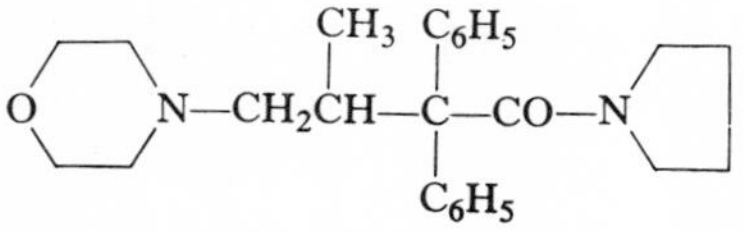

$$O \diagdown N-CH_2CH-\underset{\underset{C_6H_5}{|}}{\overset{\overset{CH_3\ C_6H_5}{|\quad\ |}}{C}}-CO-N \diagup$$

(XCVI)

Dextromoramide must be regarded as typical morphine-like analgetic. It is more potent than morphine and methadone, produces respiratory depression, and is effectively antagonized by nalorphine. Its structural similarity to methadone together with a similar spectrum of pharmacological actions indicates it should be able to satisfy the stereospecific drug-receptor complex postulated for morphine-like actions. A mutual interaction between the basic amino group, principally as the protonated species, and the amide carbonyl function may assist formation of a cyclic conformation favorable for analgetic actions.

1. Synthesis

The tertiary amides related to dextromoramide are readily prepared by the alkylation of N,N-disubstituted diphenylacetamides with tertiary aminoalkyl halides (*183, 240, 241*):

$$Am-C_nH_{2n}-X + (C_6H_5)_2CHCONR_2 \xrightarrow{\text{NaNH}_2} Am-C_nH_{2n}-C(C_6H_5)_2CONR_2$$

Unbranched butyramides are obtained from aminoethyl chlorides. Condensation with branched-chain isopropyl chlorides, capable of isomerizing via a cyclic immonium structure, produces mixtures of isomers, analogous to the mixtures of methadone- and isomethadone-type nitriles. These isomers may then be separated by differences in solubility. Proof of structure was established by unambiguous synthesis or by ultraviolet spectral analysis (*242*). Identification of the branched isomers by nuclear magnetic resonance (n.m.r.) spectra should also be possible. Unequivocal synthetic methods have been patterned after those used for methadone and isomethadone (see Scheme 9). For example, alkylation with the tosylate, $TsOCH(CH_3)CH_2Cl$, or the bromoacetal, $BrCH(CH_3)CH(OEt)_2$, may be employed in the synthesis of dextromoramide to avoid isomeric mixtures. The basic amino group is then introduced at a later step.

These tertiary amides are also obtained via the acid chlorides (*183, 241*). This method is also the principal route for secondary amides. The basic intermediates required for these procedures are methadone and isomethadone nitriles which are hydrolyzed to the acids (*183, 186, 207, 211*). The acid chlorides were obtained by treating the acids with thionyl chloride or phosphorus pentachloride at low temperatures. Above about 60°, intramolecular condensation between the acid chloride and the tertiary amine tends to produce pyrrolidones (XCVII).

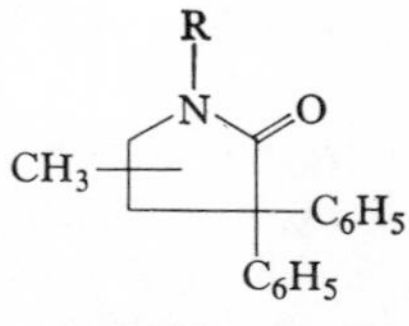

(XCVII)

The tendency to form pyrrolidones is particularly evident with the branched isomers of the isomethadone type.

243

2. Structure-Activity Relationships

Selected examples illustrating the analgetic activity of the dextromoramide family of compounds are reviewed in the second part of Table IX. The primary amide derivative (No. 13) was a clinically useful atropine-like substance, and was inactive as an analgetic agent. A number of related primary amides were also investigated for antispasmodic activity (183, 186, 240, 241), and were uninteresting as analgetics. Structural variations which improved the antispasmodic potency were, in general, changes which adversely affected analgetic activity in the methadone family. For example, the highest antispasmodic activity was usually found in the unbranched compounds, and quaternization of the tertiary amine frequently increased the antispasmodic potency. The N-ethyl derivative (No. 14) was the most active analgetic of a series (183, 241) of closely related secondary amides. It was about as potent as meperidine. Antispasmodic activity of the secondary amides was much lower than that of the corresponding primary amides, and secondary amides were also found to have oxytocic and diuretic activity (241).

The tertiary amides (Table IX, Nos. 15–18) had the best analgetic activity, and were uninteresting as antispasmodics. They were also studied as oxytocics and diuretics (241). A study of chemical structure and analgetic activity in mice indicated the highest activity was found with N,N-dimethyl (Nos. 15 and 16) and pyrrolidino amides (Nos. 17 and 18). Branched isomers related to isomethadone were more active than those related to methadone. The morpholino group was clearly the best basic moiety for analgetic activity, although piperidino, pyrrolidino, and dimethylamino groups gave active compounds. Quaternization of the tertiary amine eliminated analgetic activity. Examination of the enantiomers of racemoramide (No. 17) showed that the (+)-isomer, dextromoramide (No. 18), was approximately twice as potent as the racemate, and the (−)-isomer was virtually inactive. Thus, with minor variations, the structure-activity pattern in the dextromoramide series is similar to that of the ketone series. This work has been carried out almost exclusively by Janssen and co-workers (183, 238, 239). More recent compounds from the same workers have included a primary amide derivative with an unbranched chain and an 4-(o-methoxyphenyl)piperazin-1-yl basic moiety (243).

The wide variation in utility from clinically useful antispasmodics which presumably are nonaddicting, to the potent, narcotic analgetics of the dextromoramide family, principally by changing the substituents on an amide group, is rather striking. Primary, secondary, and tertiary amides might all be expected to form a satisfactory drug-receptor complex for some degree of morphine-like activity. Apparently, this is not possible for the primary amides.

244

3. *Pharmacological and Clinical Evaluation*

Dextromoramide (Table IX, No. 18) is the only compound in this series which has received extensive evaluation in animals (*183, 244–248*) and in man. Although dextromoramide is a morphine-like analgetic which produces physical dependence, respiratory depression, etc., there were significant quantitative differences between this drug and other morphine-like analgetics. Dextromoramide was characterized by a very short onset of action, and tolerance to the analgetic effect developed very slowly or not at all. In man, constipation was not observed, and the drug was nearly as active by oral administration as by subcutaneous injection.

Since the first clinical use of dextromoramide in 1957 (*249*), this drug has been extensively evaluated in man (*183, 250–260*), both in the United States and Europe. Doses of 5 to 10 mg, orally and parenterally, were approximately equivalent to 10 mg of morphine. In one series of trials (*251*) frequent nausea and vomiting was noted, and the side effects cast doubt upon the use of this drug in postpartum patients (*252*). Dextromoramide offered no advantage over morphine in treating post operative pain (*254*). In other trials, quite satisfactory results were obtained without serious side effects. It appears, therefore, that dextromoramide is a potent drug with actions similar to morphine and meperidine, but without particular clinical advantages over these well established agents.

D. Miscellaneous Diphenylpropylamine Types

With the intensive development of methadone, isomethadone, and other ketone derivatives as potent, morphine-like agents, a variety of other structural moieties have been investigated as replacements for the ketone function. Reduction and acylation to give the acetylmethadols, and investigation of tertiary amide analogs including dextromoramide, represent families which have been extensively evaluated and have given clinically useful drugs. A large number of additional diphenylpropylamine derivatives and analogs have been synthesized and tested for analgetic activity, and a few have shown morphine-like actions. A number of these are reviewed in Table X. These compounds have generally shown analgetic activity and other pharmacological actions which suggest that they are truly morphine-like agents. However, they have seldom been evaluated clinically. Therefore, this group of miscellaneous compounds has not achieved the importance of the well established families of ketone, alcohol, and amide derivatives discussed previously.

Synthesis of these miscellaneous diphenylpropylamine derivatives has generally followed the methods previously outlined, or are simple

245

TABLE X

MISCELLANEOUS DIPHENYLPROPYLAMINES AND DIPHENYLACETIC ACID DERIVATIVES

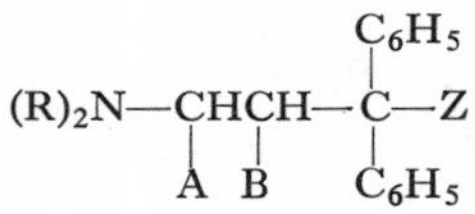

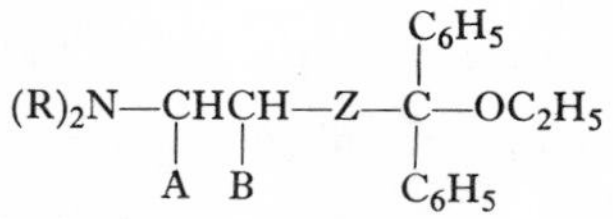

No.	$(R)_2N$	A	B	Z	Activity[a]	References

$$(R)_2N-\underset{A}{CH}\underset{B}{CH}-\underset{\underset{C_6H_5}{|}}{\overset{\overset{C_6H_5}{|}}{C}}-Z$$

	Methadone				1.0	
1.	$(CH_3)_2N$	CH_3	H	$COOC_2H_5$	0.09	207, 211, 261, 262
2.	$OC_4H_8N^b$	H	H	$COOC_2H_5$	0.25	210, 211
3.	$(CH_3)_2N$	CH_3	H	$SO_2C_2H_5$	1[183]	183, 265
4.	$C_5H_{10}N^c$	H	H	CN	0.06[183]	186, 207
5.	$C_{11}H_{20}ON_3^d$	H	H	CN (pirinitramide)	0.8	268, 269
6.	$(CH_3)_2N$	CH_3	H	$CH(NH_2)C_2H_5$	0.3[183]	183
7.	$OC_4H_8N^b$	H	CH_3	$CH_2NHCOCH_3$	0.1[183]	183
8.	$C_5H_{10}N^c$	H	H	OH (Parkiphen)	0[e]	183, 271a,b, 272
9.	$(CH_3)_2N$	CH_3	H	$OCOC_2H_5$	0.2	183, 274
10.	$C_5H_{10}N^c$	H	H	H (Aspasan)	0[e]	183, 207 271, 272

$$(R)_2N-\underset{A}{CH}\underset{B}{CH}-Z-\underset{\underset{C_6H_5}{|}}{\overset{\overset{C_6H_5}{|}}{C}}-OC_2H_5$$

	Meperidine				0.17	
11.	$(CH_3)_2N$	H	H	—OCO—	0.17	287–289
12.	$(CH_3)_2N$	H	CH_3	—OCO—	0.08	291–293
13.	$(CH_3)_2N$	H	H	—N(CH_3)CO—	0.16	303–305
14.	$C_9H_{12}N^f$	H	H	—N(CH_3)CO—	0.02(0.2[303])	303, 306, 307
15.	$(CH_3)_2N$	H	H	—OCO— (α-propargyloxy)	ca. 0.3[309]	308–310

[a] Unless otherwise noted by supersript citation of the appropriate reference, the analgetic activity, compared to methadone is taken from the Eddy hot-plate data in mice (13, 56a,b,c).

[b] OC_4H_8N = morpholino.

[c] $C_5H_{10}N$ = piperidino.

[d] $C_{11}H_{20}ON_3$ = 4-piperidino-4-carbamylpiperidin-1-yl.

[e] Has clinical antispasmodic activity.

[f] $C_9H_{12}N$ = $C_6H_5CH_2CH_2N(CH_3)$—.

transformations of intermediates already described. Therefore, a detailed review of their preparation is unnecessary.

1. Structure-Activity Relationships

The ester derivatives (Table X, Nos. 1 and 2) illustrate the findings that this type of compound, closely related to the analgetic ketone structures, has shown moderate analgetic activity (*183, 207, 211, 261, 262*). The closest analog (No. 1) of methadone was about one-half as potent as meperidine, and failed to suppress the signs of morphine abstinence in man (*13*). This type of compound also tended to show antispasmodic activity (*183*). The esters are generally obtained either directly from the nitriles or via the free acid.

Two additional ester derivatives, XCVIII and XCIX, illustrate the direction of more recent investigations. The piperidine derivative (XCVIII) is a secondary amine which is claimed to have morphine-like activity (*263*). The piperidine ring incorporates a portion of the alkylene chain in the generalized structure postulated for analgetic activity. The bisdimethyamino derivative

$$\underset{\text{(XCVIII)}}{\overset{\displaystyle C_6H_5}{\underset{\displaystyle C_6H_5}{\text{N} \atop \text{H}}\text{-CH}_2\text{CCOOC}_2\text{H}_5}} \qquad \underset{\text{(XCIX)}}{\overset{\displaystyle C_6H_5}{\underset{\displaystyle (CH_3)_2\text{NCH}_2}{(CH_3)_2\text{NCH}_2\text{CHCHCOOC}_2\text{H}_5}}}$$

(XCIX) represents a modified diphenylpropylamine structure in which one of the phenyl groups has been eliminated, and a second basic group has been introduced (*264a, b*). These compounds are claimed as analgetics.

The sulfone analog of methadone (Table X, No. 3) was obtained by the alkylation of benzhydryl ethyl sulfone by methods similar to those used for methadone (*265*). This compound shows typical morphine-like actions, including a high capacity for physical dependence in monkeys (*13*), and was tried clinically (*266*). The optical isomers were studied, and the analgetically active enantiomer has been related to D-(−)-alanine (*204*). A number of related derivatives (*265*) were also studied (1948). More recently, pharmacological studies on the enantiomers of the piperidino analog have been reported (*267*).

The nitrile intermediate (Table X, No. 4) illustrates the general finding that this type is virtually devoid of analgetic activity (*183*). This compound was less active than meperidine. A number of these nitriles showed antispasmodic activity, however. In contrast, changing the basic group to the 4-piperidino-4-carbamoylpiperidin-1-yl moiety (No. 5) produces a potent

247

morphine-like agent (*268, 269*). This compound produces respiratory depression, is effectively antagonized by nalorphine, and has high physical dependence capacity in monkeys (*56c*).

A number of amine analogs of the alkyl ketone moiety of the methadones have been prepared by reduction of the ketimines or nitriles. Only a few of these were active (*183*). Compounds 6 and 7 (Table X) illustrate examples which have analgetic activity in mice in the range of 0.5 to 1.5 times meperidine. A series of derivatives related to No. 7 with one of the phenyl groups replaced by an ethyl group have been recently described as less active than the known strong analgetics (*270*).

The tertiary alcohol compound (Table X, No. 8) is typical of a group of diphenylpropylamine derivatives which are not active as analgetics, but which have been extensively investigated as antispasmodics (*183, 271a, b, 272*). This derivative has been used clinically as an antispasmodic. It is a further example of a structure that would appear to be capable of "fitting" the postulated morphine-like receptor, but which has markedly different pharmacological and clinical actions. The somewhat analogous 1,1-diphenyl-2-dimethylaminopropanol has been recently claimed as an analgetic (*273*). This structure has an alkylene chain with only one carbon atom between the basic amine and the quaternary central carbon. Acylation of the tertiary alcohol function seems to impart analgetic activity, however. The propionoxy derivative (No. 9) was about as potent as meperidine in mice (*274*). 1,1-Diphenyl-1,2-diacetoxy-4-pyrrolidinobutane (C) is a member of a recently described series claimed to possess analgetic properties (*275*), and shows a high capacity for physical dependence in the monkey (*56a*). If this is a true morphine-like analgetic, modification of the usual concept of a two carbon alkylene chain between the basic nitrogen and the central atom bearing the aromatic ring is required. There are other hints in this direction (see Section III,E).

$$
\begin{array}{c}
\overset{\displaystyle CH_3COO}{\underset{|}{}}\ \overset{\displaystyle C_6H_5}{\underset{|}{}} \\
NCH_2CH_2CHCOCOCH_3 \\
\underset{|}{} \\
C_6H_5
\end{array}
$$

(C)

(CI) — C_6H_5, $N(CH_3)_2$

The derivative (Table X, No. 10), with a hydrogen atom in place of the ethyl ketone moiety, is devoid of analgetic activity, but it has been used clinically as an antispasmodic agent. A number of closely related compounds have also been studied as antispasmodics, and do not appear to have any morphine-like analgetic activity. Once again, the distinction between an analgetic and an antispasmodic series appears to rest on small molecular changes. However, these may be responsible for critical differences in lipid solubilities or may involve groups at a sensitive site in the molecule with varied polarity.

1-Dimethylamino-3-phenylindane (CI) is a ring-closed analog of methadone, or more specifically, of the antispasmodic agent, Aspasan (Table X, No. 10). It was described in 1956, synthesized from 3-phenyl-1-indanone by hydrogenation of the oxime followed by methylation of the primary amine with formic acid and formaldehyde (276). It was a potent analgetic in animals (ca. 1.6 times meperidine) and showed low physical dependence capacity in monkeys (13). In the clinic this compound showed codeine-like activity, sometimes with gastrointestinal symptoms. This drug, therefore, appears to qualify as a morphine-like analgetic on the basis of its pharmacological actions, but its conformational analogy with the morphine-like configuration may be somewhat more difficult than many other potent analgetic agents. Several closely related compounds were less active (276). This compound was also synthesized about the same time by another group who also studied its analgetic properties (277–279). They separated the active compound into (+)- and (−)-enantiomers (280). Interest in the compound is apparently continuing as it has been assigned the name, dimefadane (281). Additional indanamine derivatives, synthesized as analgetics, have also been reported recently (282).

Three additional structures illustrate other changes in the diphenyl propylamine analgetics which eliminate analgetic activity completely. The

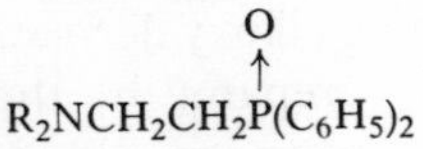

$$R_2NCH_2CH_2\overset{\overset{O}{\uparrow}}{P}(C_6H_5)_2$$

(CII)

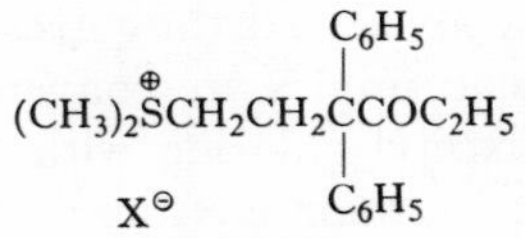

$$(CH_3)_2\overset{\oplus}{S}CH_2CH_2\overset{\overset{C_6H_5}{|}}{\underset{|}{C}}COC_2H_5$$
$$X^{\ominus} \quad C_6H_5$$

(CIII)

$$(CH_3)_2\overset{\oplus}{S}CH_2CH_2\overset{\overset{C_6H_5}{|}}{\underset{|}{C}}CH(OCOCH_3)C_2H_5$$
$$X^{\ominus} \quad C_6H_5$$

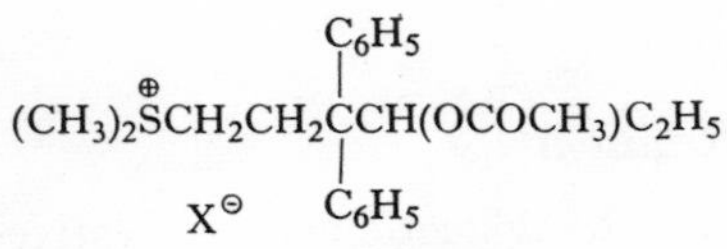

(CIV)

dialkylaminoethyl diphenylphosphine oxides (CII), synthesized by Burger and Shelver (283), are derivatives in which the quaternary carbon is replaced with phosphorus. The sulfonium analogs (CIII) and (CIV) of normethadone and the corresponding acetylmethadol, respectively, were also inactive (181).

E. ALKOXYDIPHENYLACETIC ACID DERIVATIVES

A group of basic esters and amides of alkoxydiphenylacetic acids have recently attracted interest in this type of derivative for analgetic testing. The general structure CV describes these compounds. All of the elements of the

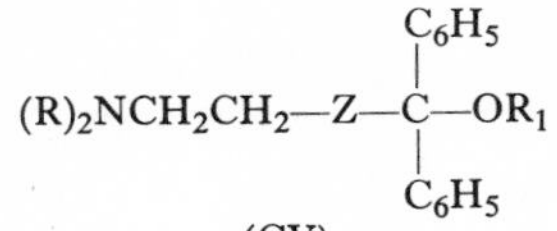

$$
\begin{array}{c}
\text{C}_6\text{H}_5 \\
| \\
(\text{R})_2\text{NCH}_2\text{CH}_2\text{—Z—C—OR}_1 \\
| \\
\text{C}_6\text{H}_5
\end{array}
$$

(CV)

generalized structure postulated for morphine-like activity (and of the diphenylpropylamine analgetics) are easily recognized, with the important difference that the alkylene chain is separated (—Z—) from the quaternary carbon by an ester (—OCO—) or amide (—NRCO—) function. Thus, the distance between the basic group and the central atom bearing the aromatic ring appears to be significantly increased, and a polar group is introduced in a position usually occupied by a hydrocarbon chain. The two carbon alkylene chain has been a feature of morphine-like analgetics which has been the least susceptible to exceptions. The distance between the basic nitrogen and the flat aromatic ring has been accepted as a rather critical dimension in forming a stereospecific drug-receptor complex for analgetic activity. Revision of this concept may be required for the alkoxydiphenylacetic acid derivatives.

These compounds are readily obtained by straightforward synthetic procedures. For example, the esters may be obtained from the appropriate basic alcohols and an alkoxydiphenylacetic acid, or the appropriate basic ester of benzilic acid is converted to the corresponding alkoxy derivative via a tertiary halide. The basic amides are conveniently prepared by the reaction of α-chlorodiphenylacetyl chloride with the appropriate diamine followed by treatment of the reaction mixture with an alcohol. Alternately, 2-ethoxy-N-methyl-2,2-diphenylacetamide is alkylated with a dialkylaminoethyl halide using sodium amide.

1. Structure-Activity Relationships

This family of alkoxydiphenylacetic acid derivatives is closely related to structures well known for their antispasmodic activity. These include the basic esters of diphenylacetic and benzilic acids, several of which have been widely used as clinical antispasmodics. 2-Dialkylaminoethyldiphenylethoxy-acetic acids were apparently synthesized as analogs of the antispasmodic benzilic ester by at least three independent laboratories (284–286), one as early as 1950. Blicke et al. (286) indicated the diethylamino analog was inactive,

250

and Klosa (*287, 288*) reported a pronounced analgetic effect, (> meperidine) for the dimethylamino analog, about the same time (1954). This introduced the development of this series as analgetic agents.

The principal analgetic compounds in this series are reviewed in the second part of Table X. The 2-dimethylaminoethyl ester (No. 11), the lead compound, is approximately equipotent with meperidine by the hot-plate procedure in mice, and showed high physical dependence capacity in monkeys (*13*). It has also been proclaimed to have addiction liability similar to morphine (*289*). These findings are typical of a morphine-like analgetic that can be expected to show a good degree of "fit" with the postulated stereospecific receptor. This compound, with four atoms between the tertiary amine and the central carbon atom bearing the aromatic ring (instead of the usual two carbon atoms), represents the principal argument for modification of the previous conclusions concerning the desirability of a two carbon alkylene chain. Most of the related derivatives appear to be less potent, and is not yet evident how well they show the concomitant pattern of other morphine-like actions such as tolerance, respiratory depression, and antagonism by nalorphine. Nonetheless, this series is important in establishing that a morphine-like configuration, as judged by the spectrum of pharmacological actions, may possibly be obtained by acyclic (or other) structures which are increasingly remote from those usually accepted as characteristic of the potent, narcotic analgetics. This compound has also been studied in Japan (*290*). The dimethylaminoisopropanol ester (No. 2) is considerably less active (ca. one-third the meperidine activity) in mice, and showed a very low capacity for physical dependence in monkeys (*56a*). Therefore, it remains to be more fully demonstrated whether this activity is truly morphine-like (with lower potency).

A number of related basic esters have also been described. The ethyl ethers were superior to methoxy and propoxy derivatives (*294*). Other alkoxy derivatives have also been studied (*295*) with the phenethyl, 2-cyanoethyl, 4-chlorobutyl and 3-hexyl ethers reported as compounds with good activity (one-third that of morphine or better). Variations in the basic alcohol have also been studied. These include 2-pyrrolidinoethanol esters (*296*), 1-ethyl-3-pyrrolidyl, and 1-methyl-3(and 4)-piperidyl esters (*297, 298*), and esters with 1-methyl-2-(hydroxymethyl)pyrrolidine (*299a, b*). All are claimed as analgetic or antispasmodic agents, but detailed pharmacological data is not available. The related compounds CVI and CVII have also been investigated as analgetics (*300–302*), representing additional changes in the basic structure of this series. Compound CVI (*300*) bears some resemblance to propoxyphene (see Section V), and CVII (*301*) has one-tenth the activity of meperidine in mice and no physical dependence capacity in monkeys (*56b*).

251

The basic amide type is illustrated by two derivatives (Table X, Nos. 13 and 14) which have received the most attention in this group. The *N*-(2-dimethylaminoethyl)amide, studied first, was approximately equal to

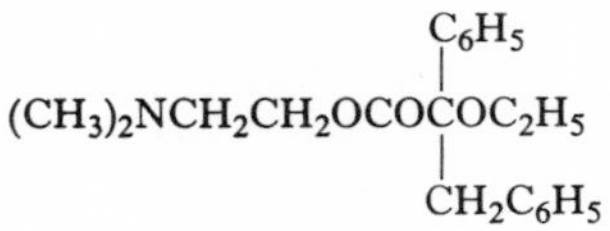

$$(CH_3)_2NCH_2CH_2OCOCOC_2H_5$$

with C_6H_5 and $CH_2C_6H_5$ substituents

(CVI)

$$N—CH_2CH_2COCOC_2H_5$$

with C_6H_5 and C_6H_5 substituents

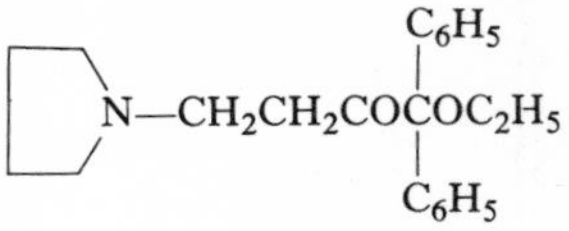

(CVII)

meperidine in mice and rats. Some tolerance developed in rats but there was no cross tolerance to morphine or meperidine (*305*). The amide containing the *N*-methylphenethylamine moiety (No. 14) was less potent (about one-half as active as codeine, or less) and is reported (*303*) to be orally effective in man (150 mg dose). It showed no physical dependence capacity in monkeys (*56c*). A number of related compounds were studied, and the *p*-aminophen-ethyl and β-2(and 4)-pyridylethyl substituents on the basic nitrogen also showed good activity (*303*).

Another member of the basic ester series has received particular attention in recent publications (*295, 308–310*). This is the α-propargyl ether deriva-tive (Table X, No. 15). It appears to be somewhat more active than the corresponding ethoxy ether, and its pharmacological actions have been studied in some detail (*295, 309, 310*). The corresponding 1-phenylpropargyl ether has been reported to be about twice as active (*295*) as No. 15. Basic amides of the propargyl ethers have also been prepared (*308*). This series of ethers derived from benzilic ester and amides therefore represents a current trend in analgetic agents related to methadone that remains to be put into better perspective with more detailed pharmacological (and perhaps clinical) data. Their importance in requiring a modified picture of the structural characteristics of the morphine-like analgetics will then be more evident.

The testing of additional compounds will also contribute to this area. For example, the 2,3-dihydro-3-benzofurancarboxylate derivative (CVIII) is a member of a series described as analgetics and hypotensors (*311*). This

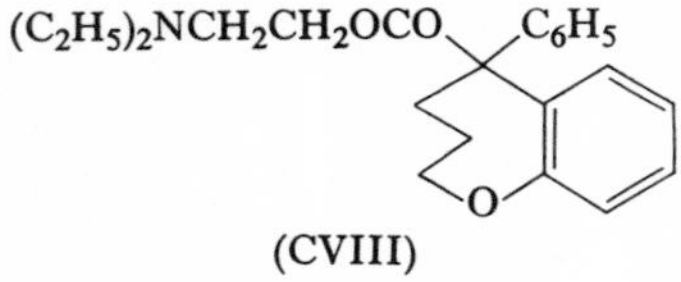

$$(C_2H_5)_2NCH_2CH_2OCO \quad C_6H_5$$

(CVIII)

compound showed weak activity by the hot-plate method in mice and did not support physical dependence in monkeys (*56c*).

IV. Dithienylbutenylamine Derivatives
(Thiambutene Family)

As part of a general program for the pharmacological investigation of aminoalkyl tertiary alcohols and derived products, a group of 3-*tert*-amino-1,1-bis(2-thienyl)-1-butenes were developed as a new series of potent analgetics by Adamson and Green in 1950 (*312*). About this time, intensive development of methadone relatives as analgetics and investigation of the antispasmodic properties of 3-*tert*-amino-1,1-diaryl-1-propanol derivatives were both prominent in work published from a number of independent groups. It was difficult to predict whether new analogs would have analgetic or antispasmodic activity, and frequently they were tested for both types of utility. The lowest homolog of the dithienylbutenylamine series is 3-di-methylamino-1,1-bis(2-thienyl)-1-butene or dimethylthiambutene (CIX).

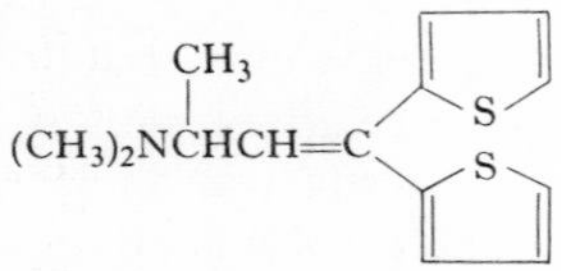

This compound was almost as potent an analgetic as morphine in animals, and showed other typical morphine-like actions such as respiratory depression. Its activity in man, together with that of several higher homologs of the tertiary amine function, was promptly confirmed. This series was thus established as another type of synthetic morphine-like agent from its pharmacological actions. However, its structural analogy with the narcotic analgetics, including morphine, was more difficult to understand. In 1956, Beckett and co-workers (*213*) included this series in their conformational analysis of potent analgetics, including the methadones, emphasizing that most of the potent analgetics of all types can approximate a morphine-like configuration (*1*).

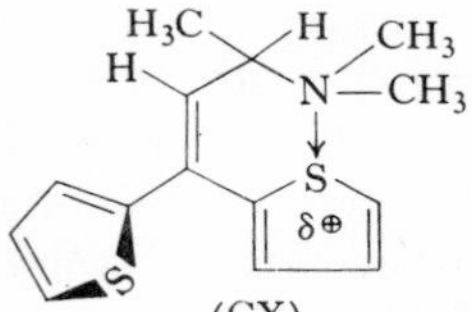

The structure CX illustrates the manner in which dimethylthiambutene may approximate a morphine-like configuration, as suggested by Beckett *et al.* (*213*). The sulfur atoms carry a partial positive charge due to resonance effects and will tend toward maximum separation (and twisting of the two thiophene rings out of the same plane) due to both steric and inductive repulsions. The double bond contributes to the rigidity of the structure, and an interaction between the basic nitrogen and the positive sulfur establishes a "piperidine-like" conformation that is favorable for association with the postulated analgetic receptor. These conclusions were supported by the

253

fact that the analog of CX with phenyl rings in place of the thiophene rings was virtually inactive as an analgetic (*213*). In this example, the inductive forces for holding the basic group in a favorable orientation for the analgetic receptor are absent.

Synthesis of the thiambutenes was straightforward and was readily accomplished from the appropriate β-aminoesters (*313*):

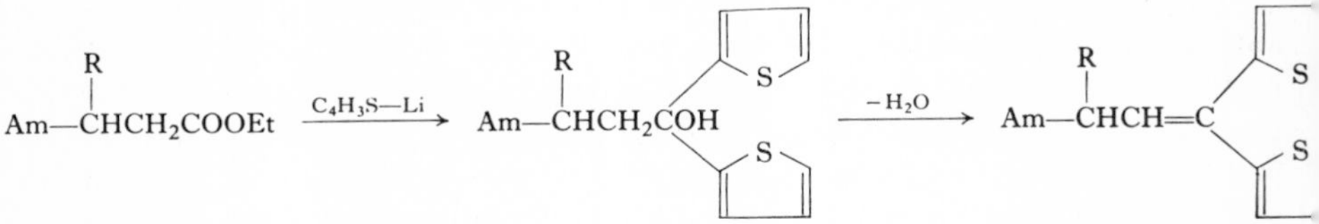

$$
\underset{\substack{| \\ \text{Am—CHCH}_2\text{COOEt}}}{\overset{\text{R}}{}} \xrightarrow{\text{C}_4\text{H}_3\text{S—Li}} \underset{\substack{| \\ \text{Am—CHCH}_2\text{COH}}}{\overset{\text{R}}{}} \xrightarrow{-\text{H}_2\text{O}} \underset{\substack{| \\ \text{Am—CHCH}}}{\overset{\text{R}}{=}}\text{C}
$$

The β-aminoesters were obtained by addition of amines to the appropriate α,β-unsaturated esters (acrylates and crotonates, etc.). Synthesis of the tertiary alcohols with thienyllithium gave good yields, but the thienyl Grignard reagent gave principally the ketone derivatives, such as 2-thienyl 2-dimethylaminopropyl ketone. Preparation of tertiary alcohols containing primary and secondary amino groups in place of the tertiary amine function gave lower yields. The dehydration step was accomplished with a mixture of hydrochloric and acetic acids or with hydrogen chloride alone, and the specific conditions sometimes had to be varied for different members of the series. For example, the thiambutenes without a branched methyl group (R = H) were readily obtained with hydrochloric and acetic acids, but these conditions had to be modified (to a shorter heating period or HCl alone) for the branched methyl compounds (R = CH₃).

1. Structure-Activity Relationships

The thiambutene analogs which have shown morphine-like actions are reviewed in Table XI. Potent analgetic activity in this series appears to be narrowly restricted to homologous analogs of the tertiary amine function. The ethylmethylamino compound (Table XI, No. 2) was the best of the di-lower alkylamino derivatives, and the pyrrolidino and piperidino analogs retained good activity. However, the morpholino derivative was considerably less active, and the hexamethyleneimino compound (*213*) was active. All of the potent derivatives in this series were much less active by the oral route in mice and saturated analogs, from hydrogenation of the double bond, also exhibited markedly reduced analgetic activity (*23*). The branched methyl group (R) was optimal. Both hydrogen and higher alkyl groups in this position were less active (*316*). Compounds in which one of the thienyl groups has

254

been replaced with phenyl have been prepared (*315*) and, apparently, are less interesting. The isomeric 4-amino-1-butene derivatives, with the basic group moved to the end of the chain, are claimed as antispasmodics and local anesthetics (*317*). The (+)-enantiomers are more active than the (−)-isomers, and (+)-dimethylthiambutene has been related to the configuration of D-(−)-alanine (*204*).

Following the initial development of this series, relatively few newer derivatives have been reported, except for work carried out in Japan where

TABLE XI

DITHIENYLBUTENYLAMINE DERIVATIVES

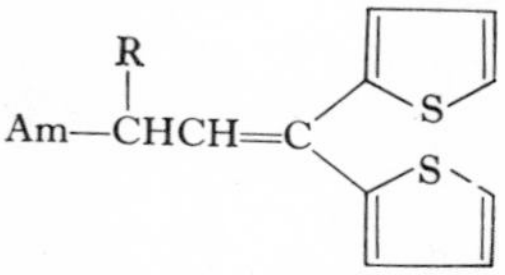

No.	Am	R		Activity[a]	References
	Morphine			1.0	
1.	$(CH_3)_2N$	CH_3 (dimethylthiambutene)		0.7 (1.0[316])	*313–316*
2.	$C_2H_5(CH_3)N$	CH_3		0.9	*313–316*
3.	$(C_2H_5)_2N$	CH_3		0.5 (1.0[316])	*313–316*
4.	C_4H_8N[b]	CH_3		0.4	*313–316*
5.	$C_5H_{10}N$[c]	CH_3		1.0	*313–316*
6.	OC_4H_8N[d]	CH_3		0.3[316]	*313–316*

[a] Unless otherwise noted by superscript citation of the appropriate reference, the analgetic activity, compared to morphine, is taken from the Eddy hot-plate data in mice (*23*).
[b] C_4H_8N = pyrrolidino.
[c] $C_5H_{10}N$ = piperidino.
[d] OC_4H_8N = morpholino.

dimethylthiambutene has been used clinically. Minor modifications of the previously outlined synthesis of dimethylthiambutene have been described (*318–320*). An isomer, 3-dimethylamino-2-methyl-1,1-bis(2-thienyl)-1-propene, of dimethylthiambutene has been claimed as an analgetic (*321*). The resolution of piperidinothiambutene has been reported (*322*). Additional variations of the thiambutene structure studied in Japan are illustrated by structures CXI (*323, 324*) and CXII (*325*). These compounds are claimed to have analgetic or antitussive activity.

255

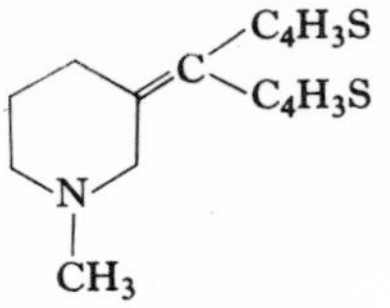

(CXI) 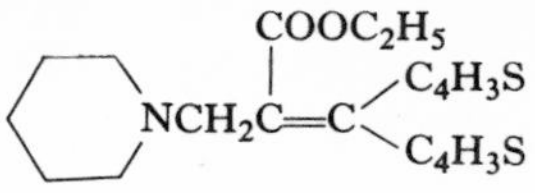   (CXII)

2. *Clinical Evaluation*

Four of the initial thiambutene derivatives were studied in humans, the first trials being reported in 1952 (7). They included the dimethylamino, ethylmethylamino, diethylamino, and pyrrolidino compounds (Table XI). The most effective of these was ethylmethylthiambutene (Table XI, No. 2), but more than 50 mg was required to equal the analgetic effect of 10 mg of morphine. It had a respiratory depressent effect and addiction liability approximately equivalent to morphine. Other members of this series were judged to be inferior due to weaker analgetic actions and concomitant side effects. Dimethylthiambutene (called Ohton) has been used clinically in Japan (7, *326*, *327*), and addiction to this drug has occurred resulting from illicit use (7). Analytical procedures have been reported, including its identification in urine (*328*, *329*).

Piperidinothiambutene (Table XI, No. 5) has been studied in Japan as a clinical antitussive agent (*330*). About 6 mg of the racemate was equivalent to a 20 mg dose of codeine, and the equivalent dose of the (+)-isomer was 3 mg. The piperidilidene compound (CXI) has also been tried as a clinical antitussive agent (*324*).

V. 3-Phenyl-3-acyloxybutylamine Derivatives (Propoxyphene Family)

Investigation of the pharmaceutical properties of 3-dialkylamino-1,1-diphenylpropanols and esters (see Table X, Compounds 8 and 9) led to a new series of morphine-like analgetics by designing esters that were more stable to hydrolysis. Esters of the 1,1-diphenyl propanols (benzhydrol esters) had been found to exhibit weak analgetic properties, but were unstable in aqueous solution. The tertiary 1,1-diphenylpropanol hydrolysis products were devoid of analgetic properties (but frequently had good antispasmodic properties). The current series of 3-phenyl-3-acyloxybutylamines were developed by Pohland and Sullivan (*331*) in 1953 by altering the diphenyl-carbinol structure, removing one phenyl group from the quaternary carbon atom, to give the general structure CXIII. They may, therefore, be considered a modification of the diphenylpropylamine analgetics. The basic

256

elements of the hypothetical morphine-like analgetic are readily apparent. The tertiary amine function, attached through a two carbon alkylene chain (usually branched) to the central carbinol carbon atom carrying one phenyl group provide the important moieties thought to be necessary for a stereospecific drug-receptor complex for morphine-like actions. A mutual interaction between the protonated basic nitrogen and the oxygen-containing

$$Am-\overset{|}{\underset{A}{C}}H\overset{|}{\underset{B}{C}}H-\overset{\overset{\displaystyle OCOR}{|}}{\underset{\underset{\displaystyle C_6H_5}{|}}{C}}-CH_2C_6H_5$$

(CXIII)

$$(CH_3)_2N-CH_2\overset{|}{\underset{\underset{\displaystyle CH_3}{|}}{C}}H-\overset{\overset{\displaystyle OCOC_2H_5}{|}}{\underset{\underset{\displaystyle C_6H_5}{|}}{C}}-CH_2C_6H_5$$

(CXIV)

ester moiety may assist in the formation of an analgetically favorable conformation in a manner similar to that described in detail for the methadone series.

4-Dimethylamino-1,2-diphenyl-3-methyl-2-propionoxybutane (CXIV), including its various stereoisomers, has been the principal compound in this series, which has been extensively evaluated and used in man. Two diastereomeric racemates were obtained, and analgetic activity was evident only in the α-racemate, which was the predominant isomer. This compound, *dl*-propoxyphene, was approximately equipotent with codeine in rats, and was capable of producing a profound morphine-like analgesia in these animals (*332*). Clinical trials followed promptly (1954), and it was found to be an effective analgetic in humans (*333*). This established the importance of this series. The (+)-α-isomer, *d*(or +)-propoxyphene, was more active than the racemate, and has now become very widely accepted as a moderately potent, orally effective analgetic drug with little or no addiction liability.

1. *Synthesis*

Synthesis of the propoxyphene series was readily accomplished by methods entirely analogous to those used for the tertiary alcohol and tertiary ester analogs of the diphenylpropylamines. These general procedures are outlined by sequence (*a*) in Scheme 11. The intermediate β-dialkylaminopropiophenones (CXV) were prepared by means of the Mannich reaction when the unbranched ethylene chain or the isomethadone-type branched chain was required. Addition of secondary amines to phenyl propenyl ketone gave the corresponding intermediates with the methadone-type branched chain. Treatment of these amino ketones with benzylmagnesium chloride gave predominantly one diastereoisomer, the α-carbinol, together with minor amounts of the β-carbinol, which was separated by solubility differences. They were

257

usually converted to the acylated derivatives (CXVI) with acetic or pro-pionic anhydride and pyridine. These acyl derivatives were quite resistant to hydrolysis. The racemic α-carbinol has been resolved by fractional crystalli-zation of the (+)-camphorsulfonic acid salt and the optically active carbinol hydrochlorides acylated to give (+)- and (−)-propoxyphene (*334*). *N*-Methyl-C^{14}-*dl*-propoxyphene has also been prepared (*335*).

An extensive series of chemical transformations have been carried out to establish the configuration of both asymmetric centers of propoxyphene (*336*). The configuration at C-3 was related to D-(−)-1-dimethylamino-2-propylbenzoate (CXVIII) by the transformations outlined in sequence (b), Scheme 11. The (−)-(CXVIII) was related to D-(−)-1-amino-2-propanol by methylation and benzoylation of the latter compound which had been previously related to D-(+)-glyceraldehyde. Thus, the isomethadone-type branched methyl group of (+)-propoxyphene (the more active isomer) is related to the same configuration as the more active isomer of isomethadone. (−)-Isomethadone was related to (R)-(−)-α-methyl-β-alanine by Beckett *et al.* (*337*), and the latter compound has the same configuration as D-(+)-glyceraldehyde. The validity of this scheme requires that the Baeyer-Villiger rearrangement of the amino ketone (CXVII) proceeds with retention of configuration, following the precedent of other rearrangements of this type. The (−)-amino ketone (CXVII) was particularly stable to racemization and has proven to be an excellent intermediate for a stereoselective synthesis of (+)-propoxyphene by reaction with benzylmagnesium chloride followed by acylation of the derived α-(+)-carbinol (*338*).

The configuration at C-2 was established by a lengthy series of transfor-mations outlined, in part, by sequence (*c*) in Scheme 11. The *N*-oxide of (+)-propoxyphene was prepared and degraded to the (+)-butene deriva-tive. Ozonolysis, hydrolysis of the propionate ester, and degradation of the methyl ketone gave (−)-2,3-diphenyl-2-hydroxypropionic acid. Esterifi-cation followed by hydrogenolysis of the benzylic carbinol with retention of configuration gave methyl (+)-2,3-diphenylpropionate. Lithium alumin-ium hydride reduction of the ester followed by formation of a tosylate and treatment with sodium iodide afforded (+)-2,3-diphenyl-1-iodopropane. Catalytic hydrogenolysis gave L-(+)-2,3-diphenylpropane (CXIX) which is related to L-(*S*)-(−)-glyceraldehyde by previous work. Thus, the two asymmetric centers in the analgetic (+)-propoxyphene can be assigned the (2S:3R)-configuration.

2. *Structure-Activity Relationships*

Relatively little structural variation in the propoxyphene molecule is permissible without loss of analgetic activity. The active derivatives are

GENERAL SYNTHESIS:

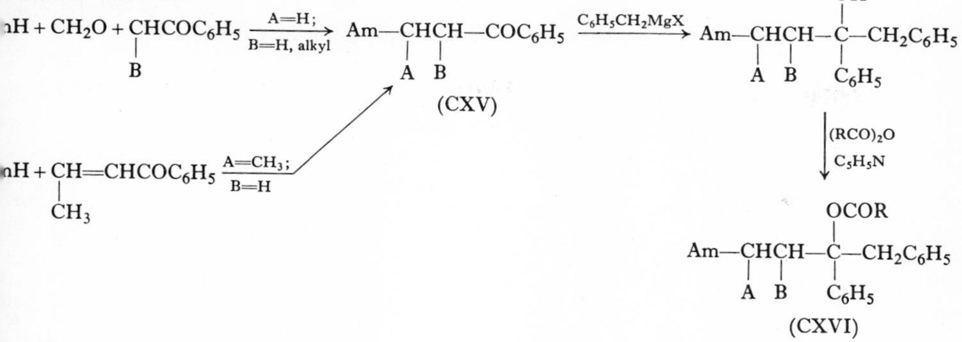

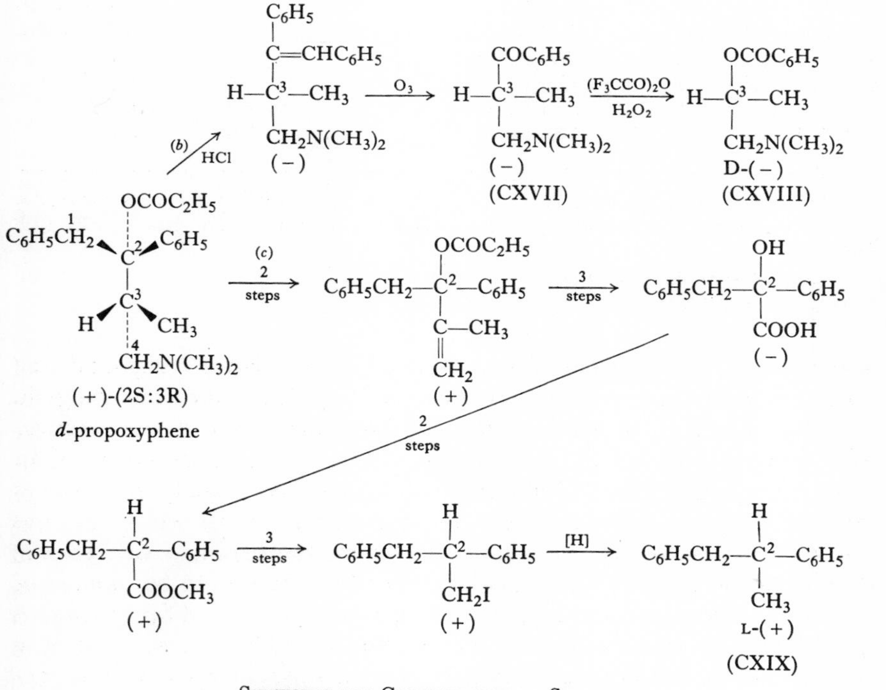

$$\text{nH} + CH_2O + \underset{\underset{B}{|}}{CHCOC_6H_5} \xrightarrow[B=H, \text{alkyl}]{A=H;} Am-\underset{\underset{A}{|}}{CH}\underset{\underset{B}{|}}{CH}-COC_6H_5 \xrightarrow{C_6H_5CH_2MgX} Am-\underset{\underset{A}{|}}{CH}\underset{\underset{B}{|}}{CH}-\underset{\underset{C_6H_5}{|}}{\overset{\overset{OH}{|}}{C}}-CH_2C_6H_5$$

(CXV)

$$\text{nH} + \underset{\underset{CH_3}{|}}{CH=CHCOC_6H_5} \xrightarrow[B=H]{A=CH_3;}$$

$$\downarrow \substack{(RCO)_2O \\ C_5H_5N}$$

$$Am-\underset{\underset{A}{|}}{CH}\underset{\underset{B}{|}}{CH}-\underset{\underset{C_6H_5}{|}}{\overset{\overset{OCOR}{|}}{C}}-CH_2C_6H_5$$

(CXVI)

$$\underset{\substack{(b) \\ HCl}}{}\quad H-\underset{\underset{CH_2N(CH_3)_2}{|}}{\overset{\overset{\overset{C_6H_5}{|}}{C=CHC_6H_5}}{\overset{|}{C^3}}}-CH_3 \xrightarrow{O_3} H-\underset{\underset{CH_2N(CH_3)_2}{|}}{\overset{\overset{COC_6H_5}{|}}{C^3}}-CH_3 \xrightarrow[H_2O_2]{(F_3CCO)_2O} H-\underset{\underset{CH_2N(CH_3)_2}{|}}{\overset{\overset{OCOC_6H_5}{|}}{C^3}}-CH_3$$

$$\qquad\qquad\qquad (-) \qquad\qquad\qquad (-) \qquad\qquad\qquad D-(-)$$

$$\qquad\qquad\qquad\qquad\qquad\qquad (CXVII) \qquad\qquad\qquad (CXVIII)$$

$$C_6H_5CH_2\overset{1}{\underset{\underset{\underset{CH_2N(CH_3)_2}{|}}{\overset{|}{\underset{H}{\diagup}\overset{|}{C^3}\diagdown CH_3}}}{\overset{\overset{OCOC_2H_5}{|}}{\underset{}{}\overset{2}{C^2}}}}C_6H_5 \xrightarrow[\text{steps}]{\substack{(c) \\ 2}} C_6H_5CH_2-\underset{\underset{\underset{CH_2}{||}}{\overset{|}{C-CH_3}}}{\overset{\overset{OCOC_2H_5}{|}}{C^2}}-C_6H_5 \xrightarrow[\text{steps}]{3} C_6H_5CH_2-\underset{\underset{COOH}{|}}{\overset{\overset{OH}{|}}{C^2}}-C_6H_5$$

$$(+)-(2S:3R) \qquad\qquad\qquad\qquad\qquad (+) \qquad\qquad\qquad\qquad (-)$$

$$d\text{-propoxyphene}$$

$$\underset{\text{steps}}{\overset{2}{\diagdown}}$$

$$C_6H_5CH_2-\underset{\underset{COOCH_3}{|}}{\overset{\overset{H}{|}}{C^2}}-C_6H_5 \xleftarrow[\text{steps}]{3} C_6H_5CH_2-\underset{\underset{CH_2I}{|}}{\overset{\overset{H}{|}}{C^2}}-C_6H_5 \xrightarrow{[H]} C_6H_5CH_2-\underset{\underset{CH_3}{|}}{\overset{\overset{H}{|}}{C^2}}-C_6H_5$$

$$\qquad (+) \qquad\qquad\qquad\qquad (+) \qquad\qquad\qquad\qquad L-(+)$$

$$\qquad\qquad\qquad\qquad\qquad\qquad\qquad\qquad\qquad\qquad (CXIX)$$

SYNTHESIS AND CONFIGURATIONAL STUDIES
SCHEME 11

reviewed in Table XII. *dl*-Propoxyphene (No. 1) was about equal to codeine in rats and somewhat less potent by the hot-plate procedure in mice. It showed low physical dependence capacity in monkeys (*13*). The (+)-isomer (No. 2) possessed all of the analgetic activity of the racemate, and the (−)-

TABLE XII

3-Phenyl-3-acyloxybutylamine Derivatives (Propoxyphene Family)

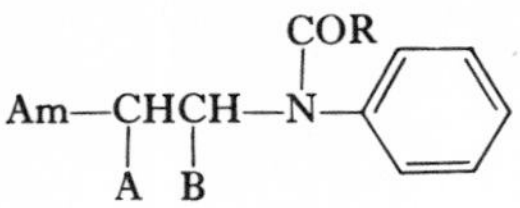

$$\text{Am—CHCH—N} \overset{\text{COR}}{\underset{\overset{|}{\text{A}}\ \ \overset{|}{\text{B}}}{\Big\langle}\ \rangle}$$

No.	Am	A	B	R	Activity[a]	References
	Meperidine				1.0	
	Codeine				0.8	
1.	$(CH_3)_2N$	H	CH_3	C_2H_5 (dl-α-; propoxyphene)	0.4 (0.7[332])	331–333, 339
2.	$(CH_3)_2N$	H	CH_3	$C_2H_5[(+)$-α]	1.3	334, 336, 338
3.	$(CH_3)_2N$	H	CH_3	$C_2H_5[(-)$-α]	0[b]	334, 340, 341
4.	$(CH_3)_2N$	H	CH_3	C_2H_5 (dl, β-)	0[331]	331
5.	$(CH_3)_2N$	H	CH_3	$CH_3[(+)$-α]	1.9	331, 339
6.	$C_4H_8N^c$	H	CH_3	C_2H_5(dl-α)	ca. 1.0[331]	331, 339
7.	$C_4H_8N^c$	H	CH_3	CH_3 (dl-α)	2.0	331, 339

[a] Unless otherwise noted by superscript citation of the appropriate reference, the analgetic activity, compared to meperidine, is taken from the Eddy hot-plate data in mice (13, 56b).

[b] Has good antitussive activity.

[c] C_4H_8N = ;pyrrolidino.

isomer (No. 3) was devoid of analgetic action. The latter compound was unique in exhibiting greater antitussive activity than either the analgetic (+)-isomer or its α-racemate (340). The β-racemate (No. 4) was inactive. The resolved (+)-α-acetoxy derivative (No. 5) was more potent than meperidine, and exhibited high physical dependence capacity in monkeys (56b). This indicates that the more potent members of this series show the signs of true morphine-like actions, including the expected side effects. Propoxyphene and related derivatives, therefore, appear to be capable of forming the stereospecific drug-receptor complex postulated for the potent analgetics. The pyrrolidino compounds (Nos. 6 and 7) represent the only variation in the amino function which retained analgetic activity. The acetoxy derivative (No. 7) was, similarly (to No. 5), more active than the propionoxy derivative and it showed intermediate physical dependence capacity in monkeys (56b). A number of closely related derivatives were less active (331, 340). These included piperidino and morpholino analogs of propoxyphene. Branched-chain analogs with an ethyl group at position (B), and analogs with the branched methyl in the position (A) corresponding to the methadone-type isomer have also been synthesized. A few compounds with substituents on the aromatic rings, such as methyl or chloro, have been prepared, but apparently are less interesting.

Several interesting new analogs of propoxyphene have been synthesized recently. The pyridyl analog (CXX), described by deStevens *et al.* (*342*), was found to be twice as potent as *d*-propoxyphene in animals. Replacement of the other phenyl group (at C-2) of propoxyphene with the 2-pyridyl group gave an inactive compound. This is probably the aromatic ring specifically involved in a morphine-like drug-receptor complex, and its alteration appears to be undesirable. Structures (CXXI) and (CXXII) represent

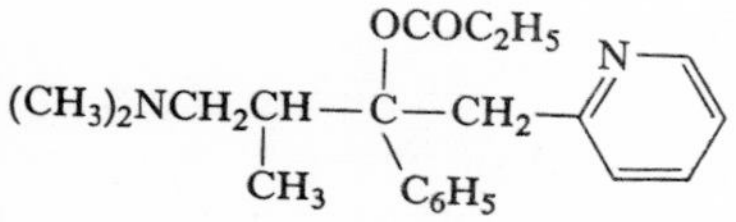

$$(CH_3)_2NCH_2CH-\overset{\overset{\displaystyle OCOC_2H_5}{|}}{\underset{\underset{\displaystyle C_6H_5}{|}}{\overset{|}{C}}}-CH_2-$$

CH₃

(CXX)

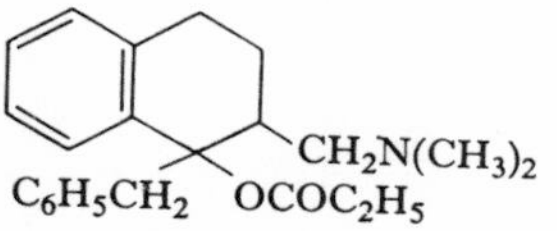

(CXXI)

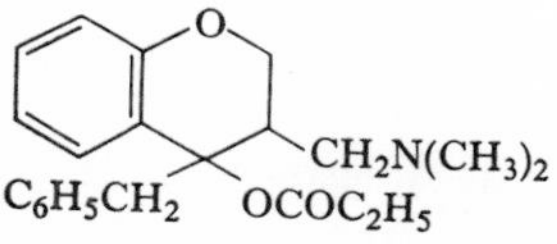

$C_6H_5CH_2$ $OCOC_2H_5$ $CH_2N(CH_3)_2$

(CXXII)

$C_6H_5CH_2$ $OCOC_2H_5$ $CH_2N(CH_3)_2$

cyclized propoxyphene analogs that have been independently investigated by two different laboratories. Patchett and Giarrusso (*343*) reported the tetrahydronaphthalene derivative (CXXI) was an analgetic agent equipotent with *d*-propoxyphene, but that the onset of tolerance was remarkably fast. Thus, this new series also appears to qualify as morphine-like, both structurally and from its pharmacological actions. The acetoxy analog of CXXI was somewhat more potent, similar to the enhancement found in the propoxyphene series. deStevens *et al.* (*342*) also studied this compound, separated the two diastereomeric racemates, and found that analgetic activity was found in only one isomer. Furthermore, these authors found the 1-(2-picolyl) analog of CXXI, obtained as only one isomer, was 5–10 times more potent than morphine by the tail-flick method. This substance exhibited high physical dependence capacity in monkeys (*56c*). The chromane derivative (CXXII) was less active (0.3–0.5 that of codeine) than CXXI (*342*, *343*), and 5- and 7-membered analogs of CXXI were less interesting than CXXI (*343*). Replacement of the 4-benzyl group in CXXII with the 4-(2-picolyl) moiety again increased the analgetic potency (to 2 times that of codeine) (*342*). This change has produced more potent compounds in three

261

different series of derivatives related to propoxyphene. Thiachromane analogs were less interesting (*342*). All of these compounds were synthesized by methods entirely analogous to procedures used for the preparation of propoxyphene (Scheme 11).

3. *Clinical Evaluation*

Propoxyphene (Table XII, No. 1) is the principal compound of this family that has been studied intensively in animals and in man. The initial clinical trials were conducted by Gruber and co-workers (*7, 333*), and they indicated 50 mg of *dl*-propoxyphene was equivalent to 32.5 mg of codeine given orally to patients with slight to moderate pain. Since then, the (+)-isomer has been the form of the drug which has generally been used for therapeutic purposes as an analgesic. However, the metabolic fate of *dl*-propoxyphene, labeled with the $C^{14}H_3N$ group, has been studied in rats and humans (*344*). The principal metabolic transformation was removal of one of the *N*-methyl groups, as evidenced by the production of $C^{14}O_2$ and the isolation of the dinitrophenyl derivative of *N*-demethylpropoxyphene from urine. The rate of metabolic demethylation of propoxyphene was considerably slower than that of meperidine.

d-Propoxyphene was as effective as codeine when equal doses were given orally for chronic pain (*7*). At the 65 mg dose, the side effects with *d*-propoxyphene were usually less than those with codeine. The addiction liability of *dl*- and *d*-propoxyphene was substantially less than that of codeine (*345*), and on this basis the drug has been exempted from opiate regulations in the United States (*346*). *d*-Propoxyphene has become very widely accepted as an orally effective, non-narcotic analgetic agent for general clinical use. The recommended dose is 32 or 65 mg orally. Following the initial clinical trials (7), a variety of reports have appeared (*347–354*), and increasingly *d*-propoxyphene has become a reference agent for comparison with newer drugs, both with respect to analgetic activity and associated side effects. *d*-Propoxyphene must be classified with the morphine-like agents, but it possesses a very practical combination of moderately potent analgetic activity without serious addiction liability hazard or other important side effects.

More recently, the (−)-isomer, or *l*-propoxyphene, has been studied as a clinical antitussive agent (*355, 356*). The (−)-isomer was more potent than the *dl*-compound, or the analgetic (+)-isomer. *l*-Propoxyphene-2-naphthalenesulfonate and *l*-propoxyphene oxide hydrochloride were also active (*356*). The recommended antitussive dose of *l*-propoxyphene is 50–100 mg of the 2-naphthalenesulfonate.

VI. Nitrogen Analog Derivatives
(Phenampromide Family)

This family of basic anilides was conceived as a flexible model of the methadone-isomethadone (or meperidine) series of analgetics in which the quaternary carbon atom and one of its attached phenyl groups was replaced by nitrogen. Such compounds retain the steric requirements postulated for the potent analgetics, and would be expected to fit the same analgetic receptor as methadone (or morphine, etc.). These structures were readily prepared, and in 1959 Wright *et al.* (*357*) described two members of a new series of basic anilides, phenampromide (CXXIII) and diampromide (CXXIV), which were selected for clinical trial on the basis of promising results in pharmacological evaluation. Phenampromide was found to approximate the

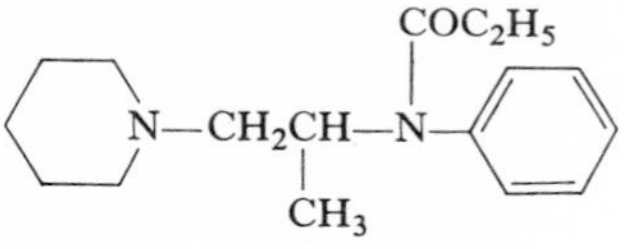

(CXXIII) 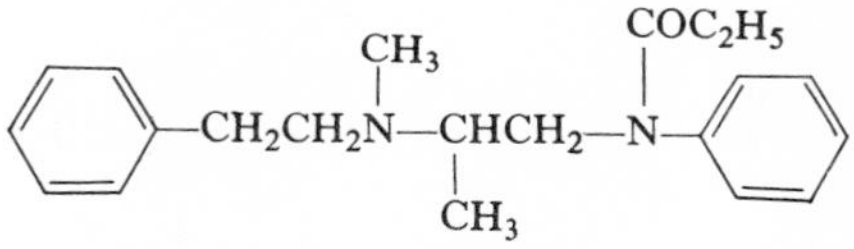   (CXXIV)

potency of meperidine in rats and diampromide approached the potency of morphine (*358*). Clinical results indicated that both compounds were narcotic-type analgetics. Both structural analogy and a spectrum of actions qualitatively similar to morphine thus established this family as belonging to the morphine-like analgetics.

The basic anilides (CXXVI) were readily obtained by acylation of the appropriately substituted ethylene and propylene diamines (CXXV) (*359*). The straight chain ethylenediamines were obtained by the well known alkylation of an aniline with a *tert*-aminoethyl chloride. Branched-chain alkylene diamines of unequivocal structure were prepared by lithium aluminium hydride reduction of amides of known structure. A number of end products containing a variety of phenalkyl groups attached to the basic nitrogen were obtained by alkylation of the common intermediate, N-(2-methylaminopropyl)propionanilide. The latter compound was obtained by hydrogenolysis of the corresponding benzylmethylamino derivative.

Resolution of phenampromide was accomplished with either (−)-malic acid or (+)-tartaric acid (*359*). Diampromide could not be resolved directly but its enantiomers were obtained by resolution of N^2-benzyl-N^2-methyl-N^1-phenyl-1,2-propanediamine and conversion to diampromide by two slightly different routes (*360*). The configurations of the analgetically less active (−)-enantiomer of diampromide and of (−)-N-(2-benzylmethylamino-propyl)propionanilide (inactive) have been related to D-(−)-alanine by

263

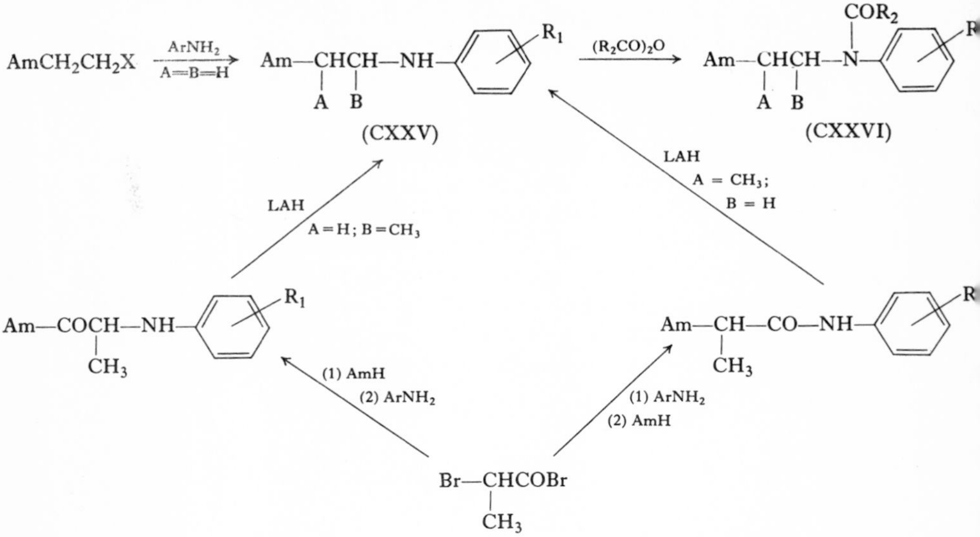

Portoghese (*361, 362*). The active enantiomers must therefore be related to L-(+)-alanine. These results were unexpected since the more active enantiomers of the methadone and thiambutene families have the D-configuration. Scheme 12 is used to establish these configurations as outlined on p. 265.

1. Structure-Activity Relationships

Structure-activity relationships in this series formed a consistent pattern, and are illustrated by the compounds reviewed in Table XIII. *dl*-Phenampromide (Table XIII, No. 1) was found to approximate the potency of codeine in mice and meperidine in rats. When the racemate was resolved, separation of activity was not complete (Nos. 2 and 3). The (+)-isomer, with lower analgetic activity, also showed good antitussive activity. Analgetic activity was particularly sensitive to changes in the alkylene chain. For example, phenampromide, with the isomethadone-type chain was a potent analgetic, but the isomeric N-(2-piperidinopropyl)propionanilide, with the methadone-type alkylene chain, was virtually devoid of analgetic activity. Optimum activity was obtained with the propionyl group in the acyl portion of the anilide moiety. Substituents on the anilide ring generally reduced activity. The aliphatic *tert*-amino group could be varied somewhat with retention of activity, but the piperidino group gave the best results. Ethyl-N-(2-ethylmethylaminoethyl)carbanilate (No .4) may be considered a nitrogen analog derivative derived from meperidine by replacing the quater-

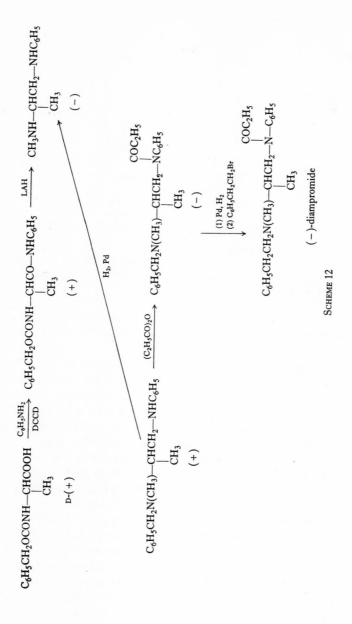

SCHEME 12

TABLE XIII

BASIC ANILIDE DERIVATIVES

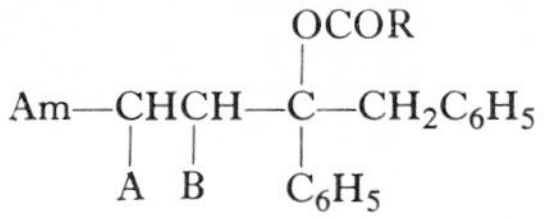

$$\begin{array}{c} \text{OCOR} \\ | \\ \text{Am—CHCH—C—CH}_2\text{C}_6\text{H}_5 \\ |\quad|\quad\;| \\ \text{A}\;\;\text{B}\quad\text{C}_6\text{H}_5 \end{array}$$

No.	Am	A	B	R	Activity[a]	References
	Meperidine				1.0	
1.	$(CH_3)_2N$	H	CH_3	C_2H_5 (dl-phenampromide)	0.7	357–359, 363
2.	$(CH_3)_2N$	H	CH_3	C_2H_5 (−)	1.1[359]	357–359, 363
3.	$(CH_3)_2N$	H	CH_3	C_2H_5 (+)	0.3[359]	357–359, 363
4.	$C_2H_5(CH_3)N$	H	H	OC_2H_5	0.1[359]	359
5.	$C_6H_5CH_2CH_2(CH_3)N$	CH_3	H	C_2H_5 (dl-diampromide)	4.0	357, 359, 364
6.	$p\text{-NH}_2C_6H_4CH_2CH_2(CH_3)N$	CH_3	H	C_2H_5	0.8[359]	359, 364
7.	$C_6H_5CH_2(CH_3)N$	CH_3	H	C_2H_5	2.3	359, 364
8.	$p\text{-ClC}_6H_4CH_2(CH_3)N$	CH_3	H	C_2H_5	1.9	359, 364
9.	$m\text{-CH}_3C_6H_4CH_2(CH_3)N$	CH_3	H	C_2H_5	5.5[359]	359, 364

[a] Unless otherwise noted by superscript citation of the appropriate reference, the analgetic activity, compared to meperidine, is taken from the Eddy hot-plate data in mice (13, 56a).

nary C-4 atom with nitrogen (and opening the piperidine ring). This series showed poor analgetic activity compared to codeine, meperidine, and the anilides.

dl-Diampromide (Table XIII, No. 5) illustrates the general finding that introduction of a phenalkyl group on the basic nitrogen significantly increased analgetic activity in many cases. This parallels the pattern found in the meperidine series. The best activity in the phenalkyl series was always found when the alkylene chain was analogous to that of methadone. A variety of phenalkyl derivatives with a considerable range of potency is illustrated by compounds 5–9 in Table XIII. Additional analogs with oxyalkyl substituents attached to the basic nitrogen, such as phenoxyalkyl and ethoxyalkyl, have also been prepared and show good activity (365).

This series of basic anilides and related derivatives has also been studied extensively in Japan (366–374). Ethanesulfonyl analogs of the acyl moiety (367, 371, 374), and replacement of the benzene ring with heterocyclic rings, including thiophene (373), thiazole (373), and pyridine (373, 375) have been described. Basic anilides with the acyl moiety derived from phenylacetic (or mandelic) acid have also been described as narcotics and analgetics (*376*). 1-(1-Methyl-2-dimethylaminoethyl)-3-phenylindole has been described as a member of a series of codeine-like analgetics (*377*). This is a nitrogen analog in which the indole nitrogen is the central atom of the generalized analgetic structure.

Two additional types of nitrogen analog derivatives are illustrated by CXXVII and CXXVIII. The 3,4-dihydro-2-quinolone derivative (CXXVII was a member of a series of cyclized basic anilide analogs which had the same

(CXXVII)   (CXXVIII)

order of antipyretic and analgetic activity as aminopyrine (*378*). This compound also had antitussive activity somewhat less than that of codeine phosphate. The basic anilide (CXXVIII), named fenatyl (or phenatyl), is the prototype of a new series developed by Janssen (*11a, b, 379*). This compound is a potent morphine-like analgetic with the usual concomitant side effects. It was found to be about 270 times more potent than morphine (when subcutaneously injected in rats), and had a more rapid onset of action and shorter duration. From its pharmacological actions it would, therefore, appear to be capable of forming an excellent complex with the stereospecific receptor postulated for analgetic actions. However, the three carbon atoms between the basic nitrogen and the tertiary anilide nitrogen are a significant modification of the usual two carbonalkylene chain found in the majority of the morphine-like analgetics. *N*-(3-Dialkylaminopropyl)anilides related to phenampromide were inactive. Fenatyl is another example which suggests that potent morphine-like actions may be found in molecules less closely related to the previously postulated structural requirements for analgetics than thought possible. This appears to be particularly true with respect to the length and composition of the alkylene chain, and may require additional modification of the optimum dimensions and arrangement of the stereospecific receptor postulated for analgetic activity. The general pharmacologic properties of fenatyl citrate have been reported (*380, 381*), and it has been studied clinically in combination with a butyrophenone (a central nervous system depressant) derivative and nitrous oxide for general anesthesia (*382*).

Both phenampromide and diampromide have been evaluated clinically in man. Although these compounds showed very low physical dependence liability in monkeys (*13,*) they were judged to be narcotic-type analgetics in man with sufficient addiction liability to warrant control as opiates (*383*). Phenampromide, 25–50 mg by injection, approached but did not equal the pain relief afforded by 10 mg. of morphine in postoperative patients (*384*). It was relatively ineffective by mouth (*385*). (+)-Phenampromide-(+)-tartrate was tried clinically as a moderate potency antitussive agent (*359*).

REFERENCES

1. A. H. Beckett and A. F. Casy, *J. Pharm. Pharmacol.* **6**, 986 (1954).
2. O. J. Braenden, N. B. Eddy, and H. Halbach, *Bull. World Health Organ.* **13**, 937 (1955).
3. O. Eisleb and O. Schaumann, *Deut. med. Wochschr.* **65**, 967 (1939).
4. F. Bergel and A. L. Morrison, *Quart. Rev.* (*London*) **2**, 349 (1948).
5. O. J. Braenden and P. O. Wolff, *Bull. World Health Organ.* **10**, 1003 (1954).
6. N. B. Eddy, H. Halbach, and O. J. Braenden, *Bull. World Health Organ.* **14**, 353 (1956).
7. N. B. Eddy, H. Halbach, and O. J. Braenden, *Bull. World Health Organ.* **17**, 569 (1957).
8. E. L. May, *in* "Medicinal Chemistry" (A. Burger, ed.), 2nd ed., p. 311. Wiley (Interscience), New York, 1960.
9. A. H. Beckett and A. F. Casy, *in* "Progress in Medicinal Chemistry" (G. P. Ellis and G. B. West, eds.), Vol. 2, p. 43. Butterworths, London, and Washington, D.C., 1962
10. N. B. Eddy, *Chem. & Ind.* (*London*), p. 1462 (1959).
11a. P. A. J. Janssen, *Brit. J. Anaesthesia* **34**, 260 (1962).
11b. P. A. J. Janssen, *Anaesthesist* **11**, 1 (1962).
12. S. Pfeifer, *Pharmazie* **17**, 189 (1962).
13. L. B. Mellett and L. A. Woods, *in* "Progress in Drug Research" (E. Jucker, ed.), Vol. 5, p. 155. Birkhäuser, Basel, 1963.
14. "The Merck Index", 7th ed., p. 646. Merck & Co., Rahway, New Jersey, 1960.
15. A. H. Beckett and A. F. Casy, *Nature* **173**, 1231 (1954).
16. O. Eisleb, *Chem. Ber.* **74**, 1433 (1941).
17. P. A. J. Janssen, U.S. Patent 3,004,977 (October 17, 1961); *Chem. Abstr.* **56**, 12861 (1962).
18. T. D. Perrine and N. B. Eddy, *J. Org. Chem.* **21**, 125 (1956).
19. R. L. Clark, A. A. Pessolano, J. Weijlard, and K. Pfister, 3rd, *J. Am. Chem. Soc.* **75**, 4963 (1953).
20. R. A. Millar and R. P. Stephenson, *Brit. J. Pharmacol.* **11**, 27 (1956).
21. J. Weijlard, O. D Orahovats, A. P. Sullivan, Jr., G. Purdue, F. K. Heath, and K. Pfister, 3rd, *J. Am. Chem. Soc.* **78**, 2342 (1956).
22. B. Elpern, L. N. Gardner, and L. Grumbach, *J. Am. Chem. Soc.* **79**, 1951 (1957).
23. N. B. Eddy and D. Leimbach, *J. Pharmacol. Exptl. Therap.* **107**, 385 (1953).
24. R. H. Thorp and E. Walton, *J. Chem. Soc.* p. 559 (1948).
25. K. Pfister, 3rd and A. A. Pessolano (to Merck), U.S. Patent 2,947,753 (August 2, 1960); *Chem. Abstr.* **55**, 12427 (1961).
26. B. Elpern (to Sterling Drug), U.S. Patent 3,109,004 (October 29, 1963).

27. P. A. J. Janssen and N. B. Eddy, *J. Med. Pharm. Chem.* **2**, 31 (1960).
28. N. V. Smirnova, A. P. Arendaruk, D. D. Smolin, and A. P. Skoldinov, *Med. Prom. SSSR* **12**, No. 7, 31 (1958); *Chem. Abstr.* **55**, 13421 (1961).
29a. Merck & Co., British Patent 815,808 (July 1, 1959); *Chem. Abstr.* **54**, 1559 (1960).
29b. Merck & Co., British Patent 815,926 (July 1, 1959); *Chem. Abstr.* **54**, 1559 (1960).
30. B. Elpern, P. Carabateas, A. E. Soria, L. N. Gardner, and L. Grumbach, *J. Am. Chem. Soc.* **81**, 3784 (1959).
31. R. Dahlbom, B. Bjorkquist, and S. Ross, *Acta Chem. Scand.* **17**, 227 (1963).
32. F. A. Cutler, Jr. and J. F. Fisher (to Merck & Co.) U.S. Patent 2,962,501 (November 29, 1960); *Chem. Abstr.* **55**, 10475 (1961).
33. C. H. Boehringer Sohn, Belgian Patent 627,675 (July 30, 1963).
34. Boehringer Ingelheim Ltd., South African Patent 62/5001 (May 15, 1963).
35. K. Pfister, 3rd (to Merck & Co.), U.S. Patent 2,966,492 (December 27, 1960); *Chem. Abstr.* **55**, 11440 (1961).
36. B. Elpern (to Sterling Drug), U.S. Patent 3,097,208 (July 9, 1963).
37. P. A. J. Janssen, A. H. M. Jageneau, P. J. A. Demoen, C. van de Westeringh, A. H. M. Raeymaekers, M. S. J. Wouters, S. Sanczuk, B. K. F. Hermans, and J. L. M. Loomans, *J. Med. Pharm. Chem.* **1**, 105 (1959).
38. P. A. J. Janssen, A. H. M. Jageneau, P. J. A. Demoen, C. van de Westeringh, J. H. M. de Cannière, A. H. M. Raeymaekers, M. S. J. Wouters, S. Sanczuk, and B. K. F. Hermans, *J. Med. Pharm. Chem.* **1**, 309 (1959).
39. P. A. J. Janssen, A. H. M. Jageneau, P. J. A. Demoen, C. van de Westeringh, J. H. M. de Cannière, A. H. M. Raeymaekers, M. S. J. Wouters, S. Sanczuk, and B. K. F. Hermans, *J. Med. Pharm. Chem.* **2**, 271 (1960).
40. A. Pohland (to E. Lilly & Co.), U.S. Patent 2,951,080 (August 30, 1960); *Chem. Abstr.* **55**, 4540 (1961).
41. R. H. Mazur, *J. Org. Chem.* **26**, 962 (1961).
42. B. Elpern, P. M. Carabateas, A. E. Soria, and L. Grumbach, *J. Org. Chem.* **25**, 2045 (1960).
43. B. Elpern (to Sterling Drug), U.S. Patent 2,901,487 (August 25, 1959); *Chem. Abstr.* **54**, 1555 (1960).
44. R. J. Anderson, P. M. Frearson and E. S. Stern, *J. Chem. Soc.* p. 4088 (1956).
45. P. M. Frearson and E. S. Stern, *J. Chem. Soc.* p. 3065 (1958).
46. B. G. Boggiano, V. Petrow, O. Stephenson, and A. M. Wild, *J. Chem. Soc.* p. 1143 (1959).
47. C. Bianchi and A. David, *J. Pharm. Pharmacol.* **12**, 449 (1960).
48. E. S. Stern and R. L. Watt (to Macfarlan & Co., Ltd.), U.S. Patent 2,960,507 (November 15, 1960); *Chem. Abstr.* **55**, 18779 (1961).
49. R. E. Lister, *Brit. J. Pharmacol.* **15**, 254 (1960).
50. P. M. Frearson, D. G. Hardy, and E. S. Stern, *J. Chem. Soc.* p. 2103 (1960).
51. P. M. Frearson and E. S. Stern, *J. Chem. Soc.* p. 3062 (1958).
52. P. M. Frearson and E. S. Stern (to Macfarlan & Co., Ltd.), British Patent 797,448 (July 2, 1958); *Chem. Abstr.* **54**, 583 (1960).
53. H. G. Morren, Belgian Patent 558,883 (July 31, 1957); *Chem. Abstr.* **54**, 1555 (1960).
54. E. Merlevede and S. Levis, *Arch. Intern. Pharmacodyn.* **115**, 213 (1958).
55. Research N.V., British Patent 941,748 (November 13, 1963).
56a. G. A. Deneau and M. H. Seevers, *Bull. Drug Addiction and Narcotics*, **No. 23**, *Addendum 1.* Natl. Acad. Sci., Natl. Res. Council, Div. Med. Sci., Washington, D.C., 1961.
56b. G. A. Deneau and M. H. Seevers, *Bull. Drug Addiction and Narcotics*, **No. 24**, *Addendum 2.* Natl. Acad. Sci., Natl. Res. Council, Div. Med. Sci., Washington, D.C., 1962.
56c. G. A. Deneau and M. H. Seevers, *Bull. Drug Addiction and Narcotics* **No. 25**, *Adden-*

dum 1. Natl. Acad. Sci., Natl. Res. Council, Div. Med. Sci., Washington, D.C., 1963.

57. C. H. Boehringer Sohn, Belgian Patents 613,759-761 (August 9, 1962); *Chem. Abstr.* **58**, 512 (1963).

58. M. Protiva, J. O. Jilek, J. Pomykacek, J. Jirkovsky, and Z. J. Vejdelek, *Collection Czech. Chem. Commun.* **28**, 2627 (1963).

59. P. A. J. Janssen, U.S. Patent 3,012,030 (December 5, 1961); *Chem. Abstr.* **56**, 12861 (1962).

60. P. A. J. Janssen, U.S. Patent 3,004,977 (October 17, 1961); *Chem. Abstr.* **56**, 12861 (1962).

61. P. A. J. Janssen, Belgian Patent 576,331 (March 31, 1959); *Chem. Abstr.* **54**, 4623 (1960).

62. F. A. Cutler, Jr. and J. M. Chemerda (to Merck & Co.), U.S. Patent 2,897,204 (July 28, 1959); *Chem. Abstr.* **54**, 584 (1960).

63. B. Elpern (to Sterling Drug), U.S. Patent, 3,093,652 (June 11, 1963).

64. A. M. J. N. Blair and R. P. Stephenson, *Brit. J. Pharmacol.* **15**, 247 (1960).

65. M. R. Bell and S. Archer, *J. Am. Chem. Soc.* **82**, 4638 (1960).

66. P. A. J. Janssen A. H. Jageneau, and J. Huygens, *J. Med. Pharm. Chem.* **1**, 299 (1959).

67. Sterling Drug, British Patent 880,139 (October 18, 1961); *Chem. Abstr.* **56**, 12860 (1962).

68. H. S. Lowrie (to G. D. Searle), U.S. Patent 3,112,308 (November 26, 1963).

69. J. R. Geigy, Irish Patent 268/63 (March 31, 1963).

70a. E. L. Way and T. K. Adler, *Bull. World Health Organ.* **26**, 261 (1962).

70b. E. L. Way and T. K. Adler, *Bull. World Health Organ.* **27**, 359 (1962).

70c. E. L. Way and T. K. Adler, *Pharmacol. Rev.* **12**, 383 (1960).

71. A. H. Beckett, A. F. Casy, and N. J. Harper, *J. Pharm. Pharmacol.* **8**, 874 (1956).

72a. J. Axelrod, *Science* **124**, 263 (1956).

72b. J. Axelrod, *J. Pharmacol. Exptl. Therap.* **117**, 322 (1956).

72c. J. Axelrod and J. Cochin, *J. Pharmacol. Exptl. Therap.* **121**, 107 (1957).

73. N. B. Eddy, L. E. Lee, Jr., and C. Harris, *Bull. World Health Organ.* **20**, 1245 (1959).

74. C. M. Helsel and H. J. Mann, *Penn. Med. J.* **63**, 1790 (1960).

75. E. H. Hanekamp, G. E. Magaletta, H. G. Lankford, and L. J. Hartnett, *Southern Med. J.* **54**, 274 (1961).

76. A. F. Pasquet, F. MacDonald, and W. James, *Can. Anaesthesia Soc. J.* **9**, 131 (1962).

77. L. J. Cass and W. S. Frederik, *Current Therap. Res.* **5**, 81 (1963).

78. T. DeKornfeld and L. Lasagna, *Federation Proc.* **18**, 382 (1959).

79. T. DeKornfeld and L. Lasagna, *J. Chronic Diseases* **12**, 252 (1960).

80. M. S. Sadove, A. K. Sen, and M. J. Schiffrin, *Current Therap. Res.* **2**, 61 (1960).

81. A. R. deC. Deacock, *Brit. J. Anaesthesia* **32**, 590 (1960).

82. D. W. Molander, *Current Therap. Res.* **2**, 370 (1960).

83. M. S. Sadove and M. J. Schiffrin, *Postgrad. Med.* **29**, 346 (1961).

84. V. L. deCiutiis, *Anesthesia Analgesia Current Res.* **40**, 174 (1961).

85. W. H. L. Dornette, M. F. Poe, J. P. Jones, and B. H. Hughes, *Anesthesia Analgesia, Current Res.* **40**, 307 (1961).

86. W. A. Abruzzi, *J. New Drugs* **1**, 230 (1961).

87. A. M. Betcher, C. Yum-San, A. N. Godholm, and J. Alter, *Anesthesia Analgesia, Current Res.* **41**, 39 (1962).

88. J. I. Pretto, *Clin. Med.* **69**, 2011 (1962).

89. J. L. Weare and N. F. Westermann, *Anesthesia Analgesia, Current Res.* **42**, 334 (1963)

90. J. De Castro and M. Dupont, *Agressologie* **3**, 77 (1962).

91. A. S. Brown, *Anaesthesist* **11**, 22 (1962).

92. W. N. Rollason and J. S. Sutherland, *Anaesthesia* **18**, 16 (1963).
93. K. A. Jensen, F. Lindquist, E. Rekling, and C. G. Wolfbrandt, *Dansk Tids. Farm.* **17**, 173 (1943); *Chem. Abstr.* **39**, 2506 (1945).
94. A. Ziering and J. Lee, *J. Org. Chem.* **12**, 911 (1947).
95. A. H. Beckett, A. F. Casy, and G. Kirk, *J. Med. Pharm. Chem.* **1**, 37 (1959).
96. S. M. McElvain and M. D. Barnett, *J. Am. Chem. Soc.* **78**, 3140 (1956).
97a. I. N. Nazarov, *Izbrannye Tr. I.N. Nazarov, Akad. Nauk SSSR* p. 588 (1961); *Chem. Abstr.* **56** 8682 (1962).
97b. N. S. Prostakov and N. N. Mikheeva *Zh. Obshch. Khim.* **31** 108 (1961); *Chem. Abstr.* **55** 22308 (1961).
97c. O. I. Sorokin *Izv. Akad. Nauk SSSR Otd. Khim. Nauk* p. 460 (1961); *Chem. Abstr.* **55**, 22310 (1961).
98. C. J. Schmidle and R. C. Mansfield, *J. Am. Chem. Soc.* **78**, 1702 (1956).
99a. F. R. Ahmed, W. H. Barnes, and G. Kartha, *Chem. & Ind.* (*London*) p. 485 (1959).
99b. G. Kartha, F. R. Ahmed, and W. H. Barnes, *Acta Cryst.* **13**, 525 (1960); *Chem. Abstr.* **54**, 19078 (1960).
99c. G. Kartha, F. R. Ahmed, and W. H. Barnes, *Acta Cryst.* **14**, 93 (1961); *Chem. Abstr.* **56**, 2969 (1962).
100. H. Gutfreund, *in* "The Enzymes" (P. D. Boyer, H. Lardy, and K. Myrbäck, eds.) 2nd ed., Vol. 1, p. 233. Academic Press, New York, 1959.
101. F. R. Ahmed, W. H. Barnes, and L. A. Masironi, *Chem. & Ind.* (*London*) p. 97 (1962).
102. A. Ziering, A. Motchane, and J. Lee, *J. Org. Chem.* **22**, 1521 (1957).
103. S. Archer, *Am. Chem. Soc., Abstr. Papers, 133rd Meeting, San Francisco, April 1958* p. 4M.
104. A. H. Beckett, A. F. Casy, and N. J. Harper, *Chem. & Ind.* (*London*) p. 19 (1959).
105. A. H. Beckett, A. F. Casy, G. Kirk, and J. Walker, *J. Pharm. Pharmacol.* **9**, 939 (1957).
106. A. Ziering, L. Berger, S. D. Heineman, and J. Lee, *J. Org. Chem.* **12**, 894 (1947).
107. N. Itoh, *Chem. Pharm. Bull.* (*Tokyo*) **10**, 55 (1962).
108. P. M. Carabateas and L. Grumbach, *J. Med. Pharm. Chem.* **5**, 913 (1962).
109. Tanabe Seiyaku Co. Ltd., Japanese Patent 14741/63 (August 13, 1963).
110. P. A. J. Janssen, Belgian Patent 578,395 (May 30, 1959); *Chem. Abstr.* **54**, 4623 (1960).
111. A. Pohland (to E. Lilly & Co.), British Patent 824,607 (December 2, 1959); *Chem. Abstr.* **54**, 7742 (1960).
112. Wellcome Foundation Ltd., British Patent 919,124 (February 20, 1963).
113a. Dr. K. Thomae, G.m.b.H., British Patent 940,534 (October 30, 1963).
113b. C. H. Boehringer Sohn, French Patent 1914M (August 12, 1963).
114. A. H. Beckett and J. V. Greenhill, *J. Med. Pharm. Chem.* **4**, 423 (1961).
115. R. T. Major and F. Dürsch, *J. Org. Chem.* **26**, 1867 (1961).
116. A. A. Patchett and F. F. Giarrusso, *J. Med. Pharm. Chem.* **4**, 385 (1961).
117. P. M. Carabateas, W. F. Wetterau, and L. Grumbach, *J. Med. Chem.* **6**, 355 (1963).
118. P. A. J. Janssen, C. van de Westeringh, A. H. M. Jageneau, P. J. A. Demoen, B. K. F. Hermans, G. H. P. van Daele, K. H. L. Schellekens, C. A. M. van der Eycken, and C. J. E. Niemegeers, *J. Med. Pharm. Chem.* **1**, 281 (1959).
119. L. O. Randall and G. Lehman, *J. Pharmacol. Exptl. Therap.* **93**, 314 (1948).
120. H. Roberts and M. A. C. Kuck, *Can. Med. Assoc. J.* **83**, 1088 (1960).
121. A. S. Keats, J. Telford, and Y. Kurosu, *J. Pharmacol. Exptl. Therap.* **130**, 218 (1960).
122. F. F. Blicke and E.-P. Tsao, *J. Am. Chem. Soc.* **75**, 3999 (1953).
123. J. Diamond and W. F. Bruce (to Am. Home Products Corp.), U.S. Patent 2,666,050 (January 12, 1954); *Chem. Abstr.* **49**, 4031 (1955).
124a. J. Seifter, D. K. Eckfeld, I. A. Letchack, E. M. Gore, and J. M. Glassman, *Federation Proc.* **13**, 403 (1954).

271

ROBERT A. HARDY, JR. AND M. GERTRUDE HOWELL

124b. J. M. Glassman and J. Seifter, *J. Pharmacol. Exptl. Therap.* **115**, 21 (1955).

125a. A. J. Grossman, M. Golbey, W. C. Gittinger, and R. C. Batterman, *J. Am. Geriat. Soc.* **4**, 187 (1956).

125b. M. Golbey, W. C. Gittinger, and R. C. Batterman, *Federation Proc.* **14**, 344 (1955).

126. J. Diamond, W. F. Bruce, and F. T. Tyson *J. Org. Chem.* **22**, 399 (1957).

127. J. Diamond, M. Dymicky, and W. F. Bruce (to Am. Home Products Corp.), British Patent 843,924 (August 10, 1960); *Chem. Abstr.* **55**, 2705 (1961).

128a. J. Diamond and W. F. Bruce (to Am. Home Products Corp.), U.S. Patent 2,740,777 (April 3, 1956); *Chem. Abstr.* **50**, 15598 (1956).

128b. J. Diamond and W. F. Bruce (to Am. Home Products Corp.), British Patent 781,002 (August 14, 1957); *Chem. Abstr.* **52**, 9230 (1958).

129. J. Diamond and W. F. Bruce (to Am. Home Products Corp.), U.S. Patent 2,775,589 (December 25, 1956). *Chem. Abstr.* **51**, 444 (1957).

130. J. Diamond, W. F. Bruce, and F. T. Tyson, *J. Med. Chem.* **7**, 57 (1964).

131. J. Malis, *Pharmacologist* **4**, 154 (1962).

132. J. Malis, M. A. Ries, and R. J. Bradley, *Federation Proc.* **22** (2, Part 1), 248 (1963).

133. T. Baum, *Pharmacologist* **5**, 244 (1963).

134. J. Diamond, W. F. Bruce, C. Gochman, and F. T. Tyson, *J. Org. Chem.* **25**, 65 (1960).

135. J. Diamond and W. F. Bruce (to Am. Home Products Corp.), U.S. Patent 2,740,780 (April 3, 1956); *Chem. Abstr.* **50**, 15600 (1956).

136. J. Diamond and W. F. Bruce (to Am. Home Products Corp.), U.S. Patent 2,740,779 (April 3, 1956); *Chem. Abstr.* **50**, 15599 (1956).

137. S. S. Walkenstein, J. A. Macmullen, C. Knebel, and J. Seifter, *J. Am. Pharm. Assoc. Sci. Ed.* **47**, 20 (1958).

138. W. J. Fitzgerald, J. J. Carrier, and L. Carlson, *Clin. Med.* **8**, 2159 (1961).

139. P. Cinelli and M. Zucchini, *Minerva Med.* **53**, 637 (1962).

140. L. J. Cass, J. T. Laing, and W. S. Frederik, *Current Therap Res.* **3**, 289 (1961).

141. F. Bergel, N. C. Hindley, A. L. Morrison, and H. J. Rinderknecht, *J. Chem. Soc.* p. 269 (1944).

142. G. F. Woods, T. L. Heying, L. H. Schwartzman, L. H. Grenell, S. M. Gasser, W. F. Rowe, and N. C. Bolgiano, *J. Org. Chem.* **19**, 1290 (1954).

143. J. F. Cavalla, J. Davoll, M. J. Dean, C. S. Franklin, and D. M. Temple, *J. Med. Pharm. Chem.* **4**, 1 (1961).

144. J. W. Kissel and J. R. Albert, *Federation Proc.* **20**, 309 (1961).

145. L. J. Cass and W. S. Frederik, *Current Therap. Res.* **3**, 97 (1961).

146. C. V. Winder, J. Wax, B. Serrano, L. Scotti, S. P. Stackhouse, and R. H. Wheelock, *J. Pharmacol. Exptl. Therap.* **133**, 117 (1961).

147. E. L. Eliel, "Stereochemistry of Carbon Compounds," p. 251. McGraw-Hill, New York, 1962.

148a. Y.-H. Wu, W. A. Gould, W. G. Lobeck, Jr., H. R. Roth, and R. F. Feldkamp, *J. Med. Pharm. Chem.* **5**, 752 (1962).

148b. Y.-H. Wu, W. G. Lobeck, Jr., and R. F. Feldkamp, *J. Med. Pharm. Chem.* **5**, 762 (1962).

149. J. F. Cavalla and J. Davoll (to Parke, Davis & Co.), British Patent 862,513 (March 8, 1961); *Chem. Abstr.* **55**, 19950 (1961).

150. Mead Johnson & Co., British Patent 874,216 (August 2, 1961); *Chem. Abstr.* **56**, 4734 (1962).

151. J. F. Cavalla, R. A. Selway, J. Wax, L. Scotti, and C. V. Winder, *J. Med. Pharm. Chem.* **5**, 441 (1962).

152. J. W. Kissel, J. R. Albert, and G. C. Boxill, *J. Pharmacol. Exptl. Therap.* **134**, 332 (1961).

153. J. R. Albert, A. G. Wheeler, H. C. Hawkins, and J. W. Kissel, *Pharmacologist* **3**, 66 (1961).

154. J. H. Weikel and J. A. LaBudde, *J. Pharmacol. Exptl. Therap.* **138**, 392 (1962).

155. L. J. Cass and W. S. Frederik, *J. Pharmacol. Exptl. Therap.* **139**, 172 (1963).

156. S. R. Splitter, *Current Therap. Res.* **3**, 472 (1961).

157. R. C. Batterman, G. J. Mowratoff, and J. E. Kaufman, *Am. J. Med. Sci.* **247**, 62 (1964).

158. A. W. D. Avison and A. L. Morrison, *J. Chem. Soc.* p. 1469 (1950).

159. B. Elpern, P. M. Carabateas, and L. Grumbach, *J. Org. Chem.* **26**, 4728 (1961).

160. B. Elpern (to Sterling Drug), U.S. Patent 3,096,335 (July 2, 1963).

161a. Dr. Karl Thomae, G.m.b.H., British Patent 882,891 (November 22, 1961); *Chem. Abstr.* **56**, 11575 (1962).

161b. Dr. Karl Thomae, G.m.b.H., French Patent M831 (October 23, 1961); *Chem. Abstr.* **58**, 9032 (1963).

162. B. Elpern (to Sterling Drug), U.S. Patent 3,043,844 (July 10, 1962); *Chem. Abstr.* **54**, 16753 (1962).

163. E. S. Stern (to J. F. Macfarlan), British Patent 841,120 (July 13, 1960); *Chem. Abstr.* **55**, 3620 (1961).

164. C. H. Boehringer Sohn, Belgian Patent 614,688 (September 5, 1962); *Chem. Abstr.* **58**, 11334 (1963).

165a. P. A. J. Janssen (to Res. Lab. Dr. C. Janssen), U.S. Patent 3,097,209 (July 9, 1963).

165b. Res. Lab. Janssen, British Patent 931,789 (July 17, 1963).

166. A. F. Casy and A. H. Beckett, *J. Pharm. Pharmacol.* **13**, 161-T (1961).

167. A. F. Casy, A. H. Beckett, G. H. Hall, and D. K. Vallance, *J. Med. Pharm. Chem.* **4**, 535 (1961).

168. A. F. Casy, A. H. Beckett, and N. A. Armstrong, *Tetrahedron* **16**, 85 (1961).

169. A. H. Beckett, Australian Patent 774/61 (February 10, 1963).

170. P. A. J. Janssen (to N. V. Res. Lab. Dr. C. Janssen), Belgian Patent 615,349 (September 20, 1962); *Chem. Abstr.* **59**, 1601 (1963).

171. S. M. McElvain and D. H. Clemens, *J. Am. Chem. Soc.* **80**, 3915 (1958).

172a. S. M. McElvain, U.S. Patent 2,892,842 (June 30, 1959); *Chem. Abstr.* **54**, 4624 (1960).

172b. S. M. McElvain, British Patent 853,814 (November 9, 1960); *Chem. Abstr.* **55**, 13451 (1961).

173. E. S. Stern, R. L. Watt, and D. G. Hardy (to J. F. Macfarlan), U.S. Patent 3,108,111 (October 22, 1963).

174. N. J. Harper and A. B. Simmonds, *J. Med. Pharm. Chem.* **1**, 181 (1959).

175. K. Schulte and H.-G. Kraft (to E. Merck, Darmstadt), U.S. Patent 3,100,205 (August 6, 1963).

176. N. J. Harper and S. E. Fullerton, *J. Med. Pharm. Chem.* **4**, 297 (1961).

177. G. Deltour, J. Mercier, R. Charlier, M. Prost, F. Binon, and P. Etzensperger, *Arch. Intern. Pharmacodyn.* **142**, 493 (1963).

178. M. Prost (to Soc. Marly), U.S. Patent 3,081,309 (March 12, 1963).

179. J. Buchi, M. Prost, H. Eichenberger, and R. Lieberherr, *Helv. Chim. Acta* **35**, 1527 (1952).

180. S. Archer (to Sterling Drug), U.S. Patent 2,777,850 (January 15, 1957); *Chem. Abstr.* **51**, 12986 (1957).

181. C. M. Hofmann, and M. J. Weiss, *J. Org. Chem.* **25**, 653 (1960).

182. T. P. Carney, *in* "Medicinal Chemistry" (F. F. Blicke and R. H. Cox, eds.), Vol. III, p. 1. Wiley, New York, 1956.

ROBERT A. HARDY, JR. AND M. GERTRUDE HOWELL

183. P. A. J. Janssen, "Synthetic Analgesics" Part 1; Diphenylpropylamines. Pergamon Press, New York, 1960.
184. E. C. Kleiderer, J. B. Rice, V. Conquest, and J. H. Williams, *Report No.* PP-981, Office of the Publication Board, Dept. of Commerce, Washington, D.C. 1945.
185. A. H. Beckett, *J. Pharm. Pharmacol.* **8**, 848 (1956).
186. M. Bockmühl and G. Ehrhart, *Ann.* **561**, 52 (1949).
187. E. M. Schultz, C. M. Robb, and J. M. Sprague, *J. Am. Chem. Soc.* **69**, 188, 2454 (1947).
188. N. R. Easton, J. H. Gardner, and J. R. Stevens, *J. Am. Chem. Soc.* **69**, 976, 2941 (1947).
189. A. A. Larsen, B. F. Tullar, B. Elpern, and J. S. Buck, *J. Am. Chem. Soc.* **70**, 4194 (1948).
190. L. C. Cheney, R. R. Smith, and S. B. Binkley, *J. Am. Chem. Soc.* **71**, 53 (1949).
191. A. H. Beckett and A. F. Casy, *J. Pharm. Pharmacol.* **7**, 204 (1955).
192. A. L. Morrison and H. Rinderknecht, *J. Chem. Soc.* pp. 1478, 1510 (1950).
193. J. Attenburrow, J. Elks, B. A. Hems, and K. N. Speyer, *J. Chem. Soc.* p. 510 (1949).
194. M. Sletzinger, E. M. Chamberlain, and M. Tishler, *J. Am. Chem. Soc.* **74**, 5619 (1952).
195. H. Ruschig and K. Schmitt, *Chem. Ber.* **88**, 875 (1955).
196. H. Ruschig and K. Schmitt (to Farbwerke Hoechst), German Patent 959,097 (February 28, 1957); *Chem. Abstr.* **53**, 11316 (1959).
197. Österreiche Stickstoffwerke A.-G., Austrian Patent 187,915 (December 10, 1956); *Chem. Abstr.* **51**, 5835 (1957).
198. R. H. Thorp, E. Walton, and P. Ofner, *Nature* **160**, 605 (1947).
199. W. R. Brode and M. W. Hill, *J. Org. Chem.* **13**, 191 (1948).
200. E. E. Howe and M. Sletzinger, *J. Am. Chem. Soc.* **71**, 2935 (1949).
201. G. Ehrhart and H. Ott (to Farbwerke Hoechst), German Patent 837,849 (May 2, 1952); *Chem. Abstr.* **51**, 14834 (1957).
202. A. A. Larsen and B. F. Tullar (to Sterling Drug) U.S. Patent 2,841,609 (July 1, 1958); *Chem. Abstr.* **53**, 2166 (1959).
203. L. Ther, E. Lindner, and G. Vogel, *Deut. Apotheker-Ztg.* **103**, 514 (1963); *Chem. Abstr.* **59**, 15819 (1963).
204. A. H. Beckett and A. F. Casy, *J. Chem. Soc.* p. 900 (1955).
205. A. H. Beckett and N. J. Harper, *J. Chem. Soc.* p. 858 (1957).
206a. B. D. Tiffany (to Upjohn), U.S. Patent 2,862,968 (December 2, 1958); *Chem. Abstr.* **53**, 16082 (1959).
206b. Upjohn Co., British Patent 793,226 (April 9, 1958); *Chem. Abstr.* **54**, 2278 (1960).
207. E. Walton, P. Ofner, and R. H. Thorp, *J. Chem. Soc.* p. 648 (1949).
208. P. Ofner, E. Walton, A. F. Green, and A. C. White, *J. Chem. Soc.* p. 2158 (1950).
209. A. H. Beckett and A. F. Casy, *J. Chem. Soc.* p. 3076 (1957).
210. D. J. Dupré, J. Elks, B. A. Hems, K. N. Speyer, and R. M. Evans, *J. Chem. Soc.* p. 500 (1949).
211. M. E. Speeter, W. M. Byrd, L. C. Cheney, and S. B. Binkley, *J. Am. Chem. Soc.* **71**, 57 (1949).
212. M. Ehrlenbach and A. Sieglitz, British Patent 685,616 (January 7, 1953); *Chem. Abstr.* **48**, 3396 (1954).
213. A. H. Beckett, A. F. Casy, N. J. Harper, and P. M. Phillips, *J. Pharm. Pharmacol.* **8**, 860 (1956).
214. B. B. Brodie and C. A. M. Hogben, *J. Pharm. Pharmacol.* **9**, 345 (1957).
215. L. B. Mellett and L. A. Woods, *Pharmacologist* **1**, 77 (1959).
216. H. Kaneto and L. B. Mellett, *Pharmacologist* **2**, 98 (1960).
217. D. E. Ames, *J. Chem. Soc.* p. 2780 (1960).

274

218. S. L. Shapiro, H. Soloway, and L. Freedman, *J. Org. Chem.* **24**, 129 (1959).
219. A. A. Patchett and F. F. Giarrusso, *J. Med. Pharm. Chem.* **4**, 403 (1961).
220. C. C. Scott, E. B. Robbins, and K. K. Chen, *J. Pharmacol. Exptl. Therap.* **93**, 282 (1948).
221. R. H. Thorp, *Brit. J. Pharmacol.* **4**, 98 (1949).
222. A. E. Light and R. V. Fanelli, *Toxicol. Appl. Pharmacol.* **2**, 504 (1960).
223. H. F. Fraser and H. Isbell, *Bull. Narcotics, U.N. Dept. Social Affairs* **14**, 25 (1962); *Chem. Abstr.* **58**, 14607 (1963).
224. E. Cope and P. O. Jones, *Brit. Med. J.* p. 211 (1959, **1**).
225. A. B. Dobkin and V. G. Criswick, *Anesthesiology* **22**, 398 (1961).
226. E. Zolata and X. Giotes, *Arch. Latrikon Epistimon* **18**, 367 (1962); *Chem. Abstr.* **57**, 12640 (1962).
227. J. W. Mostert and S. O. Rencken, *S. African Med. J.* **37**, 826 (1963).
228. A. H. Beckett and W. H. Linnell, *J. Pharm. Pharmacol.* **2**, 418, 427 (1950).
229. E. L. May and E. Mosettig, *J. Org. Chem.* **13**, 459, 663 (1948).
230. M. E. Speeter, L. C. Cheney, and S. B. Binkley, *J. Am. Chem. Soc.* **72**, 1659 (1950).
231. N. B. Eddy, E. L. May, and E. Mosettig, *J. Org. Chem.* **17**, 321 (1952).
232. E. L. May and N. B. Eddy, *J. Org. Chem.* **17**, 1210 (1952).
233. A. Pohland, H. R. Sullivan, and H. M. Lee, *Am. Chem. Soc., Abstr. Papers, 136th Meeting, Atlantic City, September 1959* p. 15-0.
234. A. Pohland (to E. Lilly), U. S. Patent 3,021,360 (February 13, 1962); *Chem. Abstr.* **57**, 4594 (1962).
235. Farbwerke Hoechst, Irish Patent 340/63 (April 15, 1963).
236. R. Baltzly, P. B. Russell, and N. B. Mehta (to Burroughs Wellcome), U.S. Patent 3,098,076 (July 16, 1963).
237. C. M. Gruber, Jr. and A. Baptisti, Jr., *Clin. Pharmacol. Therap.* **4**, 172 (1963).
238. P. A. J. Janssen, *J. Am. Chem. Soc.* **78**, 3862 (1956).
239. P. A. J. Janssen and A. H. Jageneau, *J. Pharm. Pharmacol.* **9**, 381 (1957).
240. L. C. Cheney, W. B. Wheatley, M. E. Speeter, W. M. Byrd, W. E. Fitzgibbon, W. F. Minor, and S. B. Binkley, *J. Org. Chem.* **17**, 770 (1952).
241. R. B. Moffett and B. D. Aspergren, *J. Am. Chem. Soc.* **79**, 4451, 4457, 4462 (1957).
242. P. A. J. Janssen, unpublished results (see ref. *183*).
243. N. V. Research Labs. Dr. C. Janssen, French Patent M1766 (April 8, 1963).
244. D. K. deJongh and E. G. van Proosdij-Hartzema, *J. Pharm. Pharmacol.* **9**, 730 (1957).
245. E. G. van Proosdij-Hartzema and D. K. deJongh, *Acta Physiol. Pharmacol. Neerl.* **5**, 398 (1957); *Chem. Abstr.* **55**, 25059 (1961).
246. P. A. J. Janssen and A. H. Jageneau, *J. Pharm. Pharmacol.* **10**, 14 (1958).
247. G. A. Krüger and Ph. Orth, *Anaesthesist* **8**, 11 (1959); *Chem. Abstr.* **53**, 9454 (1959).
248. P. Nanni-Costa, *Acta Anesthesiol.* **11**, 217 (1960); *Chem. Abstr.* **55**, 26227 (1961).
249. R. Soupault, J. Caroli, M. Renon, Th. Schops, and A. Charbonnier, *Therapie* **12**, 898 (1957); *Chem. Abstr.* **53**, 11660 (1959).
250. D. A. Cahal, *Brit. J. Pharmacol.* **13**, 30 (1958).
251. D. J. J. Martinez and N. M. R. O. de Martinez, *Semana Med.* (*Buenos Aires*) **113** 1169 (1958); *Chem. Abstr.* **53**, 9476 (1959).
252. L. Lasagna, T. DeKornfeld, and P. Safar, *J. Chronic Diseases* **8**, 689 (1958).
253. B. Calesnick, *J. Chronic Diseases* **10**, 58 (1959).
254. A. S. Keats, J. Telford, and Y. Kurosu, *J. Pharmacol. Exptl. Therap.* **130**, 212 (1960).
255. A. L. Kolodny, *Antibiot. Med. Clin. Therapy* **7**, 695 (1960).

256. R. O. Bauer, S. M. Free, and E. H. Bowen, Jr., *J. Pharmacol. Exptl. Therap.* **131**, 373 (1961).

257. J. M. Kapferer, *Anaesthesist* **10**, 101 (1961).

258. M. Gavend and M.-R. Gavend, *Compt. Rend. Soc. Biol.* **155**, 1977 (1961).

259. S. G. F. Matts, *Practitioner* **188**, 524 (1962).

260. M. Sabathie, *Anaesthesist* **11**, 20 (1962).

261. J. H. Gardner, N. R. Easton, and J. R. Stevens, *J. Am. Chem. Soc.* **70**, 2906 (1948).

262. A. Pohland, F. J. Marshall, and T. P. Carney, *J. Am. Chem. Soc.* **71**, 460 (1949).

263. Aspro-Nicholas, Ltd., British Patent 939,019 (October 9, 1963).

264a. H. G. Morren (to Union chimique belg. S.A.), U.S. Patent 2,832,776 (April 29, 1958); *Chem. Abstr.* **52**, 14687 (1958).

264b. H. G. Morren, British Patent 808,960 (February 11, 1959); *Chem. Abstr.* **54**, 3321 (1960).

265. M. M. Klenk, C. M. Suter, and S. Archer, *J. Am. Chem. Soc.* **70**, 3846 (1948).

266. A. S. Keats and H. K. Beecher, *J. Pharmacol. Exptl. Therap.* **105**, 109, 210 (1952).

267. K. Kubota, and T. Kaku, *Yakugaku Zasshi* **81**, 186 (1961); *Chem. Abstr.* **55**, 15736 (1961).

268. P. A. J. Janssen, Belgian Patent 606,850 (August 2, 1961); *Chem. Abstr.* **56**, 12862 (1962).

269. P. A. J. Janssen, *J. Pharm. Pharmacol.* **13**, 513 (1961).

270. K. Schmitt and E. Lindner, *Arch. Pharm.* **295**, 744 (1962); *Chem. Abstr.* **58**, 6784 (1963).

271a. D. W. Adamson, *J. Chem. Soc.* p. 1445 (1949).

271b. D. W. Adamson, *Nature* **164**, 500 (1949).

272. A. W. Ruddy and J. S. Buckley, Jr., *J. Am. Chem. Soc.* **72**, 718 (1950).

273. S. Shigematsu (to Tanabe Drug), Japanese Patent 6363 (August 17, 1957); *Chem. Abstr.* **52**, 12916 (1958).

274. T. D. Perrine, *J. Org. Chem.* **18**, 898 (1953).

275. A. Schlesinger and S. M. Gordon (to Endo Labs. Inc.), U.S. Patent 2,954,383 (September 27, 1960); *Chem. Abstr.* **55**, 5432 (1961).

276. J. A. Barltrop, R. M. Acheson, P. G. Philpott, K. E. MacPhee, and J. S. Hunt, *J. Chem. Soc.* p. 2928 (1956).

277. H. Richter and M. Schenck, (to Schering A.G.), German Patent 946,058 (July 26, 1956); *Chem. Abstr.* **52**, 18356 (1958).

278. H. Richter and M. Schenck (to Schering A.G.), German Patent 951,628 (October 31, 1956); *Chem. Abstr.* **53**, 322 (1959).

279. M. Schenck and H. Richter (to Schering A.G.), British Patent 793,853 (April 23, 1958); *Chem. Abstr.* **52**, 20107 (1958).

280. H. Richter and B. Acksteiner (to Schering A.G.), German Patent 1,098,511 (February 2, 1961); *Chem. Abstr.* **55**, 21492 (1961).

281. Council on Drugs, *J. Am. Med. Assoc.* **184**, 227 (1963).

282. T. Takahashi, H. Fujimura, and K. Okamura, *Yakugaku Zasshi* **82**, 1597 (1962); *Chem. Abstr.* **59**, 611 (1963).

283. A. Burger and W. H. Shelver, *J. Med. Pharm. Chem.* **4**, 225 (1961).

284. A. Wander A.-G., British Patent 641,571 (August 16, 1950); *Chem. Abstr.* **45**, 2506 (1951).

285. F. Adickes (to C. H. Boehringer Sohn), German Patent 894,846 (October 29, 1953); *Chem. Abstr.* **52**, 12917 (1958).

286. F. F. Blicke, J. A. Faust, and H. Raffelson, *J. Am. Chem. Soc.* **76**, 3161 (1954).

287. J. Klosa, *Arch. Pharm.* **287**, 321 (1954); *Chem. Abstr.* **50**, 17209 (1956); *Chem. Abstr.* **51**, 13311 (1957).

288. J. Klosa, *Arch. Pharm.* **288**, 42 (1955); *Chem. Abstr.* **51**, 13819 (1957).

289. *Federal Register* **24**, 37 (January 3, 1959); *Chem. Abstr.* **53**, 5589 (1959).

290. T. Teshigawara, Japanese Patent 2326 (May 21, 1962); *Chem. Abstr.* **58**, 7871 (1963).

291. T. Krugmann and M. Krugmann (to Krugmann & Co.), British Patent 878,068 (September 27, 1961); *Chem. Abstr.* **56**, 12806 (1962).

292. G. Gillissen and J. Kaufmann, *Arzneimittel-Forch.* **11**, 988 (1961); *Chem. Abstr.* **56**, 6608 (1962).

293. J. Klosa, *J. Prakt. Chem.* **16**, 258 (1962); *Chem. Abstr.* **58**, 7862 (1963).

294. S. S. Liberman and A. I. Polezhaeva, *Farmakol. i. Toksikol.* **26**, 656 (1963).

295. H. Hueller, E. Schultz, and W. Scheler, *Acta Biol. Med. Ger.* **10**, 357 (1963); *Chem. Abstr.* **59**, 15797 (1963).

296. F. L. Chubb, G. Frangatos, and J. Nissenbaum, *Can. J. Chem.* **38**, 1231 (1960); *Chem. Abstr.* **55**, 2563 (1961).

297. F. P. Doyle, M. D. Mehta, and R. Ward (to Beecham Res. Labs. Ltd.), British Patent 886,437 (January 10, 1962); *Chem. Abstr.* **56**, 14245 (1962).

298. J. Klosa and G. Delmar, *J. Prakt. Chem.* **16**, 71 (1962); *Chem. Abstr.* **57**, 16544 (1962).

299a. F. P. Doyle and M. D. Mehta (to Beecham Res. Labs. Ltd.), British Patent 861,377 (February 22, 1961); *Chem. Abstr.* **55**, 24792 (1961).

299b. F. P. Doyle and M. D. Mehta (to Beecham Res. Labs. Ltd.), British Patent 886,436 (January 10, 1962); *Chem. Abstr.* **57**, 7234 (1962).

300. K. Ogiu, H. Fujimura, G. Shino, and Y. Yamakawa, Japanese Patent 3221 (April 30, 1959); *Chem. Abstr.* **54**, 13069 (1960).

301. A. Schlesinger and S. M. Gordon (to Endo Labs. Inc.), U.S. Patent 3,073,842 (January 15, 1963); *Chem. Abstr.* **59**, 1652 (1963).

302. H. Fujimura and Y. Yamakawa, *Yakugaku Zasshi* **80**, 333 (1960); *Chem. Abstr.* **54**, 18433 (1960).

303. J. Krapcho and C. F. Turk, *J. Med. Chem.* **6**, 547 (1963).

304. W. A. Lott and J. Krapcho (to Olin Mathieson), U.S. Patent 2,862,965 (December 2 1958); *Chem. Abstr.* **53**, 7215 (1959).

305. G. L. Hassert, J. J. Piala, J. C. Burke, and B. N. Craver, *Federation Proc.* **20**, 211 (1961)

306. J. Krapcho (to Olin Mathieson), U.S. Patent 2,944,700 (August 1, 1961); *Chem. Abstr.* **57**, 11117 (1962).

307. B. N. Craver, J. C. Burke, J. Krapcho, and L. L. Monroe, *Biochem. Pharmacol.* **12** (Suppl.), 6 (1963).

308. J. Klosa (to Rhein Chemie G.m.b.H.), Belgian Patent 617,668 (August 31, 1962); *Chem. Abstr.* **58**, 6755 (1963).

309. D. Kupke, *Naturwissenschaften* **50**, 127 (1963).

310. D. Kupke and S. Geissler, *Arzneimittel-Forsch.* **13**, 312 (1963); *Chem. Abstr.* **59**, 6865 (1963).

311. H. E. Zaugg, R. W. DeNet, and R. J. Michaels, Jr., Belgian Patent 618,672 (December 7, 1962); *Chem. Abstr.* **59**, 3897 (1963).

312. D. W. Adamson and A. F. Green, *Nature* **165**, 122 (1950).

313. D. W. Adamson, *J. Chem. Soc.* p. 885 (1950).

314. D. W. Adamson (to Burroughs Wellcome), U.S. Patent 2,561,899 (July 24, 1951); *Chem. Abstr.* **46**, 3085 (1952).

315. D. W. Adamson (to Burroughs Wellcome), British Patent 657,301 (September 19, 1951); *Chem. Abstr.* **46**, 9611 (1952).

316. A. F. Green, *Brit. J. Pharmacol.* **8**, 2 (1953).

317. P. A. Barrett and S. Wilkinson (to Wellcome Foundation Ltd.), British Patent 683,977 (December 10, 1952); *Chem. Abstr.* **48**, 2779 (1954).

318. T. Kametani and Y. Akazawa, *J. Pharm. Soc. Japan* **73**, 649 (1953); *Chem. Abstr.* **48**, 5175 (1954).

319. I. Hirao and H. Hatta, *J. Pharm. Soc. Japan* **73**, 1058 (1953); *Chem. Abstr.* **48**, 12026 (1954).

320. I. Hirao, *Japan J. Pharm. Chem.* **25**, 575 (1953); *Chem. Abstr.* **49**, 1003 (1955).

321. N. Sugimoto *et al.* (to Tanabe Drug), Japanese Patent 3922 (May 28, 1956); *Chem. Abstr.* **51**, 16563 (1957).

322. R. Kimura and T. Yabuuchi, *Chem. Pharm. Bull. (Tokyo)* **7**, 171 (1959); *Chem. Abstr.* **54**, 22625 (1960).

323. K. Okumara, T. Tanaka, S. Saito, H. Kugita, and N. Sugimoto, *Tanabe Seiyaku Kenkyu Nempo* **3** (2), 30 (1958); *Chem. Abstr.* **53**, 10214 (1959).

324. Y. Kase, T. Yuizono, Y. Yamasaki, T. Yamada, S. Io, M. Tamiya, and I. Kondo, *Chem. Pharm. Bull. (Tokyo)* **7**, 372 (1959); *Chem. Abstr.* **54**, 22625 (1960).

325. N. Shigematsu and G. Hayashi, *Yakugaku Zasshi* **81**, 421 (1961); *Chem. Abstr.* **55**, 17618 (1961).

326. S. Yamamoto, *Nippon Yakurigaku Zasshi* **53**, 475 (1957); *Chem. Abstr.* **52**, 15739 (1958).

327. K. Ogiu, H. Takagi, and S. Yamamoto, *Nippon Yakurigaku Zasshi* **54**, 1 (1958); *Chem. Abstr.* **53**, 572 (1959).

328. S. Nishiyama, H. Kitsunezuka, and G. Niwase, *Eisei Kagaku* **4**, 29 (1957); *Chem. Abstr.* **51**, 10313 (1957).

329. M. Kanda, K. Mimura, M. Ishikawa, S. Yoshi, and M. Okamura, *Kagaku To Sosa* **10**, 62 (1957); *Chem. Abstr.* **52**, 12041 (1958).

330. R. Kimura, M. Ogawa, and T. Yabuuchi, *Chem. Pharm. Bull. (Tokyo)* **7**, 175 (1959); *Chem. Abstr.* **54**, 22625 (1960).

331. A. Pohland and H. R. Sullivan, *J. Am. Chem. Soc.* **75**, 4458 (1953).

332. E. B. Robbins, *J. Am. Pharm. Assoc. Sci. Ed.* **44**, 497 (1955).

333. C. M. Gruber, *J. Lab. Clin. Med.* **44**, 805 (1954).

334. A. Pohland and H. R. Sullivan *J. Am. Chem. Soc.* **77**, 3400 (1955).

335. A. Pohland, H. R. Sullivan, and R. E. McMahon, *J. Am. Chem. Soc.* **79**, 1442 (1957).

336. H. R. Sullivan, J. R. Beck, and A. Pohland, *J. Org. Chem.* **28**, 2381 (1963).

337. A. H. Beckett, G. Kirk, and R. Thomas, *J. Chem. Soc.* p. 1386 (1962).

338. A. Pohland, L. R. Peters, and H. R. Sullivan, *J. Org. Chem.* **28**, 2483 (1963).

339. A. Pohland (to E. Lilly), U.S. Patent 2,728,779 (December 27, 1955); *Chem. Abstr.* **50**, 13997 (1956).

340. J. A. Miller, Jr., E. B. Robbins, and D. B. Meyers, *J. Pharm. Sci.* **52**, 446 (1963).

341. V. C. Stephens (to E. Lilly), U.S. Patent 3,065,261 (November 20, 1962); *Chem. Abstr.* **58**, 11173 (1963).

342. G. deStevens, A. Halamandaris, P. Strachan, E. Donoghue, L. Dorfman, and C. F. Huebner, *J. Med. Chem.* **6**, 357 (1963).

343. A. A. Patchett and F. F. Giarrusso, *J. Med. Pharm. Chem.* **4**, 393 (1961).

344. H. M. Lee, E. G. Scott, and A. Pohland, *J. Pharmacol. Exptl. Therap.* **125**, 14 (1959).

345. H. F. Fraser and H. Isbell, *Bull. Narcotics, U.N. Dept. Social Affairs* **12**, 9 (1960). *Chem. Abstr.* **55**, 25039 (1961).

346. Federal Register **27**, 2770 (March 24, 1962); *Chem. Abstr.* **57**, 4769 (1962).

347. J. W. Marrs, W. W. Glas, and J. Silvani, *Am. J. Pharm.* **131**, 271 (1951).

348. S. M. Chernish and C. M. Gruber, Jr., *Antibiot. Med. Clin. Therapy* **7**, 190 (1960).

349. R. Reiss and A. H. Aufses, Jr., *Arch. Surg.* **82**, 429 (1961).

350. M. S. Sadove, M. J. Schiffrin, and S. M. Ali, *Am. J. Med. Sci.* **241**, 103 (1961).
351. G. M. Howard, J. Levy, and J. Dougherty, *N. Y. State J. Med.* **61**, 3285 (1961).
352. V. K. Stoelting, R. K. Stoelting, and C. M. Gruber, Jr., *Anesthesiology* **23**, 21 (1962).
353. H. W. Hyatt, Sr., *New Engl. J. Med.* **267**, 710 (1962).
354. H. L. Verhulst, *New Engl. J. Med.* **268**, 56 (1963).
355. H. A. Bickermann, E. German, B. M. Cohen, and S. E. Itkin, *Am. J. Med. Sci.* **234**, 191 (1957).
356. C. M. Gruber, Jr. and C. H. Carter, *Am. J. Med. Sci.* **242**, 443 (1961).
357. W. B. Wright, Jr., H. J. Brabander, and R. A. Hardy, Jr., *J. Am. Chem. Soc.* **81**, 1518 (1959).
358. A. C. Osterberg and C. E. Rauh, *Pharmacologist* **1**, 78 (1959).
359. W. B. Wright, Jr., H. J. Brabander, and R. A. Hardy, Jr., *J. Org. Chem.* **26**, 476, 485 (1961).
360. W. B. Wright, Jr. and R. A. Hardy, Jr., *J. Med. Chem.* **6**, 128 (1963).
361. P. S. Portoghese and D. L. Larson, *J. Pharm. Sci.* **51**, 1115 (1962).
362. P. S. Portoghese, *J. Pharm. Sci.* **51**, 1197 (1962).
363. W. B. Wright, Jr. and H. J. Brabander (to Am. Cyanamid Co.), U.S. Patent 3,016,382 (January 9, 1962); *Chem. Abstr.* **57**, 16485 (1962).
364. W. B. Wright, Jr., R. A. Hardy, Jr., and H. J. Brabander (to *Am.* Cyanamid Co.), U.S. Patent 2,944,081 (July 5, 1960); *Chem. Abstr.* **54**, 22496 (1960).
365. W. B. Wright, Jr. (to Am. Cyanamid Co.), U.S. Patent 3,005,850 (October 24, 1961); *Chem. Abstr.* **56**, 3352 (1962).
366. T. Kikuchi, T. Takashima, and H. Takagi, *Nippon Yagurigaku Zasshi* **57**, 585 (1961); *Chem. Abstr.* **59**, 2082 (1963).
367. N. Shigematsu, *Yakugaku Zasshi* **81**, 423 (1961); *Chem. Abstr.* **55**, 17618 (1961).
368. N. Shigematsu, *Yakugaku Zasshi* **81**, 815 (1961); *Chem. Abstr.* **55**, 24754 (1961).
369. N. Shigematsu (to Tanabe Seiyaku Co., Ltd.), Japanese Patent 5940 (June 25, 1962); *Chem. Abstr.* **59**, 1601 (1963).
370. K. Suzuki, K. Kigasawa, K. Fukawa, and T. Uchibori (to Grelan Pharm. Co., Ltd). Japanese Patent 2263 (March 18, 1963); *Chem. Abstr.* **59**, 11329 (1963).
371. G. Hayashi, N. Shigematsu, and Y. Kowa, *Yakugaku Zasshi* **83**, 62 (1963).
372. K. Kigasawa, H. Sugahara, M. Hiiragi, and K. Fukawa, *Yakugaku Zasshi* **83**, 696 (1963).
373. K. Okumura, G. Hayashi, and N. Sugimoto, *Yakugaku Zasshi* **83**, 900 (1963).
374. N. Shigematsu and G. Hayashi (to Tanabe Seiyaki Co., Ltd.), Japanese Patent 10,770 (August 10, 1962); *Chem. Abstr.* **59**, 10068 (1963).
375. Farbenfabriken Bayer, British Patent 939,947 (October 16, 1963).
376. H. Zellner (to Donau-Pharmazie G.m.b.H.), Austrian Patent 221,508 (June 12, 1962); *Chem. Abstr.* **57**, 11115 (1962).
377. Dumex A/S, Canadian Patent 662,750 (May 7, 1963).
378. Y. Kase, T. Yuizono, and M. Muto, *J. Med. Chem.* **6**, 118 (1963).
379. P. A. J. Janssen, C. J. E. Niemegeers, and J. G. H. Dony, *Arzneimittel-Forsch.* **13**, 502 (1963).
380. J. Yelnosky and J. F. Gardocki, *Federation Proc.* **22**, 188 (1963).
381. J. F. Gardocki and J. Yelnosky, *Toxicol. Appl. Pharmacol.* **6**, 48 (1964).
382. M. C. Holderness, P. E. Chase, and R. D. Dripps, *Anesthesiology* **24**, 336 (1963).
383. *Federal Register* **25**, 10387 (October 29, 1960); *Chem. Abstr.* **55**, 2017 (1961).
384. T. J. DeKornfeld and L. Lasagna, *Anesthesiology* **21**, 159 (1960).
385. L. Lasagna, *Am. J. Med. Sci.* **242**, 620 (1961).

CHAPTER VI

Isoquinoline Analgetics

A. BROSSI,* H. BESENDORF,** L. A. PIRK,*

and A. RHEINER, Jr.**

RESEARCH DEPARTMENTS OF *HOFFMANN-LA ROCHE INC., NUTLEY, NEW JERSEY
AND **F. HOFFMANN-LA ROCHE & CO., A.G., BASLE, SWITZERLAND

I. Introduction

The hypothesis of Schaumann (1), as previously discussed in detail in Chapter V, that the analgetic potency of Eisleb's (2) piperidine derivative, meperidine (Demerol®) (I) is associated with a distinct structural similarity to morphine (II), greatly stimulated the search for new centrally active analgetics. The development of drugs such as the morphinanes, benzomorphanes, piperidines of the meperidine-type and the open-chain compounds of the methadone-type is intimately associated with this concept. This hypothesis, which postulates that a quaternary carbon atom, a benzene

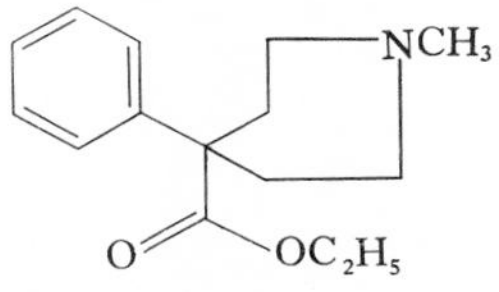

(I) 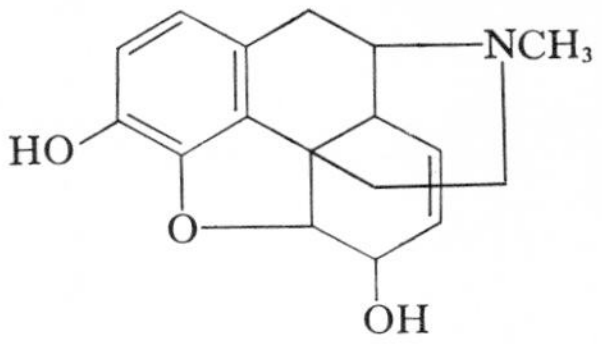   (II)

nucleus attached to the quaternary carbon, and a tertiary amino group separated from that carbon by two methylene groups are essential for analgetic activity, became almost an inviolable law for many of those working in this field. More recent developments, however, have disclosed that this assumption is not entirely justified, and it has been suggested by Braenden et al. (3), Eddy (4), and others (5) that some aspects of this concept should be changed. Therefore, it is indeed surprising to note that 1-aralkylisoquinolines and their partially or fully hydrogenated derivatives, both structurally and biogenetically related to morphine, have not been more thoroughly investigated in this respect. It is quite possible that compounds of this type were overlooked because the primary goal was to discover analgetics more potent than morphine. The 1-aralkylisoquinolines and their derivatives seemed to offer little hope of success since certain well-known representatives, such as papaverine and the related opium alkaloids, do not exert any analgetic effects. When we initiated our analgetic program, aimed at finding new centrally active analgetics characterized by markedly lower addictive properties, we recognized this gap and, therefore, began a systematic study of the various isoquinolines which had been prepared in our laboratories in recent years. Also included in our program from its inception was the search for antitussive compounds, since it is well known that a close structural relationship exists between many analgetics and antitussives. Our entire studies are presented later in detail. For completeness, this review also includes a literature survey of isoquinoline analgetics and antitussives.

II. Isoquinoline Alkaloids

The tetrahydroisoquinoline alkaloids appear to be devoid of pain-relieving properties. This is evident from the literature (6) and from our own work, in which certain representatives (III–V) of this class were tested. Furthermore, we also retested papaverine (VI), papaveraldine (VII), and ($\pm$)-laudanosine (VIII)—1-benzylisoquinolines (*6–8*) which are even more

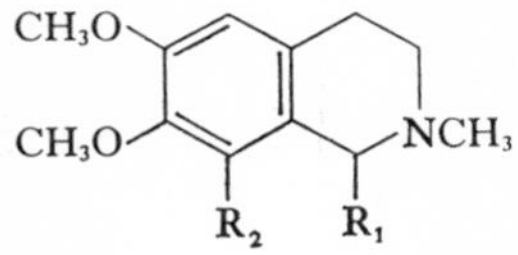

CH$_3$O
CH$_3$O
NCH$_3$
R$_2$ R$_1$

(III) ($\pm$)-carnegine   R$_1$=—CH$_3$;R$_2$=—H
(IV) ($\pm$)-pellotine   R$_1$=—CH$_3$;R$_2$=—OH
(V) ($\pm$)-N-methylcalycotomine R$_1$=—CH$_2$OH;R$_2$=—H

closely related structurally to morphine than III, IV, and V—and confirmed that they do not have any distinct analgetic efficacy. However, it would be worthwhile to extend this testing program and include some of the optically active and partially O-demethylated alkaloids of type IX, which have been isolated recently from menispermaceous plants (*9–12*).

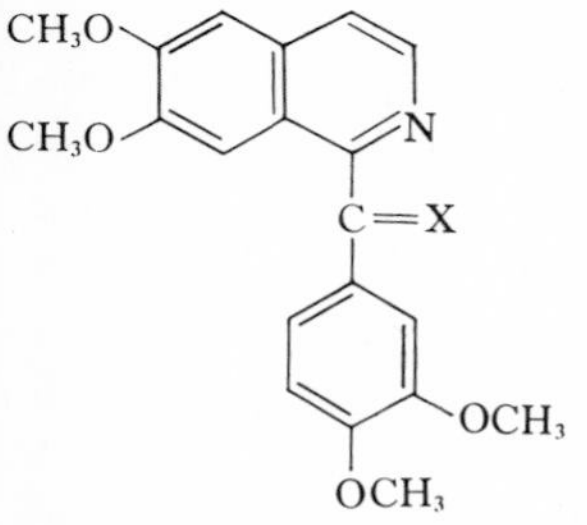

CH$_3$O
CH$_3$O
N
C=X
OCH$_3$
OCH$_3$

CH$_3$O
CH$_3$O
N—CH$_3$
CH$_2$
OCH$_3$
OCH$_3$

RO
RO
N—CH$_3$
CH$_2$
R$_1$
OR

(VI) X = —H$_2$
(VII) X = =O

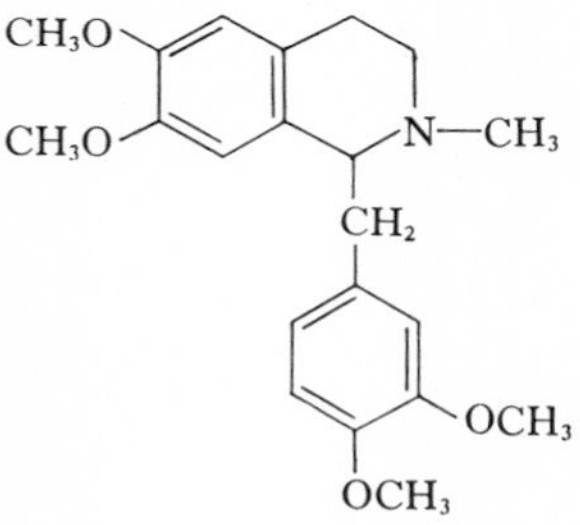

(VIII)

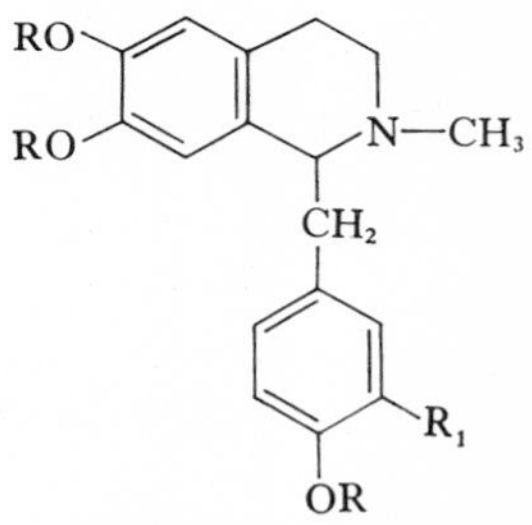

(IX) R = —H or —CH$_3$
(but different)
and R$_1$ = —H or —OCH$_3$

The only alkaloids representing a simple isoquinoline structure which warrant interest—not so much for their weak analgetic activity as for their antitussive properties—are the phthalide isoquinoline alkaloids (*13–15*). The most interesting members of this group studied so far are the two naturally occurring alkaloids, ($\pm$)-α-narcotine, also called α-gnoscopine (X), and its (−) enantiomer (*7, 13, 16*). Both ($\pm$)-narcotine isomers, α- as well as β-gnoscopine, and the four optically active stereoisomers, of still unknown absolute configuration (*17*), have been prepared (*13*). Since it is well established that a close interrelationship exists between central analgetic activity and configuration, the fact that little is known about the activity of the unnatural racemate or its optical antipodes, is a serious void in our overall knowledge of this field. It might also be added that nothing in this respect

283

TABLE I

ANALGETIC EFFECTIVENESS OF DIFFERENT DRUGS

(ED_{50} IN MG/KG IN MICE)

	Gross (45)		Hardy et al. (53)	Siegmund et al. (54)		LD$_{50}$ Mice (mg/kg)		
	subcutaneous	oral	subcutaneous	subcutaneous	oral	subcutaneous	oral	intravenous
Morphine[a]	4	30	5[b]	0.8	—	280	—	170
Codeine[a]	18	40	35	5.5	—	140	250	56
Pethidine[a]	10	—	44[b]	3.0	10	—	—	44
Propoxyphene[a]	15	32	—	3.5	—	125	180	25
Methopholine[a] (47)	18	38	40	5	12	180	180	35
Acetylsalicylic acid	—	>300	—	—	100	—	700	—
Phenacetin	—	>300	—	—	120	—	2200	—
α-(−)-Narcotine[a]	>100 (inact.)	—	—	—	—	>3500[b]	—	83[b]

[a] All values are calculated for the free base.
[b] These values were taken from the literature and are not necessarily comparable.

is known concerning the other members of this group (15), (±)-adlumidine, (±)-bicuculline, (±)-adlumine, and (±)-corlumine.

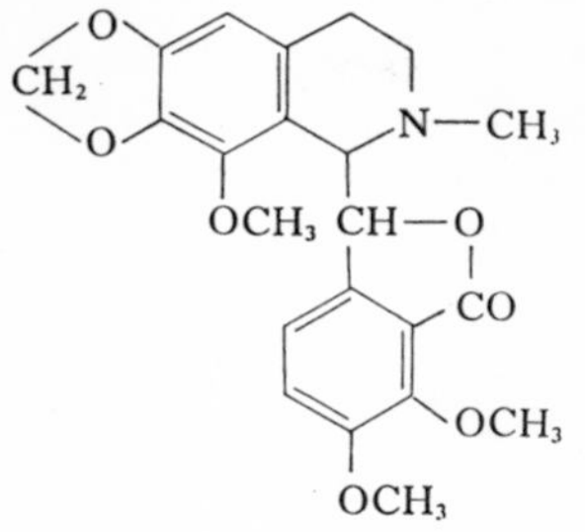

(X)

The analgetic activity of α-(−)-narcotine seems to be decidely less than that of codeine (Table I) (7, 18), whereas its antitussive effect (Table II) is of the same order as that of codeine (16, 19–21).

TABLE II

ANTITUSSIVE PROPERTIES OF DIFFERENT DRUGS AS COMPARED WITH CODEINE

	Cat[a] (intravenous)	Guinea pig[b] (intravenous)	Dog (oral)	LD_{50} mice (mg/kg, intravenous)
Codeine phosphate	1	1	1	80
Narcotine	0.2	ca. 0.4	ca. 0.5	150
Romilar®	1	ca. 0.25	ca. 1	33
Methopholine (47)	0.4	ca. 0.7	ca. 0.1	35
Compound LVIII	ca. 0.8	ca. 0.7	<0.01	70
Compound (−)-LVIII	2	ca. 0.7	ca. 0.3	49
Compound LX	ca. 1	ca. 0.5	ca. 0.5	50

[a] Method of Domenjoz (55).
[b] The measured values scatter considerably (56).

III. Synthetic Isoquinoline Derivatives

Current standard texts on medicinal chemistry (22) and up-to-date reviews on synthetic analgetics (5, 23–25) do not mention that simple isoquinolines are being used in clinical practice as analgetics. However, three types of compounds developed recently should be mentioned here. The first of these are the cotarnine derivatives of type (XI) (26), studied by

Hungarian scientists (27), which are said to be as active as codeine. Reports regarding human pharmacology have not appeared since this statement was published. A representative of the second type is the lactam corydaldine (XII), which was prepared by a new synthesis (28) and tested in our laboratories. It exhibited analgetic properties in different so-called rheumatic tests (25, 29), but the results in human pharmacology were disappointing. We therefore shall restrict our review of synthetic isoquinolines to those

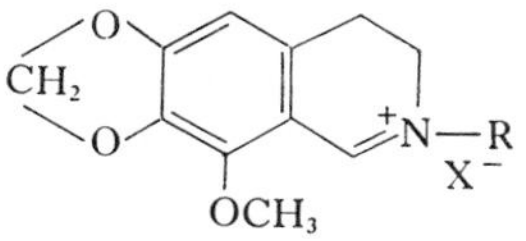

R = —alkyl, —aralkyl, —aryl

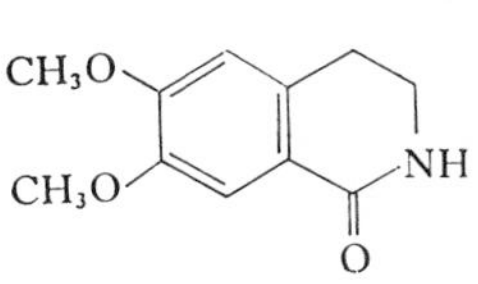

which, like codeine and morphine, exhibit definite central analgetic effects in humans. By doing so, we can omit many isoquinolines which are mentioned in patents. These were mainly prepared as intermediates for the synthesis of morphinanes and morphanes and were simply induced in the literature under the general title of this subject.

We can now discuss the third, and most interesting series of synthetic isoquinoline analgetics, which were developed during the period 1958–1962 in the laboratories of Hoffmann-La Roche in Basle. Among this group of partially hydrogenated 1-aralkyl-substituted isoquinolines, we find many which show high analgetic activity, the most active ones being much more potent than morphine. The development of this new group of analgetics and antitussives and the intensive studies to which they have been subjected has, in addition, led to new ideas regarding structural relationships among centrally active analgetics. This series will, therefore, be discussed in detail.

A. 1-Phenethyl-Substituted 1,2,3,4-Tetrahydroisoquinolines

During studies in the field of ipecac alkaloids, new procedures for the synthesis of 1-phenethyl-substituted isoquinoline derivatives were evolved (28), which offered possibilities for wide structural variations. This fact stimulated our interest in systematically developing this group of compounds related to either laudanosine (VIII) or papaverine (VI).

German patents (30), issued during 1935–1940, describing isoquinolines of types XIII, XIV, and XV, suggested to us from the very beginning that analgetics might be found among our compounds.

The 1-aralkyl-substituted isoquinolines mentioned by the German authors were mostly secondary amines. Having in mind one of Schaumann's concepts, which at present is still valid, we immediately directed our efforts

286

toward the synthesis of tertiary amines of this group. The interesting results reported by our pharmacologists, who indeed found central analgetic activity in this series, prompted us to expand our program in many directions.

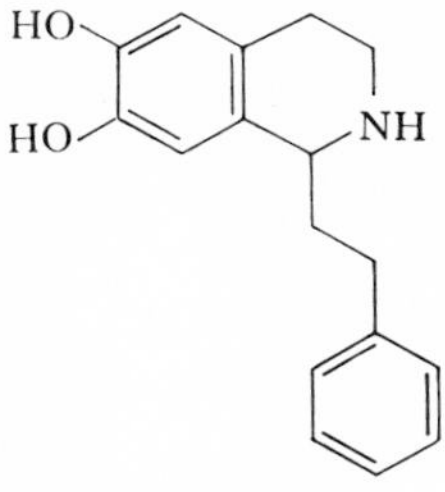

(XIII)

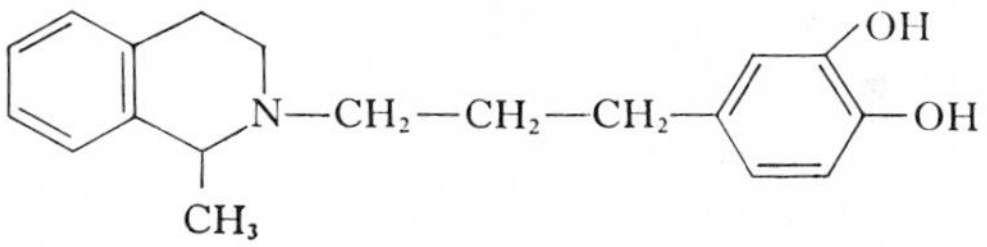

(XIV)

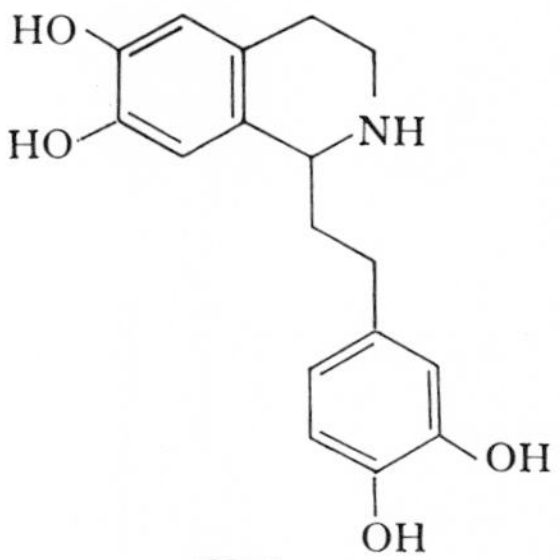

(XV)

1. *Syntheses*

The three convenient syntheses of 1-phenethyl-substituted 1,2,3,4-tetra-hydroisoquinolines worked out in our laboratories are outlined in Figs. 1–3.

a. Acetophenone approach (Figure 1, Method A). In the first scheme (*31*), readily available 2-acyl-*N*-acetphenethylamines, of which the 4,5-dimethoxy derivative (XVI) (*28, 31, 32*) is a prototype, are used as starting materials. Condensation with an appropriate aromatic aldehyde, for example *p*-chlorobenzaldehyde, leads to the chalcone derivative (XVII). The latter compound, after heating with dilute hydrochloric acid or a mixture of hydrochloric acid and acetic acid, is converted directly to the intensely colored 1-*p*-chlorostyryl-substituted 3,4-dihydroisoquinoline (XVIII) as the hydrochloride in excellent yield. The chromophore of this system can be detected easily by ultraviolet spectroscopy. An obvious advantage of this method is the ease with which a large variety of 1-styryl-substituted dihydro-isoquinolines of type XVIII can be prepared by reacting the easily available alkoxy-, aralkoxy-, or alkyl-substituted 2-acyl-*N*-acetphenethyl-amines (*28, 31*) with differently substituted aromatic aldehydes. Catalytic hydrogenation of XVIII yields, after absorption of two moles of hydrogen, the substituted 1-phenethyltetrahydroisoquinoline derivative (XIX), which

287

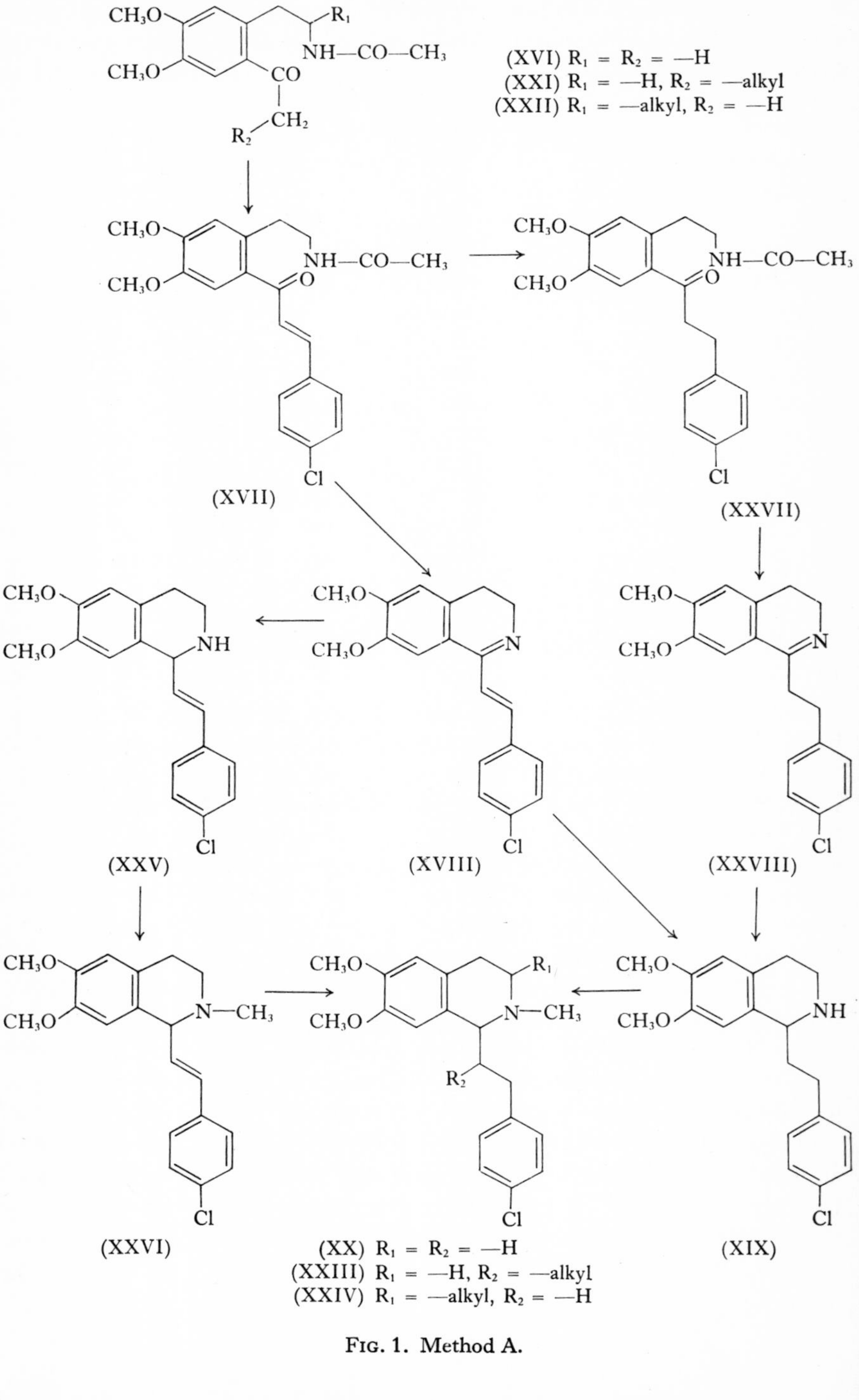

$$(XVI) \quad R_1 = R_2 = -H$$
$$(XXI) \quad R_1 = -H, R_2 = -alkyl$$
$$(XXII) \quad R_1 = -alkyl, R_2 = -H$$

(XVII)

(XXVII)

(XXV)

(XVIII)

(XXVIII)

(XXVI)

$$(XX) \quad R_1 = R_2 = -H$$
$$(XXIII) \quad R_1 = -H, R_2 = -alkyl$$
$$(XXIV) \quad R_1 = -alkyl, R_2 = -H$$

(XIX)

FIG. 1. Method A.

on N-methylation, is converted to the tertiary amine (XX). By this route, tetrahydroisoquinolines of type XXIII and XXIV with alkyl residues in the phenethyl side chain (XXIII) or in the heterocyclic ring moiety (XXIV), can also be prepared by starting with the properly substituted 2-acyl derivatives of type XXI or XXII, respectively. Due to the presence of two asymmetric centers in XXIII or XXIV, two racemic diastereomers of each of these compounds are possible.

The tertiary amine (XX) can also be obtained by the following modification of the synthesis: reduction of the hydrochloride of XVIII, by means of sodium borohydride in alcohol, yields the 1-styryl-substituted tetrahydroisoquinoline derivative (XXV); N-methylation of the free base (XXV) with formic acid and formalin yields XXVI, which, after catalytic hydrogenation of the double bond located in the styryl side chain, gives XX identical with the saturated tertiary amine prepared by the other route.

As a third possibility, the chalcone (XVII) can be hydrogenated to the diphenylpropanone derivative (XXVII) which, by heating with dilute hydrochloric acid, is cyclized to the 3,4-dihydroisoquinoline derivative (XXVIII). Reduction of (XXVIII), either by catalytic hydrogenation or with sodium borohydride, yields the secondary amine (XIX), an intermediate in the first synthesis.

A list of differently substituted 1-phenalkyl-*N*-methyl-1,2,3,4-tetrahydroisoquinolines prepared by these modifications is given in Tables III–VII. Data regarding their analgetic activity are also included. The analgetic potency of reference compounds is shown in Table I, whereas in Table II the antitussive activity of several representatives is compared with that of standard drugs.

b. Starting from quaternary 1-methylisoquinolinium compounds (Fig. 2, Method B). Quaternary salts of 1-methyl-3,4-dihydroisoquinolines such as XXIX, as well as 1-methylisoquinolines, such as XXX which are known to have an especially activated methyl group (*33*), can be condensed directly with an appropriate aromatic aldehyde, thereby offering a second approach to 1-phenethyl-substituted isoquinoline derivatives. Thus, from the methobromide XXIX and *p*-chlorobenzaldehyde in methanol at room temperature, using piperidine as a catalyst, XXXI was obtained. This quaternary salt proved to be identical with the methobromide prepared for comparison from the styryl-substituted dihydroisoquinoline XVIII (Fig. 1) and methyl bromide. Sodium borohydride reduction of the methobromide (XXXI) and catalytic hydrogenation of the 1-styryl-substituted base (XXVI) yielded the same tertiary amine (XX) which had already been obtained by method A.

In general, route B does not offer any advantages over route A.

TABLE III

DIFFERENTLY SUBSTITUTED 1-PHENETHYL-2-METHYL-6,7-DIMETHOXY-1,2,3,4-TETRAHYDROISOQUINOLINES OF THE GENERAL FORMULA

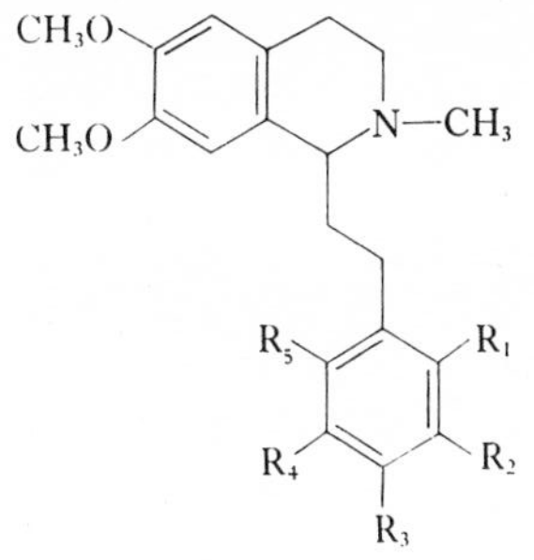

R_1	R_2	R_3	R_4	R_5	Melting point (°C)		Method	LD_{50} mice (mg/kg intravenous)	Activity[a]
					Base	Salt			
—Cl	—	—	—	—	—	HBr 164°	A	25	>0.3
—	—Cl	—Cl	—	—	96°	—	A	70	0.6
—	—Cl	—	—	—	—	HCl 112°	A	35	0.4
—Cl	—Cl	—Cl	—Cl	—	112°	—	A	50–100	inact.
—Cl	—	—Cl	—	—	107°	—	A	50	ca. 0.3
—	—NO₂	—NO₂	—	—	—	HCl 117°	C	25	ca. 2.5
—NO₂	—	—	—	—	92°	—	C	10	20
—OCH₃	—	—	—	—	78°	—	C	12.5	1.6
—Cl	—Cl	—Cl	—Cl	—Cl	122°	—	A	35	>0.6
—Cl	—Cl	—Cl	—Cl	—Cl	121°	—	A	>1000 oral	inact.
—Cl	—	—Cl	—Cl	—	117°	—	A	25	≪0.5
—	—Cl	—Cl	—Cl	—	—	HCl 160°	A	60–120	0.5

[a] Activity = analgesia in mouse tail flick test (Gross) (45) compared to codeine (base) = 1 after subcutaneous application.

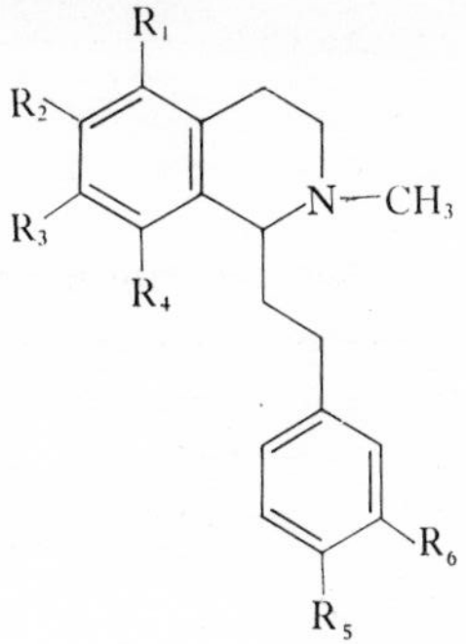

R1	R2	R3	R4	R5	R6	Melting point (°C)		Method	LD$_{50}$ mice (mg/kg) intravenous	Activity[a]
						Base	Salt			
—OCH$_3$	—OCH$_3$	—	—	—Cl	—	—	HCl 188°	C	27	inact.
—	—OCH$_3$	—OCH$_3$	—OCH$_3$	—Cl	—	—	HBr 95°	A	50	ca. 0.2
—	—OAc	—OAc	—	—Cl	—	—	Oxalate 152°	Acetylation	70	inact.
—	—OCH$_3$	—	—	—Cl	—	—	HCl 178°	—	50	inact.
—	—OH	—OH	—	—Cl	—	—	HCl 172°	Hydrolysis	70	inact.
—	—O—CH$_2$—O—		—	—NO$_2$	—	112°	—	C	18	<0.3
—	—OC$_2$H$_5$	—OC$_2$H$_5$	—	—Cl	—	—	Oxalate 103°	A	35	inact.
—	—OCH$_3$	—	—	—NO$_2$	—	116°	—	C	35	5.5
—OH	—OCH$_3$	—	—	—Cl	—	—	Oxalate 211°	C	ca. 40	inact.
—	—CH$_3$	—CH$_3$	—	—Cl	—Cl	—	HBr 208°	A	180[b] / >200[c]	inact.
—	—O—CH$_2$—O—		—	—Cl	—	—	HCl 98°	A	70	inact.
—	—OH	—OCH$_3$	—	—Cl	—	—	HCl 235°	C	50	0.4
—	—OCH$_3$	—OH	—	—Cl	—	—	HCl 183°	C	50	0.7

[a] See Table III.   [b] Oral.   [c] Subcutaneous.

291

TABLE V

DIFFERENTLY SUBSTITUTED 1-PHENETHYL-1,2,3,4-TETRAHYDROISOQUINOLINES OF THE GENERAL FORMULA[a]

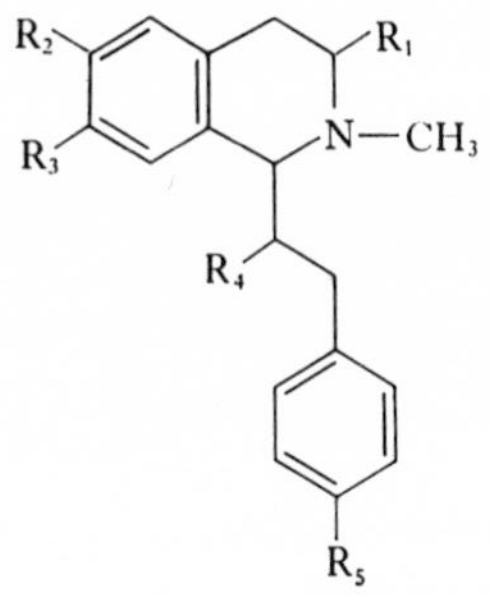

R_1	R_2	R_3	R_4	R_5	Method	Melting point (°C)—Salt		LD$_{50}$ mice (mg/kg, intravenous)	Activity[b]
—CH$_3$	—OCH$_3$	—OCH$_3$	—H	—Cl	A	HBr	192°	35	inact.
—CH$_3$	—CH$_3$	—CH$_3$	—H	—Cl	A	HCl	212°	50	inact.
—H	—OCH$_3$	—OCH$_3$	—CH$_3$	—NO$_2$	C	Sulfosalicylate	207°	70[c]	10
—H	—OCH$_3$	—OCH$_3$	—CH$_3$	—Cl	A	HBr	192°	35	0.9

[a] The compounds tested represent one of the two possible diastereomers.
[b] See Table III.
[c] Subcutaneous.

292

TABLE VI

DIFFERENTLY N-SUBSTITUTED 1-PHENETHYL-6,7-DIMETHOXY-1,2,3,4-TETRAHYDROISO-
QUINOLINES OF THE GENERAL FORMULA

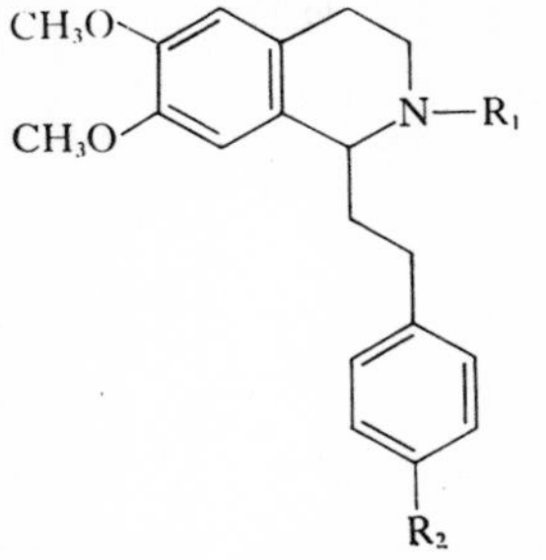

| | | Melting point (°C) | | LD$_{50}$ Mice (mg/kg | |
R$_1$	R$_2$	Base	Salt	intravenous)	Activity[a]
—CH$_2$—CH=CH$_2$	—Cl	—	HCl 210°	140	inact.
—CH$_2$—CH=CH$_2$	—NO$_2$	—	HCl 82°	70	inact.
—CH$_2$—CH$_3$	—Cl	78°		37	inact.
—CH$_2$—CH$_2$—Ph	—Cl	—	Oxalate 194°	100	inact.
—CH$_2$—CH=C(CH$_3$)CH$_3$	—Cl	58°	—	700[b]	inact.
—CH$_2$—CH$_2$—N(C$_2$H$_5$)C$_2$H$_5$	—Cl	—	HBr 195°	70	inact.

[a] See Table III.
[b] Oral value.

Nevertheless, as outlined in Fig. 2, it proved to be important for the synthesis of the tertiary amine (XXXIV).

   c. *Bischler-Napieralski procedure* (*Fig. 3, Method C*). The third and probably most convenient approach to the synthesis of 1-phenethyl-substituted tetrahydroisoquinolines, studied in our laboratories, employs methods well known in isoquinoline chemistry (*31*). The synthesis starts with phenethyl-amines (XXXV, R$_1$ = H) or phenylisopropylamines (XXXV, R$_1$ = methyl) substituted in the aromatic ring with alkoxy-, aralkoxy, alkylenedioxy, or

TABLE VII

DIFFERENTLY SUBSTITUTED 1-ω-PHENYLALKYL-2-METHYL-6,7-DIMETHOXY-1,2,3,4-TETRAHYDROISOQUINOLINES OF THE FORMULA

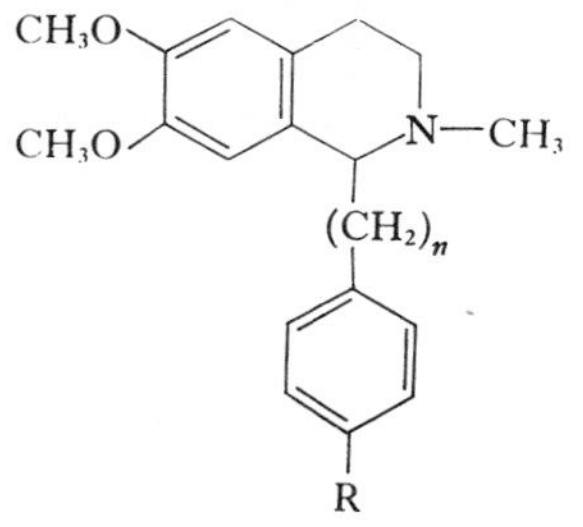

n	R	Melting point (°C) —Salt	LD$_{50}$ Mice (mg/kg intravenous)	Activity[a]
3	—Cl	HBr 160°	50	< 0.3
1	—Cl	HBr 163°	29	inact.
3	—NO$_2$	HBr 195°	35	1.1
1	—H	HBr 206°	15	inact.
3	—H	HCl 181°	20	inact.
1	—NO$_2$	HCl 205°	82 s.c.	0.5

[a] See Table III.

alkyl residues, with at least one of these substituents being attached in 3 position. By condensation of these amines with substituted dihydrocinnamic acids, the amides (XXXVI) are easily obtained. These are then cyclized to 3,4-dihydroisoquinoline derivatives of type XXXVII by the method of Bischler and Napieralski. The dihydroisoquinolines can either be converted into the N-methylated amines, such as XLI, by methods already mentioned (Fig. 1) or by reducing their quaternary salts (XXXVIII) with sodium borohydride. The Bischler-Napieralski procedure can also be extended to phenethylamides of substituted cinnamic acids which yield, after cyclization, the 1-styryl-substituted 3,4-dihydroisoquinolines of type XXXIX, already described in the literature (Fig. 1) (34). A distinct advantage of this approach is the fact that tertiary amines of type XLI substituted with nitro groups in the phenethyl moiety, can also be prepared (35). These derivatives are difficult to obtain by use of the two methods previously mentioned. For this purpose nitro-substituted dihydroisoquinolines (XXXVII) are first either reduced to XL with sodium borohydride or quaternized to the metho-

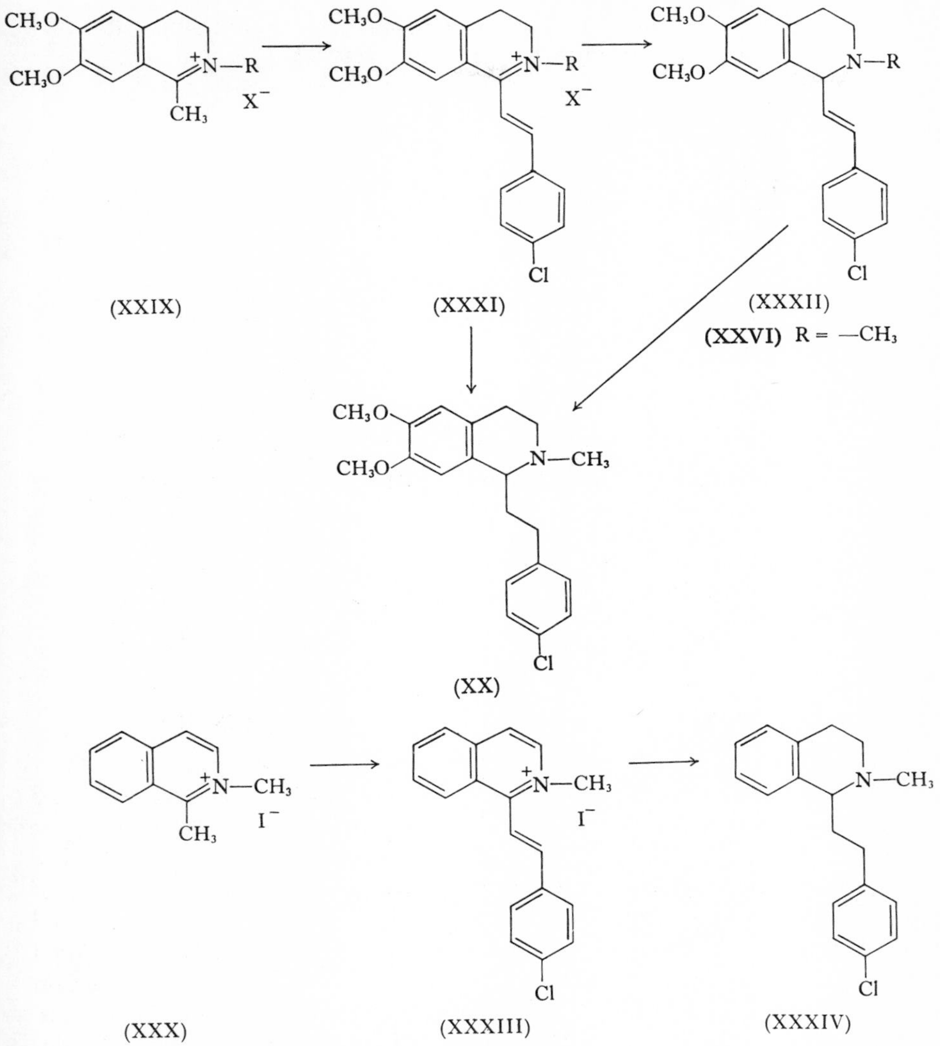

FIG. 2. Method B.

sulfates of XXXVIII with dimethyl sulfate. Heating XL with formic acid and formalin, or treating the quaternary salts (XXXVIII) with sodium borohydride, leads to the common N-methyl tertiary amine XLI. Nitro-substituted derivatives of type XLI, prepared by this route are also incorporated in Tables III–VII.

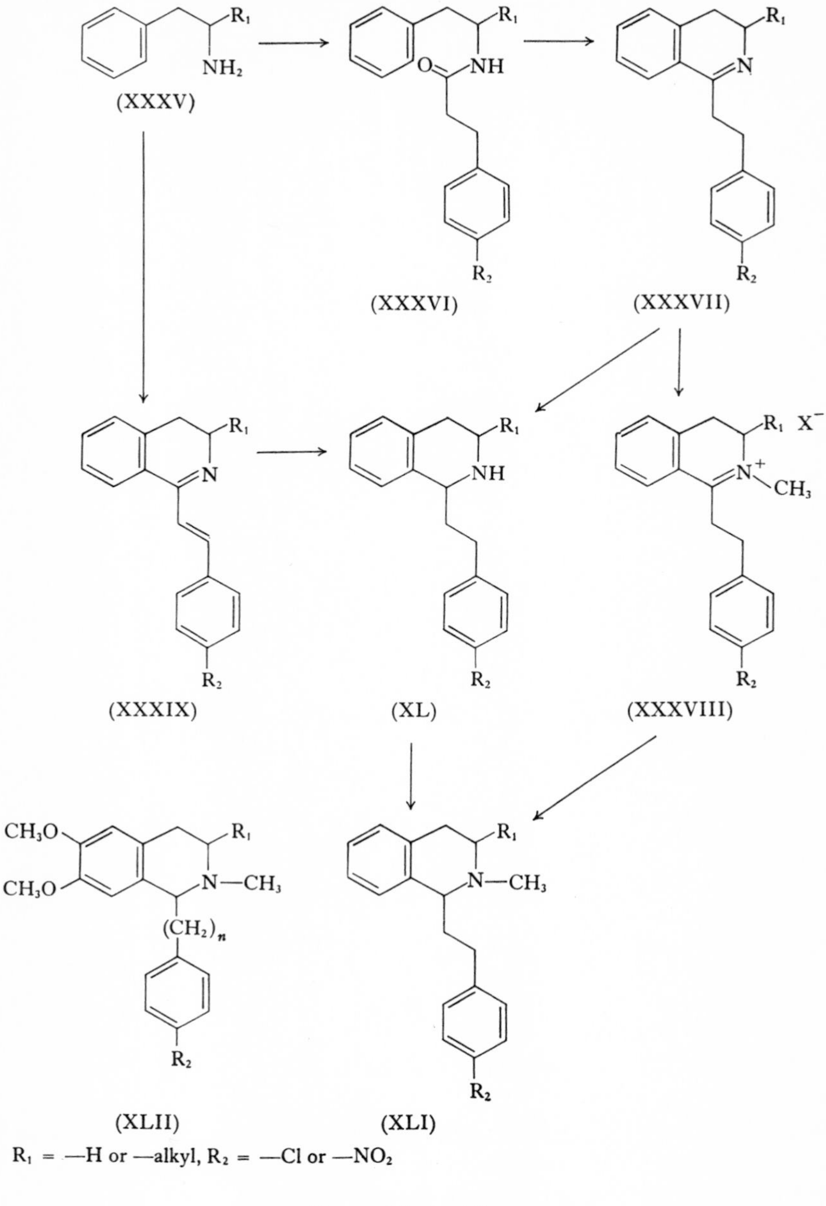

FIG. 3. Method C.

R_1 = —H or —alkyl, R_2 = —Cl or —NO_2

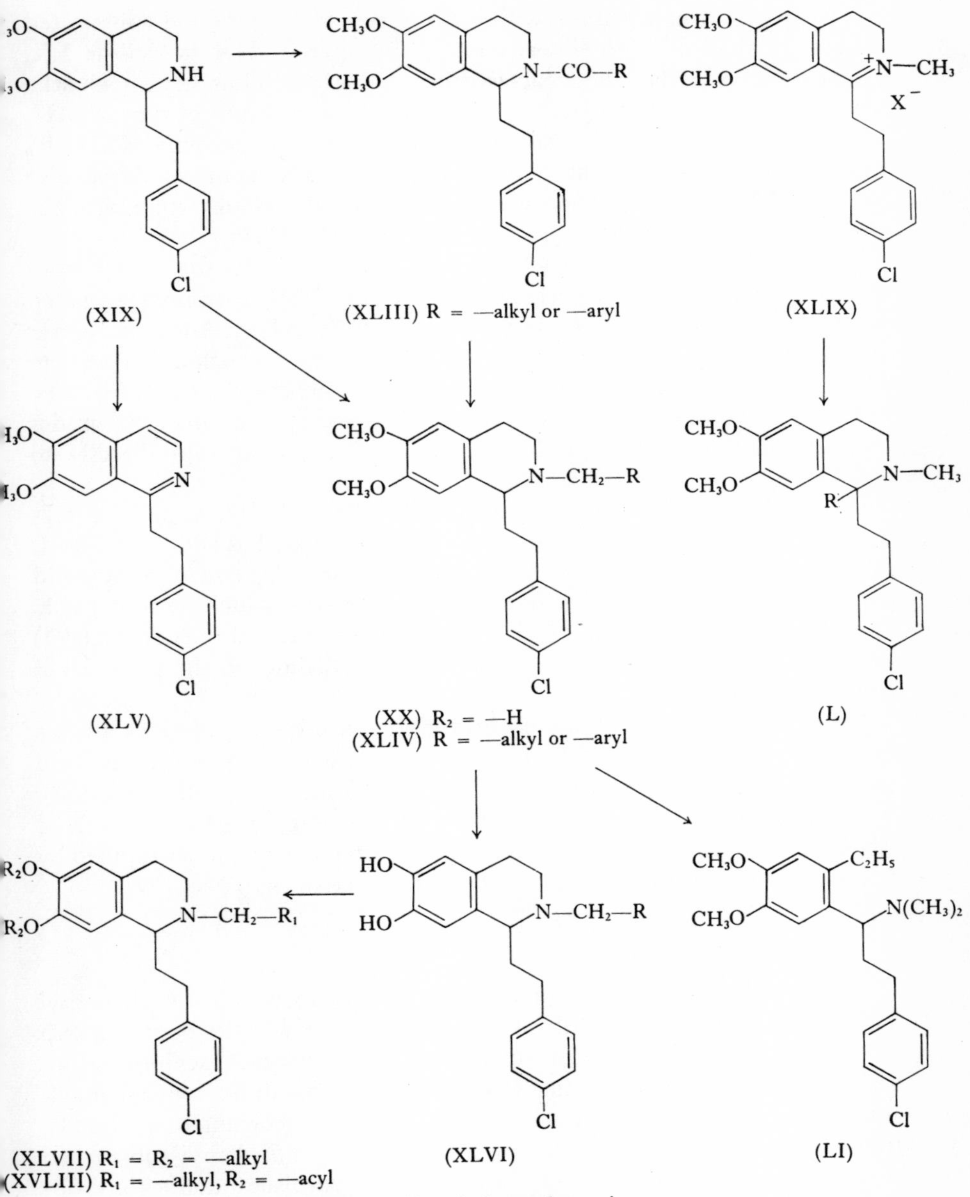

FIG. 4. Chemical transformations.

2. Chemical Transformations (Fig. 4)

Two types of compounds within the series of 1-phenethyl-substituted 1,2,3,4-tetrahydroisoquinolines, namely the amines XIX as well as XX, can be used for further chemical transformations (31). Thus, acylation of the secondary amines (XIX) yields neutral N-acyl derivatives of type XLIII, which can be converted easily into tertiary amines of type XLIV by reduction with lithium aluminium hydride. The latter compounds can also be prepared from the secondary amines XIX by direct alkylation with the corresponding alkyl halides by conventional methods (36).

The secondary amines, such as XIX, on heating in the presence of dehydrogenation catalysts such as palladium or nickel, are dehydrogenated to 1-phenethylisoquinoline derivatives of type XLV. An even better approach to this interesting group of isoquinolines, which are related to papaverine, starts with substituted β-methoxyphenethylamines (37). The latter, by reaction with dihydrocinnamic acids and cyclization of the amides thus obtained with phosphorus oxychloride, are converted directly to substances of this type.

6,7-Dialkoxy homologs of XX or XLIV, like XLVII, as well as 6,7-diacyloxy derivatives such as XLVIII, can be prepared as shown in Fig. 4. Heating 6,7-dimethoxy-substituted amines with 48% hydrobromic acid yields the corresponding 6,7-dihydroxy amines XLVI, which are susceptible to O-acylation or O-alkylation. For O-alkylation, the o-diphenols (XLVI) are reacted either with diazoalkanes or with alkylhalides in the presence of sodium hydroxide.

Other derivatives which are useful for chemical transformations are the quaternary salts of type XLIX. They react easily with Grignard reagent and thus yield directly 1,1-disubstituted tetrahydroisoquinolines of type L (38).

Hofmann degradation of quaternary salts of tertiary amines, such as XX, yields, after hydrogenation, phenethyl-substituted benzylamines typified by LI, which constitutes a new series of centrally active analgesics (39).

3. Homologs and Isomers

a. Homologs (Fig. 3). Tetrahydroisoquinolines in which the phenethyl side chain carries an alkyl substituent β with respect to the phenyl group can be prepared either from substituted 2-propionyl-N-acylphenethyl-amines (or higher acyl homologs) as already mentioned, or from α-benzyl-substituted alkane carboxylic acid phenethylamides according to method C. By the same procedure, and starting with appropriate β-phenyl-substituted alkane carboxylic acid phenethylamides, tetrahydroisoquinolines are obtained in which the phenethyl side chain is substituted with an alkyl group α with respect to the phenyl group. In these cases, due to the presence of two asymmetric centers, two racemic stereoisomers are theoretically possible.

1-Benzyl-substituted tetrahydroisoquinolines of type (XLII, $n = 1$) belonging to the laudanosine series, as well as its homologs (XLII, $n > 2$), can be prepared easily by processing the requisite ω-phenyl-substituted alkane

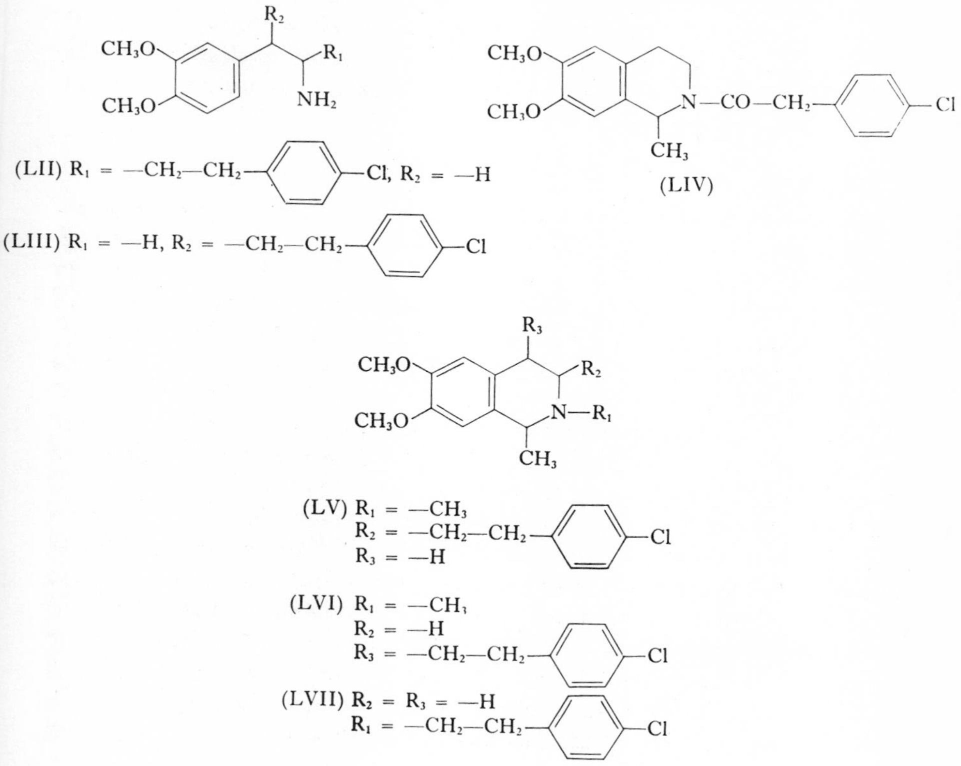

(LII) R_1 = —CH_2—CH_2—⟨⟩—Cl, R_2 = —H

(LIII) R_1 = —H, R_2 = —CH_2—CH_2—⟨⟩—Cl

(LIV)

(LV) R_1 = —CH_3
      R_2 = —CH_2—CH_2—⟨⟩—Cl
      R_3 = —H

(LVI) R_1 = —CH_3
      R_2 = —H
      R_3 = —CH_2—CH_2—⟨⟩—Cl

(LVII) R_2 = R_3 = —H
       R_1 = —CH_2—CH_2—⟨⟩—Cl

FIG. 5.

carboxylic acid phenethylamides according to method C. The analgetic activities of the compounds mentioned in this section are presented in Tables V and VII. Tetrahydroisoquinolines, carrying in 1 position a lower pyridylalkyl residue instead of a phenalkyl group, have recently been mentioned in a patent application (40). Thus far, nothing is known concerning their analgetic effectiveness.

b. *Isomers* (*Fig. 5*). The tetrahydroisoquinolines LV and LVI, both of which are homologous with XX, were prepared by conventional methods.

299

The intermediate phenethylamines LII and LIII, when subjected to acetylation, cyclization, hydrogenation, and finally to N-methylation, yielded LV and LVI. The isomeric N-p-chlorophenethyl-substituted derivative (LVII) was easily prepared by reducing the amide LIV with lithium aluminium hydride.

None of these p-chlorophenethyl-substituted tertiary tetrahydroisoquinoline derivatives exhibited analgetic properties. Since structures LV and LVI each have two asymmetric centers, and since it was not established whether the amines represent one stereoisomer or a mixture of two stereoisomers, the results are incomplete.

4. Resolution

In a racemic mixture of analgetics of different classes having one asymmetric center, the analgetic activity was always found to be associated with only one of the two enantiometers (5, 41). We were, therefore, also very much interested in studying the relationship between configuration and activity in our series of 1-phenethyl-substituted tetrahydroisoquinolines. Resolution within the series was achieved easily by conventional methods (31, 35, 39). The tertiary amines were either resolved directly, or the corresponding secondary amines were separated and then converted into optically active tertiary amines by N-methylation. In the four examples mentioned as being the most interesting representatives, the enantiomers of XX, LVIII, and LIX showing (−) $[\alpha]_D$ values and the enantiometer of LX having a (+) $(\alpha)_D$ value, exhibited twice as much analgetic activity as their corresponding racemates. Since, in all four examples under discussion, it was also possible to obtain the analgetically inactive enantiomers in a state of optical purity, the specificity with respect to configuration within this series of compounds is clearly established. It must be emphasized that for such studies, optical purity is an absolute necessity, since the picture can be changed completely if the active isomers are contaminated with even small amounts of inactive material.

Dehalogenation of (−)-LVIII, (+)-LX, or (−)-XX resulted in the formation of the same optically active dechloroderivative, namely (−)-LXI (42). The identical product was also obtained from (−)-LIX by reduction and deamination (42). The four compounds in question have, therefore, the same absolute configuration. Since (−)-XX has been chemically correlated with (+)-calycotomine (43)—a substance of known absolute configuration—the correct absolute configuration of all of these analgetics has been established as shown in their formulas.

Only one of the two enantiometers is responsible for the analgetic activity. Studies directed toward converting the unwanted optically active isomer

300

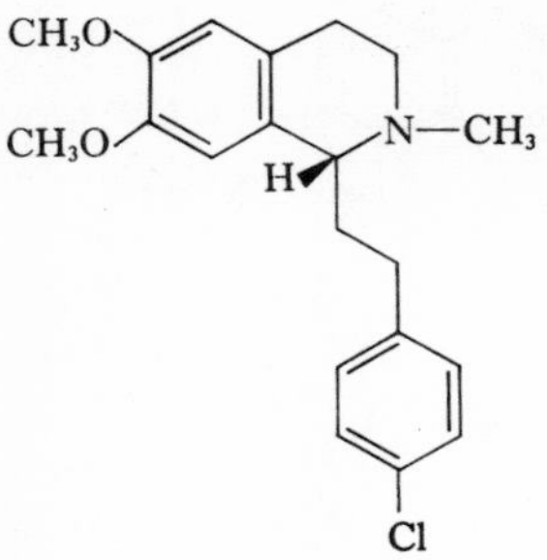

[(−)-XX]

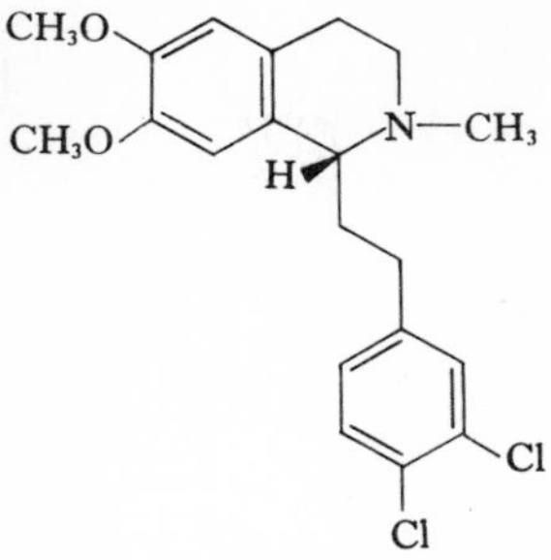

[(−)-LVIII]

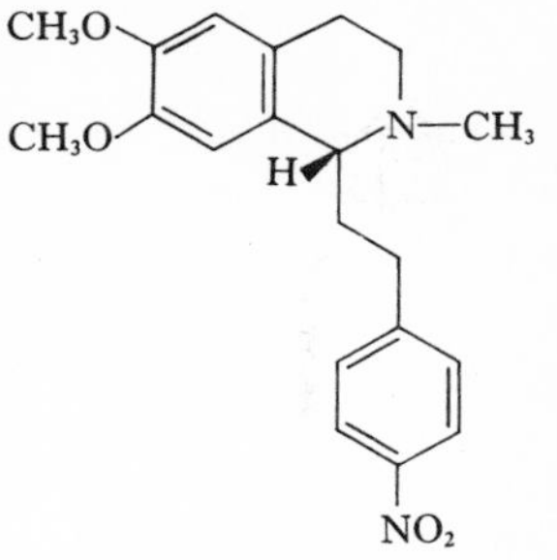

[(−)-LIX]

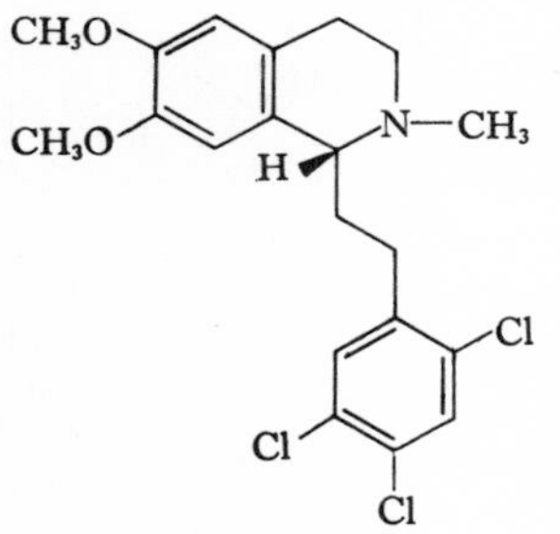

[(+)-LX]

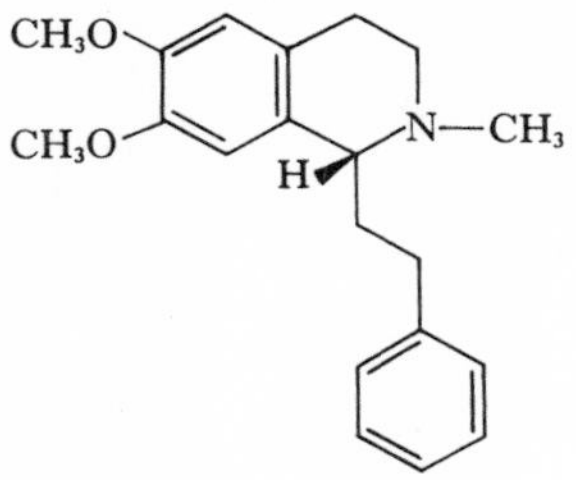

[(−)-LXI]

back into the racemate, which could then be resolved again, were therefore initiated. With secondary amines, this can, for instance, be achieved by subjecting the unwanted optically active secondary amines to oxidation with hypochlorite followed by catalytic hydrogenation (44). With tertiary amines such as (+)-XX, this was accomplished by oxidation with mercuric acetate in acetic acid solution, followed by catalytic hydrogenation, as shown in the following flowsheet. The racemic compound XX is obtained in excellent yield, and the over-all process represents, therefore, an almost stereospecific synthesis for (−)-XX.

5. Structure-Activity Relationships

a. Analgetic activity. All the isoquinolines discussed below were tested for analgetic activity in mice, after subcutaneous and oral administration, by the method of Gross (45). Effectiveness was determined by comparison with codeine. Only those compounds which showed activity at levels below the toxic dose were considered to be of importance. The toxicity (LD_{50}) was determined in mice by the intravenous route. The list of compounds to be discussed can be shortened considerably, since it was found that 3,4-dihydroisoquinolines of type XXVIII, *sec*-tetrahydroisoquinolines of type

301

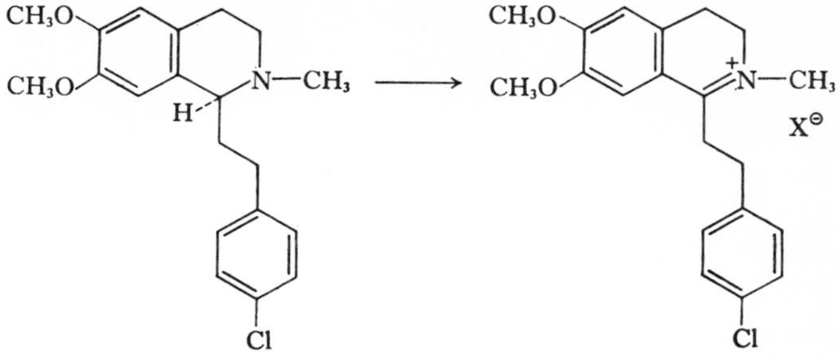

[(+)-XX]

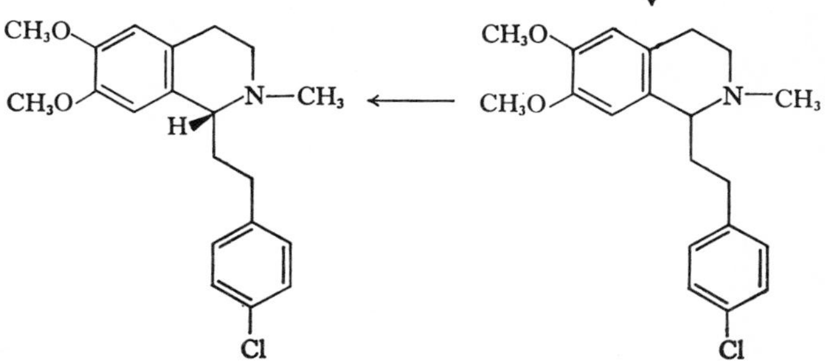

[(−)-XX]   (XX)

XIX, isoquinolines of type XLV, as well as 1-styryl-substituted tetra-hydroisoquinolines of type XXVI, were completely devoid of analgetic effectiveness.

It was recognized early that the presence of least one halogen- or nitro-residue in the phenyl residue is essential for activity of 1-phenethyl-substi-tuted *N*-methyltetrahydroisoquinolines, and, therefore, all further chemical changes within the molecule were carried out on an active model. Shortening or lengthening of the substituted 1-phenethyl side chain led to compounds of minor interest (Table VII). The studies carried out with respect to N-substitution were extremely interesting (Table VI). Only the N-methylated derivatives were found to be active. Replacing the N-methyl group by another alkyl group, by an *N*-phenethyl or by an *N*-allyl residue led to compounds which showed neither enhanced activity nor antagonistic pro-perties. This clearly distinguishes the tetrahydroisoquinoline analgetics from the morphines, morphinanes, benzomorphans, and pethidines. The sensi-tivity of the analgetic activity with respect to substitution within the aromatic ring A (Table IV) was also quite unexpected. Only compounds substituted at the 6,7 positions with either methoxyl or methyl groups exhibited analgetic effects. It is interesting that the 6,7-desmethoxy-, the 6,7-methylenedioxy-, and the 6,7,8-trimethoxy-substituted analogs showed no noteworthy activity. Partially demethylated compounds, which were isolated as metabolites, will be discussed later. It is also interesting to note that the only compound we prepared with a quaternary carbon atom, namely compound (L), exerted only weak analgetic properties.

We shall now discuss the relationship between analgetic activity and constitution within the group of compounds which have been the basic skeleton found to be essential for analgetic activity, namely the 1-phenethyl-substituted 2-methyl-6,7-dimethoxy-1,2,3,4-tetrahydroisoquinolines of the accompanying formula. With respect to substitution on the phenyl group,

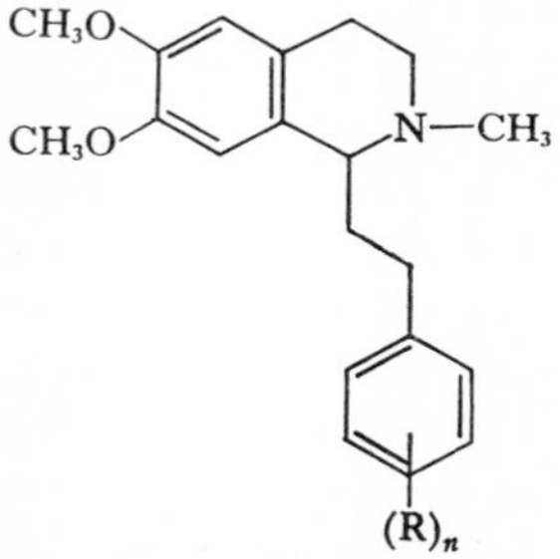

R = halogen or nitro

the most active compound prepared was the p-nitro derivative, followed by the m-nitro-, p-fluoro-, p-chlor-, and p-bromo-derivatives. Shifting the chloro group into the *ortho* or *meta* position or the nitro group into the *ortho* position yielded compounds of minor interest (Table III). Introduction of additional halogens did not lead to compounds with enhanced analgetic activity, but rather to compounds which were more active as antitussives. These will be discussed under this topic.

With respect to alkyl substitution within the heterocyclic ring moeity or within the phenethyl side chain (Table V), it must be noted that some of these compounds display considerable activity, but at this time no definite statement can be made as to which compound is the best.

Among all the compounds studied so far, the analgetic effectiveness has always been found to be associated with only one of the two enantiometers, and, in so far as the studies have progressed, all the active isomers have the same absolute configuration and belong to the (R)-series (42).

Studies of the physical dependence capacity of several racemates and their enantiomers, carried out by Deneau and Seevers (46), led to the

303

conclusion that the degree of addictiveness is commensurate with that of analgetic activity. The most interesting compound was 1-*p*-chlorophenethyl-2-methyl-6,7-dimethoxy-1,2,3,4-tetrahydroisoquinoline (XX) (*47*). The analgetic activity of this substance, as will be discussed later in detail, is similar to that of codeine, but its addictiveness is of such a low order that it can be considered academic. As soon as the analgetic activity was enhanced, as in the case of the *p*-nitro analog, addiction was found. Since both enantiomers of XX show distinct spasmolytic effects, it was deemed preferable to choose the racemic compound for clinical trials, despite the fact that technical syntheses of the analgetically active (−) isomer are available.

b. Antitussives (Table II). All antitussives found so far in this series exhibit analgetic effects of varying degrees. Moreover, antitussive activity is always associated with the enantiomer which also exhibits analgetic properties. In this respect, tetrahydroisoquinolines are distinctly different from morphinans.

Within this series, the basic skeleton, which is essential for antitussive activity, is identical with that which is also essential for analgesic activity. Careful studies have shown, however, that different substitution in the phenyl residue of the phenethyl side chain does not show close parallelism between optimal antitussive and analgetic activity. Optimal antitussive activity, associated with distinct analgetic properties as exhibited by codeine, was found in the 3,4-dichloroderivative, with the (−) enantiomer being responsible for the activity. Optimal antitussive properties with only significant analgetic effects are exhibited by the (±)-2,4,5-trichloro derivative. Substitution with chlorine in other positions did not produce compounds which seem to be of greater interest. Clinical trials will determine to what extent the antitussive effects observed in animals occur also in humans.

6. *Methopholine* (*47*)

From the many compounds prepared and tested, (±)-1-*p*-chlorophenethyl-2-methyl-6,7-dimethoxy-1,2,3,4-tetrahydroisoquinoline (XX) was selected for evaluation as an analgetic in humans.

This compound was tested in the form of its crystalline free base under the code number Ro 4-1778/1 and in the form of its water-soluble hydrochloride as Ro 4-1778.

Physicochemical properties of methopholine. The free base crystallizes in colorless plates. It is insoluble in water and melts at 110°. Of its salts, the hydrochloride is unsuitable for pharmaceutical compositions, since it is hygroscopic and tends to retain solvents. Much more convenient for this purpose are the acid phosphate (m.p. 126° C), the acid sulfate (m.p. 167° C),

304

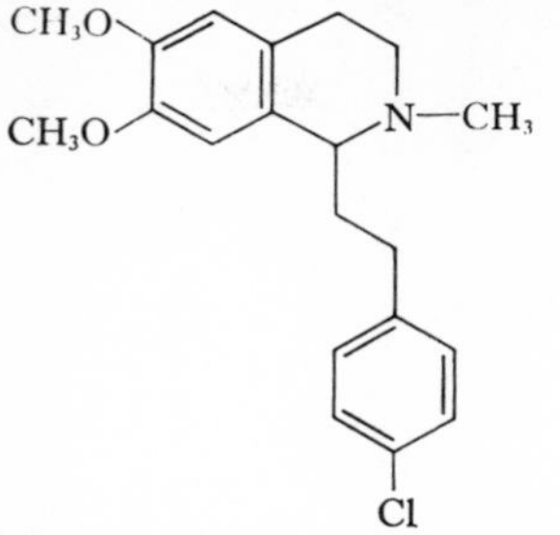

(XX)

or the fumarate (m.p. 143° C). The salts and the free base are stable at room temperature and also when they are submitted to the usual stability tests.

For the characterization of methopholine, the picrate (m.p. 125° C) or the methobromide (m.p. 202° C) are convenient.

As a test for the purity of the drug, the ultraviolet spectrum with the $\lambda_{max.}$ at 282 mμ, characteristic for a 6,7-dimethoxy-1,2,3,4-tetrahydroisoquinoline chomophore, is not very suitable. The analytical methods using paper chromatography and thin layer chromatography, which have been worked out, are preferred.

By application of these techniques, it was found that most likely the three compounds XIX, LXII, and LXIII could be the impurities of methopholine.

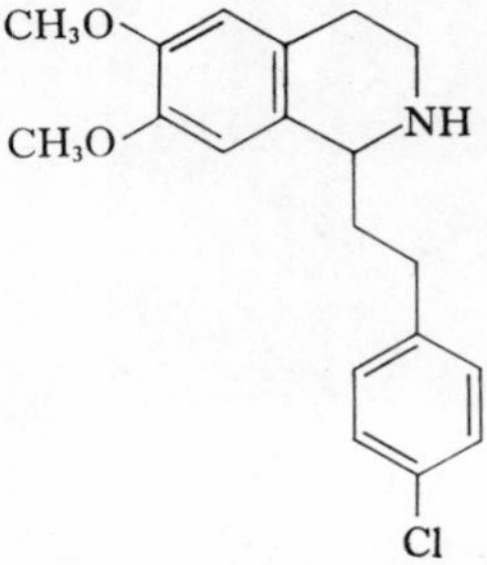

(XIX) 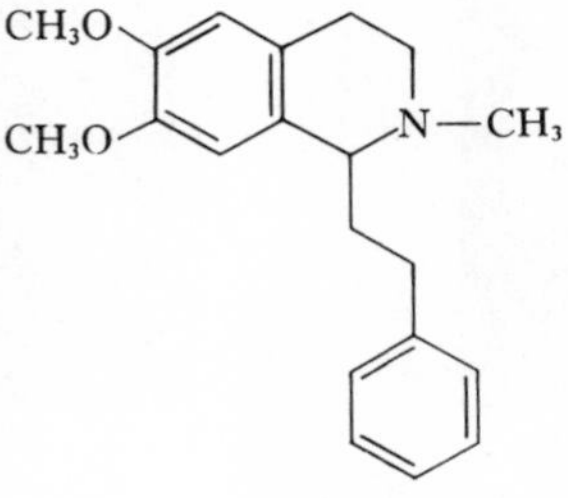   (LXII) 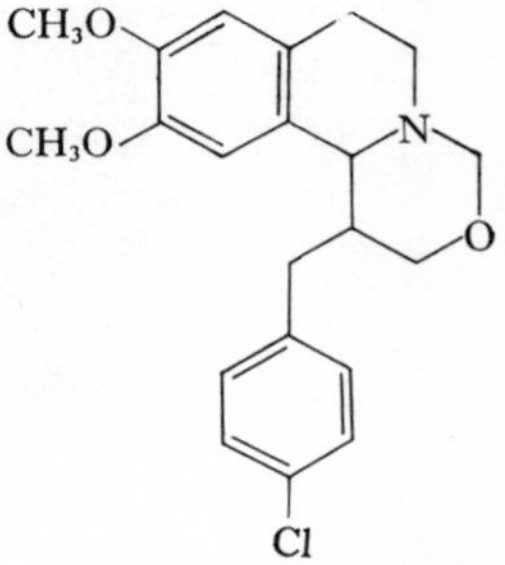   (LXIII)

The secondary amine XIX, the penultimate compound in the methopholine synthesis, may be present because of incomplete N-methylation, whereas the dechloro tertiary amine LXII may be formed during the catalytic hydrogenation step. The most interesting compound, which was encountered in the first batches of unpurified methopholine, is the 1-*p*-chlorobenzyl-substituted derivative (LXIII) (*48*). This contaminant was formed from the 3,4-dihydroisoquinoline (XXVIII) due to the presence of formalin as demonstrated by the synthesis shown on page 306.

305

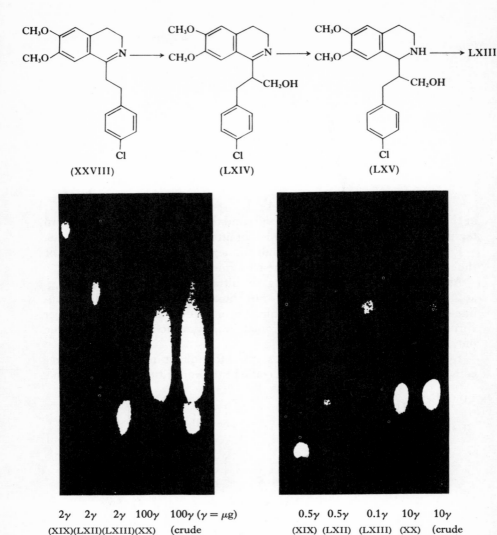

$$(XXVIII) \longrightarrow (LXIV) \longrightarrow (LXV) \longrightarrow LXIII$$

2γ	2γ	2γ	100γ	100γ (γ = μg)
(XIX)	(LXII)	(LXIII)	(XX)	(crude methopholine)

0.5γ	0.5γ	0.1γ	10γ	10γ
(XIX)	(LXII)	(LXIII)	(XX)	(crude methopholine)

Paper Chromatogram^a   Thin Layer Chromatogram^b

Fig. 6. ^a Descending on Whatman No. 4 paper buffered to pH 3.0. Substances brought on paper, while eluent (benzene–*n*-butanol 19:1) is already creeping downwards. Duration: 1.5 hours. Development by spraying with a diluted solution of cerium(IV) sulfate in trichloroacetic acid and sulfuric acid. After drying, observation of the fluorescence at 365 mμ. The tetrahydroisoquinolines which are not fluorescent per se are dehydrogenated by Ce(IV) to the corresponding 3,4-dihydro derivatives. ^b Ascending on Silica Gel-G in acetone-ethanol 9:1 for 1/2 hour. Development as described under *a*.

The product thus obtained (LXIII) proved to be identical with the impurity detected by thin layer chromatography. That these contaminants can be avoided or eliminated by purification of the intermediates as well as the final product is clearly demonstrated in Fig. 6, which shows a thin layer chromatogram of pure and impure methopholine (49).

B. 1-Phenethyl-Substituted 1,2,3,4,5,6,7,8-Octahydroisoquinolines

The interesting pharmacological activities exhibited by the series of 1,2,3,4-tetrahydroisoquinolines mentioned before, initiated studies aimed at the synthesis of other partially hydrogenated isoquinoline derivatives. Starting with the cyclohexenylethylamine derivative (LXVI), Schnider and Walter synthesized many compounds typified by LXVII and LXVIII via the Bischler-Napieralski method (procedure C) already described, for the synthesis of the corresponding 1,2,3,4-tetrahydroisoquinolines (50).

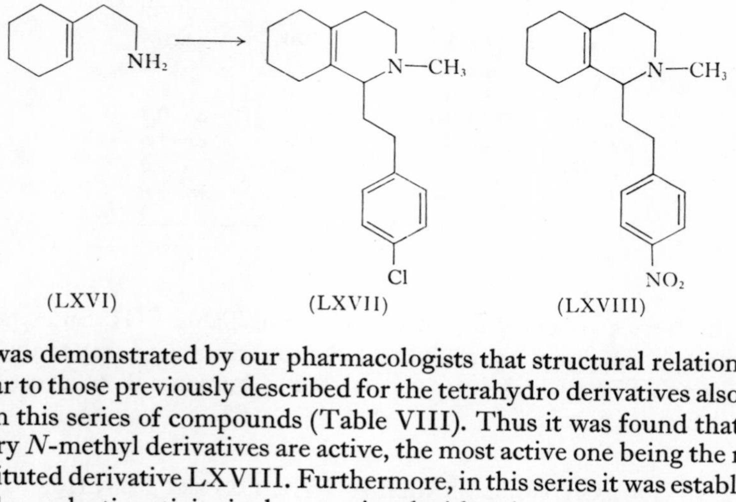

(LXVI)   (LXVII)   (LXVIII)

It was demonstrated by our pharmacologists that structural relationships similar to those previously described for the tetrahydro derivatives also exist within this series of compounds (Table VIII). Thus it was found that only tertiary N-methyl derivatives are active, the most active one being the nitro-substituted derivative LXVIII. Furthermore, in this series it was established that the analgetic activity is also associated with only one of the enantiomers of the racemate. The close relationship between octahydro- and tetrahydro-isoquinolines is also evident from the finding that on both series, the racemate as well as both of the enantiomers, exerts distinct spasmolytic properties.

In both groups of isoquinoline derivatives, the length of the 1-aralkyl substituent has a similar influence on the activity. However, in the octahydro series the p-nitro-n-phenylpropyl derivative is slightly more active than the p-nitrophenethyl compound, but the n-butyl homolog is inactive. As a group, the octahydroisoquinoline derivatives exhibit less analgetic activity than the tetrahydroisoquinoline series. Some representatives of the

307

TABLE VIII

SUBSTITUTED 1-PHENETHYL-2-METHYL-1,2,3,4,5,6,7,8-OCTAHYDROISOQUINOLINES (*35*) OF THE GENERAL FORMULA

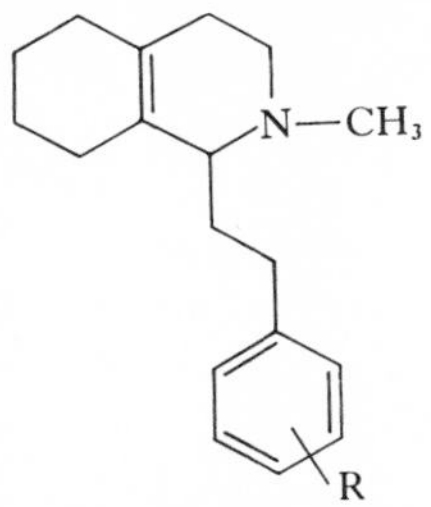

R	Optically	LD$_{50}$ Mice subcutaneous	Activity[a]
—H	inactive	220	inactive
4-Cl	inactive	350	ca. 0.1
2-NO$_2$	inactive	350	1.0
3-NO$_2$	inactive	500	ca. 0.3
4-NO$_2$	inactive	190	ca. 1.6
4-NO$_2$	(—)-base	125	< 1.0
4-NO$_2$	(+)-base	250	ca. 3.0

[a] See Table III.

octahydro series are compared with codeine in Table VIII. Since none of the octahydroisoquinolines appeared to be superior in any way to the tetrahydroisoquinolines which have been tested in humans, their investigation was not further pursued.

C. 1,2,3,4-TETRAHYDROISOQUINOLINES WITH OXYGEN FUNCTIONS IN THE PHENETHYL SIDE CHAIN (FIG. 7) (*51*)

Later it was found that substituted acetophenone derivatives can be condensed easily with quaternary salts of 3,4-dihydroisoquinolines, resulting directly in substituted 1-phenacyl-2-alkyl-1,2,3,4-tetrahydroisoquinolines in high yield. By this procedure, the 1-*p*-chlorphenacyl-2-methyl-6,7-dimethoxytetrahydroisoquinoline derivative (LXX) was obtained from the methosulfate (LXIX) and *p*-chloroacetophenone. It was hoped that this simple synthesis could provide a new procedure for obtaining 1-phenethyl-substituted tetrahydroisoquinolines. This did not materialize, however, because during catalytic hydrogenation these 1-phenacyl derivatives readily

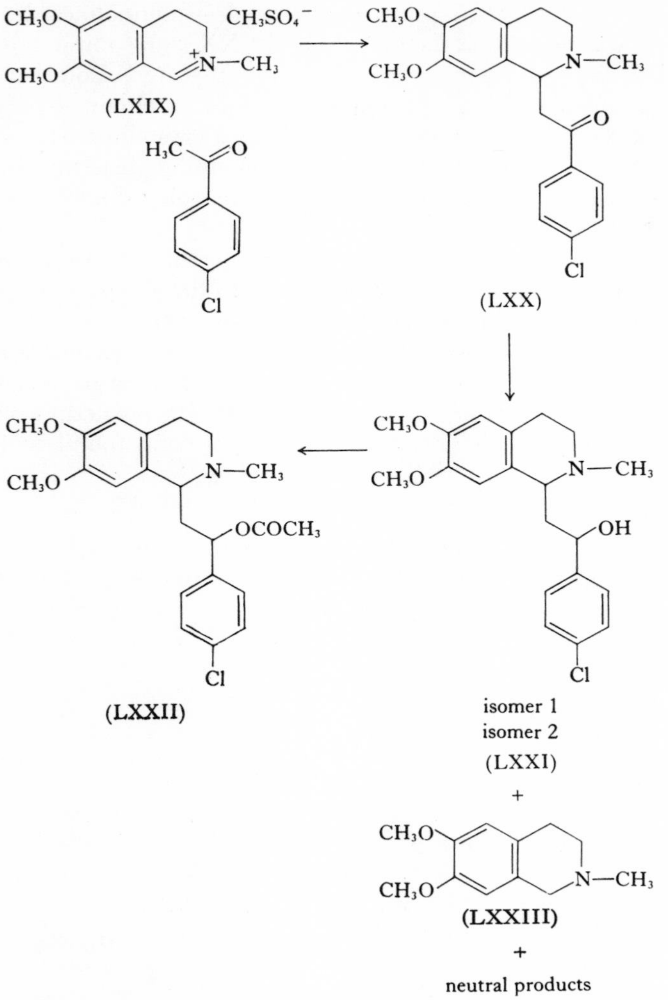

FIG. 7. 1,2,3,4-Tetrahydroisoquinolines with oxygen functions in the 1-phenethyl side chain.

undergo fragmentation. The tetrahydroisoquinoline derivative (LXXIII), p-chloroacetophenone and/or the corresponding carbinol, were the only products isolated.

The phenacyl-substituted compound (LXX) still possessed an analgetic activity in animals at a level similar to the corresponding phenethyl-substituted derivative. This suggested, therefore, a more detailed study with this

309

new series of oxygenated 1-phenethyltetrahydroisoquinolines. In pursuing this task, it was found that the reduction of LXX with sodium borohydride yields, in addition to fragmentation products, two stereoisomeric carbinols (LXXI) (isomers 1 and 2). Both isomers could be obtained pure. It was shown that one of these isomers, obtained as a crystalline base, has much stronger analgetic properties than the corresponding phenethyl-substituted derivative, whereas the other (obtained as an amorphous base) was about ten times less active.

Many members of this series were prepared by the same procedure, and it was shown that those isomers which belong to the series of isomer 1 constitute a new group of highly centrally active analgetics.

The studies with regard to stereochemical considerations are not yet complete. Activity-structure relationships exist for the oxygenated compounds, similar to those previously described for the phenethyl-substituted tetrahydroisoquinolines. The most active compound found so far is the

TABLE IX

DIFFERENTLY SUBSTITUTED 1-PHENETHYL-2-METHYL-6,7-DIMETHOXY-1,2,3,4-TETRAHYDRO-ISOQUINOLINES SUBSTITUTED IN THE PHENETHYL SIDE CHAIN WITH A HYDROXY GROUP

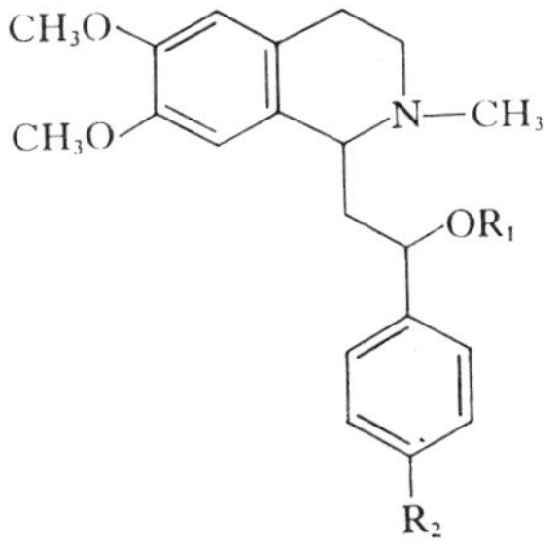

	R_1	R_2	Melting point (°C) Base	Salt	LD_{50} mice (mg/kg intravenous)	Activity[a]
Isomer 1	—H	—Cl	118°	—	25	ca. 7
Isomer 2	—H	—Cl	—	Oxalate 118°	35	0.7
Isomer 1	—H	—NO$_2$	152°	—	7	45
Isomer 2	—H	—NO$_2$	—	HBr 128°	25	ca. 3
Isomer 1	—CO—CH$_3$	—Cl	—	HCl 232°	35	ca. 2.0
Isomer 1	—CO—CH$_2$—CH$_3$	—Cl	—	HCl 231°	53	ca. 2.0

[a] See Table III.

p-nitro derivative which, as the racemate, is many times more active than morphine. The corresponding *p*-chloro derivative, by contrast, exerts activity of the same order as morphine. Esters of isomer 1, such as LXXII, are less active, but the activity is of longer duration. The *N*-allyl derivatives, which have been prepared thus far, have not shown antagonistic properties. From the pharmacological data available at present, it can be concluded that this series of compounds exhibits a spectrum of pharmacological properties similar to the phenethyl-substituted tetrahydroisoquinolines, but with a higher degree of effectiveness. A few examples are mentioned in Table IX. The analgetics tested thus far showed high physical dependence capacity in monkeys (*52*), and it can be assumed that they are very addictive. Whether or not this series of new analgetics can compete with morphine or other addictive analgetics can be determined only when the results of their clinical evaluation in humans are available.

IV. Metabolism of 1-*p*-Chlorophenethyl-2-methyl-6,7-dimethoxy-1,2,3,4-tetrahydroisoquinoline[1]

Studies of the metabolic fate of methopholine (Versidyne®) (*47*) were carried out spectrofluorometrically and by means of methopholine C^{14}-labeled in the 3 position.

The technique for the spectrofluorometric determination of this drug and some of its free and conjugated metabolites in blood and urine were described by Schwarz and Rieder (*57*).

Schwartz *et al.* (*58*) identified in man and rabbit the following four metabolites of methopholine (Fig. 8):

Metabolite I (XIX), the *N*-desmethyl analog of methopholine;
Metabolite II (LXXIV), the 6-*O*-desmethyl derivative of methopholine;
Metabolite III (LXXV), the *N*-desmethyl-6-*O*-desmethyl derivative of methopholine;
Metabolite IV (LXXVI), the 1,2-dehydrogenated derivative of metabolite III.

Metabolite I was found in its free form in small quantities in blood and urine. The other three metabolites were excreted in their conjugated forms in the urine, with metabolite II forming the major portion of the four

[1] All investigations herein reported were carried out in the Chemical Pharmacology Departments of F. Hoffmann-La Roche & Co., A.G., Basle, Switzerland (J. Rieder and D. E. Schwartz) and Hoffmann-La Roche Inc., Nutley, New Jersey, U.S.A. (L. D'Arconte, B. A. Koechlin, F. Rubio, and P. Stefko).

metabolites; metabolite III occurred in more limited amounts and metabolite IV was excreted only in small quantities.

Following oral administration of a single 120 mg dose of methopholine to humans (3 subjects), the total urinary excretion of the drug and its 4 metabolites, over a 2–3 day period, was found to range from 42.9 to 66% [1] with the excretion of metabolite II ranging from 33.5 to 50.6% and of metabolites

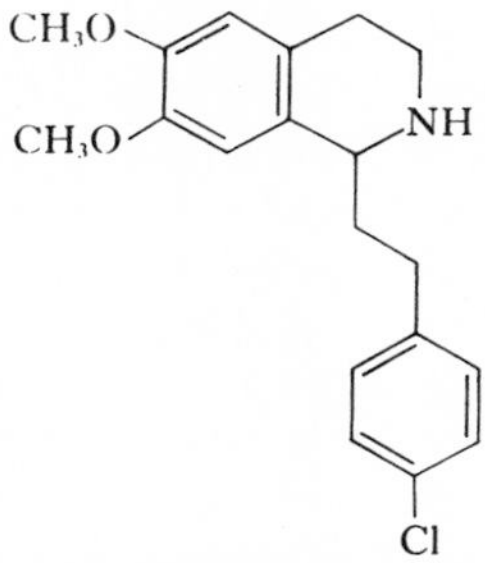

(XIX) Metabolite I

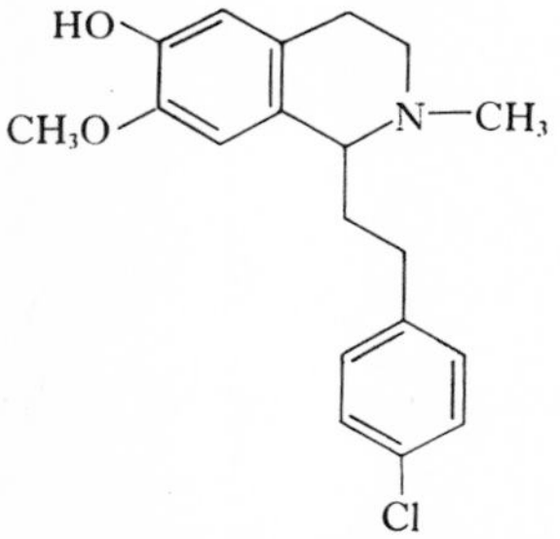

(LXXIV) Metabolite II 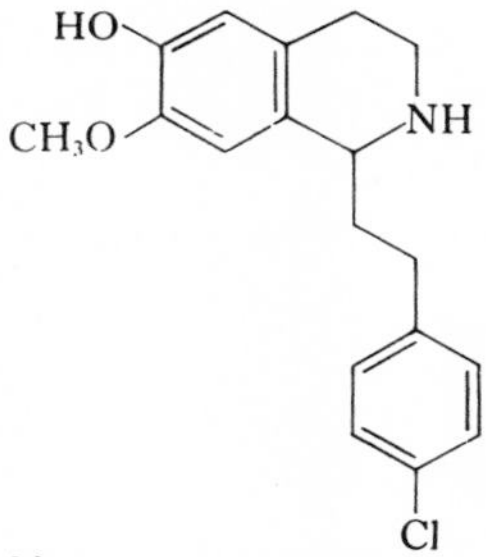   (LXXV) Metabolite III 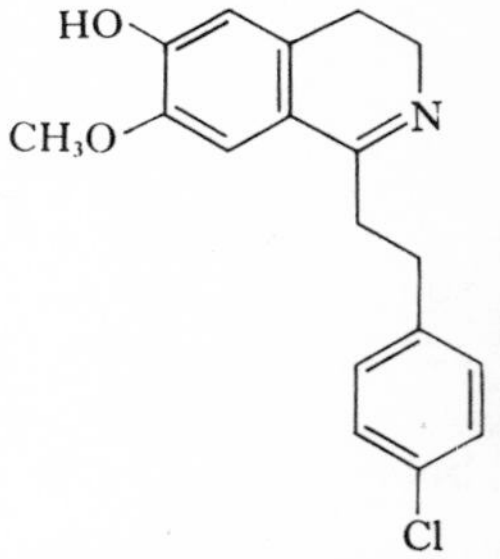   (LXXVI) Metabolite IV

FIG. 8. Main metabolites of methopholine in animals and humans.

III + IV, from 9.4 to 15.2% (only 0.2% appeared as methopholine + metabolite I). Similarly, in the rabbit, following intraperitoneal injection of 20 mg/kg, the total urinary excretion of methopholine and its 4 metabolites was 54.5% over a 3-day period, and the proportion between methopholine and the metabolites resembled that observed in man.

In contrast, in the dog only 1.4% and 2.7% were excreted in the urine as metabolites II, III, and IV, over a 3-day period, following intraperitoneal and oral administration respectively of 10 mg/kg of methopholine.

The average urinary excretion of the combined metabolites II, III, and

[1] All percentages given are in terms of the administered dose.

IV[1] in man, rabbit, and dog amounted, in this sequence, to 54.7, 54, and 2% of the administered dose of methopholine.

Koechlin et al. (59) administered orally single 120 or 180 mg doses of methopholine to humans (7 experiments in 5 subjects) and determined, spectrofluorometrically, the urinary excretion of this drug and its metabolites over a 12- to 24-hour period. Expressed in terms of the administered dose and calculated as methopholine the total amounts recovered ranged from 13.6 to 32%. These figures were 17.7 to 40% if the quantities excreted were calculated in terms of the main metabolite (LXXIV). The fact that this group of investigators reported generally lower urinary excretion values than the former group may be explained by the difference in the procedures used and the prevailing experimental conditions.

These workers also studied urinary excretion in monkeys which were treated chronically with methopholine at 3 dose levels. It was found that, independent of the dose, the 24-hour excretion amounted to approximately 4% of the daily dose and that the methopholine was eliminated mainly as the conjugate of metabolite II.

The same group (60) found in the dog that 1.3% of the administered dose of methopholine was recovered as fluorometrically measurable metabolites (mostly as the conjugate of metabolite II) in the urine aspirated from the bladder of an animal, sacrificed 4 hours after intravenous injection of 10 mg/kg of Ro 4-1778, the hydrochloride of methopholine.

Thus, it appears that whereas man excretes in the urine a very considerable portion (up to 66%) of the administered dose of methopholine, the dog excretes only a very small portion (up to 2.7%).

Koechlin et al. (60) also determined, at 30-minute intervals for 4 hours, the amounts of methopholine metabolites excreted in the bile of the dog for which the urinary excretion after intravenous injection of 10 mg/kg of Ro 4-1778 was assessed (see above). The 4-hour recovery from the bile was found to be 23.5% of the administered dose, again as the conjugated metabolite II. Thus, the rate of excretion of the drug in the bile was approximately 15 times higher than that in the urine in this species. These results are consistent with the findings that, in contrast to man and rabbit, the dog excretes methopholine metabolites predominantly in the feces (see below) and not in the urine, as shown above. Thus, the route of excretion of methopholine in man and rabbit on the one hand, and in the dog on the other, is very definitely different.

Schwartz and Rieder (61) studied the route of excretion of methopholine, following single dose administration, by radiometric techniques in several

---

[1] These 3 metabolites account for almost the entire quantities of methopholine and its degradation products recovered in the urine of man and rabbit.

animal species (rabbit, rat, and dog) and in man. The route of administration, the doses of C^{14}-labeled methopholine and the amounts of metabolites found in urine and feces, within the days indicated, and expressed as per cent of the administered doses, are shown in Table X.

As is seen, rabbit and man excrete the radioactivity primarily in the urine and much smaller portions of the administered dose are eliminated in the feces. Conversely, in rat and dog, the main route of the drug's excretion is via the feces, with comparatively small amounts being eliminated in the urine. Thus, the findings in the urinary excretion studies of methopholine by means of radioactive tracer techniques are in agreement with those obtained by the use of spectrofluorometric methods.

In another phase of their metabolic studies, these investigators sacrificed the animals used for the above elimination studies and determined distribution of radioactivity in the blood and various organs. Suffice it to say here that these studies revealed marked differences in radioactivity ratios (radioactivity in organ: radioactivity in blood) among the 3 animal species following oral administration of methopholine. These ratios were much higher in the dog than in the rabbit and rat for the liver and intestinal wall and higher in the rabbit than in the dog and rat for the kidney. The high residue concentration of metabolites of methopholine peculiar to the dog's liver and intestinal wall, may well explain in part the gastroenteritis, peritoneal adhesions, and hepatic changes observed in dogs which received high doses of methopholine for a 60-week period (see Section V,B).

A. CHEMISTRY OF THE METABOLITES (58, 62)

For the synthesis of the metabolites LXXIV and LXXV, 3-benzyloxy-4-methoxyphenethylamine (63) was condensed with p-chlorodihydrocinnamic acid and the resulting amide (m.p. 153°C) cyclized according to method C. Sodium borohydride reduction followed by catalytic O-debenzylation yielded LXXV and after N-methylation LXXIV was obtained (Fig. 8).

For the synthesis of the metabolite LXXVI, 3-hydroxy-4-methoxyphenethylamine (64) was condensed with p-chlorodihydrocinnamic acid to give the amide (m.p. 141°C) which was cyclized directly according to the aforementioned procedure.

B. PHARMACOLOGY OF THE METABOLITES

With respect to pharmacology, only the analgetic activity of the main metabolite, the tertiary amine LXXIV, requires comment since the other metabolites are inactive.

The analgetic activity of LXXIV (ED_{50} mouse 54 mg/kg administered

314

TABLE X

EXCRETION PATTERN OF C14-LABELED METHOPHOLINE IN RABBIT, RAT, DOG, AND MAN

Species	Rabbit		Rat	Dog		Man	
						Patient M.O.	Patient E.S.
Route of administration	Oral	Intraperitoneal	Oral	Oral	Intraperitoneal	Oral	Oral
Dose of methopholine[a] given	10 mg/kg	10 mg/kg	4 mg/kg	5 mg/kg	5 mg/kg	40 mg	120 mg
Days of collection	3	3	3	3	3	4½	5½
Specimen	urine feces	urine feces	urine feces	urine feces	urine feces	urine feces	urine feces
Excretion in per cent of dose	77.8 12.8	93.0 6.0	15.8 79.6	17.0 64.2	18.7 59.9	48.1[b] 15.3[b]	66.3 17.6
Total excretion in per cent of dose	90.6	99.0	95.4	81.2	78.6	63.4[b]	83.9

[a] The drug was given orally as the base and intraperitoneally as the hydrochloride.
[b] This patient failed to collect one urine and stool specimen each during the 4½ days of the experiment.

315

subcutaneously) is decidedly lower than that of methopholine. It follows that Versidyne itself must be mainly responsible for its analgetic efficacy.

V. Pharmacological Findings with 1-p-Chlorophenethyl-2-methyl-6,7-dimethoxy-1,2,3,4-tetrahydroisoquinoline[1]

A. ANALGESIA

Comparing the analgetic effectiveness of methopholine and codeine, Besendorf et al. (65) administered both agents to mice, rats, and rabbits by various routes. They found that approximately equal subcutaneous doses produced a 50% prolongation of reaction time to a heat stimulus in mice and rats. When mice were treated orally and the same test method was used, the ED_{50} values of the two anodynes were again about equal, but by this route approximately twice the subcutaneous doses were required. It was also noted that in mice 10 mg/kg methopholine, given subcutaneously, or 40 mg/kg administered orally, completely abolished the writhing reaction to chemically induced peritoneal pain, while in this assay, codeine was not fully effective at these doses. However, the ED_{50} values of these drugs, injected subcutaneously, were about equal in this test. Studies in rabbits showed that by the intravenous route, methopholine was considerably more potent than codeine in terms of the dose required for a 50% elevation of pain threshold on electrical stimulation of the tooth pulp. The onset of effect of methopholine was generally rapid and the duration of activity slightly shorter than that of codeine.

Using his hot plate method in mice, Eddy (66) found the analgetic effectiveness of Ro-4-1778, the hydrochloride of methopholine, to be almost three times that of codeine, but Baruth and Randall (67) and Randall (25) reported methopholine and codeine to be of the same order of activity by this test.

Table XI lists the methods employed and the actual findings in these investigations.

Using the inflamed rat foot method of Randall and Selitto (72), Baruth and Randall (67) found that with subcutaneous doses of 12.5 to 50 mg/kg of methopholine there was an increase in the pain threshold, in both the normal and the inflamed foot, comparable to that seen with codeine. These findings were confirmed by Besendorf et al. (65).

[1] With the exception of a small number of studies, all investigations herein reported were carried out in the Pharmacology Departments of F. Hoffmann-La Roche & Co., A.G., Basle, Switzerland (H. P. Bächtold, B. Pellmont, K. Reber, K. Schärer, and A. Studer) and Hoffmann-La Roche Inc., Nutley, New Jersey, U.S.A. (R. E. Bagdon, R. Banziger, H. Baruth, J. Courter, G. A. Heise, C. Impellizzeri, E. F. Keith, H. J. McConnell, R. A. Moe, L. O. Randall, E. Schwartz, P. L. Stefko, and G. Zbinden).

DeSalva and Monteleone (73) found methopholine to be effective in delaying the onset of an electrically-induced skin twitch in rabbits and increasing the voltage requirements for the twitch response to occur.

Separation of analgesia and sedation in methopholine was demonstrated in rats by McConnell (74) by means of continuous avoidance tests in which the

TABLE XI

ANALGETIC ACTIVITY OF METHOPHOLINE AND CODEINE

Animal species	Method	Route of administration	ED_{50} (mg/kg)[a]	
			Methopholine	Codeine (as free base)
Mouse	Tail flick method by Gross (45)	subcutaneous	18	18
		oral	38	40[b]
	Writing reaction by Siegmund et al. (68)	subcutaneous	5[b]	5.5[b]
		oral	12[b]	
	Hot plate method by Eddy and Leimbach (69)	subcutaneous	5[c]	14[c]
Rat	Dorsal heat method by Ercoli and Lewis (70)[d]	subcutaneous	40	35
		oral	55[b]	
Rabbit	Tooth pulp method by Ruckstuhl (71)	intravenous	4.4	7.4

[a] If not indicated otherwise, values are from Besendorf et al (65).
[b] Values by Besendorf et al., but not included in Reference 65.
[c] Values by Eddy (66).
[d] Modification of method by Hardy, Goodell, and Wolff (53).

rat adjusted the intensity of shock to its feet by pressing a lever. Ro 4-1778, the hydrochloride of methopholine produced analgesia (that is, it permitted rats to endure greater intensity of electrical shock) at approximately one-half the dosage required to produce sedation. With morphine, on the other hand, analgesia was invariably accompanied by a like degree of sedation.

B. TOXICITY

LD_{50} values of Versidyne by different routes of administration in mice, rats, and rabbits were determined by Besendorf et al. (65), as shown in Table XII, which also lists comparative data for codeine and findings in

317

dogs. As can be seen, the acute toxicity of methopholine and codeine is approximately of the same order.

The toxicity of methopholine in the mouse was characterized by excitation, and lethal doses produced convulsions and respiratory failure. In the rat and rabbit, mild sedation was observed. In the cat 30 mg/kg, given intraperitoneally, failed to produce morphine-type excitation which is characteristic for this species.

TABLE XII

ACUTE TOXICITY OF METHOPHOLINE AND CODEINE

		LD_{50} (mg/kg)[a]	
Animal species	Route of administration	Methopholine	Codeine (as free base)
Mouse	subcutaneous	180	140
	oral	180	250[b]
	intravenous	70[b]	56[b]
	intraperitoneal	70[b]	
Rat	subcutaneous	400	500
	oral	400[c]	—
	intraperitoneal	100[b]	—
Rabbit	intravenous	30	34
Dog	oral	295[c]	—

[a] If not indicated otherwise, values are from Besendorf et al. (65).

[b] Values by Besendorf et al., but not included in Reference 65.

[c] Values by Banziger.

The acute toxicity of methopholine, administered intraperitoneally to newborn mice and rats, was found by Pellmont to be practically identical with that determined for mature animals.

Chronic toxicity studies with methopholine were carried out in rats, dogs, and monkeys. Reber and Studer administered the drug, suspended in gum arabic, intraperitoneally to rats. They gave single doses of as much as 15 mg/kg five times per week for eight weeks, followed by gradual increases up to 125 mg/kg during the last four weeks of the 6 months' experiment.

Except for cessation of growth at 40 mg/kg and a weight loss at 85 mg/kg, untoward reactions were not observed.

In an 18 months' chronic toxicity study, Schärer administered methopholine to rats as a dietary admixture in concentrations of 0.05, 0.1, and 0.2%, corresponding to a daily drug intake of 30–60, 60–110, and 100–200 mg/kg. Hematological investigations, urinalyses, hepatic and renal function tests, and histopathological examinations failed to show any methopholine-induced toxic effects. The only changes noted in the treated animals were pigmentation in the tubuli of the outermost renal cortex and reduction in the resistance to infections.

In another long-term experiment in rats, including reproduction studies, Schwartz and Bagdon gave methopholine as a dietary admixture, allowing for a daily drug intake of 100 mg/kg, to a parent and first generation group for 34 and 29 weeks, respectively. The drug administration, initiated 4 weeks prior to breeding, did not influence fertility significantly and congenital malformations did not result; also other abnormalities were not observed either in the parent animals or their offspring.

Bagdon *et al.* carried out chronic toxicity studies in dogs which received daily methopholine doses of 10, 20, and 40 mg/kg by mouth for 9 months. The only adverse effect was occasional emesis in the animals given the highest dose. When these experiments were extended to over one year (60 weeks), the findings in liver function tests suggested hepatic impairment in one dog each at 20 and 40 mg/kg, which upon autopsy exhibited periportal fibrosis. Furthermore, in these animals and in two additional dogs (one at 20 and one at 40 mg/kg), gastroenteritis, peritonitis, and peritoneal adhesions were observed. Popper (75) thought that the inflammatory, fibrotic, and scarring changes observed in the livers of these dogs were not of a primary nature, but secondary to the enteritis and peritonitis which, in turn, were sequelae of the modality of drug administration, i.e., the high daily quantities given in one dose over a very prolonged period.

The findings that daily intravenous injections of methopholine to dogs for over one month failed to produce significant toxicity (see below) supports the opinion that the fibrotic changes in "chronic" dogs were the result of the drug's irritant action of the gastrointestinal tract. Moreover, the oral administration of methopholine to monkeys for one year (see below) and to rats for 18 months (see above) was tolerated well without the occurrence of significant methopholine-induced histopathological changes. Thus, the changes observed in "chronic" dogs appear to be species specific. Finally, it was established that the dog, in contrast to man, excretes methopholine mainly in the feces and that high concentrations of methopholine metabolites are found in the dog's liver and intestinal wall (see Section IV). These findings may explain the gastrointestinal and hepatic changes observed in "chronic" dogs.

Bagdon found that daily intravenous administrations of 5 mg/kg of methopholine to dogs for periods ranging from 50 to 35 days did not produce fibrotic changes in the parenchymal organs of the peritoneal cavity. Similarly, histological examination of many other organs did not reveal histopathological changes.

Woodard Research Corporation (76) carried out a chronic toxicity study in monkeys. Daily doses of 10, 20, and 40 mg/kg of methopholine, administered orally for one year, were tolerated very well. However, one animal, receiving the highest dose level, died suddenly during the 43rd experimental week. Elevated transaminase values were obtained for this monkey at the point of death, but alkaline phosphatase remained normal. Histopathological examination of the liver revealed congestion and hepatic cell vacuolation. Popper (75) was of the opinion that the liver injury was not of the type usually produced by hepatotoxic substances. The cause of the animal's death could not be determined. Hemograms, blood urea nitrogen, and urinalyses remained within normal limits for all animals, as did the liver function tests except for the one monkey which died. It was concluded that changes attributable to methopholine administration were not produced.

C. Physical Dependence Capacity

It was found by Besendorf et al. (65) that the analgetic effectiveness of methopholine did not decrease when they administered the drug intramuscularly to rats five times weekly for three weeks. Bagdon failed to observe abstinence signs in dogs which had received daily methopholine doses of 40 mg/kg, increased to 70 mg/kg, for 23 to 27 weeks and were then abruptly withdrawn from this drug. Deneau and Seevers (77), who studied the effects of Ro-4-1778, the hydrochloride of methopholine, on abstinence signs of monkeys addicted to morphine and withdrawn from this narcotic, estimated the physical dependence capacity of the experimental drug to be "very low."

D. Other Pharmacological Properties

Besendorf et al. (65) reported that methopholine, in contrast to codeine, antagonized barium chloride-induced spasm of the isolated rabbit intestine. This spasmolytic action was approximately one-fifth to one-half that of papaverine. The intravenous injection of 1 mg/kg of methopholine did not have any effect on the movement of the small intestine of the rabbit *in vivo*, but 5 mg/kg decreased both tone and amplitude.[1] In the dog such a decrease

[1] These latter observations are not included in reference 65.

of contractions of the small intestine was not observed, according to Stefko.

Besendorf *et al.* (*65*)[1] found that in the narcotized rabbit, 4 mg/kg doses of methopholine, given intravenously, had a respiratory depressing effect which was antagonized by 0.1 mg/kg of Lorfan® [(−)-3-hydroxy-*N*-allyl-morphinan] tartrate, administered by the same route. They also reported that methopholine, given intravenously, exerted a hypotensive and brady-cardic action. As for antitussive effectiveness, this was found to be one-fifth that of codeine in the cat against cough induced by ammonia inhalation.

Baruth and Randall (*67*) reported that methopholine, administered sub-cutaneously, alleviated edema produced by injection of yeast in the rat's foot. Methopholine also reduced temperature in the inflamed foot and decreased temperature slightly in the normal foot, but, according to Randall (*25*), did not have anti-inflammatory activity as measured on kaolin-induced inflam-mation of the rat's foot and did not decrease rectal temperature. Generally speaking, the drug lacks anti-inflammatory and antipyretic properties.

VI. Clinical Experience with 1-*p*-Chlorophenethyl-2-methyl-6,7-dimethoxy-1,2,3,4-tetrahydroisoquinoline

Of the many derivatives of 1-phenethyl-2-methyl-1,2,3,4-tetrahydro-isoquinoline prepared and tested pharmacologically, methopholine (*47*) (trademark Versidyne) was selected for clinical evaluation, as mentioned in Section III, A,6. This choice was made because the analgetic potency of this drug in experimental animals was found to be of the order of codeine (see Section V,A), yet, unlike codeine, its prolonged use in man does not lead to physical dependence.

Methopholine was usually administered orally. For a very few studies, which required parenteral drug administration, Versidyne was used as the water-soluble hydrochloride or citrate. Since the predominant action of the drug was found to be analgesia, it seemed desirable to undertake some trials in combination with other agents which provide anti-inflammatory and anti-pyretic action and sedation, if desired. Therefore for these studies, metho-pholine was combined with aluminium aspirin; with aspirin, phenacetin, and caffeine (APC); and with aluminium aspirin, methyprylon, and caffeine.

A. HUMAN PHARMACOLOGY

1. *Chronic Tolerance*

Brandman (*78*) carried out chronic tolerance trials in 50 subjects who did not require analgetic medication, and who, with very minor deviations,

---

[1] These observations, but not the dosages, are included in reference *65*.

received methopholine orally in daily doses of 240 mg for 6 months. Laboratory studies were carried out for each patient as follows: a leukocyte count, hemoglobin determination, and urinalysis every week; a complete hemogram at frequent, predetermined intervals; and a transaminase determination initially and after 3 and 6 months of drug administration. In addition, for 10 of these subjects, the following studies were perfomed initially and after 3 and 6 months of treatment: electrocardiograms, electroencephalograms, protein-bound iodine tests, and measurements of blood cholesterol and blood sugar levels. Pulse rates and blood pressure readings were recorded for all patients at weekly intervals.

Significant changes were not observed in any of these parameters. The author concluded that methopholine does not have "side effects on the central nervous system, gastrointestinal tract, cardio-respiratory system and the skin..." and "does not have any untoward effects in daily doses of 240 mg given over a period of one-half year."

In the second part of this study, Brandman (79) administered daily methopholine doses of 360 mg, with very minor deviations, to the same 50 subjects for another 6-month period. Tests, similar to those carried out previously, were made. As in the first phase, aberrations were not observed in any of the parameters studied. Brandman concluded that "daily Versidyne® doses of 360 mg can be taken with impunity for very prolonged periods."

2. Respiration and Circulation

Foldes et al. (80) studied the effects of 1 mg/kg methopholine, administered intravenously, on respiration and circulation in 36 surgical patients anesthetized with Pentothal® Sodium and nitrous oxide-oxygen.

Twenty of these patients (Group I), who were premedicated with pentobarbital sodium, Demerol® HCl, and scopolamine, received methopholine alone; twelve (Group II) were given 0.02 mg/kg Lorfan tatrate intravenously, 7 minutes after injection of methopholine, and four (Group III) received 0.02 mg/kg Lorfan, 5 minutes before the administration of methopholine. In Groups II and III, Demerol was omitted from the premedication. Determinations of respiratory rates, minute and tidal volumes, and of pulse rates and blood pressures led the investigators to conclude that 1 mg/kg methopholine, administered intravenously to anesthetized patients, produced respiratory depression which was about the same as or less than that observed following supplementation with equianalgetic doses of narcotics. Furthermore, methopholine administered alone, or in conjunction with Lorfan, caused only moderate changes in pulse rate and blood pressure.

322

3. *Addiction Liability and Tolerance*

Fraser *et al.* (*81*) studied the addiction liability of methopholine at the Addiction Research Center, U.S. Public Health Service Hospital, Lexington, Kentucky. They carried out single dose experiments in nontolerant post-addicts and in partially tolerant subjects; 24-hour substitution experiments in subjects stabilized on morphine and withdrawn from this narcotic; and direct addition experiments in nontolerant postaddicts. The addictiveness of methopholine was compared with that of morphine sulfate, codeine phosphate, and *d*-propoxyphene HCl in single-blind or double-blind fashions, with placebo medication being employed for control purposes. The study included 104 subjects of whom 39, 25, and 40 were given the drugs by the oral, intramuscular, and intravenous route, respectively. Almost invariably patients were used as their own controls in crossover experiments. Thus, these investigations included "every criterion customarily used—degree and quality of morphine-like subjective effects, ability to suppress symptoms of abstinence from morphine, and severity of abstinence reaction after prolonged chronic administration."

The authors found that methopholine "is a compound of very little or no addictiveness" and that it has ". . . even less addictiveness than *d*-propoxyphene."

B. ANALGESIA

1. *Effectiveness of Parenteral Administration*

Methopholine is not generally available in an injectable form. However, as previously stated, a limited number of methopholine studies were carried out by the parenteral route and, for completeness, the published reports dealing with the drug's parenteral administration are summarized below.

Sadove *et al.* (*82*) and Sadove and Bruce (*83*) administered methopholine parenterally to postoperative cases. In the former study, 15 patients received 10–40 mg doses intravenously. Pain relief, which lasted up to one hour, was achieved with 30–40 mg doses. In the other study, 30–120 mg doses given intravenously or intramuscularly to 11 patients provided analgesia for more than two hours in some subjects. Intravenous injections and injections into the deltoid were painful, but intragluteal injections were generally tolerated without pain.

Foldes *et al.* (*80*) compared the effectiveness of methopholine and Demerol, administered intravenously to 20 surgical patients each, for supplementation of Pentothal-nitrous oxide-oxygen anesthesia. These workers observed that 1 mg/kg of methopholine and 0.5 mg/kg of Demerol were about equianalgetic and that the duration of the methopholine effect was longer than of the Demerol effect. Another difference was that methopholine was not accompanied by a hypnotic effect, which, however, was exhibited by Demerol.

Swerdlow *et al.* (*84*) found methopholine unsuitable for supplementation of Pentothal-nitrous oxide-oxygen anesthesia in 26 surgical patients. The discrepancy between the findings by these workers and by Foldes *et al.* (*80*) can undoubtedly be explained by the fact that the latter group used considerably higher doses.

2. *Effectiveness of Oral Administration*

The analgetic effectiveness of methopholine and/or methopholine combinations was evaluated in a series of double-blind studies by Sadove *et al.* (*82, 85*), Sadove and Bruce (*83, 86*), Chilton *et al.* (*87*), Moore *et al.* (*88*), Adels and Rogers (*89*), Koslin (*90*), and Cass and Frederik (*91*). With exception of the investigations by Chilton *et al.* (*87*) and by Koslin (*90*), these studies were carried out in hospitalized patients.

Sadove *et al.* (*85*) determined analgesia scores in 40 postsurgical, orthopedic cases following administration of 20 and 40 mg methopholine, 30 mg codeine, and placebo medication. These authors concluded that, on a milligram for milligram basis, methopholine appeared to be equal to codeine in analgetic potency.

In the other study (*82*), these workers compared 30 and 60 mg methopholine, 32 and 65 mg *d*-propoxyphene, 30 and 60 mg codeine sulfate, and placebo medication in 43 postsurgical, orthopedic patients with skeletal-muscular pain. They found that at the higher doses all three drugs were about equianalgetic, as were 30 mg doses of methopholine and codeine. However, 32 mg doses of *d*-propoxyphene were less effective than 30 mg methopholine.

The study of Sadove and Bruce (*83*) included 35 postsurgical, orthopedic patients who received 60 mg of methopholine and/or *d*-propoxyphene and placebo medication. The difference in the frequency of pain relief produced in the 22 patients who were given both active drugs was significant statistically in favor of methopholine.

Sadove and Bruce (*86*) compared also the effectiveness of 30, 60, and 120 mg methopholine, of 30 mg methopholine with 325 mg aspirin,[1] and of 30 mg methopholine with 325 mg aspirin,[1] 50 mg methyprylon, and 30 mg caffeine in 34 patients with pain following gynecological surgery. Satisfactory analgesia resulted from all medications with the exception of the 30 mg dose of methopholine alone. The addition of the other agents increased the effectiveness of 30 mg methopholine to that of 60 or 120 mg of methopholine given alone.

[1]As Aluminum Asprin.

Chilton *et al.* (*87*) evaluated 60 mg methopholine, 60 mg codeine sulfate, 65 mg *d*-propoxyphene and placebo medication in 501 patients with pain after minor oral surgical procedures. No statistically significant difference between the effectiveness of codeine and methopholine was found, but codeine was significantly more effective than *d*-propoxyphene or placebo.

Moore *et al.* (*88*) compared the potency of 60 mg methopholine and 50 mg Demerol in 212 postsurgical patients. They found both drugs to be about equally effective in marked and moderate pain, but the incidence of complete relief in severe pain was higher with Demerol than with methopholine. However, this difference was not significant statistically.

Adels and Rogers (*89*) treated 70 patients with various types of pain in the immediate postpartum period with 60 mg methopholine, 60 mg methopholine combined with 417 mg aluminum aspirin and placebo medication. The authors concluded that both active drugs are valuable agents for the relief of postpartum pain.

Koslin (*90*) administered two analgetic combinations to 443 patients with pain following minor oral surgical procedures. One of these combinations contained 60 mg methopholine, 325 mg aspirin,[1] 50 mg methyprylon, and 30 mg caffeine, and the other *d*-propoxyphene, aspirin, phenacetin, and caffeine in the quantities provided by Darvon® Compound 65. When all patients, regardless of severity of pain and degree of relief, were considered together, the incidence of relief was about the same for both drugs. However, when those patients were considered who derived complete relief, it was found that the differences in effectiveness of the methopholine combination over the *d*-propoxyphene combination were highly significant statistically for all individual doses when the pain was marked and for some of the doses when pain was moderate, but a significant difference in the performance of the two drugs did not exist in patients who had severe pain initially.

Cass and Frederik (*91*) compared in 34 patients with chronic pain of various etiologies, the effectiveness of 60 mg methopholine; 60 mg methopholine, 227 mg aspirin, 162 mg phenacetin, and 32.4 mg caffeine; 227 mg aspirin, 162 mg phenacetin, and 32.4 mg caffeine; 15 mg codeine, 227 mg aspirin, 162 mg phenacetin, and 32.4 mg caffeine; and placebo medication. Statistical analysis of the results revealed the following.

Methopholine-APC,[2] codeine-APC, methopholine (plain) and APC (plain) were all significantly better than placebo medication.

There was no significant difference between the efficacy of methopholine-APC and codeine-APC on the one hand and between the efficacy of methopholine (plain) and APC (plain) on the other.

[1] As Aluminum Aspirin.
[2] Now known as Versidyne® Compound.

325

Both methopholine-APC and codeine-APC were significantly better than either methopholine (plain) or APC (plain).

In all these double-blind studies, the incidence of side effects attributable to methopholine and its combinations was minimal and the few reactions encountered were entirely inconsequential. It is noteworthy that methopholine did not produce constipation or sedation and that nausea was an extremely rare occurrence.

Good clinical results with methopholine combinations and/or methopholine in nonblind studies were reported by Brandman (78), Elia (92), Ryan (93), Hoffmann (94), Muras (95), Thomas et al. (96), and Brodsky (97). The patients treated in these investigations suffered from a variety of acute pain problems, chronic pain due to arthritic and related disorders, headaches, pain following oral surgical procedures, postoperative pain, dysmenorrhea, and a variety of orthopedic conditions.

VII. Conclusions

The analgetic properties of various 1-phenethyl-substituted 1,2,3,4-tetrahydroisoquinolines as described in this review suggest that, contrary to previous conceptions, the quaternary carbon atom is not an essential feature of centrally active analgetics. However, the presence of a tertiary amine function is still required and the observation that only one of the two enantiomers is responsible for the analgetic properties remains valid. These prerequisites hold for most of the known centrally active analgetics containing one asymmetric carbon atom.

In our group of compounds, the N-allylnor derivatives are devoid of antagonistic properties. Furthermore, N-substituents which, in other groups of analgetics, cause considerable increase in activity, do not show this behavior in the series of 1-phenethyl-substituted 1,2,3,4-tetrahydroisoquinolines. This clearly demonstrates the hazard of making general statements regarding structure-activity relationships.

Several analgetics were found which are more active than methopholine, but they are all addictive. Whether or not any of these compounds would be of practical value as an analgetic in man can be determined only by clinical trials. Since a large number of such drugs are already available, and since the steps preparatory to marketing a potent analgetic are involved and time-consuming, the advisability of developing any of these compounds further seems questionable. On the other hand, it is conceivable that some of the materials listed may be of interest for other reasons.

With the synthesis of methopholine, a considerable dissociation between analgesia and every aspect of addictiveness has been achieved. When given orally, the analgetic effectiveness of methopholine is equal to codeine and at least equal to d-propoxyphene (Darvon), on a weight basis. Sixty mg methopholine and 50 mg Demerol are approximately equianalgetic for relief of marked to moderate postoperative pain. In patients with severe pain, however, the incidence of complete relief is somewhat higher following Demerol administration.

Unlike codeine, methopholine does not produce sedation or constipation and daily doses of 360 mg can be given for prolonged periods without adverse effects on hematopoiesis or hepatic or renal function. Patients do not develop tolerance to the analgetic effect of methopholine and its prolonged use does not lead to physical dependence. Therefore, methopholine is not subject to narcotic control.

The analgetic effectiveness of methopholine is increased by the addition of aluminum aspirin or APC or aluminum aspirin, methyprylon, and caffeine.

It is concluded that methopholine is a safe analgetic, well suited for the treatment of mild to moderately severe pain.

ACKNOWLEDGMENTS

We are especially indebted to Mr. H. Roth, Dr. R. Silberschmidt, Dr. A. Hürlimann, Dr. A. Vetterli, Dr. M. Walter, Dr. H. Bruderer, and Dr. O. Schnider of F. Hoffmann-La Roche & Co., A.G., Basle, Switzerland, and also to Dr. R. E. Bagdon, Dr. B. A. Koechlin and Dr. A. I. Rachlin of Hoffmann-La Roche Inc., Nutley, New Jersey, for their help in one way or another during these studies.

REFERENCES

1. O. Schaumann, *Arch. Exptl. Pathol. Pharmakol.* **196**, 109 (1940); *Pharmazie* **4**, 364 (1949).
2. O. Eisleb, *Ber.* **74**, 1433 (1941).
3. O. J. Braenden, N. B. Eddy, and H. H. Halbach, *Bull. World Health Organ.* **13**, 937 (1955).
4. N. B. Eddy, *Chem. & Ind. (London)* **47**, 1462 (1959).
5. A. H. Beckett and A. F. Casy, *in* "Progress in Medicinal Chemistry" (J. P. Ellis and G. B. West, eds.), Vol. 2, p. 43. Butterworths, London, 1962; P. A. J. Janssen, *J. Pharm. Pharmacol.* **13**, 513 (1961); S. Pfeifer, *Pharmazie* **17**, 189 (1962).
6. T. A. Henry, "The Plant Alkaloids," 4th ed., p. 154. McGraw-Hill (Blakiston), New York, 1949; L. Reti, *in* "The Alkaloids" (R. H. F. Manske and H. L. Holmes, eds.), Vol. IV, pp. 7 and 23. Academic Press, New York, 1954; K. W. Bentley, *Endeavour* **23**, 97 (1964).
7. H. Krueger, N. B. Eddy, and M. Sumwalt, "The Pharmacology of the Opium Alkaloids," Part 2, p. 1007. U.S. Govt. Printing Office, Washington, D.C., 1943.
8. A. Burger, *in* "The Alkaloids" (R. H. F. Manske and J. H. Holmes, eds.), Vol. IV, p. 29. Academic Press, New York, 1954.

A. BROSSI, H. BESENDORF, L. A. PIRK, A. RHEINER, JR.

9. H. G. Boit, "Ergebnisse der Alkaloid-Chemie bis 1960," p. 216. Akademie-Verlag, Berlin, 1961.
10. B. Frydman, R. Bendisch, and V. Deulofeu, *Tetrahedron* **4**, 342 (1958).
11. K. W. Gopinath, T. R. Govindachari, and N. Viswanathan, *Chem. Ber.* **92**, 1657 (1959).
12. M. Tomita and J. Kunitomo, *J. Pharm. Soc. Japan* **82**, 734 (1962).
13. J. Stanek and R. H. F. Manske, *in* "The Alkaloids" (R. H. F. Manske and H. L. Holmes, eds.), Vol. IV, p. 167. Academic Press, New York, 1954; J. Stanek, *ibid.*, Vol. VII, p. 433, 1960.
14. T. A. Henry, "The Plant Alkaloids," 4th ed., p. 200. McGraw-Hill (Blakiston), New York, 1949.
15. H. G. Boit, "Ergebnisse der Alkaloid-Chemie bis 1960," p. 354. Akademie-Verlag, Berlin, 1961; cf. Y. Ota, N. Endo and M. Hirasawa, *Chem. and Pharm. Bull. (Japan)* **12**, 569 (1964).
16. K. W. Bentley, "The Alkaloids," p. 62. Wiley (Interscience), New York, 1957.
17. For the absolute configuration of nat. hydrastine, compare M. Ohta, H. Tani, and S. Morozumi, *Tetrahedron Letters* 859 (1963); cf. M. Ohta, H. Tani, S. Morozumi, S. Kodaira, and K. Kuriyama *Tetrahedron Letters* 1857 (1963); A. R. Battersby and H. Spencer, ibid. p. 11 (1964).
18. J. Szegi, J. Rausch, K. Magda, and J. Nagy, *Chem. Abstr.* **54**, 15663 (1960).
19. K. Takagi, H. Fukuda, and M. Sato, *J. Pharm. Soc. Japan* **81**, 266 (1961).
20. I. Källqvist and B. Melander, *Arzneimittel-Forsch.* **7**, 301 (1957).
21. H. A. Bickerman, E. German, B. M. Cohen, and S. E. Itkin, *Am. J. Med. Sci.* **234**, 191 (1957).
22. E. L. May, *in* "Medicinal Chemistry" (A. Burger, ed.) 2nd ed., p. 311. Wiley (Interscience), New York, 1960; "Merck Index", 7th ed. Merck & Co., Rahway, New Jersey, 1960; C. C. Pfeiffer, *in* "Pharmacology in Medicine" (V. A. Drill, ed.), Part V, Sect. 17. McGraw-Hill, New York, 1954.
23. H. Krueger, *in* "The Alkaloids" (R. H. F. Manske, ed.), Vol. V, p. 1. Academic Press, New York, 1955.
24. L. B. Mellett and L. A. Woods, *in* "Progress in Drug Research" (E. Jucker, ed.), Vol. V, p. 155. Birkhäuser, Basle, Switzerland, 1963.
25. L. O. Randall, *in* "Physiological Pharmacology" (W. S. Root and F. G. Hofmann, eds.), Vol. 1, pp. 390–394. Academic Press, New York, 1963.
26. D. Beke, C. Szántay, and M. Bárczai-Beke, *Ann. Chem.* **636**, 150 (1960).
27. B. Kelentey, E. Stenszky, and F. Czollner, *Pharmazie* **15**, 111 (1960).
28. A. Brossi, J. Würsch, and O. Schnider, *Chimia (Aarau)* **12**, 114 (1958).
29. A. K. Reynolds and L. O. Randall, "Morphine and Allied Drugs." Univ. of Toronto Press, Toronto, 1957.
30. Tropon-Werke, D.R.P. 726,173; 728,326; and 732,502.
31. A. Brossi, H. Besendorf, B. Pellmont, M. Walter, and O. Schnider, *Helv. Chim. Acta* **43**, 1459 (1960).
32. Hoffmann-La Roche Inc., U.S.P. 3,067,203 (1962).
33. R. C. Elderfield, "Heterocyclic Compounds," Vol. 4, p. 450. Wiley, New York, 1952.
34. Y. Tomimatsu, *J. Pharm. Soc. Japan* **77**, 7 (1957).
35. M. Walter, A. Besendorf, and O. Schnider, *Helv. Chim. Acta* **46**, 1127 (1963).
36. A. Grüssner, J. Hellerbach, and O. Schnider, *Helv. Chim. Acta* **40**, 1232 (1957).
37. R. P. Evstigneeva and N. A. Preobrazhensky, *Tetrahedron* **4**, 236 (1958).
38. J. Knabe and A. Schepers, *Arch. Pharm.* **295**, 481 (1962).
39. A. Rheiner, Jr. and A. Brossi, *Helv. Chim. Acta* **45**, 2590 (1962).

40. Ciba, U.S.P. 3,133,926 (1964).
41. A. H. Beckett and N. J. Harper, *J. Chem. Soc.* p. 858 (1957).
42. A. Rheiner, Jr., *Experientia*, **20**, 488 (1964).
43. A. Brossi and F. Burkhardt, *Helv. Chim. Acta* **44**, 1558 (1961).
44. Wellcome Foundation, Australian Patent 2383 (1963).
45. F. Gross, *Helv. Physiol. Pharmacol. Acta* **5**, C31 (1947).
46. G. A. Deneau and M. H. Seevers, personal communication (1963).
47. (±)-1-*p*-Chlorphenethyl-2-methyl-6,7-dimethoxy-1,2,3,4-tetrahydroisoquinoline (code number Ro 4-1778/1), generic name methopholine, trademark "Versidyne ®".
48. Dr. A. Vetterli and Dr. H. Bruderer, F. Hoffmann-La Roche & Co., A.G., Basle, Switzerland. Unpublished results.
49. These thin layer chromatograms were kindly submitted by Dr. H. R. Bolliger, F. Hoffmann-La Roche & Co., A.G., Basle, Switzerland.
50. M. Walter, H. Besendorf, and O. Schnider, *Helv. Chim. Acta* **44**, 1546 (1961).
51. To published in *Helv. Chim. Acta*.
52. G. A. Deneau and M. H. Seevers, personal communication (1964).
53. J. D. Hardy, H. Goodell, and H. G. Wolff, *Am. J. Physiol.* **133**, 316 (1941).
54. E. Siegmund, R. Cadmus, and G. Lu, *Proc. Soc. Exptl. Biol. Med.* **95**, 729 (1957).
55. R. Domenjoz, *Arch. Exptl. Pathol. Pharmakol.* **215**, 19 (1952).
56. C. A. Winter and L. Flataker, *J. Exptl. Med.* **101**, 17 (1955).
57. D. E. Schwartz and J. Rieder, *Clin. Chim. Acta* **6**, 453 (1961).
58. D. E. Schwartz, H. Bruderer, J. Rieder, and A. Brossi, *Biochem. Pharmacol.* **13**, 777 (1964).
59. B. A. Koechlin, F. Rubio, and L. D'Arconte, personal communication (1963).
60. B. A. Koechlin, F. Rubio, and P. Stefko, personal communication (1963).
61. D. E. Schwartz and J. Rieder, personal communication (1963).
62. All the compounds mentioned were prepared by Dr. H. Bruderer of F. Hoffmann-La Roche, A.G., Basle, Switzerland.
63. M. Tomita and T. Nakano, *J. Pharm. Soc. Japan* **72**, 1256 (1952).
64. K. E. Hamlin and F. E. Fischer, *J. Am. Chem. Soc.* **75**, 5119 (1953).
65. H. Besendorf, B. Pellmont, H. P. Bächtold, K. Reber, and A. Studer, *Experientia* **18**, 446 (1962).
66. N. B. Eddy, personal communication (1961).
67. H. Baruth and L. O. Randall, *Federation Proc.* **21** (2), 323 (1962).
68. E. Siegmund, R. Cadmus, and G. Lu, *Proc. Soc. Exptl. Biol. Med.* **95**, 729 (1957).
69. N. B. Eddy and D. G. Leimbach, *J. Pharmacol. Exptl. Therap.* **107**, 385 (1953).
70. N. Ercoli and M. N. Lewis, *J. Pharmacol. Exptl. Therap.* **84**, 301 (1945).
71. K. Ruckstuhl, Dissertation, Bern, Switzerland (1939); cf. A. Fleisch and M. Dolivo, *Helv. Physiol. Pharmacol. Acta* **11**, 305 (1953).
72. L. O. Randall and J. J. Selitto, *Arch. Intern. Pharmacodyn.* **111**, 409 (1957).
73. S. J. DeSalva and V. J. Monteleone, *Federation Proc.* **22** (1), 248 (1963).
74. H. McConnell, *Federation Proc.* **21** (2), 418 (1962).
75. H. Popper, personal communication (1963).
76. Woodard Research Corporation, personal communication (1963).
77. G. A. Deneau and M. H. Seevers, personal communication (1961).
78. O. Brandman, *Am. J. Med. Sci.* **242**, 694 (1961).
79. O. Brandman, personal communication (1962).
80. F. F. Foldes, J. Moore, and I. M. Suna, *Am. J. Med. Sci.* **242**, 682 (1961).

329

A. BROSSI, H. BESENDORF, L. A. PIRK, A. RHEINER, JR.

81. H. F. Fraser, W. R. Martin, A. B. Wolbach, and H. Isbell, *Clin. Pharmacol. Therap.* **2**, 287 (1961a); *Federation Proc.* **20**, 310 (1961b); H. F. Fraser, G. D. Van Horn, W. R. Martin, A. B. Wolbach, and H. Isbell, *J. Pharmacol. Exptl. Therap.* **133**, 371 (1961c).

82. M. S. Sadove, M. J. Schriffrin, and S. M. Ali, *Am. J. Med. Sci.* **241**, 103 (1961).

83. M. S. Sadove and D. L. Bruce, *Current Therap. Res.* **3**, 201 (1961).

84. M. Swerdlow, J. L. Milligan, and I. P. McEwan, *Anesthesia Analgesia Current Res.* **39**, 553 (1960).

85. M. S. Sadove, S. M. Ali, and M. J. Schriffrin, *Illinois Med. J.* **117**, 425 (1960).

86. M. S. Sadove and D. L. Bruce, *Current Therap. Res.* **3**, 507 (1961).

87. N. W. Chilton, A. Lewandowski, and J. R. Cameron, *Am. J. Med. Sci.* **242**, 702 (1961)

88. J. Moore, F. F. Foldes, and G. M. Davidson, *Am. J. Med. Sci.* **244**, 337 (1962).

89. M. J. Adels and S. F. Rogers, *Am. J. Obstet. Gynecol.* **84**, 952 (1962).

90. A. J. Koslin, *J. Oral Surg., Anesthesia Hosp. Dental Serv.* **21**, 414 (1963).

91. L. J. Cass and W. S. Frederik, *Am. J. Med. Sci.* **246**, 550 (1963).

92. J. C. Elia, *Headache* **2**, 138 (1962).

93. R. T. Ryan, *Headache* **11**, 203 (1963).

94. M. M. Hoffman, *Dental Digest* **69**, 21 (1963).

95. O. Muras, *Orientacion Med.* **11**, 234 (1962).

96. M. Thomas, G. C. Tandan, and N. P. Singh, *Indian J. Anaesthesia* **10**, 230 (1962).

97. A. E. Brodsky, *Am. J. Orthoped.* **5**, 198 (1963).

CHAPTER VII

Pyrazole Derivatives

WALTER KROHS[1]

FORMERLY RESEARCH CHEMIST OF FARBWERKE HOECHST A.G.;
MEMBER OF THE ASSOCIATION OF GERMAN CHEMISTS

[1] *Present address*: Waldstr. 43, Bad Soden im Taunus, Germany.

I. Introduction[1]

A. HISTORICAL SURVEY

The discovery of the antipyretics and analgesics that belong to the group of pyrazolones is intimately connected with the attempts to clarify the constitution of the specific malaria remedy and antipyretic, quinine. On breaking down the quinine molecule it became possible to isolate quinoline and methoxyquinoline, and since it was found that antipyretic and antiseptic properties could be ascribed to quinoline, chemists again and again referred to this substance in the course of their syntheses as the basic structure required to obtain a compound having the characteristics of quinine. Even though this conception subsequently underwent many changes, it is valid —as far as its antimalarial action is concerned—to this day. The notion that it would be of significance for the achievement of therapeutically valuable antipyretics and analgesics, however, proved to be erroneous. But this error became the means by which the synthesis of pharmaceuticals was to reap a rich harvest.

Since the quinoline molecule had a high hydrogen content, and it was furthermore conjectured that this hydrogen is bound to the quinoline part, the synthesis of hydrogenated quinoline derivatives was attempted first. O. Fischer created kairine (I), Königs made kairoline (II), and Skraup, noting the methoxy group in the quinine molecule which is not contained in the very much less active cinchonine, synthesized thalline (III). Pharma-

(I) (II) (III)

cological and clinical investigation of the three compounds appeared to confirm the suppositions of those who had synthesized them. The substances exhibited an extraordinarily powerful antipyretic action but on closer examination it was shown that they were by no means harmless febrifuges. Because of their dangerous side reactions they soon had to be withdrawn

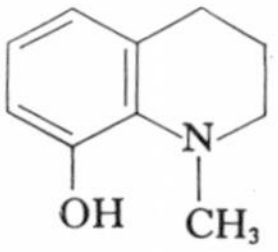

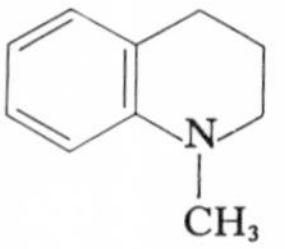

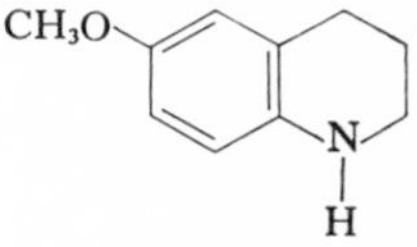

[1] *Important notice:* The denotations used in this article also include registered trademarks. Insofar as they are known after a careful check, they have been identified the first time mentioned in the text by the symbol ®. This does not, however, signify that they are registered in all countries in which this article may appear in print. In cases where denotations appear which have not been identified by the symbol ® but are actually registered trademarks, this article cannot be taken as evidence of the fact that they are generic or that they have lost their character as trademarks in the meantime.

from the pharmaceutical market. But they did not disappear without first having provided several revealing glimpses into the interrelation between constitution and biological action.

Thus, the introduction of an OH group into the hydrogenated molecule brought about more rapid action (I). This was, however, of a more fleeting nature, a disadvantage which was compensated by protecting the OH group with the formation of a methoxyl group (III). Methylating the nitrogen atom (I, II) proved to be an artifice of great significance in pharmacological syntheses. It reappears in the syntheses of the pyrazolone series, where it leads to substances whose therapeutic value is yet unknown.

Later, Emil Fischer referred to the vast field of application of the aromatic hydrazines, especially in relation to the chemistry of sugars. On the other hand, acetoacetic ester were obtained by the autocondensation of ethyl acetate. Ludwig Knorr then was asked by Fischer to bring about a reaction between the two substances phenylhydrazine and acetoacetic ester (*1*). In this reaction he succeeded in isolating a substance which he considered to be a quinoline-like compound in which the ring that contained the nitrogen atom and was condensed with the benzene nucleus was reminiscent of the hydrogenated state of the kairine and thalline molecules. Knorr called the substance he had found methoxyquinizine and attributed to it (*2*) the structural formula shown (IV).

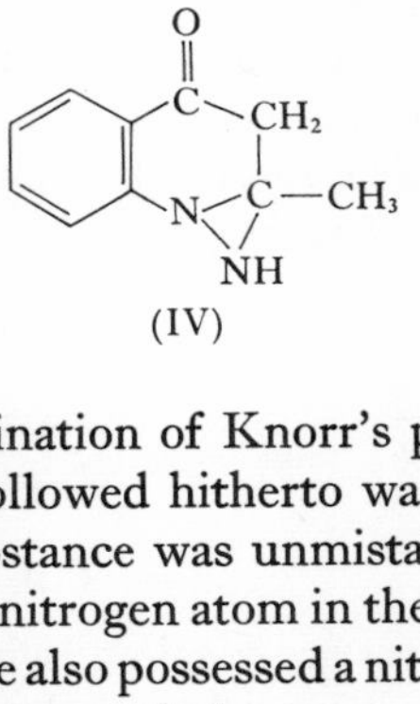

(IV)

The pharmacological examination of Knorr's product by Filehne showed that the line of approach followed hitherto was not without promise; the antipyretic action of the substance was unmistakable. The favorable effect attained by methylating the nitrogen atom in the kairine group had not been forgotten. Methoxyquinizine also possessed a nitrogen atom whose hydrogen was obviously replaceable by a methyl group.

The attempt to methylate it was successful but resulted in a substance of completely different physical properties. In contrast to the unmethylated product it was distinctly basic and extremely soluble in water. The detailed pharmacological analysis which was also conducted by Filehne revealed that the substance had very valuable pharmacological properties. It was strongly

333

antifebrile in action and at the same time relatively nontoxic, so that clinical evaluation could be considered.

Clinical studies confirmed what had already been found by pharmacological experiment, excellent antipyretic action without the dangerous toxicity of the representatives of the kairine group. On the contrary, the side reactions were confined to very moderate limits and, in view of the otherwise beneficial effect on the various forms of fever, it was accepted unhesitatingly. Under the name Antipyrine®, for which we shall use the generic name phenazone in this chapter, the supposed dimethyloxyquinizine made its debut on the pharmaceutical market in 1883, and was destined not to disappear from it again.

B. 1-Phenyl-3-methyl-2-pyrazoline-5-one

$$H_2C \underset{4}{\overset{}{-}} \underset{3}{\overset{}{C}}-CH_3$$

$$OC_5 \quad _1 \quad _2N$$

$$N$$

$$C_6H_5$$

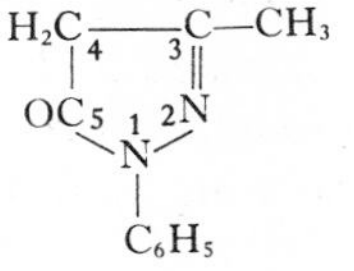

(V)

The resulting manifold reactions manifested by phenazone could no longer be reconciled with a methylated methoxyquinizine. After working on this problem for several years, Knorr found that the ring formation during condensation of phenylhydrazine with acetoacetic ester had taken place in a different way from that originally assumed (3). Initially the phenylhydrazone of acetoacetic ester is formed while still cold. On warming, it closes to form a ring structure with the elimination of a molecule of alcohol. Knorr named it pyrazolone. Scheme (1) shows the reaction.

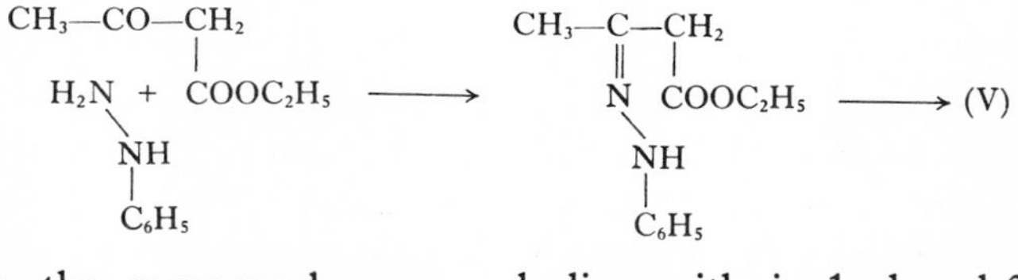

$$\begin{array}{ccc} CH_3-CO-CH_2 & & CH_3-C-CH_2 \\ H_2N + COOC_2H_5 & \longrightarrow & N \quad COOC_2H_5 \longrightarrow (V) \quad (1) \\ NH & & NH \\ C_6H_5 & & C_6H_5 \end{array}$$

Thus, the compound we are dealing with is 1-phenyl-3-methyl-2-pyrazoline-5-one, and since it has become the basic substance from which many other products are derived, it is often called "technical pyrazolone." Even today, it is manufactured on a large scale by the classic method of Knorr from phenylhydrazine and acetoacetic ester. It is essential for the quality of the product that only a slight excess of phenylhydrazine be used. Too great an excess of this reaction component acts as an oxidizing agent

334

and results in the formation of 4,4′-bis-(1-phenyl-3-methyl-2-pyrazoline-5-one) (VI) (*4*).

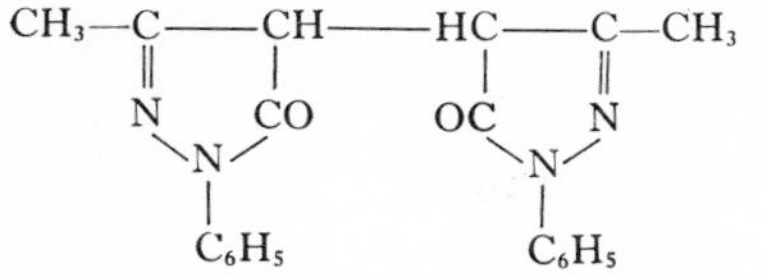

$$CH_3-C\underline{\quad\quad}CH\underline{\quad\quad}HC\underline{\quad\quad}C-CH_3$$

N   CO   OC   N

N   N

C_6H_5   C_6H_5

(VI)

C. MEDICAL SIGNIFICANCE OF THE PYRAZOLE DERIVATIVES

By the synthesis of technical pyrazolone, Knorr had opened up the field of pyrazolone chemistry which in the following years was to become exceptionally fruitful both in the pharmaceutical field as well as in dyestuffs chemistry. The great clinical success of phenazone inspired chemists to make further efforts in respect to new syntheses which were aimed at creating more effective preparations or to widen their sphere of application. To this day, after 80 years, this development has not been concluded and one can but marvel how one single chemical reaction, viz. the condensation of phenylhydrazine with acetoacetic ester, could have touched off such an avalanche.

Many new pyrazolone preparations of great value to medicine, which will be dealt with in the following sections, were synthesized. The synthesis of phenylbutazone took place in 1946. This is a pyrazolidinedione derivative which was to embark upon its triumphal march soon after, and so inspired chemists to new efforts in this interesting field.

Originally tried as a febrifuge, it was soon demonstrated clinically that the pyrazole derivatives possess valuable therapeutic properties which became of great importance to their application. It was, moreover, soon recognized that, in addition, they possess an analgetically active component. They thus belong to the group of mild analgesics which are distinguished by low toxicity and good tolerability. A few of the pyrazole derivatives in addition exhibit good spasmolytic action. This property in conjunction with the analgesic action had led to their application in colics in extremely severe painful conditions. The antiphlogistic action of many pyrazole derivatives is, however, of particular significance. Remedies were thus presented to the physician for the treatment of diseases associated with rheumatoid conditions which are so widely spread today.

If one considers the many-sided modes of action exhibited by the pyrazole derivatives one need not be astonished to find that they have attained such great significance in medicine and that chemists are inspired again and again to perform new syntheses.

335

II. Pyrazolone-5-one Derivatives

A. ANTIPYRIN®

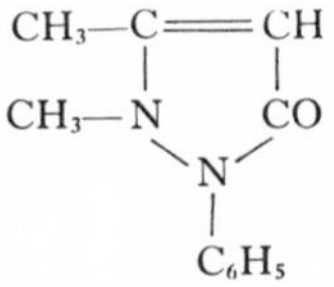

$$CH_3-C\!=\!=\!CH$$
$$CH_3-N \quad CO$$
$$N$$
$$C_6H_5$$

1-Phenyl-2,3-dimethyl-3-pyrazoline-5-one

(VII)

1. Synthesis and Constitution

By methylating compound V with methyl iodide in methanol at 100°–120° C, Knorr (5) obtained 1-phenyl-2,3-dimethyl-3-pyrazoline-5-one (VII) which was introduced to therapeutics under the name Antipyrine. As already stated earlier on, the generic name phenazone will be used in this chapter. Knorr (6) interpreted the methylation as the joining of methyl iodide to the nitrogen atom in the 2-position forming a quaternary compound and subsequent splitting off of hydrogen iodide to form the corresponding salt of phenazone (Eq. 2).

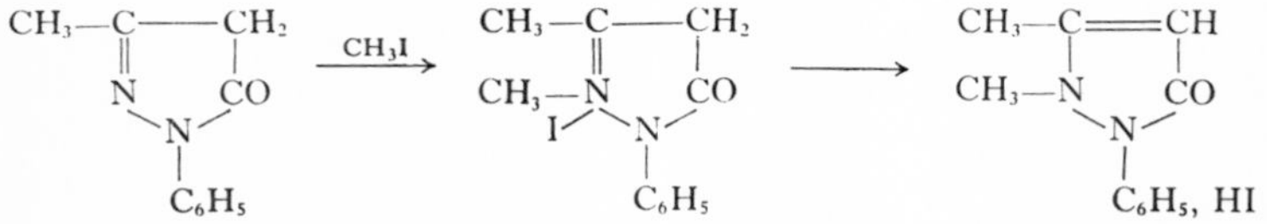

$$CH_3-C\!-\!-\!-\!CH_2 \quad \xrightarrow{CH_3I} \quad CH_3-C\!-\!-\!-\!CH_2 \quad \longrightarrow \quad CH_3-C\!=\!=\!CH \qquad (2)$$
$$N \quad CO \qquad\qquad CH_3-N \quad CO \qquad\qquad CH_3-N \quad CO$$
$$N \qquad\qquad\qquad I \quad N \qquad\qquad\qquad N$$
$$C_6H_5 \qquad\qquad\qquad C_6H_5 \qquad\qquad\qquad C_6H_5, HI$$

Michaelis (7) opposed the structural formula of phenazone as elaborated by Knorr, and suggested the so-called phenol betaine formula (VIII) which Knorr (8) had previously discussed but had discarded.

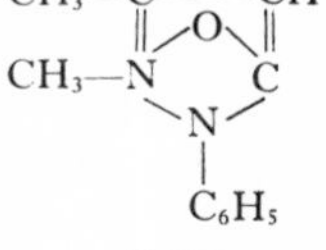

$$CH_3-C\!-\!-\!-\!CH$$
$$O$$
$$CH_3-N \quad C$$
$$N$$
$$C_6H_5$$

(VIII)

Both scientists attempted to prove the validity of their respective formulas by many new reactions but did not succeed in settling the question. In 1940, the Japanese Kitamura (9) took up the problem anew. Basing his findings on the modern conception of the mesomerism of organic ring systems, and after conducting further experiments, he came to the conclusion that a state of oscillation exists in the phenazone molecule which therefore occurs in the following three forms

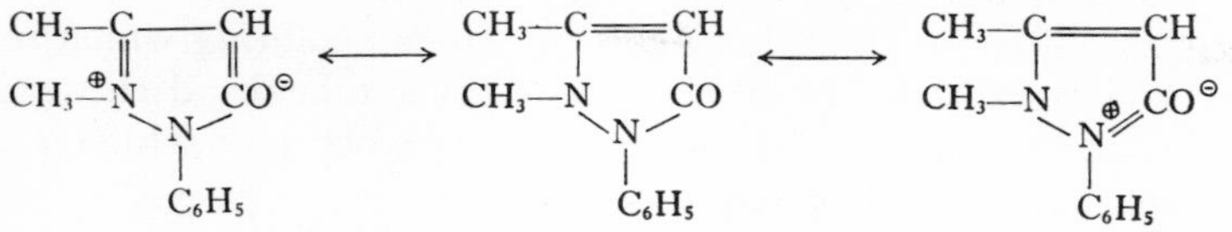

In his theoretical studies on the mesomerism of phenazone, Duquénois (*10*) arrived at the same result as Kitamura.

See references *11* and *12* for discussions of manufacturing processes for phenazone.

2. Chemical and Physical Properties

Phenazone, which is extremely readily soluble in water, possesses the capacity to act as adjuvant for drugs that are sparingly soluble in water. This property is frequently made use of. According to Gancia (*13*), the dissolution of up to 20% dimethylaminophenazone was achieved with the help of a 25% phenazone solution. Farbenfabriken Bayer (*14*) state that the use of phenazone is required to prepare a Conteben® solution which, according to Polster (*15*), is suitable for intracavitary injection, and according to Unholtz (*16*) can be used for the resistance test of tuberculin bacilli. Further substances which could be brought into solution with the help of phenazone are: salicylamide, phenacetin, and *p*-aminobenzoic acid ester (*17*); quinine hydrochloride, sulfanilamide, and sulfapyridine (*18*); quinidine hydrochloride (*19*); arsenobenzene (*20*); morphine hydrochloride (*21*); and barbituric acids (*22*).

Phenazone is a weak base which forms salts with inorganic and organic acids, among which the citrate and salicylate salts deserve special mention since they are frequently made use of in combinations of pharmaceuticals. Its complex compounds of chloralhydrate and butyl chloralhydrate were used as soporifics at one time.

3. Qualitative and Quantitative Tests

Many papers have been published which describe reactions that serve as tests for the determination of phenazone. Only a few of the most important will be mentioned here. An aqueous solution in a concentration of $1:100,000$ gives an intensive brown coloring with ferric chloride; an emerald green coloring in a concentration of $1:10,000$ is obtained by the addition of sodium nitrite in the presence of acids (*23*). These two color reactions serve

337

as a test for phenazone in urine. For this purpose a few cm^3 urine are admixed with ammonia and then shaken with chloroform. After separating, drying, and evaporating the chloroform, the residue is dissolved in water. The addition of ferric chloride gives a brown-red coloring which remains stable when heated. If, on the other hand, 30% acetic acid and a little sodium nitrite are added, a characteristic green coloring is obtained which is caused by the formation of 4-nitrophenazone.

The green color reaction can also be utilized for the qualitative test for phenazone in the presence of dimethyl aminophenazone (24). One method for the photometrical determination of phenazone is based on the color reaction with 3-methyldiaminobenzaldehyde (25). The absorption maximum of the salmon-pink compound is at 513 mμ, the determinable limit at 0.03 mg. Ruggieri (26) reports on a method of determining phenazone by potentiometrical titration with 0.1 N perchloric acid that is also suitable to test its purity. Phenazone can be determined in plasma by the photometry of 4-nitrosophenazone (at 350 mμ) which is formed by adding sodium nitrite and sulfuric acid (27).

4. Toxicity

Compared to other therapeutic drugs, phenazone is only slightly toxic. Hale (28) found that the minimum lethal dose for guinea pigs administered orally was 1.4 gm/kg. Fromherz (29) established that the lethal dose administered orally to mice was also between 1.5 and 1.6 gm/kg. The same values, namely 1.25 gm/kg were found by Koppányi and Liberson (30) in experiments with cats. The mean lethal dose (LD$_{50}$) administered orally to cats was recently determined by Krop et al. (31) and found to be 600–800 mg/kg. The lethal dose of phenazone cannot be given accurately for humans. If one assumes, however, that it lies within the same limits as found by animal experiment, it is indeed very high.

5. Fate in the Organism

Brodie and Axelrod (32) recently examined the fate of phenazone in the human organism. The substance is completely absorbed by the gastrointestinal tract and is evenly distributed throughout the body fluids immediately after. Only 5% is excreted in the urine, the remainder being transformed within the organism. Absorption is very rapid, since excretion via the urine which can be checked by the ferric chloride test already begins 10–20 minutes after oral administration. Transformation within the organism, on the other hand, is slow. After a single therapeutic dose plasma levels are maintained for 15 hours and longer, whereby the corresponding values for acetanilide and phenacetin are surpassed by far. In the course of one hour these values decline by only 1–12%. According to Schweissinger (*33*) the reason for the protracted excretion of the phenazone administered intravenously and rectally is to be sought in the fact that a portion is absorbed by the liver by way of the stomach and intestine and is slowly converted there. Soberman *et al.* (*34*) were also able to confirm these results in the examinations they conducted. They found that the average amount converted per hour is 6% and varies between 1–12% from person to person. Over a period of 12 hours, however, this portion is constant in individual persons. Huchard (*35*) observed that after administering 2 gm phenazone, it was still present in the urine after 36–48 hours. Such experiments on the time taken for excretion of a drug are of great importance with regard to the problem of accretion. The protracted excretion of phenazone does not appear to have had any harmful effect.

About 25% of the phenazone administered is oxidized in the organism to 4-hydroxyphenazone (IX) and, coupled with glucuronic and sulfuric acid,

$$CH_3-C=\!\!=\!\!C-OH$$
$$CH_3-C \quad CO$$
$$N$$
$$C_6H_5$$

(IX)

it is excreted rapidly while the remainder is broken down in an unknown manner. Halberkann and Fretwurst (*36*) found that of 4 gm phenazone taken, 0.1003 gm (2.5%) was excreted unchanged in the urine and 1.0025 gm (23.1%) as 4-hydroxyphenazone bound to glucuronic acid. Unchanged phenazone was found not only in urine but also in the saliva and perspiration.

6. *Clinical Significance*

On the strength of animal experiments by which the good antefebrile action and low toxicity of phenazone had been established, clinical trials were now begun. It was soon shown by these trials that phenazone possessed antipyretic properties as well as being a good analgesic. In view of the great advantages it offered over the preparations used hitherto, the medical profession made use of it with great success not only in all febrile conditions but also in cases of lesser pain, and above all in migraine and headaches. Phenazone was put to the test when a severe influenza epidemic broke out in Germany shortly after its appearance on the pharmaceutical market in 1888.

Phenazone is rarely used alone today. But it enjoys great popularity in Germany as an analgesic component in compounded preparations.

Caffeine, phenacetin, and dimethylaminophenazone (Pyramidon®) are the substances which head the list of those preferred for use in combination with phenazone. It frequently finds use as a salicylate or citrate salt in such a combination. The extensive and interesting experiments conducted by Zwintz (37) showed that phenazone salicylate is a good antipyretic and antirheumatic which does not exhibit any deleterious side reactions on the heart. Very recently Herxheimer and Stresemann (38) found that it is effective in the treatment of asthma.

B. ISOPROPYLPHENAZONE

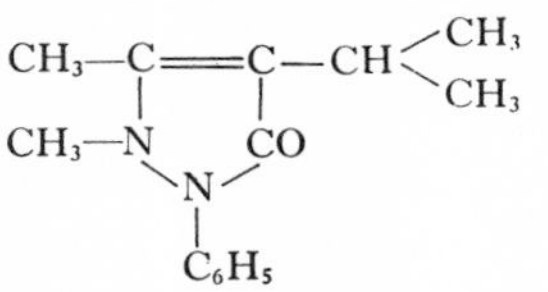

$$CH_3-C{=\!=\!=}C-CH{<}^{CH_3}_{CH_3}$$
$$CH_3-N\quad CO$$
$$\diagdown N\diagup$$
$$|$$
$$C_6H_5$$

1-Phenyl-2,3-dimethyl-4-isopropyl-3-pyrazoline-5-one

(X)

1. *Synthesis*

Substitution in the 4-position gained great importance in the further development of the pyrazolone derivatives. In the manufacture of phenazone, 4-methylphenazone (XI) had been isolated as a by-product which

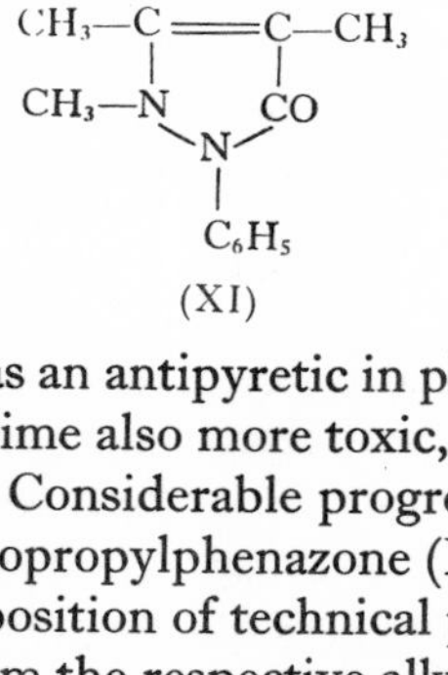

$$CH_3-C{=\!=\!=}C-CH_3$$
$$CH_3-N\quad CO$$
$$\diagdown N\diagup$$
$$|$$
$$C_6H_5$$

(XI)

proved to be more effective as an antipyretic in pharmacological trials, than phenazone, but at the same time also more toxic, and was consequently not introduced as a therapeutic. Considerable progress was made, however, in 1931 by the synthesis of 4-isopropylphenazone (X).

The CH_2 group in the 4-position of technical pyrazolone (V) reacts with aldehydes and ketones to form the respective alkylated compounds (Eq. 3).

$$CH_3-C{-\!\!-\!\!-}CH_2 \qquad\qquad CH_3-C{-\!\!-\!\!-}C{=}C{<}^{R_1}_{R_2} + H_2O \qquad (3)$$
$$N\quad CO + OC{<}^{R_1}_{R_2} = \qquad N\quad CO$$
$$\diagdown N\diagup \qquad\qquad\qquad \diagdown N\diagup$$
$$|\qquad\qquad\qquad\qquad\qquad |$$
$$C_6H_5 \qquad\qquad\qquad\qquad\qquad C_6H_5$$

If pyrazolone is hydrogenated catalytically in a solvent in the presence of aldehydes or ketones, the 4-alkyl pyrazolones are obtained at once by the adding of H_2 to the intermediate alkylated compound.

4-Isopropylphenazone is prepared by catalytic hydrogenation of technical pyrazolone in a Ni contact process using an excess of acetone (39) or the equivalent amount of acetone and methanol as the solvent (40); the resulting 1-phenyl-3-methyl-4-isopropyl-2-pyrazoline-5-one is then methylated to isopropylphenazone by fusing with dimethyl sulfate for 3 hours at 125° C (Eq. 4) (41).

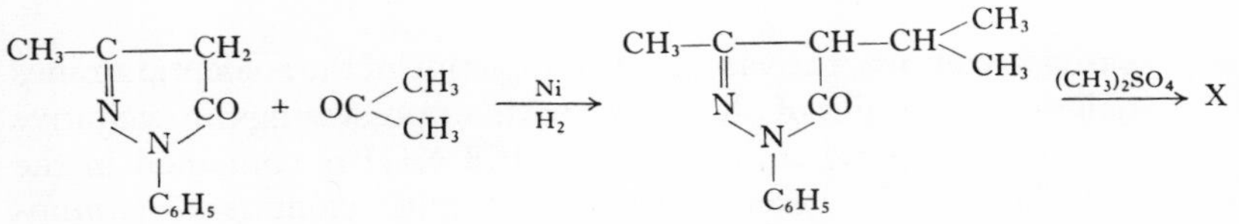

$$CH_3-C{\overset{||}{\underset{N}{}}}CH_2 \quad + \quad OC{<}{\overset{CH_3}{\underset{CH_3}{}}} \quad \xrightarrow[H_2]{Ni} \quad CH_3-C{\overset{||}{\underset{N}{}}}CH-CH{<}{\overset{CH_3}{\underset{CH_3}{}}} \quad \xrightarrow{(CH_3)_2SO_4} X \quad (4)$$

Detailed manufacturing instructions containing a critical survey of the individual processing stages and discussion of the sources of error were published by Jansen (42), who also described a more suitable method of methylation in alkaline solution with dimethyl sulfate at 20 to 35° C.

2. Chemical and Physical Properties

Isopropylphenazone forms molecular compounds with 5,5-disubstituted barbituric acids, a property also possessed by many other pyrazolone derivatives (43); however, only those barbituric acids enter into such a reaction that possess only saturated or at most one unsaturated substituent, such as diethyl, phenylethyl, isopropylethyl, and isopropyl-(β-bromoalkyl) barbituric acid. Allional ®is a therapeutic belonging to this series. It is a combination of isopropylphenazone and allylisopropylbarbituric acid. The clinical importance of such molecular structures will be dealt with in a later chapter in the discussion of Veramon®.

A further derivative of isopropylphenazone must be mentioned here. 1-Phenyl-2-methyl-3-bromomethyl-4-isopropyl-3-pyrazoline-5-one (XII) is obtained by bromination, in which the bromine atom is very reactive. By

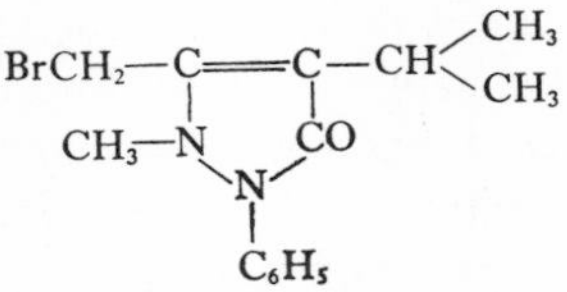

$$BrCH_2-C{=}C-CH{<}{\overset{CH_3}{\underset{CH_3}{}}}$$

(XII)

341

reacting XII with γ-phenyl-β-amino(N-methyl)propane, 1-phenyl-2-methyl-3-[N-methyl-(α-methyl-β-phenyl)ethylaminomethyl]-4-isopropyl-3-pyrazoline-5-one (XIII) is obtained (44).

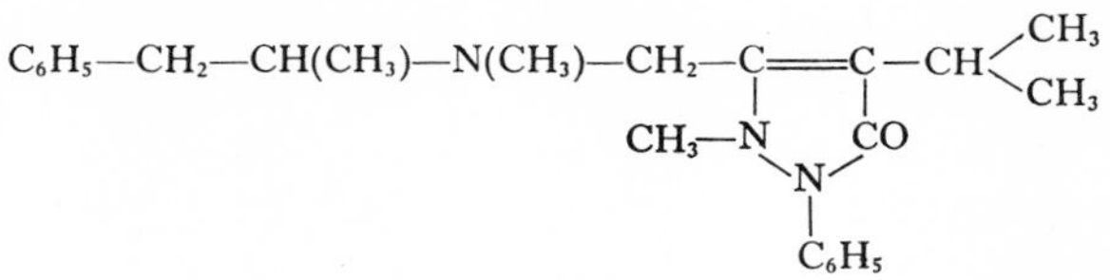

$$C_6H_5-CH_2-CH(CH_3)-N(CH_3)-CH_2-C{=\!=\!=}C-CH\diagdown{CH_3}^{CH_3}$$

$$CH_3-N \qquad CO$$
$$N$$
$$C_6H_5$$

(XIII)

It was prepared to combine the vasoconstrictor action of the analeptic amines with the analgesic properties of phenazone without possessing the excitative component of the analeptic amines. Compound XIII is contained in the preparation "Gewodin" together with isopropylphenazone, p-acetamino-phenol and caffeine.

3. Toxicity and Action

According to Fromherz (45), isopropylphenazone is half as toxic in mice as in cats and rabbits and twice as toxic as dimethylaminophenazone. Analogous to the other pyrazolones, toxic dosages result in stimulation of the

TABLE I

LETHAL DOSE OF ISOPROPYLPHENAZONE ADMINISTERED ORALLY AS AGAINST DIMETHYLAMINOPHENAZONE (IN GM/KG)

Animal	Isopropyl-phenazone	Dimethylamino-phenazone
Mouse	2.0	0.8
Rabbit	0.5	1.25
Cat	0.15–0.2	0.3–0.4

central nervous system and cramp. According to Fromherz, the antipyretic effect of isopropylphenazone is double and the spasmolytic effect 4 times that of dimethylaminophenazone. These findings were confirmed by Orestano (46), who discovered that isopropylphenazone, when administered in small doses, is twice as effective as dimethylaminophenazone. In large doses, on the other hand, the effect of dimethylaminophenazone was greater. Bauer (47) examined the analgesic effect of isopropylphenazone in mice.

Employing the hot-plate method he found it to be about equally powerful in action, but of shorter duration than that of dimethylamino phenazone.

4. Clinical Significance

Isopropylphenazone is a good antipyretic and analgesic. It is a component of many combination products of which the best-known are Saridon® and Melabon®.

C. 4-FORMYLPHENAZONE

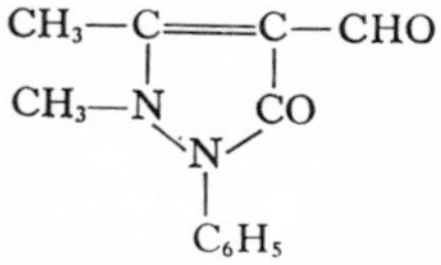

$$CH_3—C{=\!=}C—CHO$$
$$CH_3—N \quad CO$$
$$\diagdown N \diagup$$
$$|$$
$$C_6H_5$$

1-Phenyl-2,3-dimethyl-4-formyl-3-pyrazoline-5-one

(XIV)

1. Synthesis

Work on the substitution of phenazone in the 4-position has been continued in recent years. Bodendorf et al. (48) succeeded in synthesizing 4-formylphenazone (XIV) which is also frequently called phenazone aldehyde. They obtained it by heating 1-phenyl-2,3-dimethyl-4-[β,β,β-trichloro-α-hydroxyethyl]-3-pyrazoline-5-one (XV)—which had been obtained by condensing chloralhydrate to phenazone (49)—in cold-saturated potassium carbonate solution, chloroform being eliminated (Eq. 5).

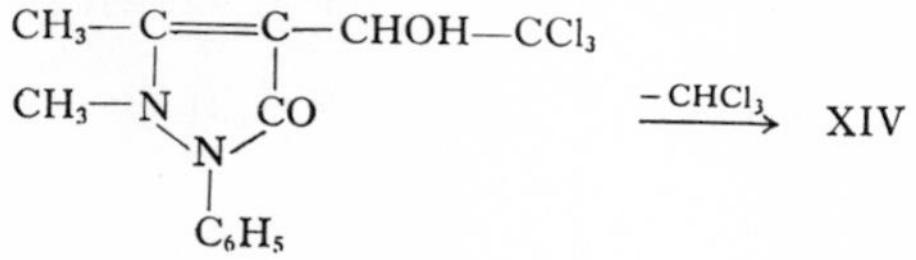

$$CH_3—C{=\!=}C—CHOH—CCl_3$$
$$CH_3—N \quad CO \qquad \xrightarrow{-CHCl_3} \quad XIV \qquad (5)$$
$$\diagdown N \diagup$$
$$|$$
$$C_6H_5$$
$$(XV)$$

It is claimed that better yields are obtained by splitting the trichloro compound (XV) by heating with 30% potassium carbonate solution at 80–85° C and driving off the chloroform formed by the use of CO_2 or N_2 (50). Other processes use phenazone as the starting material which is reacted with n,n-dialkyl or n-aryl-n-alkylformamides at 60–65° C in the presence of phosgene (51) or phosphorus oxychloride (52), and the reaction mixture is then decomposed with water to form formylphenazone (Eq. 6).

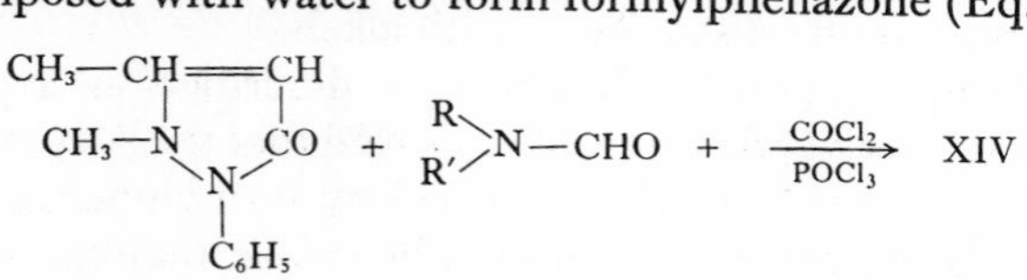

$$CH_3—CH{=\!=}CH$$
$$CH_3—N \quad CO \quad + \quad \begin{matrix} R \\ R' \end{matrix}{\diagdown}N—CHO \quad + \quad \xrightarrow[POCl_3]{COCl_2} \quad XIV \qquad (6)$$
$$\diagdown N \diagup$$
$$|$$
$$C_6H_5$$

343

2. Chemical and Physical Properties

On heating formylphenazone with 10% caustic soda solution or allowing it to stand with a large excess of 3/4 N caustic soda solution for 1–2 days, it is rearranged to form 1-phenyl-2-methyl-4-acetyl-3-pyrazoline-5-one (XVI) in accordance with the mechanism (53) shown (Eq. 7).

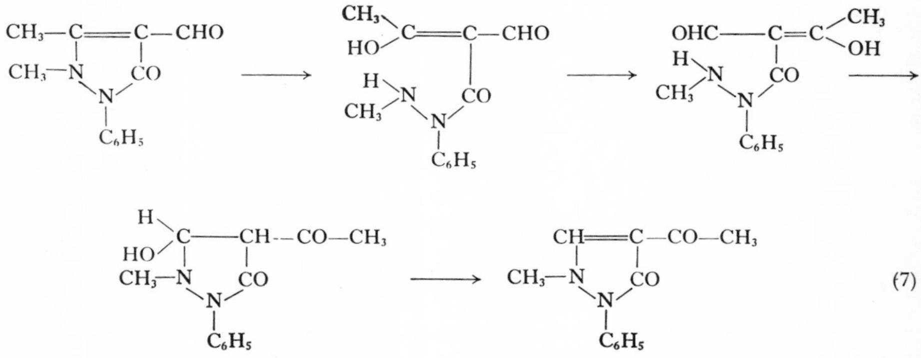

$$
\begin{array}{ccc}
\underset{\substack{| \\ CH_3-N \quad CO \\ \diagdown N \diagup \\ | \\ C_6H_5}}{CH_3-C\!\!=\!\!C-CHO}
& \longrightarrow &
\underset{\substack{H \diagdown \quad | \\ \quad N \quad CO \\ CH_3 \diagup \diagdown N \diagup \\ | \\ C_6H_5}}{\overset{CH_3 \diagdown}{\underset{HO \diagup}{C}}\!\!=\!\!C-CHO}
& \longrightarrow &
\underset{\substack{H \diagdown \quad | \\ \quad N \quad CO \\ CH_3 \diagup \diagdown N \diagup \\ | \\ C_6H_5}}{OHC-\!\!-C\!\!=\!\!C\!\!<\!\!{}^{CH_3}_{OH}}
& \longrightarrow
\end{array}
$$

$$
\begin{array}{ccc}
\underset{\substack{| \quad\; | \\ CH_3-N \quad CO \\ \diagdown N \diagup \\ | \\ C_6H_5}}{\overset{H \diagdown}{\underset{HO \diagup}{C}}-\!\!-CH-\!\!-CO-\!\!-CH_3}
& \longrightarrow &
\underset{\substack{| \quad\; | \\ CH_3-N \quad CO \\ \diagdown N \diagup \\ | \\ C_6H_5}}{CH\!\!=\!\!C-\!\!CO-\!\!CH_3}
& \qquad (7) \\
& & (\mathrm{XVI})
\end{array}
$$

Passerini and Losco had isolated compound XVI in 1940 (54) by reacting 1-phenyl-4-methylpyrazoline-5-one with phenylisonitrile, methylating the anil formed, and subsequently dissociating with alkali. They mistook this compound for formylphenazone. Bodendorf et al. (48) explained that the reaction took place in accordance with the mechanism shown (Eq. 8), in

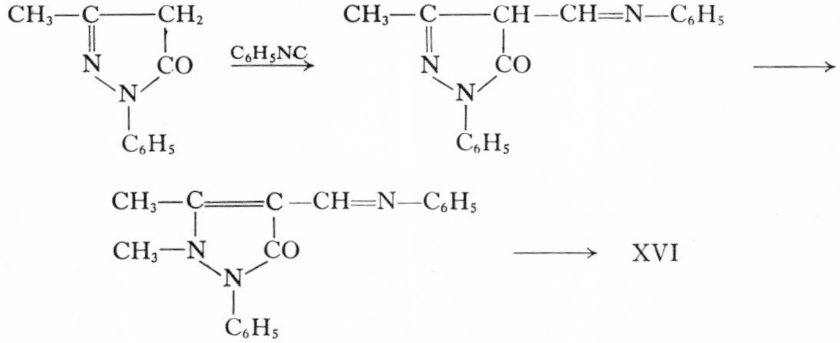

$$
\underset{\substack{\| \quad\; | \\ N \quad CO \\ \diagdown N \diagup \\ | \\ C_6H_5}}{CH_3-C-\!\!-CH_2}
\xrightarrow{C_6H_5NC}
\underset{\substack{\| \quad\; | \\ N \quad CO \\ \diagdown N \diagup \\ | \\ C_6H_5}}{CH_3-C-\!\!-CH-\!\!CH\!\!=\!\!N-\!\!C_6H_5}
\longrightarrow
$$

$$
\underset{\substack{| \quad\;\; | \\ CH_3-N \quad CO \\ \diagdown N \diagup \\ | \\ C_6H_5}}{CH_3-C\!\!=\!\!C-\!\!CH\!\!=\!\!N-\!\!C_6H_5}
\longrightarrow \quad \mathrm{XVI} \qquad (8)
$$

which transformation of the intermediate formylphenazone takes place in the last phase of the reaction by dissociation with alkali.

In the relevant literature, formylphenazone is described as a yellow colored substance. Ledrut et al. (55), however, proved that the preparations contained up to 4% impurities which are formed by formylphenazone in condensation and oxidation processes. Formylphenazone may be isolated chromatographically in the form of colorless crystals from these products. Colorless product may, on the other hand, be prepared directly if phenazone is formylated with dimethylformamide and phosphorus oxychloride according to Eq. (6) if the temperature is maintained at 60–65° C and the reaction takes place in an anhydrous solvent or mixture of solvents such as chloroform/toluene.

3. *Toxicity and Action*

Formylphenazone is slightly more toxic than phenazone but its febrifugal and analgesic properties are more marked (*56*). Compared to dimethylaminophenazone the relation between toxicity and analgesic action is a little more favorable in formylphenazone but, on the other hand, it does not possess the powerful antiphlogistic action of dimethylaminophenazone. According to van Cauwenberge *et al.* (*57*), formylphenazone and its salicylate are less antiinflammatory than phenazone.

D. TARUGAN®

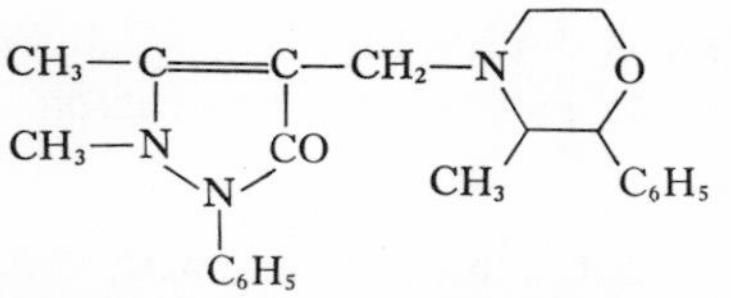

$$CH_3-C=\!=\!C-CH_2-N$$
$$CH_3-N \quad CO$$
$$N$$
$$C_6H_5$$

with morpholine ring bearing CH_3 and C_6H_5

4-(2′-Phenyl-3′-methylmorpholinomethyl)-1-phenyl-2,3-dimethyl-3-pyrazoline-5-one

(XVII)

1. *Synthesis and Properties*

Compound XVII is formed by Mannich-condensation of phenazone in alcoholic solution with 3-methyl-2-phenylmorpholine and formaldehyde (*58*). This compound, together with dimethylaminophenazone and salicylamide, is a compound of the combination preparation "Rosimon-new"®. The hydrochloride and ascorbic acid salt of compound XVII are readily soluble in water and permit the preparation of highly concentrated, stable aqueous solutions. Excellent yields of the hydrochloride are obtained in a one-phase process if the Mannich-condensation mentioned above is carried out in *a* medium acidified with hydrochloric acid (*59*).

2. *Toxicity and Action*

According to Hengen *et al.* (*59*), the LD_{50} of XVII is 115 mg/kg in subcutaneous administration, and the LD_{50} (mean cramp inducing dose) 80 mg/kg. Table II gives the toxicity in oral administration. The values for dimethylaminophenazone found by Wilhelmi (*60*) are included for

345

comparison. Administered orally, XVII is thus considerably more toxic than dimethylaminophenazone.

TABLE II

LD 50 OF XVII ADMINISTERED ORALLY (IN MG/KG)
COMPARED TO DIMETHYLAMINOPHENAZONE

Preparation	Mouse	Rat
XVII	250	250
Dimethylaminophenazone	830	930

Delayed toxicity was not observed by Hengen *et al.*, indicating rapid detoxification of the substance in the organism. Its analgesic effect was tested in mice by the method of Wolff-Hardy, comparing it to dimethylaminophenazone, phenacetin, and salicylamide. This revealed that the analgesic action of XVII is 2–3 times that of dimethylaminophenazone, about 15 times that of phenacetin, and about 12 times that of salicylamide. Its antiinflammatory effect is double that of dimethylaminophenazone in the treatment of edema in rats' paws caused by dextron.

3. *Clinical Application*

Richard (*61*) conducted clinical trials with "Rosimon new" on 100 patients. The action of the antiinflammatory component was particularly marked. After administering it for a few days, complete freedom from pain was attained in rheumatic conditions, and inflammatory processes were rapidly eliminated. The use of opiates was obviated to a great extent, particularly also in postoperative stadia. No damage of any kind, no signs of intolerability or habit-forming tendencies were observed. Stomach tolerability was good. Control tests did not reveal toxic influences of any kind.

E. 4-AMINOPHENAZONE

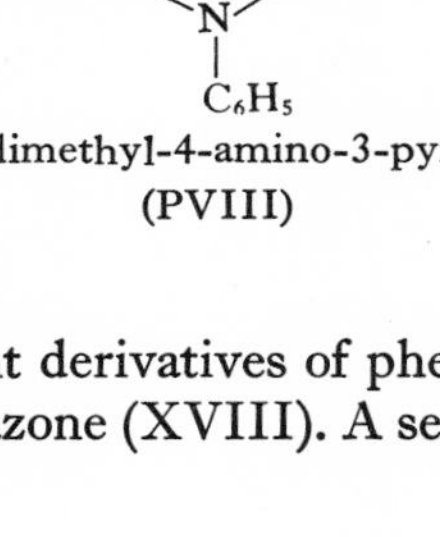

$$CH_3-C\!=\!\!=\!\!C-NH_2$$
$$CH_3-N\quad CO$$
$$N$$
$$|$$
$$C_6H_5$$

1-Phenyl-2,3-dimethyl-4-amino-3-pyrazoline-5-one
(PVIII)

1. *Synthesis*

By far the most important derivatives of phenazone are those which are derived from 4-aminophenazone (XVIII). A section is devoted to it in this chapter because it constitutes an important intermediate for the synthesis of therapeutic preparations, plays an important part as a metabolite of dimethylaminophenazone, and will combine with many therapeutic compounds that contain a phenolic OH group which enables photometric determinations to be made.

The technical manufacturing process of 4-aminophenazone is by the reduction of 4-nitrosophenazone (XIX) which is obtained by nitrosation of phenazone in a solution of sulfuric acid (62) by reacting with sodium hydrogen sulfite, whereby 4-sulfaminophenazone (XX) is formed. By the process introduced by Scheitlin (63) it is then converted to the 4-amino compound by boiling with dilute sulfuric acid (Eq. 9). It is not necessary to isolate the

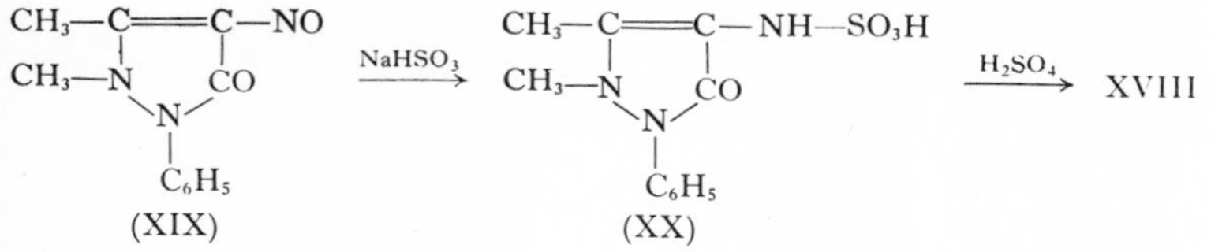

$$
\begin{array}{ccc}
\underset{\substack{\text{CH}_3-\text{C}===\text{C}-\text{NO} \\ \text{CH}_3-\text{N} \quad \text{CO} \\ \diagdown \text{N} \diagup \\ | \\ \text{C}_6\text{H}_5 \\ \text{(XIX)}}}{} & \xrightarrow{\text{NaHSO}_3} &
\underset{\substack{\text{CH}_3-\text{C}===\text{C}-\text{NH}-\text{SO}_3\text{H} \\ \text{CH}_3-\text{N} \quad \text{CO} \\ \diagdown \text{N} \diagup \\ | \\ \text{C}_6\text{H}_5 \\ \text{(XX)}}}{} & \xrightarrow{\text{H}_2\text{SO}_4} & \text{XVIII} \quad (9)
\end{array}
$$

individual intermediates because the reaction mixtures obtained are immediately used for further processing. Caustic soda solution is then added in excess and the mixture stirred in the presence of benzene until the 4-amino phenazone has separated.

2. Properties and Chemical Behavior

4-Aminophenazone is readily soluble in water. According to Strunz and Körber (64) it is a suitable solvent for dimethylaminophenazone. Its aqueous solution is turned violet red by oxidizing agents such as permanganate, ferric chloride, or platinum chloride (65).

Quantitative photometric determination of various therapeutic compounds which possess a phenolic hydroxyl group is based on a condensation process by which it reacts with 4-aminophenone in the presence of potassium hexacyanoferrate(III) as the oxidizing agent (66). The process is based on a reaction discovered by Emerson (67) which represents a special case of the indophenol reaction. It proceeds as shown in the accompanying scheme (Eq. 10). The practicability of this process was demonstrated by the

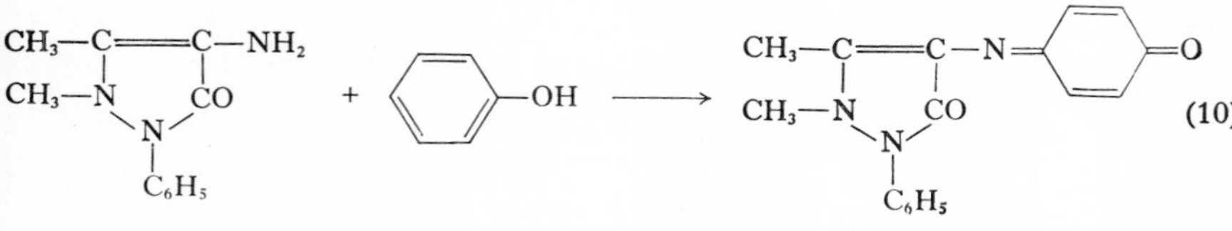

$$
\underset{\substack{\text{CH}_3-\text{C}===\text{C}-\text{NH}_2 \\ \text{CH}_3-\text{N} \quad \text{CO} \\ \diagdown \text{N} \diagup \\ | \\ \text{C}_6\text{H}_5}}{} \quad + \quad \underset{}{\text{⟨⟩-OH}} \quad \longrightarrow \quad \underset{\substack{\text{CH}_3-\text{C}===\text{C}-\text{N}==\text{⟨⟩}==\text{O} \\ \text{CH}_3-\text{N} \quad \text{CO} \\ \diagdown \text{N} \diagup \\ | \\ \text{C}_6\text{H}_5}}{} \quad (10)
$$

347

production of a large number of therapeutic compounds and formulations, Hiskey and Levin (*68*) worked out a colorimetric determination of phenyl-ephrin by this method wherein isolation of the drug is not required. They obtained a red coupling product which possesses an absorption maximum at 500 mμ. Johnson and Savidge (*69*) used this process on salol, salicylamide, and a number of other phenols by which dyestuffs soluble in chloroform were obtained and which could be evaluated photometrically. Yavorksii (*70*) determined 27 organomedical products by this method. Haslinger and Strunz (*71*) worked out a process employing the Emerson reaction for the colorimetric determination of 4-aminophenazone alongside dimethylamino-phenazone in serum which permits measurements of 0.2 mg% to 10 mg% and higher to be made. The dyestuff formed by the reaction of *p*-dimethyl-aminocinnamic aldehyde with 4-aminophenazone and perchloric acid is suitable, according to Strell and Reindl (*72*), for the qualitative and quanti-tative determination of 4-aminophenazone as a decomposition product of dimethylaminophenazone in the urine. The authors worked out an exact method using a Beckman apparatus as well as a rapid method using a dip stick colorimeter. The polymethine dyestuff formed exhibits a clearly defined absorption zone in the visible area.

Prior chromatographic removal of "Rubazonsäure," a further red-colored separation product of dimethylaminophenazone in the urine, is not necessary for the rapid determination process since it is not the intensity of the solution coloring that is measured in the spectroscope but solely the extinction of the polymethine dyestuff.

It should be mentioned finally also that 4-aminophenazone is suitable for the testing of blood circulation in the extremities, as was demonstrated in experiments on dogs by Huckabee and Walcott (*73*). This method has several advantages: rapidity and simplicity of colorimetric analysis and accuracy of the determination even in small blood or plasma quantitities (0.1 ml), together with the rapid achievement of equilibrium in the blood and tissues.

3. *Toxicity and Behavior in the Organism*

4-Aminophenazone is only slightly toxic. This circumstance is of impor-tance inasmuch as it is a metabolite of dimethylaminophenazone. It is considerably less toxic than phenazone. Frogs tolerate injection of 150 mg into the dorsal lymph pouch without any untoward manifestations (*74*). Doses of 250 mg merely have a paralyzing effect but do not act as exciters as do most pyrazolones and bring about death only after prolonged periods. Administered under the same conditions, phenazone already causes death in doses of 50 mg. The toxicity of 4-aminophenazone is about one-third that of

348

phenazone also in warm blooded animals (75). 1 gm/kg administered sub-cutaneously to a rabbit weighing 3 kg was tolerated without any noticeable change in the condition of the animal; 2 gm/kg administered subcutaneously resulted in death after 26 hours, whereas 0.6–0.8 gm/kg phenazone was lethal. Halberkann and Fretwurst (76) found in another experiment that 35.5% of the 4-aminophenazone they had taken was excreted in the urine unchanged and 25.1% was excreted as 4-acetylaminophenazone.

F. Pyramidon®

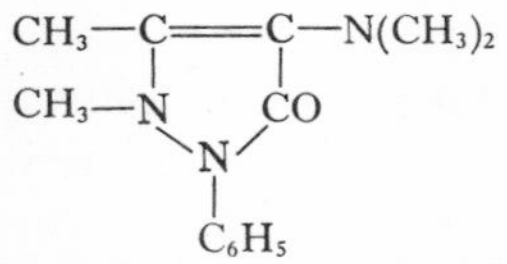

$$CH_3-C=C-N(CH_3)_2$$
$$CH_3-N \quad CO$$
$$N$$
$$C_6H_5$$

1-Phenyl-2,3-dimethyl-4-dimethylamino-3-pyrazoline-5-one
(XXI)

1. History

The dimethylamino group plays an important part in synthetic chemistry on the formation of dyestuffs and therapeutic drugs. Methylation of the nitrogen atom in the kairine group as well as in the manufacture of phenazone was of particular importance in the synthesis of therapeutic compounds and thus paved the way for considerably more effective preparations. Based on the knowledge of these facts the pharmacologist Filehne, who carried out the first animal experiments with phenazone and detected its good antifebrile effect, suggested that the dimethylamino group be joined to the phenyl radical of the phenazone in the *para* position, that is, to synthesize 1-(4'-dimethylaminophenyl-2,3-dimethyl-5-pyrazolone (XXII).

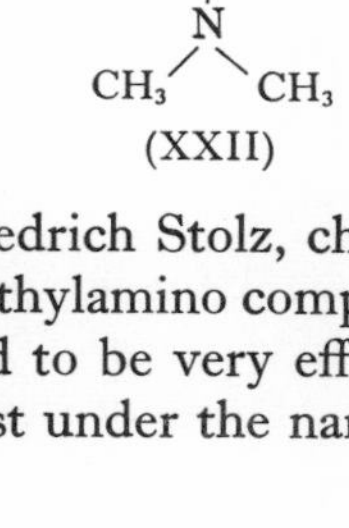

$$CH_3-C=CH$$
$$CH_3-N \quad CO$$
$$N$$

$$N$$
$$CH_3 \quad CH_3$$
(XXII)

By this time, however, Friedrich Stolz, chemist at Farbwerke Hoechst, had already found the 4-dimethylamino compound XXI which he gave to Filehne for testing. It proved to be very effective and was placed on the market by Farbwerke Hoechst under the name of Pyramidon® in 1897.

349

The generic name dimethylaminophenazone will be used for Pyramidon in this chapter. (It is frequently called Amino-pyrine in the literature. Since this name is, however, registered in many countries as a trade mark, it will not be used in this article.)

Compound XXII was also synthesized later. Pharmacological tests, however, revealed that it is far more toxic than dimethylaminophenazone, although its antipyretic action is equal, and clinical evaluation was therefore out of the question.

2. Synthesis

The first synthesis of dimethylaminophenazone was carried out by methylating aminophenazone (XVIII) with methyl iodide in methanol (77). Formaldehyde and formic acid are used to methylate aminophenazone. This process is not only inexpensive but offers the advantage of very high yields without side reactions of any magnitude being encountered. Equation (11) represents the reaction in which only water and carbon dioxide are formed.

$$R—NH_2 + 2HCHO + 2HCOOH = R—N(CH_3)_2 + 2H_2O + 2CO_2 \tag{11}$$

The technical process for the manufacture of dimethylaminophenazone has been developed into a fine art in the course of time (12). The starting product used is 1-phenyl-3-methyl-2-pyrazoline-5-one (V), which is formed by the condensation of phenylhydrazine with acetoacetic ester; the intermediate products formed in subsequent reactions are not isolated. The process is as follows: after methylating phenylmethylpyrazolone by fusion with dimethyl sulfate, the crude phenazone is salted out by adding an excess of concentrated caustic soda solution; it is separated in the form of an oil and then dissolved in water. The aqueous phenazone solution is acidified with sulfuric acid and mixed with sodium nitrite whereby nitrosophenazone (XIX) is formed. The nitrosophenazone is not separated from the reaction mixture and is reduced directly by sodium hydrogen sulfite to sulfaminophenazone (XX) which is subsequently converted to 4-aminophenazone (XVIII) by boiling with an excess of sulfuric acid while passing air through the mixture. After neutralizing with caustic soda solution, and clarifying the solution with charcoal, formic acid is admixed and the mixture boiled for 8 hours. It is then neutralized once more with caustic soda solution, and after adding the required amount of formaldehyde, it is boiled for a further period of 10 hours. When the mixture has cooled, the dimethylaminophenazone formed is dissolved in benzene and then purified by recrystallization in alcohol. The yield is equal to the amount of phenazone separated in the form of an oil in the first stage of the process.

3. Chemical and Physical Properties

Dimethylaminophenazone is relatively sparingly soluble in water. At room temperature its solubility in water is 5.5%. The series of color reactions that it will enter into is known. Some of these are specific for dimethyl-

350

aminophenazone and can be used for its identification. A synopsis is contained in the treatise of Kobert (78) and Jung (79).

Thévenon and Rolland (80) utilized the color reaction of dimethylaminophenazone with hydrogen peroxide to detect blood in the urine, feces, and in pathological exudates: 3–4 ml urine that has not been filtered or the filtrate of a small sample of feces in 3–4 ml water are mixed with an equal volume of alcoholic dimethylphenazone solution (2.5 gm substance in 50 ml 90% alcohol) to which 6–8 drops acetic acid in a dilution of 1:2 are added, and, finally, 5–6 drops 12 volume per cent hydrogen peroxide solution are also added, while shaking. If considerable amounts of blood are present, the mixture turns intensively violet in color; if small amounts are present, it turns a bluish-violet color which reaches its greatest intensity after 15 minutes.

4. Preparation of Aqueous Solutions of High Concentration

In view of the fact that parenteral application of large amounts of dimethylaminophenazone had proved of value in the treatment of rheumatic diseases, and because its relatively low solubility rendered this mode of treatment rather difficult, ways were sought to prepare the solutions in the higher concentrations necessary for this purpose.

a. Salts and double compounds. Higher concentrations of dimethylaminophenazone are possible by converting it to salts and double compounds. In this way a molecular compound (81) readily soluble in water is formed with salicylamide-O-acetic acid, which is excellently tolerated in oral and parenteral administration and in which the toxicity of the pyrazolone part is reduced by one-half. In Polinal®, phenazone-4-carboxylic acid–diethylaminoethyl ester and salicylamide glycolic acid ether are used to solubilize dimethylaminophenazone. The firm of Knoll A.G. (82) prepared a mixture of dimethylaminophenazone, calcium salicylate, and anhydrous caffeine or methylaminoheptane salicylate whose solubility in water is 50%.

b. Additives which act as solubilizers. It is also possible to dissolve larger quantities of dimethylaminophenazone by adding substances which act as solubilizers. This property of phenazone (13) has already been mentioned. A 25% solution of it will dissolve 20% dimethylaminophenazone. A second solubilizer, ethylurethane, may be used in addition to phenazone (83). By combining these two substances a twofold effect is achieved: the total amount of solubilizer required is reduced, and the stability of the solution is increased.

Apart from phenazone, 4-aminophenazone (XVIII), which is readily soluble in water, slightly toxic, and hardly active physiologically, has proved very effective in the preparation of highly concentrated solutions of

351

dimethylaminophenazone. It is thus possible to dissolve a fused mixture of 25 gm dimethylaminophenazone and 25 gm aminophenazone in 100 cc water (84).

Only two substances, however, have attained greater significance as solubilizers of dimethylaminophenazone, namely, 1,2-diphenyl-4-*n*-butyl-3,5-pyrazolidinedione (Butazolidin®) and 1,4-diphenyl-3,5-pyrazolidinedione (Phenopyrazon®), compounds which will be dealt with in a later section because of their own specific therapeutic action. Each of their salts will hold 15% dimethylaminophenazone in solution. The combination preparations are on the market under the names Irgapyrin® and Osadrin®.

5. Detection and Determination

The methods of detecting and determining dimethylaminophenazone are so numerous that they cannot be dealt with in detail here.

a. Qualitative determination. A method of detection by adsorption analysis in which not only dimethylaminophenazone but also Metamizol and 4-aminophenazone in quantities down to 0.005 mg can be detected, is described by Madaus and Meyer (85). In this test, typical crimson rings are formed in the presence of Flaveserin A (prepared by boiling a small amount of physostigmine with caustic alkalis) in a Frankonit-KL column in a medium that is acidified with hydrochloric acid. This method may also be employed for mixed preparations and molecular compounds. Runge *et al.* (86) found that many bases will form precipitates with 4,4′-dichlorophenyldisulfide, whose melting points are more suitable for identification purposes than are those of picrates and perchlorates. Dimethylaminophenazone forms a characteristic double compound with XXIII; this has a melting point of 167–168°C.

$$Cl—C_6H_4—SO_2 \diagdown$$
$$NH$$
$$Cl—C_6H_4—SO_2 \diagup$$

(XXIII)

The reaction with silver nitrate may also be employed for its identification. For this purpose, a solution is prepared by dissolving 1 gm of the substance to be tested in 16 ml water. This solution must be clear and colorless. A few drops of silver nitrate solution are added and a strong violet coloring occurs initially. After a short while, metallic silver is deposited in the form of a grayish-black precipitate.

b. Quantitative determination. A frequently used quantitative method of determining dimethylaminophenazone is based on its property to form dimethylamine on heating with aqueous caustic alkalis (87). The method was improved by Jaworski and Romanjak (88).

Titration in glacial acetic acid or anhydrous dioxan with 0.1 N $HClO_4$ is a suitable test for purity by pharmaceutical standards (89).

A number of papers have been published on the determination of dimethylaminophenazone in mixtures of pharmaceutical substances but these will not be referred to in detail here (90).

c. Determination in body fluids. Pulver (91) developed a process for its determination in serum, plasma, and liquor. He observed a new color reaction which is based on the fact that dimethylaminophenazone forms a stable compound of intensive golden yellow color in aqueous solution of pH 4–6 in the presence of small amounts of sulfaminic acid with diazotized *p*-nitraniline. This color reaction is suitable for colorimetric determination. The margin of error is ±10%.

Lohss and Kallee (*92*) modified Pulver's method, which was, however, not suitable for urine testing. The color producing component used by them was not *p*-nitraniline but sulfanilic acid in an acidic medium in the presence of a nitrite; a water soluble dye is formed.

Haslinger and Strunz (*93*) found, however, that Pulver's method also reacts to 4-aminophenazone, a metabolite of dimethylaminophenazone in the human body. In order to eliminate this source of error, they acetylated the aminophenazone contained in the serum and then proceeded with Pulver's test.

Weirich (*94*) devised a simple test method for the qualitative determination of excreted products which are found in the urine after medication with dimethylaminophenazone. After mixing the reddish colored urine with 2% ferric chloride solution it turns dark brown to dark violet in color. In a supernatant 1% iodide solution, at first a violet and later a reddish brown color ring is formed.

6. *Fate in the Organism*

In contrast to phenazone, a few per cent of which is excreted unchanged in the urine, it was not possible to detect dimethylaminophenazone as an excreted product. After administration of this drug, the human urine is colored red. The dye upon which this coloring is based was identified as "Rubazonsäure" (XXIV), 1-phenyl-4-[1-phenyl-5-oxo-3-methylpyrazolinylidene-(4)-amino]-3-methylpyrazolone-(5), by Jaffe (*95*). The forma-

(XXIV)

tion of this dye, in which up to 3% of the drug taken could be isolated, indicates that only a small fraction of dimethylaminophenazone is demethylated in the organism in such a way that the three methyl groups joined to the two N atoms are removed while the methyl group attached to the carbon atom is unaffected. Ammonia is split off in the linking together of two pyrazolone rings to form "Rubazonsäure." The urine of dogs is not colored red after the administration of dimethylaminophenazone. This coloring is only formed by oxidation due to air exposure. Jaffe assumes that 1-phenyl-3-methyl-4-amino-2-pyrazoline-5-one (XXV) is the substance excreted in the urine of dogs. This is the compound from which Knorr obtained "Rubazonsäure" earlier on. Jaffe succeeded in isolating a further metabolite in the urine of dogs, namely, up to 6% of phenazoneurea (XXVI).

The formation of this urea can probably be explained by the fact that the

CH₃—C——CH—NH₂ ... structure (XXV)

CH₃—C=C—NH—CO—NH₂ ... structure (XXVI)

$$\text{CH}_3-\underset{\underset{\underset{C_6H_5}{|}}{N}}{\overset{C}{\underset{\diagdown}{\parallel}}}-\underset{\underset{N}{\diagup}}{\overset{\text{CH}-\text{NH}_2}{\underset{\text{CO}}{|}}}$$

(XXV)

$$\text{CH}_3-\underset{\underset{\underset{C_6H_5}{|}}{N}}{\overset{\text{CH}_3-\text{N}}{\underset{\diagdown}{\diagup}}}$$

(XXVI)

demethylation process taking place in the organism, which is probably by oxidation, occurs only partly at the amino nitrogen. After subcutaneous injection in dogs, cats and rabbits, Kobert (96) detected excretion products in the kidneys, saliva glands, and in the mucous membranes of the stomach and small intestine.

Halberkann and Fretwurst (97) recently examined the excretion products of dimethylaminophenazone in the human organism. Apart from small quantitities of " Rubazonsäure," they found 22.8% 4-aminophenazone and 28.9% 4-acetylaminophenazone, calculated on the amount of dimethyl-aminophenazone. The excretion peaks for the two last named substances were reached on the first day, whereas excretion was completed over 4–5 days. The authors consider 4-acetylaminophenazone to be particularly suitable in toxicology for the detection of dimethylaminophenazone poisoning. They succeeded only with great difficulty in isolating phenazone in minute quantities which had been found as an excretion product in the urine of dogs.

Hennig and Weiler (98) also describe a method by which " Rubonaz-säure," 4-aminophenazone, and 4-acetylaminophenazone can be determined quantitatively in the urine.

Brunner and Haslinger (99) administered dimethylaminophenazone intramuscularly with 4-aminophenazone as solubilizer. Within 2 hours of application they found a dimethylaminophenazone level in the blood of 5.5 mg%, but after 12 hours the drug was not traceable any more. Using phenyl-butazone-sodium as a solubilizer they could not detect dimethylamino-phenazone in the blood for any longer period of time. The contrary results of Pulver are explained by the above authors as stemming from the fact that 4-aminophenazone is included in the quantities found by him.

Chen *et al.* (100) even observed that the transformation of dimethyl-aminophenazone in the human organism is accelerated by phenylbutazone. The blood level of dimethylaminophenazone drops more rapidly while that of its metabolites rises if it is administered together with phenylbutazone.

7. *Toxicity and Action*

Dimethylaminophenazone is 3 times as toxic in rabbits as phenazone (101) In his antipyresis tests on rabbits and humans Filehne found that the onset of action of dimethylaminophenazone is more gradual than that of phena-zone. It is also milder, has a longer lasting effect, and is more easily graded. Filehne had already observed that it has a reliable analgesic effect under varying conditions of application. It was established later that it also possesses good spasmolytic and excellent anti-inflammatory properties. The significance of dimethylaminophenazone and its use in diseases of the most diverse nature is based on its manifold effects in which it is hardly exceeded by any other therapeutic substance.

The mean lethal dose of dimethylaminophenazone was determined more recently (Table III) by Wilhelmi (60) and von Rechenberg (102). The

TABLE III

LD$_{50}$ OF DIMETHYLAMINOPHENAZONE (IN MG/KG)

	Mouse		Rat		Rabbit
	intravenously	orally	intravenously	orally	intravenously
Wilhemi	210	830	144	930	125
von Rechenberg	148	748	140	1030	156

experiments of Rühmke (103) revealed that the LD$_{50}$ on intravenous injec-tion of a 1% solution of dimethylaminophenazone in physiological salt solution was lower than when injecting a 0.5% solution.

The general action of toxic doses is characterized by excitation of the central nervous system. In warm blooded animals, cramp as well as numb-ness of the sensorium dominate the conditions arising from the toxic effect. Epileptiform spasms occur in the extremities, for example in the cervical and masticatory muscles. Strong saliva flow and an accelerated breathing rate are further side effects.

8. Veramon®

Double compounds which dimethylaminophenazone forms with sopori-fics, in particular those of the barbituric acid series, have proved eminently suitable in the therapy of pain conditions. The first preparation of this series to be put on the market was Veramon. It consists of a molecular compound of dimethylaminophenazone and 5,5-diethylbarbituric acid (104) to which a further molecule of dimethylaminophenazone has been added.

According to Pfeiffer (105), the complex of the two substances (XXVII) is brought about by the hydrogen atoms of the NH groups of diethylbarbituric

355

acid forming loose bonds with the carbonylic oxygen of dimethylamino-phenazone. To prove this assumption, Pfeiffer states that molecular com-

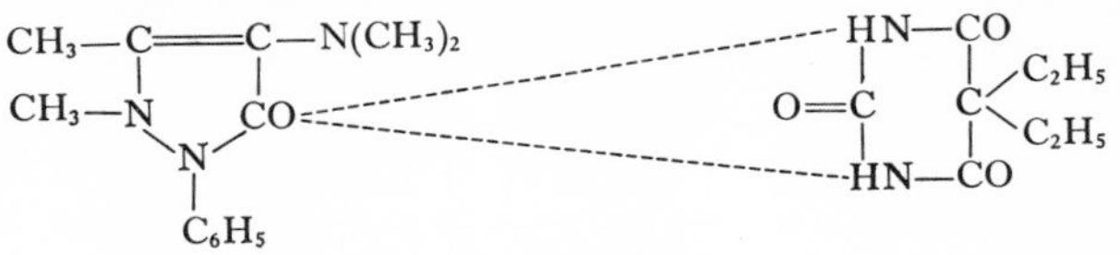

$$
\begin{array}{cc}
CH_3-C{=\!\!=}C-N(CH_3)_2 & \quad\quad HN-CO \\
| \quad\quad | & \quad\quad\quad | \quad\quad | \diagup C_2H_5 \\
CH_3-N \quad\quad CO & O{=}C \quad\quad C\diagdown \\
\quad N & \quad\quad\quad | \quad\quad | \diagdown C_2H_5 \\
| & \quad\quad\quad HN-CO \\
C_6H_5 &
\end{array}
$$

(XXVII)

pounds are not formed if the hydrogen atoms joined to the nitrogen of the diethylbarbituric acid are replaced by alkyl radicals.

Pharmacological tests (*106*) revealed that Veramon possesses extremely valuable properties. The analgesic action of dimethylaminophenazone is enhanced by the combination with the soporific while the hypnotic action of diethylbarbituric acid is lessened. Because of its rapid action, Veramon soon became very popular as an analgesic for pain of a less severe nature, especially in dental practice.

In the comparative determination of lethal doses of dimethylamino-phenazone, diethylbarbituric acid and Veramon tested by oral administration in rabbits (Table IV) it was found that diethylbarbituric acid is 4 times

TABLE IV

LETHAL DOSES OF DIMETHYLAMINOPHENAZONE, DIETHYL-
BARBITURIC ACID AND VERAMON ADMINISTERED ORALLY TO
RABBITS (IN GM/KG)

Dimethylaminophenazone	Diethylbarbituric acid	Veramon
0.7–0.8	0.3–0.4	1.2–1.4

as toxic as Veramon (*107*). The lethal dose thus calculated for adults is at least 20 gm Veramon, since the lethal dose of diethylbarbituric acid is 5–6 gm in humans. Observations on the taking of excessive doses of Veramon are in agreement with these findings.

When Veramon poisoning is encountered, the adverse effects on the central nervous system caused by the dimethylaminophenazone subside rapidly so that finally a poisoning by diethylbarbituric acid alone is in evidence (*108*).

Before Veramon appeared on the market, a compound of dimethylaminophenazone and the soporific butylchloral hydrate under the name of Trigemin® had already been introduced as a therapeutic drug *(109)*. A further number of soporifics were later combined with dimethyl aminophenazone. A few are named here:

5,5-diallylbarbituric acid, Cibalgin® *(104)*;
5-phenyl-5-ethylbarbituric acid *(104, 110)*;
5-isopropyl-5-allyl-barbituric acid *(111)*;
5-*sec*-butyl-5-bromoallyl-barbituric acid ,Doralgin® *(112)*;
5-isobutyl-5-allyl-barbituric acid, Optalidon® *(113)*;
5-ethyl-5-crotyl-barbituric acid *(114)*;
Magnesium, calcium, and strontium 5,5-diethyl- and 5-phenyl-5-ethylbarbiturates *(115)*;
β,β,γ-trichlorobutyl alcohol *(116)*;
trichloroethylurethane, Compral® *(110, 116)*;
bromodiethylacetylurea *(110)*;
diethylallylacetamide, Arantil®.

9. *Pyracortin*®

More recently, the new corticosteroids such as prednisone have been employed in the therapy of rheumatic diseases because of their superior action and tolerability.

If prednisone is combined with dimethylaminophenazone which also has an effect on rheumatoid conditions, albeit on a different basis, the integrated action of the two therapeutic substances becomes so powerfully synergetic that complete rheumatic action is attained by subliminal doses. Pyracortin, which is such a combined preparation, contains 0.75 mg prednisone and 150 mg dimethylaminophenazone per tablet; Pyracortin "forte" contains double this dose.

Of the numerous clinical papers published on the use of Pyracortin *(117)*, a few will be mentioned here. Blumencron *(118)*, reports, for instance, that the preparation was well tolerated and that no unpleasant or allergic side reactions were observed. The great value of the combination product lies in the fact that a fully effective treatment using only a small prednisone dose can be given over prolonged periods. Treiber *(119)* was very successful in the treatment of Bekhterev's disease over long periods with Pyracortin "forte," particularly with regard to pain which had not been achieved when other forms of medication had been used. Kleinschmidt *(120)* reports that the most favorable results in the effective treatment of primary and secondarily chronic types of polyarthritis may be expected with Pyracortin therapy.

357

10. *Clinical Significance of Dimethylaminophenazone*

Because of its manifold modes of action, dimethylaminophenazone is used in Germany for the treatment of the most diverse diseases. As an antipyretic it may be used successfully in all acute febrile conditions, not only in pneumonia, angina, measles, typhoid, and erysipelas, but also in influenza and all illnesses associated with the common cold. Small repeated doses of dimethylaminophenazone given during the course of a day suffice to bring about a rapid reduction of fever in tuberculosis. In erysipelas it has a beneficial effect on the elevated temperature and the inflammatory processes.

There are many uses of dimethylaminophenazone as an analgesic. It can be administered in surgery where lesser pain is encountered. It brings relief in many cases of painful tumour, sarcomas, and inoperable carcinoma. In tonsilectomies its antiphlogistic action in addition—possibly in combination with penicillin—promotes healing without complications setting in and by its obdurating action on the vasa prevents the spreading of bacteria. In gynecology, dimethylaminophenazone eliminates complaints associated with menstruation and has also proved of value in the treatment of after-pains. It also finds application in pediatrics, in difficult, painful cutting of teeth, and in dentistry in the treatment of neuralgic pain and for the prevention of pain after extractions.

The antineuralgic and antispasmolytic action of dimethylaminophenazone is reliable in trigeminal neuralgias, headaches, and migraine of various origins. Because of its spasmolytic action it is beneficial in the treatment of bronchial asthma.

Dimethylaminophenazone has proved particularly valuable because of its excellent antiinflammatory, analgesic, and antifebrile action in all acute and chronic rheumatoid complaints and in rheumatoid conditions in children.

G. NOVALGIN®

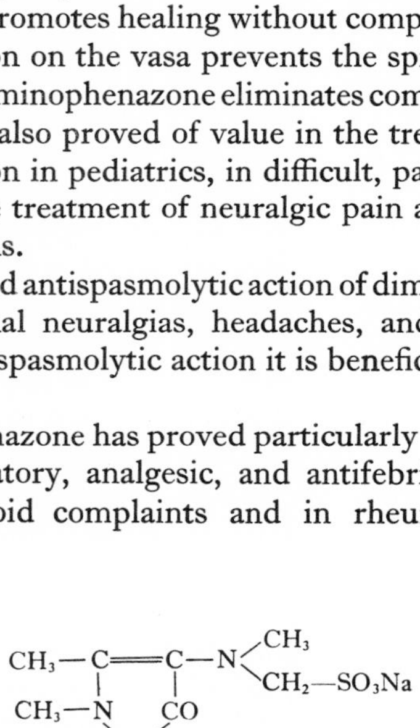

Sodium-1-phenyl-2,3-dimethyl-3-pyrazoline-5-one-4-methylamino methanesulfonate
(XXVIII)

1. *General*

Parenteral application of dimethylaminophenazone is rendered difficult because of its low solubility in water. As described in Section II,F,4, readily soluble salts of solvents had to be used in order to obtain solutions

358

in higher concentrations. All these processes, however, engender certain disadvantages and intravenous application in particular is difficult. By altering the molecular structure of dimethylaminophenazone, the attempt was made to obtain new compounds which are readily soluble in water and at the same time retain the valuable therapeutic properties.

The first success in this respect was achieved by reacting 4-amino-phenazone with formaldehyde and sodium hydrogen sulfite (*121*), whereby sodium-1-phenyl-2,3-dimethyl-3-pyrazoline-5-one-4-aminomethanesulfonate (XXIX) is formed. This substance is very readily soluble in water and makes intravenous injection possible. For some time it found application in the treatment of rheumatic diseases under the name of Melubrin®.

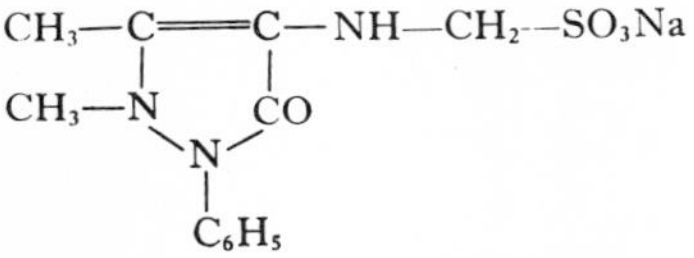

$$CH_3-C\!\!=\!\!\!=\!\!C-NH-CH_2-SO_3Na$$
$$CH_3-N \qquad CO$$
$$N$$
$$C_6H_5$$

(XXIX)

Compound XXVIII was prepared in order to get even closer to the constitution of dimethylaminophenazone. It actually brought about a considerable improvement of Melubrin and was introduced as a therapeutic drug under the trade name of Novalgin and the generic name metamizol.

2. Synthesis

Metamizol is made by heating 4-methylaminophenazone (XXX) in the presence of formaldehyde and sodium hydrogen sulfite (*122*) (Eq. 12).

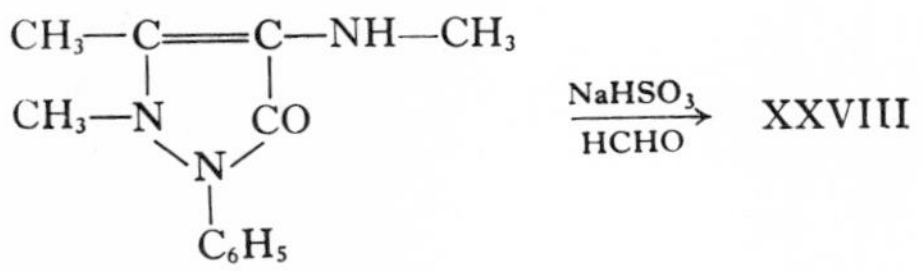

$$CH_3-C\!\!=\!\!\!=\!\!C-NH-CH_3$$
$$CH_3-N \qquad CO \qquad \xrightarrow[\text{HCHO}]{\text{NaHSO}_3} \quad XXVIII \qquad (12)$$
$$N$$
$$C_6H_5$$

(XXX)

Compound XXX is prepared in almost quantitative yield by the method of Decker (*123*). It consists in first obtaining 4-benzalaminophenazone by reacting 4-aminophenazone with benzaldehyde and then adding dimethyl sulfate to Schiff's base at 100° C. The quaternary compound obtained is split into 4-methylaminophenazone, methyl sulfuric acid, and benzaldehyde on the addition of hot water (Eq. 13).

As shown in Eq. (12), the sodium salt is obtained immediately. If, on the

359

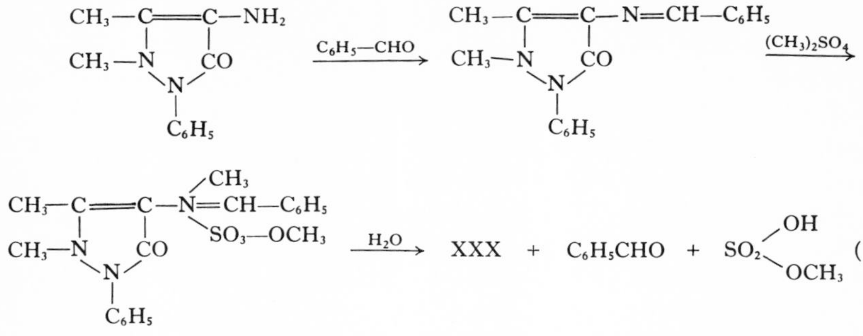

$$CH_3-C{=\!=\!=}C-NH_2$$
(with CH_3-N and CO bridged by $N-C_6H_5$ ring)

$\xrightarrow{C_6H_5-CHO}$

$$CH_3-C{=\!=\!=}C-N{=\!=}CH-C_6H_5$$
(with CH_3-N and CO bridged by $N-C_6H_5$ ring)

$\xrightarrow{(CH_3)_2SO_4}$

$$CH_3-C{=\!=\!=}C-N{=\!=}CH-C_6H_5 \quad \left(\begin{array}{c}CH_3\\SO_3-OCH_3\end{array}\right)$$
(with CH_3-N and CO bridged by $N-C_6H_5$ ring)

$\xrightarrow{H_2O}$ XXX + C_6H_5CHO + $SO_2\begin{array}{c}OH\\OCH_3\end{array}$ (13)

other hand, the alcoholic solution of methylaminophenazone is admixed with alcoholic formaldehyde, and the calculated amount of SO_2 is passed through, with cooling, the methanesulfonic acid liberated thereby will crystallize after a short while (*124*). Inorganic and organic bases form salts with this acid. The calcium and the quinine salt deserve special mention in this connection because they have proved of great value in many infectious diseases as the components of "Novalgin-Chinin."

3. *Properties*

Metamizol is readily soluble in water. Its aqueous solution is neutral and it can be applied intravenously in a concentration of 50% without causing damage to tissues. A number of color reactions are known which, according to Jung (*79*), are particularly suitable to distinguish it from Melubrin.

4. *Determination and Behavior in the Organism*

The quantitative test for metamizol is carried out iodometrically by titration using 0.1 N iodine solution in 1 N hydrochloric acid and using starch solution as the indicator. Végh et al. (*125*) worked out a photometric method of determination by which 0.5% Melubrin can be detected as impurities in metamizol. These authors also describe a chromatographic process which enables 0.5% phenazone and 4-aminophenazone to be detected as impurities.

The determination of metamizol in serum is carried out by the method which Lohse and Kallee (*92*) devised for the purpose of the rapid colorimetric determination of dimethylaminophenazone (Section II,F,5,*c*). Experiments conducted by Halberkann and Fretwurst (*126*) revealed that 22.6% metamizol is excreted in the human urine as 4-aminophenazone and 27.5% as 4-acetylaminophenazone, together with small amounts of "Rubazonsäure" (XXIV).

5. *Toxicity and Action*

According to experiments made by E. Lindner (of Hoechst A.G.), the lethal dose of a 10% solution of metamizol injected intravenously was 2 gm/kg in mice. Death was by paralysis of respiratory function, cramp was not noted. In comparison, dimethylaminophenazone, injected intravenously as a 1% solution, is lethal in a dose of 160 mg/kg. The animals are seized by violent cramps and die. Metamizol is thus only one-tenth as toxic as dimethylaminophenazone. In his investigations on the analgesic and antiin-flammatory action of metamizol, Lindner was able to prove similar relations to dimethylaminophenazone. It was about one-tenth as active but the duration of its effectiveness was longer in the antiphlogistic test. The spasmolytic properties of dimethylaminophenazone are also retained to a high degree by metamizol. Gordonoff and Bosshard (*127*) claim that their experiments with rabbits on the analgesic action of metamizol revealed that it is enhanced and prolonged by the addition of choline.

Because of its extraordinary low toxicity, its good general tolerability, and the absence of associated cramp, metamizol can be administered in relatively high doses. Because of this, an increase in its therapeutic action over that of dimethylaminophenazone is achieved, and above all, there is an improvement in its analgesic and spasmolytic effect.

6. *Combination Preparations*

This enhanced action is of special value in the therapy of colic, both in human and veterinary medicine, where metamizol can to a great extent replace opiates in the treatment of severe spasms of pain. Administered by mixed injection, a small addition of morphine and papaverine is highly effective in cases of very severe pain or acute spastic conditions in the abdomen.

Based on this knowledge, combination preparations have been developed which contain small quantities of highly effective spasmolytics which serve to support the action of metamizol. Among these are, for example, the following: Avafortan®, consisting of metamizol and α-[*n*-(β-diethylamino-ethyl)]-aminophenylacetic acid isoamylester (XXXI). Baralgin®, consisting

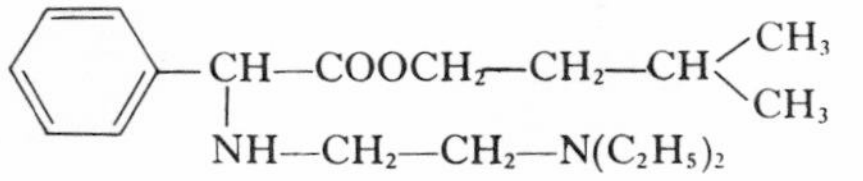

(XXXI)

of Novalgin, *p*-β-piperidinoethoxy-2'-carbmethoxybenzophenone/hydro-chloride (XXXII) and diphenyl-2-(β-piperidinoethyl)acetamidebromo-ethylate (XXXIII). Buscopan compositum®, consisting of metamizol and

361

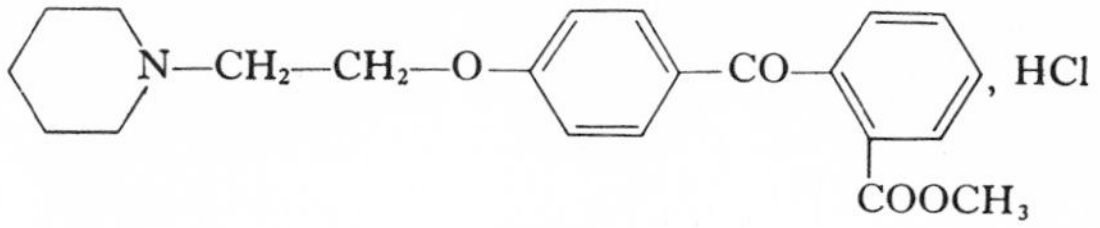

(XXXII)

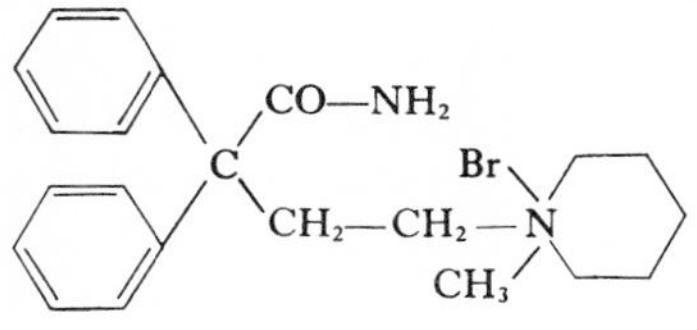

(XXXIII)

hyoscin-*N*-butylbromide (XXXIV). Helophlegan®, consisting of metamizol and hyoscyomine (XXXV). Pelerol®, consisting of metamizol, piperylone, and "Tropenzilium" (see Section II,K).

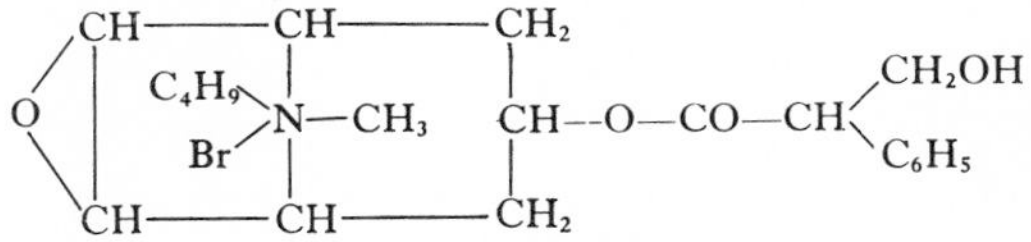

(XXXIV)

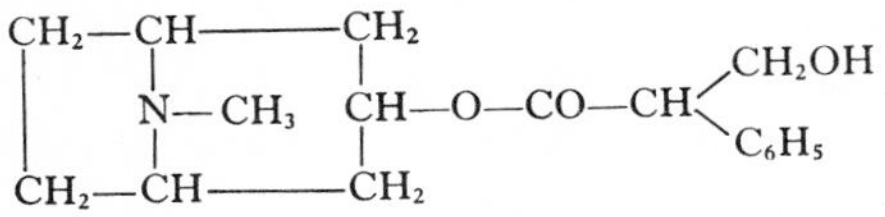

(XXXV)

The analgesic action of metamizol is increased if branched alkyl radicals instead of the methyl group are introduced at the nitrogen atom in the 4-position (*128*). For this reason a combination of sodium-1-phenyl-2,3-dimethyl-3-pyrazoline-5-one-4-isobutylaminomethanesulfonate (XXXVI)

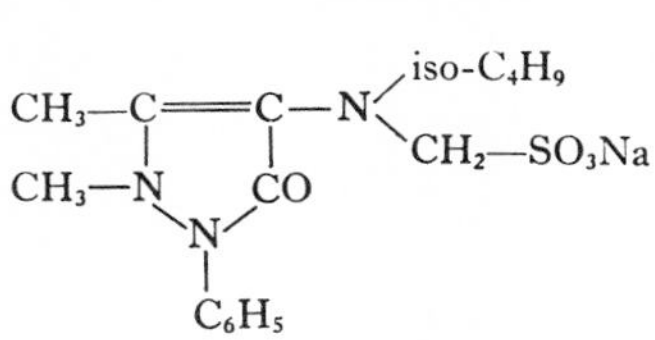

(XXXVI)

and compounds XXXII and XXXIII were introduced as a veterinary medicament under the name of Melufin®.

362

Gardan® is a combination preparation containing Pyramidon and Novalgin in equimolar quantities which has proved to be very useful in the treatment of influenza. It is more effective than the individual components. The reason for this is probably to be found in the fact that the body cells can absorb a larger amount of the active ingredients of the combination in a certain period than of twice the amount of either.

According to experiments of Laubender and Schlarb (*129*) on isolated cross-striated muscles of *Rana temporaria*, metamizol increases the effectiveness of salicylamide by approximately the power of ten in contractions resulting from potassium chloride, acetylcholine, nicotine, or sodium rhodanide. These authors are of the opinion that the combination of the two changes probably enables the therapeutic concentrations of salicylamide to be built up more rapidly at the required places than would be the case with salicylamide alone.

7. *Clinical Significance*

Like demethylaminophenazone, metamizol is a good antipyretic, analgesic, spasmolytic, and antirheumatic. By being able to inject it intravenously in large dosages without having to fear undesirable side reactions, particularly the danger of cramp, it is possible to attain a powerful analgesic effect so that even those conditions of pain can be treated which would otherwise require the administration of preparations containing opiates.

In less acute complaints parenteral application can be dispensed with and oral or rectal administration will achieve the desired results.

Apart from its analgesic action it is primarily its marked spasmolytic property which has led to the application on a large scale of metamizol in renal and biliary colics.

Conditions arising from angina pectoris can often be improved rapidly by intravenous administration of metamizol. This treatment is also responsible for the prevention of such attacks.

Metamizol has been employed successfuly in the control of birth pains. Oral, as well as intravenous or intramuscular administration of metamizol will considerably reduce dilation and expulsion pain. Favorable results have also been achieved in the treatment of spastic menstruation complaints.

The action of metamizol medication in neuralgic pain is rapid. Metamizol is of special value in the treatment of traumatic pain. In postoperative treatment the use of opiates is frequently obviated. Pain arising from burns, fractures, tonsilectomies, as well as from dental and other operations is rapidly alleviated.

The powerful analgesic action of metamizol is also revealed by its effect

363

on pain in inflammatory processes. Its combined analgesic and antiphlogistic action does not only relieve the symptoms but it also has a curative effect.

In rheumatic polyarthritis, rheumatic fever, and chronic rheumatism of the joints, the intravenous injection of metamizol rapidly alleviates pain and reduces swelling and temperature. Because of its excellent tolerability, metamizol may be used in therapy with massive doses without concern over troublesome side reactions.

Metamizol has not only proved of great value in human medicine but also in veterinary practice. Because of its analgesic and antispasmodic properties it is used to a great extent in veterinary medicine as an effective remedy for colic. In acute overdistension of the stomach the animal can be calmed down by administering metamizol and rupture is avoided if the stomach is emptied at the same time by gastric suction. Because of its antispasmodic action on the involuntary muscles it is practically the ideal medium for use in blockages of the pharynx, because the foreign body which is wedged in the throat will then either slide down of its own accord or may be pushed down by means of an esophageal probe.

H. 1-PHENYL-2,3-DIMETHYL-4-ISOPROPYLAMINO-3-PYRAZOLINE-5-ONE

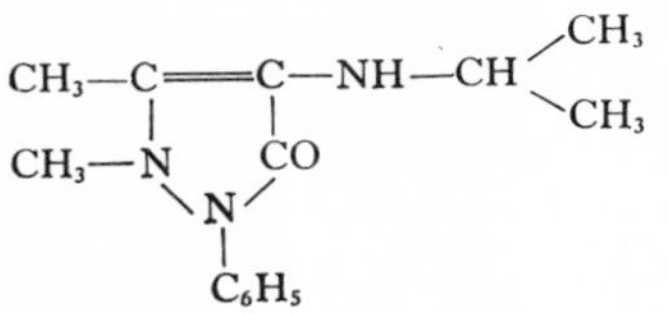

$$CH_3-C=C-NH-CH\begin{array}{c}CH_3\\CH_3\end{array}$$
$$CH_3-N\quad CO$$
$$N$$
$$C_6H_5$$

(XXXVII)

1. Synthesis

According to Skita (*130*), 4-isopropylaminophenazone (XXXVII) is formed by hydrogenating 4-aminophenazone in acetone solution using palladium as the catalyst. It is, together with phenylbutazone (Phebuzine®), a component of the combination preparation Tomanol®.

2. Pharmacological Properties

Schoetensack *et al.* (*131*) subjected XXXVII to a very searching pharmacological examination. They found that in addition to equal antipyretic, analgesic, and antiphlogistic properties, it exhibits a soothing effect on the central nervous system which is in contrast to dimethylaminophenazone and phenylbutazone. If applied in combination with XXXVII, the stimulating or convulsive effect of the two latter drugs is either restricted or even eliminated. Administered intravenously, XXXVII has a hypotensive action while dimethylaminophenazone and phenylbutazone have the opposite effect. The opposing actions of the two components in the combination preparation Tomanol therefore cancel out to a large extent.

3. *Distribution in the Organism and Excretion*

Richarz *et al.* (*132*) have reported on the distribution of XXXVII in the organism and its excretion. Experiments on rats showed that Isopyrin is rapidly distributed evenly throughout the organism after oral and parenteral administration. After intramuscular and intravenous injection of 150 mg/kg it could be detected in the blood after 10 hours.

Determination in the blood and organs was carried out by a method similar to that given by Brodie and Axelrod (*133*) for dimethylaminophenazone. Its spectrophotometrical determination in the blood resulted in the finding of 75% of the 4-aminophenazone and 30% of the 4-acetylaminophenazone present which are included in the total concentration of both substances in the serum. It is, however, so minute that the XXXVII concentration measured is at most too high by 0.3 mg%.

It was noted that not much more than 3% of the excretion products of XXXVII could be identified in rats. About 1.5% are excreted unchanged and 1.9% on average in the form of 4-aminophenazone and 4-acetylamino-phenazone. After acidifying the urine, a small quantity of "Rubazonsäure" (XXIV) could be identified in the urine.

I. NICOPYRON®

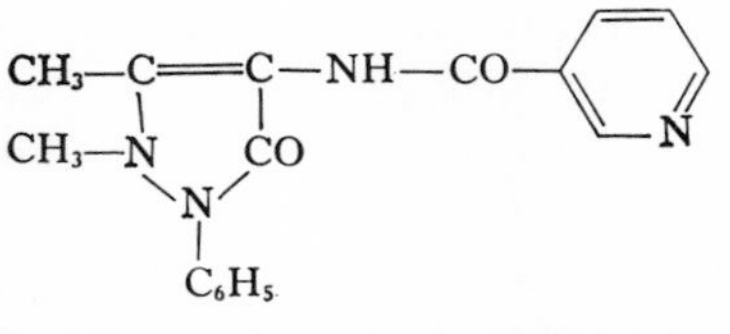

CH₃—C═══C—NH—CO—[pyridine ring]—N
CH₃—N   CO
      N
      C₆H₅

1-Phenyl-2,3-dimethyl-4-(pyridine-3'-carboxylic acidamino)-3-pyrazoline-5-one
(Nicotinic acidamidophenazone)

(XXXVIII)

More recently, a derivative of 4-aminophenazone has been put on the market which is substituted in the 4-position by the nicotinic acid radical. It is Nicopyron (XXXVIII).

1. *Synthesis and Properties*

Nicopyron is made by reacting nicotinic acid halides with 4-amino-phenazone (*135*). According to Stoltenberg (*135*), Nicopyron is obtained in a yield of 85–95% if the sodium salt of nicotinic acid is reacted in benzene with thionyl chloride and the acid chloride formed is reacted in benzene with 4-aminophenazone without cooling or using an acid-binding medium. After distilling off the solvent, the residue is dissolved in water and the reaction product is precipitated with caustic soda solution. Nicopyron is sparingly soluble in water. It can be determined spectrophotometrically (136). In 0.1 N hydrochloric acid, it possesses a maximum at 250.5 mμ and a minimum as 233–234 mμ in the ultraviolet.

2. Toxicity and Pharmacological Properties

The acute toxicity of Nicopyron in mice compared to phenazone is shown in the Table V (137). Thus Nicopyron is less toxic in mice than phenazone.

TABLE V

ACUTE TOXICITY OF NICOPYRON IN MICE AS COMPARED TO PHENAZONE (IN GM/KG)

	LD_{50} intraperitoneal	LD_{100} intraperitoneal	LD_{100} subcutaneous
Nicopyron	1.28	1.8	—
Phenazone	—	1.25	1.0–1.2

Reincke (138) compares the toxicity of Nicopyron and phenazone by using the allyl alcohol test according to Eger (139). Nicotinic acid amide inhibits the damaging effect of allyl alcohol on the liver. Since Nicopyron constitutes a compound of nicotinic acid amide and phenazone, Reincke employed Eger's test for his comparative study. This revealed that phenazone does not inhibit the deleterious effect on the liver while Nicopyron brings about an inhibitive effect equal to that of nicotinic acid amide. This toxicity coincides with that of other pyrazolone derivatives in that it produces clonic cramp which occurs a few hours after injection.

The analgesic effect of Nicopyron was determined according to a method by Fleisch and Dolivo (140). It proved to be more powerful than phenazone, and, contrary to phenazone, its analgesic effect was not terminated after 180 minutes had elapsed (137).

3. Fate in the Organism

Since Nicopyron is split into nicotinic acid and 4-aminophenazone by acid hydrolysis, Schmitt and Harwerth (141)—after carrying out the required hydrolysis of the serum sample and adjusting to pH 5.0 by the use of

VII. PYRAZOLE DERIVATIVES

acetate buffer solution—carried out the 4-aminophenazone determination in accordance with Emerson's method, as described in Section II,E,2. On administering a single oral dose of 750 mg Nicopyron, the maximum blood levels were already reached after the first hour and at the latest after the second hour. This indicates that the medicament is absorbed rapidly by the gastrointestinal tract. After 6–7 hours, a drop in the Nicopyron content of the serum becomes more or less pronounced. The tests conducted after 24 hours revealed that individual differences exist with regard to speed of decomposition and excretion. By administering 2 dragees 3 times a day (= a daily dose of 1500 mg), a relatively constant Nicopyron content could be maintained in the blood over longer periods. The maximum level in the blood was not reached until 8 hours after insertion of a suppository of 400 mg Nicopyron. Absorption is thus distinctly retarded as compared to other modes of application.

4. Clinical Significance

Hartert (*142*) reports that he gave treatment in cases of ulcus cruris, varicosclerosation, thromboses of the superficial veins of the leg, and chronically inflamed adnexal tumors by administering Nicopyron both orally and rectally, and that good results were achieved on account of its antiphlogistic, analgesic and mildly spasmolytic effect. In conditions of severe inflammation treatment was initiated by intramuscular injection of phenylbutazone.

Ballús y Roca (*143*) also found that Nicopyron is an effective and well tolerated analgesic and antirheumatic of low toxicity. It is, however, not specific for severe cases of polyarthritis and arthrosis deformans. Tests carried out by Zwerenz (*144*) on patients suffering from chronic poly-arthritis, arthroses, and spondyl arthroses showed that Nicopyron is well tolerated by nearly all patients and that it exhibited a surprisingly good analgesic and slightly sedative action. Side effects due to toxicity were not found in a single case.

5. Combination with Prednisone

As in the case of the pyrazole derivatives, a mixture of Nicopyron and prednisone was also prepared. It was marketed under the name of Nico-pred®. According to Schmidt (*145*) it is an excellent antirheumatic of medium to good tolerability and can be used in nearly all rheumatic diseases. Even degenerative processes of longer standing were improved with con-tinuous treatment. Schmidt and Pape (*146*) have reported on the treatment with Nicopyron and Nicopred of attendant rheumatic symptoms encountered in 918 tuberculous patients. Both preparations proved to be not only very effective against rheumatism but above all exhibited great tolerability.

6. *Nicopyron for Injection*

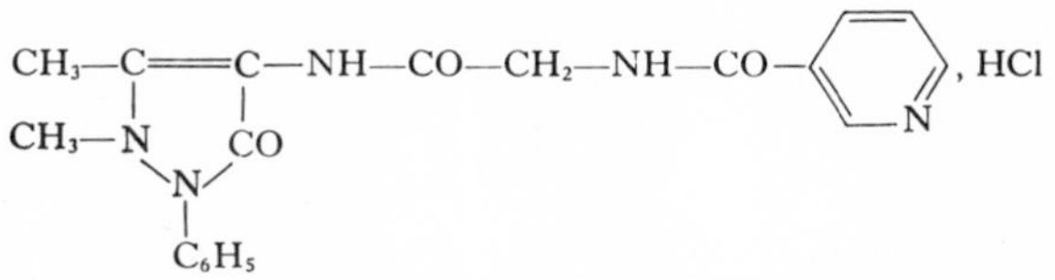

$$CH_3-C=\!=\!C-NH-CO-CH_2-NH-CO-\bigcirc\!N,\ HCl$$

1-Phenyl-2,3-dimethyl-4-(N-nicotinoylaminoacetyl- amino)-3-pyrazoline-5-one-hydrochloride

(XXXIX)

Since Nicopyron is very sparingly soluble in water and is not suitable for parenteral application, derivatives have been sought which are readily water soluble and at the same time possess its excellent therapeutic properties. Compound XXXIX is such a preparation.

a. Pharmacology. According to Eder *et al.* (*147*), compound XXXIX is only one tenth as toxic as phenylbutazone and dimethylaminophenazone (Table VI). Its analgesic action determined by the hot-plate method is less

TABLE VI

LD_{50} OF XXXIX AFTER SUBCUTANEOUS APPLICATION IN MICE AS COMPARED TO PHENYLBUTAZONE AND DIMETHYL-AMINOPHENAZONE IN (MG/KG)

XXXIX	Phenylbutazone	Dimethylaminophenazone
3750	245	263

than that of phenylbutazone and dimethylaminophenazone while it is found to be equal when determined by electrostimulus.

In protein edema, 400 mg/kg were nearly as effective as 200 mg/kg dimethylaminophenazone and considerably more so than 200 mg/kg phenylbutazone, while in formalin edema the antiphlogistic effect of the controls is not attained on administering 400 mg/kg. In chronic inflammations caused by subcutaneous implantation of small saturated cotton wool balls in rats, 5 mg/kg phenylbutazone and 20 mg/kg, XXXIX had approximately the same effect, the toxicity being one tenth that of XXXIX.

Antipyretic tests showed that 400 mg/kg XXXIX, 50 mg/kg phenylbutazone, and 100 mg/kg dimethylaminophenazone had practically the same effect.

b. Fate in the organism. To determine the content of XXXIX in the blood, Schmitt and Harwerth (*141*) administered 750 mg intramuscularly as a single daily dose on three consecutive days; 1–2 hours after the injection the blood levels reached a maximum but soon decreased rapidly. The preparation could not be detected in measurable quantities in the serum 24 hours after the injection. It is probably decomposed and excreted rapidly because of its great solubility in water.

c. Clinical significance. Dziuba (*148*) treated 89 patients suffering from rheumatic diseases and degenerative affections of the joints, with XXXIX and, because of its good analgesic ,antiphlogistic, and antipyretic action, it was reported to be very successful in most cases.

J. PIPERYLON®

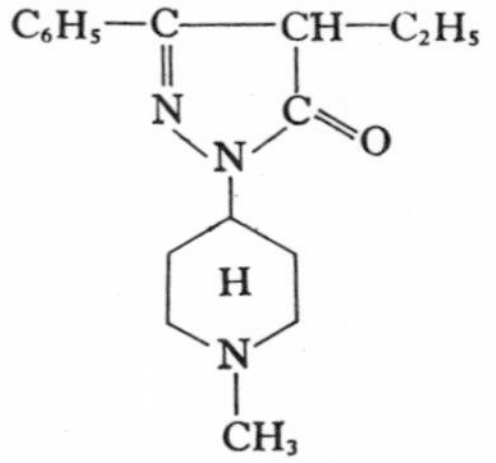

1-[*n*-Methylpiperidyl-(4')]-3-phenyl-4-ethyl-2-pyrazoline-5-one

(XL)

All therapeutics discussed so far possess a phenyl group in the 1-position of the pyrazole ring. Divergent from this, new compounds have been found recently which are not derived from phenylhydrazine but from the *n*-alkyl-piperidylhydrazines. Piperylon (XL) is a representative of this class. It is obtained by the condensation of 1-methyl-piperidylhydrazine-(4) with α-ethylbenzoylacetic acid ester (*149*) and is a mild spasmoanalgesic having analgesic properties of medium strength and has a pronounced selective spasmolytic effect on the bladder.

Together with "Tropenzilium" (6-methoxytropinebenzylic acid ester–bromoethylate) and metamizol, Piperylon is a constituent of the combination preparation Pelerol® (see Section II,G,6), which finds application in the treatment of spasms and colics in the gastrointestinal tract and the urinary passages, and also as parturifacient in normal and delayed birth.

K. OBSERVATIONS ON THE CONSTITUTION AND ACTION OF THE PYRAZOLINE-5-ONE DERIVATIVES

The relation between chemical constitution and pharmacological action is of extreme importance to the chemist engaged in the synthesis of

369

medicaments. The synthesist must not proceed aimlessly and leave to chance the possibility as to whether a compound he has made possesses the desired action, but he must formulate a hypothesis by which success may be expected in all probability. And yet, in view of the vast number of medicaments at our disposal, real success still depends on chance because it is very difficult indeed to obtain substances of more suitable properties and increased effectiveness.

If the pyrazolone derivatives are scrutizinized from this aspect, it may be stated to begin with that the carbonyl group is absolutely necessary for their pharmacological effectiveness as analgesics. It may be situated in the 5-position and also in the 3-position. However, the 3-pyrazolones have a somewhat weaker effect, are more difficult to obtain, and have not been subjected to extended clinical trials, so that they have never attained any practical significance.

It is also of importance that both nitrogen atoms in the ring are substituted, Piperlyon (XL) being the only exception to this among the many compounds which are manufactured. The introduction of a methyl group in the 2 position has been of the greatest value and methylation of the nitrogen atom has, moreover, always played an important part in the synthesis of therapeutics.

Nearly all drugs of the pyrazolone series possess a phenyl group in the 1-position. It is, however, not absolutely necessary for pharmacological effectiveness. The nitrogen atoms in the ring, are, for instance, substituted by methyl in the so-called isopyrazoles while the phenyl group is in the 3-position without any appreciable reduction in effectiveness taking place. If the phenyl group in the 1-position in dimethylaminophenazone is substituted by cyclohexyl or benzyl, very effective compounds are obtained. The cyclohexyl derivative has a more powerful antipyretic and antiphlogistic action, whereas the benzyl derivative has a stronger analgesic effect than dimethylaminophenazone. Substitution in the 4-position has an appreciable influence on the effectiveness. Phenazone does not possess a substituent in the 4-position. It was not until other groups were introduced at this point that better and more effective preparations were obtained. The dimethylamino group forms the optimum possibility, perhaps because chance would have it that this preparation, viz., dimethylaminophenazone, should possess such an extensive broad spectrum of action. In this case also the methyl groups substituted at the nitrogen atoms have the most favorable effect, whereas the introduction of other groupings did not result in compounds of greater pharmacological effectiveness.

Branched alkyl groups in the 4-position bring about increased effectiveness as compared to the parent substance. Thus isopropylphenazone is particularly effective, and compound XXXVI—in which isobutyl replaces the methyl group in metamizol—is a more powerful analgesic than metamizol. Also isopyrin, 4-isopropylaminophenazone, must be mentioned in this connection. By introducing an isopropyl group no increase in effectiveness is attained but this preparation possesses valuable properties which are lacking in the other 4-amino derivatives. Finally, it must be emphasized that in all effective preparations of the pyrazolone series the 3-position is also substituted. In this case also it is the methyl group which is encountered almost without exception. Higher and branched alkyls also produce effective compounds, but such preparations have not been introduced because of the difficulties engendered in large-scale preparation.

III. 3,5-Pyrazolidinedione Derivatives

A. BUTAZOLIDIN®

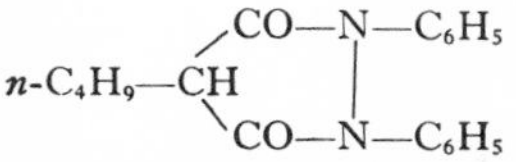

$$n\text{-}C_4H_9\text{—}CH \overset{\displaystyle /CO\text{—}N\text{—}C_6H_5}{\underset{\displaystyle \backslash CO\text{—}N\text{—}C_6H_5}{|}}$$

1,2-Diphenyl-4-n-butyl-3,5-pyrazolidinedione

(XLI)

Since the appearance of metamizol on the pharmaceutical market, work on the syntheses of pyrazolone derivatives could not register any successes for many years. Then, towards the end of the forties, Geigy of Switzerland succeeded in producing a new therapeutic compound which was destined to attain exceptional significance for the treatment of rheumatic diseases. It is Butazolidin (XLI). The generic name phenylbutazone has been generally accepted for it, and this is the description that will be used in this section.

1. *Synthesis*

Among the many processes for the manufacture of phenylbutazone (*150*) only a few will be selected. Its first synthesis (Eq. 14) was carried out by heating n-butylmalonic acid ethylester with hydrazobenzene and sodium alcoholate (*151*).

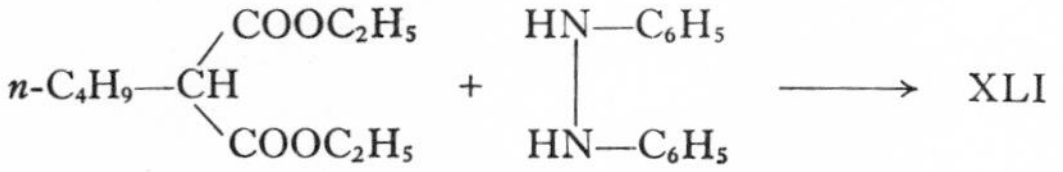

$$n\text{-}C_4H_9\text{—}CH \overset{\displaystyle /COOC_2H_5}{\underset{\displaystyle \backslash COOC_2H_5}{}} \quad + \quad \overset{\displaystyle HN\text{—}C_6H_5}{\underset{\displaystyle HN\text{—}C_6H_5}{|}} \quad \longrightarrow \quad XLI \qquad (14)$$

Another method (Eq. 15), which obviates the preparation of butylmalonic acid ester, consists in first reacting malonic acid diethylester with hydrazobenzene to obtain 1,2-diphenyl-3,5-pyrazolidinedione (XLII).

371

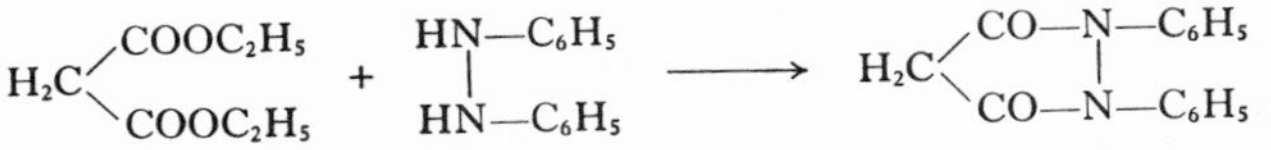

$$H_2C \overset{COOC_2H_5}{\underset{COOC_2H_5}{\Big\langle}} \;+\; \overset{HN-C_6H_5}{\underset{HN-C_6H_5}{\Big|}} \;\longrightarrow\; H_2C \overset{CO-N-C_6H_5}{\underset{CO-N-C_6H_5}{\Big\langle}} \qquad (15)$$

$$(XLII)$$

Similar to technical pyrazolone (V), the CH_2 group of compound XLII reacts with aldehydes to form alkylide derivatives, water being given off. If this condensation is carried out in conjunction with catalytic hydrogenation, the desired alkyl compound can be obtained in one processing operation. Based on this method, phenylbutazone is formed if XLII is subjected to catalytic hydrogenation in the presence of crotonic aldehyde (Eq. 16); an intermediate product, the crotylidene compound, is formed (*152*).

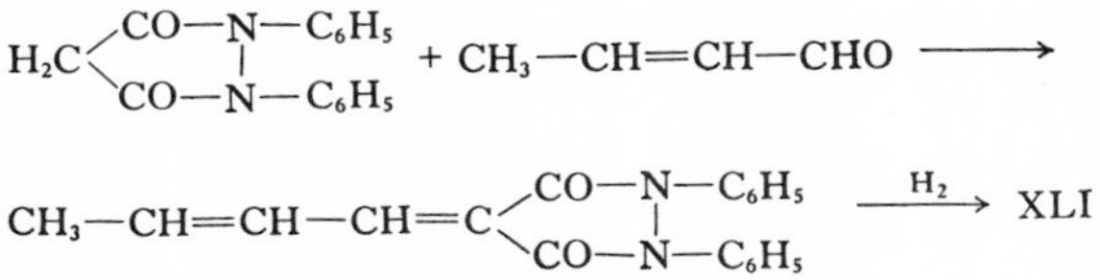

$$H_2C \overset{CO-N-C_6H_5}{\underset{CO-N-C_6H_5}{\Big\langle}} \;+\; CH_3-CH{=}CH-CHO \;\longrightarrow$$

$$CH_3-CH{=}CH-CH{=}C \overset{CO-N-C_6H_5}{\underset{CO-N-C_6H_5}{\Big\langle}} \quad\overset{H_2}{\longrightarrow}\quad XLI \qquad (16)$$

The Byk Gulden-Lomberg G.m.b.H. discovered an interesting method for the preparation of phenylbutazone (*153*). Carboxylic acid-*n,n'*-diphenylhydrazides may be reacted with carbonic acid diethylester in the presence of an alkaline condensation medium such as sodium amide to 1,2-diphenyl-3,5-pyrazolidinedione derivatives which are substituted in the 4-position. If the reaction is carried out with *n*-capronic acid diphenylhydrazide, phenylbutazone is obtained (Eq. 17).

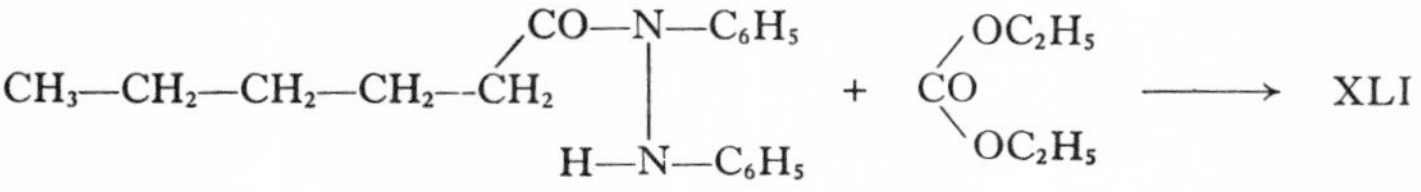

$$CH_3-CH_2-CH_2-CH_2-CH_2 \overset{CO-N-C_6H_5}{\underset{H-N-C_6H_5}{\Big|}} \;+\; CO \overset{OC_2H_5}{\underset{OC_2H_5}{\Big\langle}} \;\longrightarrow\; XLI \qquad (17)$$

2. *Properties*

By introducing the second carbonyl group into the pyrazole nucleus, phenylbutazone becomes distinctly acidic in character and will form water soluble salts with bases. As such it exists as a negatively charged enolic ion which may be considered as an intermediate of the three formulas which are depicted herewith.

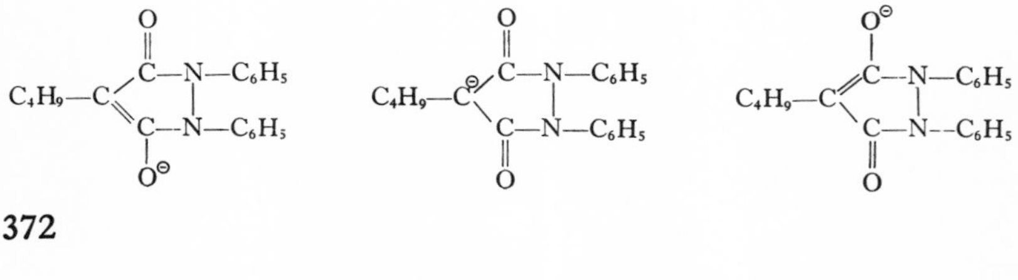

$$C_4H_9-C \overset{\overset{O}{\|}}{\underset{\underset{O^\ominus}{\|}}{\underset{C-N-C_6H_5}{\Big\langle}}} \qquad C_4H_9-C \overset{\overset{O}{\|}}{\underset{\underset{O}{\|}}{\overset{\ominus}{\Big\langle}}} \overset{C-N-C_6H_5}{\underset{C-N-C_6H_5}{}} \qquad C_4H_9-C \overset{\overset{O^\ominus}{|}}{\underset{\underset{O}{\|}}{\Big\langle}} \overset{C-N-C_6H_5}{\underset{C-N-C_6H_5}{}} \qquad (18)$$

372

This property is evinced by the spectroscopic behavior of phenylbutazone. In weakly acid methane solution, its dicarbonyl form shows a maximum at 240 mμ in the ultraviolet, and as a result of additional conjugation changes to 264 mμ on the addition of alkaline solutions. The infrared spectrum indicates that phenylbutazone must be present in its dicarbonyl form in the absence of base.

As already mentioned in Section II,F,4,*b*, aqueous solutions of phenyl-butazone-sodium act as solvents for dimethylaminophenazone, a property which is made use of in the combination preparation Irgapyrin which contains 15% each of Butazolidin-sodium and dimethylaminophenazone in aqueous solution.

3. *Identification and Assay*

Breugelmans and Braun (*154*) described methods which serve to identify phenylbutazone. It is based on a color reaction by heating with concentrated sulfuric acid and potassium nitrate. For the quantitative determination, phenylbutazone can be dissolved in 94–96% ethanol or acetone and titrated with 0.1 N caustic soda solution (*154*). The accuracy of this test is 99.5%. It can be determined spectrometrically in 0.1 N caustic soda solution on account of its maximum at 264 mμ.

Breugelmans and Braun have given detailed methods by which to determine phenylbutazone in combination preparations, for instance in mixtures with acetylsalicylic acid, phenacetine, phenazone, dimethylaminophen-azone, metimazole, caffein, phenylcinchoninic acid, and cycloheptenyl-ethylbarbituric acid.

Deffner and Deffner (*155*) reported on how to separate and determine phenylbutazone quantitatively in pharmaceutical preparations. By their method, phenylbutazone solution is mixed with FeCl$_3$ and α,α'-dipyridyl solution, and the colorimetric determination carried out at 520 mμ. In the presence of other substances which are oxidized by FeCl$_3$, it is recommended that paper chromatographic separation be employed. This paper chromato-gram can be developed by FeCl$_3$, α,α-dipyridyl, or Ehrlich's reagent.

4. *Determination in Body Fluids and Tissues*

The methods of determining phenylbutazone described so far, cannot be applied as they stand to tracing it and its decomposition products in the living organism. Pulver (*156*) was the first to work out a method which permits reasonably accurate quantitative tests to be carried out for phenyl-butazone in body fluids. It is based on the saponification of phenylbutazone with *p*-toluenesulfonic acid; hydrazobenzene is formed first, which is then converted to benzidine under the action of the acid (Eq. 19).

$$C_4H_9-CH\underset{CO-N-C_6H_5}{\overset{CO-N-C_6H_5}{\Big\langle}} \longrightarrow \underset{HN-C_6H_5}{\overset{HN-C_6H_5}{\Big|}} \longrightarrow H_2N-\text{⟨benzene⟩}-\text{⟨benzene⟩}-NH_2$$

(19)

The benzidine is diazotized, joined to *n,n*-dimethyl-α-naphthylamine, and the resulting dye determined colorimetrically. This method is not very specific, its margin of error is $\pm 15\%$.

The method by Burns *et al.* (*157*) is more accurate. For this purpose, phenylbutazone is extracted from the plasma by using heptane, is dissolved in caustic soda solution and is determined photometrically at 264 mμ in the ultraviolet. This method is very precise but possesses the disadvantage that the two metabolites of phenylbutazone are included in the amounts found. This disadvantage is avoided in the spectrophotometric method of Herrmann (*158*) by which phenylbutazone and its metabolite I (XLIII) can be determined side by side. This method is based on the fact that both compounds can be determined quantitatively together. In a second process, the metabolite is extracted selectively from the ethylene chloride solution by a phosphate buffer of pH 8, and the phenylbutazone which remains can then be measured.

The method of Burns *et al.* was developed by Fuchs (*159*) for use on the micro scale, and a specification was worked out for a margin of error of $\pm 3\%$, using 0.2 ml serum.

5. *Fate in the Organism*

A particularly large number of papers have been published on the fate of phenylbutazone in the organism. Because of the great importance of this drug for the treatment of rheumatic diseases requiring extensive medication, many authors have studied its absorption, distribution, transformation, and excretion.

a. Absorption. After oral administration, phenylbutazone is absorbed rapidly, probably in the small intestine because of the favorable pH that exists in this organ. It is therefore advisable to cover the dragees with a coating which is soluble in the small intestine, in order to protect the mucous membrane of the stomach. Concentration in the blood already reaches a maximum after only 2 hours (*157*). In oral administration in low dosage (800 mg phenylbutazone on the first day and 200 mg on the following days) maximum concentration in the blood is reached after 3 days and a constant level can be maintained in the blood over long periods (*160*).

Brodie *et al.* (*161*) assume that absorption of phenylbutazone is retarded after intramuscular administration because of localization at the place of injection. The good therapeutic effects, however, which are attained by intramuscular injection, disprove this assumption. In high oral or intra-muscular application, concentration in the blood reaches a limit which is not exceeded. The explanation is that only part of the phenylbutazone is bound to the plasma protein when high doses are given while the rest is broken down and excreted more rapidly (161).

Rectal absorption is less, but nevertheless so high that the lowest thera-peutically effective limit of 5 mg% in the blood is reached and exceeded (162). Administered subcutaneously, phenylbutazone is absorbed only very slowly from aqueous solutions and ointments.

b. Distribution. In order to be able to judge the state in which phenyl-butazone is present in the organism, its solubilities at various pH values are of importance and are given in Table VII (163). The rapid increase in

TABLE VII

Solubility of Phenylbutazone at Various pH
Values (in mg%)

Solvent	pH	Solubility
Phosphate buffer $M/15$	7.0	188
Phosphate buffer $M/15$	6.0	34.5
Acetoacetate buffer $M/10$	4.7	3.6
Acetoacetate buffer $M/10$	4.1	2.3
Acetoacetate buffer $M/10$	3.5	1.9
Distilled water		1.5

solubility at pH values of 6.0 and higher indicates that the enolic form is already formed in neutral to weakly acid reaction and that phenylbutazone is present in this form at the pH value of the blood.

The results obtained regarding its distribution in the organism are ex-plained by the different solubilities of phenylbutazone at varying pH values; the drug is concentrated in the aqueous phase while the concentrations found in the body fat and organs rich in lipoids are minute. According to investigations by Burns *et al.* (157), the larger portion of the phenylbutazone administered is bound to the plasma protein, and the other tissues as well as the organs contain far lower concentrations. The plasma level does not, however, stand in any relation to the dosage. On administering 1600 mg per day of drug it is only slightly higher than in dosages of 800 mg per day, and it also varies considerably from individual to individual. Pulver *et al.* (164) assume that phenylbutazone is loosely bound to the hydrate envelope of the proteins. As a result of diffusion and rediffusion experiments, Wunderly

375

(165) arrived at the same conclusion and found that the protein binding of phenylbutazone was of an extremely loose nature which seemed to indicate that adsorption in the hydrate envelope of the proteins is feasible. Of the plasma proteins, chiefly the albumins combine with phenylbutazone; Wunderly was able to demonstrate that phenylbutazone bonding power is less if the albumin fraction in the blood is lowered because of illness. The portion of the drug bound to the plasma protein is very high and amounts to between 94 and 99% (164). All other organs which were examined had a considerably lower phenylbutazone content. In Table VIII are shown the values which Pulver et al. (164) obtained 6 hours after intravenous injection in rats (75 mg/kg) and oral application in rabbits (200 mg/kg).

TABLE VIII

DISTRIBUTION OF PHENYLBUTAZONE IN RABBITS AND RATS
(IN MG%)

Organ	Rabbit			Rat mean value of 4 animals
	1	2	3	
Plasma	35	40	29	11.8
Liver	8.3	9.1	5.6	8.3
Kidney	14.1	15.3	19.7	5.4
Heart	8.8	9.3	8.7	2.7
Melt	3.0	5.6	4.8	2.3
Muscles	2.2	3.8	2.7	0.9
Spinal cord	2.3	1.7	4.4	1.3
Brain	1.5	1.5	0.7	2.3
Fat	2.6	1.9	1.9	—

On the other hand, Heise and Kimbel (166) found a maximum concentration of phenylbutazone in the brain of albino rats after a single increased dose. This concentration was switched to the heart muscle after a further increase. The authors believe that the bonding power of plasma protein does not suffice in high doses and that the excess is therefore absorbed by other organs. Wilhelmi and Pulver (167) were able to prove that the concentration found in the inflamed tissue was 2–4 times as high as in the normal tissue, which indicates that phenylbutazone has a special affinity for tissue altered by inflammatory processes.

Harwerth and Wöhler (168) conducted experiments on the distribution of phenylbutazone in guinea pigs using a substance which in the C-1 position of the side chain was marked by C^{14}, a pure β-emitter. After 3 hours, the content was found to be highest in the kidneys, liver, suprarenal gland, lungs, and heart muscle. But also the pancreas and stomach contained relatively high concentrations of phenylbutazone. The values obtained after 24 hours were reduced throughout. In the plasma proteins a maximum of activity was detected in the albumin fraction. Of note in these findings was the high content of phenylbutazone in the bile which reached a maximum value of 110 mg% in one animal. This would tend to indicate—as reasoned by the authors—that excretion of phenylbutazone takes place via liver and bile into the intestine. But since it is known also that only small amounts of phenylbutazone are found in the stool, the possibility of reabsorption from the intestine should also be considered. In contrast to the high concentrations found in the blood, other body fluids such as saliva and gastric juices contain only small amounts of phenylbutazone. Also fluid analyses conducted on humans as well as animals did not bring forth positive results: the drug enters the fetal circulation only in minute quantities and only traces are found in the milk of stilling mothers (*169*).

c. Decomposition and excretion. Only traces of the phenylbutazone administered are excreted unchanged in the urine of man (*157*), which indicates that it is decomposed almost completely in the human organism. Its decomposition varies considerably from individual to individual and is found to lie between 10% and 35% daily, the mean being about 20%. It takes place far more rapidly in animals than in man. The biological half-life period of phenylbutazone is as follows: man, 72 hours; dog and rat, 6 hours; guinea pig, 5 hours; rabbit, 3 hours.

von Rechenberg (*170*) does not deem it to be impossible that an enzyme stage develops a varying intensity in the phenylbutazone decomposition which differs according to the species as well as the individual, and that the fluctuations observed in blood levels and decomposition can thus be explained.

Burns *et al.* (*171*) were able to isolate two metabolites in the human urine. Metabolite A, which was found in yields of 3% of the phenylbutazone administered, is 1-*p*-hydroxyphenyl-2-phenyl-4-*n*-butyl-3,5-pyrazolidinedione (XLIII).

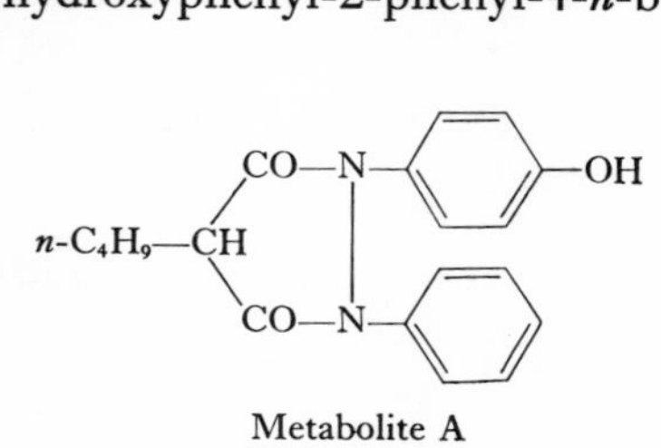

Metabolite A
(XLIII)

377

This compound also possesses the powerful antiinflammatory properties of phenylbutazone and was consequently marketed as a therapeutic drug under the name of Tanderil® and will therefore be dealt with in a later section. Mention should, however, be made here of the fact that Wilhelmi (*172*) believes metabolite A possibly to be chiefly responsible for the action of phenylbutazone inasmuch as within a certain period of administration of phenylbutazone to humans, considerably higher concentrations of metabolite A are found in the plasma than of unchanged phenylbutazone. Metabolite B, which was found in yields of 5% of the phenylbutazone administered, is 1,2-diphenyl-4-γ-hydroxybutyl-3,5-pyrazolidinedione (XLIV).

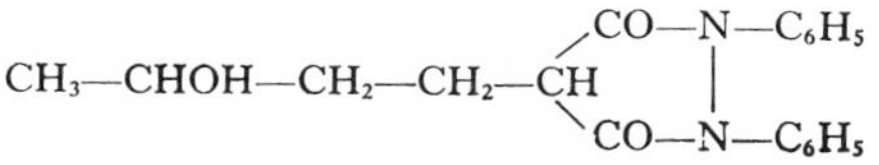

$$CH_3-CHOH-CH_2-CH_2-CH \begin{array}{c} CO-N-C_6H_5 \\ | \\ CO-N-C_6H_5 \end{array}$$

Metabolite **B**

(XLIV)

The organism thus makes use of hydroxylation for the transformation of phenylbutazone. Metabolite B is optically active, melts at 156–158° C, and shows a maximum in the ultraviolet at 262 mμ. It was compared with the synthetically produced racemic form having a melting point of 150–161° C and it was found that the ultraviolet and infrared spectra coincided. Its synthesis was described by Denss *et al.* (*173*). γ-Ethylenedioxybutylmalonic acid ethylester is reacted with hydrazobenzene and sodium methylate to form γ-ethylenedioxyphenylbutazone (XLV) Eq. (20).

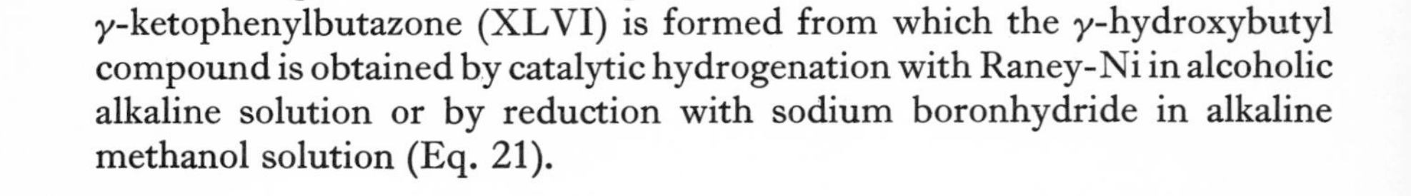

$$CH_3-C-CH_2-CH_2-CH\begin{array}{c}COOC_2H_5\\ \\COOC_2H_5\end{array} \quad + \quad \begin{array}{c}HN-C_6H_5\\ | \\HN-C_6H_5\end{array} \longrightarrow CH_3-C-CH_2-CH_2-CH\begin{array}{c}CO-N-C_6H\\ | \\CO-N-C_6H\end{array}$$

$$\begin{array}{c}O \quad O\\ | \quad | \\CH_2-CH_2\end{array} \qquad\qquad\qquad\qquad \begin{array}{c}O \quad O\\ | \quad | \\CH_2-CH_2\end{array}$$

(XLV)   (20)

After boiling for 18 hours with *p*-toluenesulfonic acid in acetone solution, γ-ketophenylbutazone (XLVI) is formed from which the γ-hydroxybutyl compound is obtained by catalytic hydrogenation with Raney-Ni in alcoholic alkaline solution or by reduction with sodium boronhydride in alkaline methanol solution (Eq. 21).

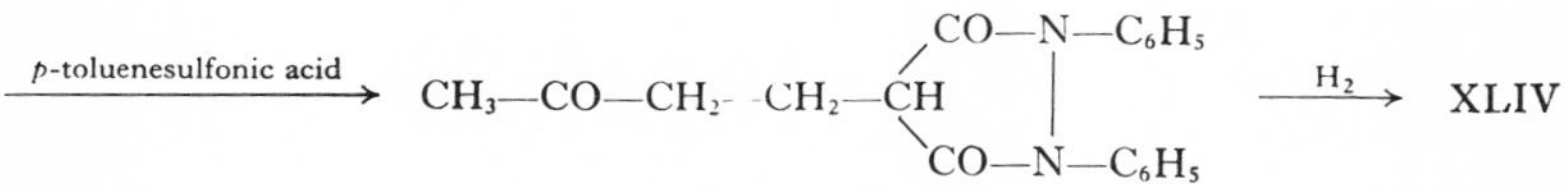

$$\xrightarrow{\textit{p}\text{-toluenesulfonic acid}} CH_3-CO-CH_2-CH_2-CH\begin{array}{c}CO-N-C_6H_5\\ | \\CO-N-C_6H_5\end{array} \xrightarrow{H_2} XLIV$$

(XLVI)   (21)

The hydroxybutyl compound is almost completely inactive pharmacologically and merely exhibits certain uricosuric properties (174). Its biological half-life period, measured after administration of the synthetic racemic preparation, is 10 hours, and 15% of the quantity administered is excreted unchanged.

d. *Toxicity and pharmacological action.* The acute toxicity of phenylbutazone has been determined by various authors (Table IX). The mani-

TABLE IX

LD_{50} OF PHENYLBUTAZONE IN MICE, RATS, AND RABBITS (IN MG/KG)

Author	Mouse		Rat			Rabbit	
	Intra-venous	Oral	Intra-venous	Oral	Intra-peri-toneal	Sub-cuta-neous	Intra-venous
Wilhelmi (172) Wilhemi and Currie (175)	112	680	150	1000	—	—	146
Schoetensack (176)	110	—	—	—	—	—	—
Hazleton et al. (177)	123	—	—	—	215	—	—
Horákova et al. (178)	130	—	—	—	—	—	—
Adami (179)	—	—	—	—	—	270	—

festations of poisoning after toxic doses coincide with those of other pyrazole derivatives and consist in conditions of excitation and tonic-clonic cramp. The general pharmacology will not be discussed here since it has been dealt with comprehensively by von Rechenberg (180). Only a few of its pharmacological properties will be mentioned here. Attention must be drawn above all to its excellent antiphlogistic action which has made it the ideal medium to be used for the treatment of rheumatic diseases. Phenylbutazone is a more effective febrifuge in coli fever of rabbits than dimethylaminophenazone (60), but it is inferior in its analgesic action.

6. Combination Preparations

a. *Irgapyrin®.* Phenylbutazone-sodium had at first been introduced to the market as a solubilizer of dimethylphenazone in the combination preparation Irgapyrin. When the valuable therapeutic properties of phenylbutazone were, however, discovered, Irgapyrin faded somewhat into the background. In Irgapyrin the two drugs complement one another in such a way that

379

synergism of action is partially attained while a reciprocal lowering of toxicity also takes place.

Tables X and XI depict the mean lethal and mean cramp doses in comparison to phenylbutazone and dimethylaminophenazone as found in experiments by Wilhelmi (60). The tables show that dimethylaminophenazone reduces the toxicity of phenylbutazone in the combination

TABLE X

LD$_{50}$ OF IRGAPYRIN, PHENYLBUTAZONE, AND
DIMETHYLAMINOPHENAZONE (IN MG/KG)

Preparation	Mouse		Rat		Rabbit
	Intravenous	Oral	Intravenous	Oral	Intravenous
Irgapyrin	250	700	160	1375	145
Phenylbutazone	102	650	98	770	145
Dimethylaminophen-azone	210	830	144	930	125

TABLE XI

MEAN CRAMP DOSE OF IRGAPYRIN, PHENYLBUTAZONE, AND DI-
METHYLAMINOPHENAZONE (IN MG/KG)

Preparation	Rabbit (intravenous)	Rat (oral)	Mouse (intravenous)
Irgapyrin	101.7	1370	93.8
Phenylbutazone	158	875	95.5
Dimethylaminophenazone	56	800	97.1

preparation. In rabbits and rats the mean cramp dose of Irgapyrin is distinctly higher than that of dimethylaminophenazone; in mice, on the other hand, it is practically equal for all three preparations tested.

b. Ircodenyl®. On account of their antispasmodic properties the soporifics phenylethylbarbituric acid and cycloheptenylethylbarbituric acid have a detoxifying effect on pyrazole compounds. In intravenous doses of 100 mg/kg, Irgapyrin causes tonic-clonic cramp in rabbits which could be partly inhibited and partly eliminated by prior intravenous injection of 30–50 mg/kg of the sodium salt of the barbituric acids named. Even 10 mg/kg cycloheptenylethylbarbituric acid were sufficient to suppress cramp in 4 out of 5 animals.

Further experiments on rats conducted by Wilhelmi (60) revealed that an antitoxic effect may be attributed to the barbituric acids in Irgapyrin poisoning. After prior administration of various quantities of the above named barbituric acids, and though cramp was not suppressed completely, the animals could be kept alive in spite of lethal doses of Irgapyrin having been given.

This knowledge was made use of in the combination preparation Ircodenyl which consists of a mixture of phenylbutazone, dimethylaminophenazone, cycloheptenylethylbarbituric acid, and codeine phosphate. With this preparation, Anders et al. (181) were able to cut out pain to the greatest possible extent, obviate post-operative edema, psychic restlessness and irritation to the throat leading to coughing and retching after tonsilectomies, combined with a lowering of postoperative bleeding whereby the prerequisites for a rapid healing effect without complications were given.

The combination of phenylbutazone, dimethylaminophenazone, and cyclohexenylethylbarbituric acid without codeine phosphate is registered as a trade mark under the name of Meliobal®.

c. *Delta-butazolidin®*. In Section II,F,9 which deals with Pyracortin, it has already been pointed out that the application of a combination of dimethylaminophenazone with prednisone has a favorable effect on rheumatic diseases because of the synergistic action of the two components.

The same experience was had with a combination preparation of Delta-butazolidin, which consists of a mixture of phenylbutazone and prednisone. According to Fiegel and Kelling (182), an increase in effectiveness by the use of this preparation over and above the purely additive action takes place, presumably as a result of the inhibition of prednisone inactivation by phenylbutazone. By the help of this combination it is often possible to maintain the improvement attained by high initial corticosteroid doses in acute and chronic rheumatic diseases, the analgesic effect being particularly reliable. Reisenhofer (183) also found that treatment was successful while good tolerability was encountered on average. Side reactions were not noted by him, and in the opinion of this author, Delta-butazolidin may be used by general practitioners for application within the compass of complete courses in the treatment of rheumatic arthritis, while exercising constant supervision on the patient.

d. *Tomanol®*. This is a further combination preparation containing phenylbutazone and XXXVII in the ratio 1: 2. In Section II,H,2, where XXXVII is discussed, it was stated that this pyrazole derivative—in contrast to dimethylaminophenazone and phenylbutazone—calms down

381

the central nervous system and lowers the blood pressure so that the opposite actions upon the circulatory system of the two components in the combination preparation Tomanol cancel out to a high degree (*131*, *132*).

Clinical investigations by Ross *et al.* (*184*) on febrile rheumatic diseases revealed that a preparation of powerful action has been produced by combining XXXVII with phenylbutazone. Within 3–5 days of beginning with the therapy, the subfebrile temperature had become normal in 12 out of 18 patients, swellings at the joints had receded, and improvement in active and passive mobility was noted. According to Schmid (*185*) the advantages of Tomanol are the less frequent administration necessary and concomitant reduced dosages required (one-third to one-half), its greater tolerability in intramuscular and intravenous injection, and the lesser extent of its side reactions in general. The dosage recommended is either one ampoule twice weekly, or 3×1 dragee daily, administered orally. Schmid is of the opinion that since such a small dosage is sufficient, the only explanation can be that the phenylbutazone action is amplified by the high XXXVII content (two-thirds) which was made possible because of the relatively less toxic property of XXXVII and because of its being a specific agent as well. Since it could be determined also that phenylbutazone disappears only slowly from the blood after the administration of Tomanol, its therapeutic dose of 5 to 10 mg% is generally reached by the dosage stated above, whereas more frequent and higher doses of Irgapyrin would be necessary to achieve the required levels. Tomanol is indicated not only in rheumatoid diseases but above all in influenza infections and superficial thrombophlebitis.

7. *Clinical Significance of Phenylbutazone*

Because of its antipyretic, analgesic, and antiphlogistic properties, phenylbutazone is eminently suitable for diseases arising from rheumatoid affections and related conditions of pain. Its excellent therapeutic properties exceed those of all medicaments of the pyrazole series.

The best and most certain results are achieved in acute polyarthritis, and even in acute attacks of arthritis itself suprisingly good results could be attained. Thus pain and swellings subside within minutes of intramuscular injection and within a few hours of oral administration. In primary chronic polyarthritis phenylbutazone develops an effectiveness which places it alongside the best medicaments in use, and sometimes even surpasses them.

In the treatment of spondyloarthritis ankyclopoietica (Bekhterev's disease), phenylbutazone has had a revolutionary effect. It replaces X-ray therapy, to which severe damage of the hematopoesis and a large number of cases of leukemia have been ascribed recently. Of the other forms of arthritis, the diseases accompanied by acute inflammation respond better than the chronic degenerative types, a result that has already been found in the case of other antirheumatics. The antiphlogistic properties of phenylbutazone have a beneficial effect also on superficial thrombophlebitis. In these properties it is clearly superior to the anticoagulants and horse chestnut preparations.

Because of its antiphlogistic and antipyretic properties phenylbutazone can be applied successfully in many other inflammatory and febrile conditions, as for instance in lymphogranulomatosis, exudative pleuritis, ophthalmological inflammations, and acute infections. In myocardial infections it is as effective as the anticoagulants.

An interesting property will be mentioned in conclusion: it is extremely toxic to the common louse. Lice that suck the blood of patients who are under phenylbutazone treatment perish.

B. Tanderil®

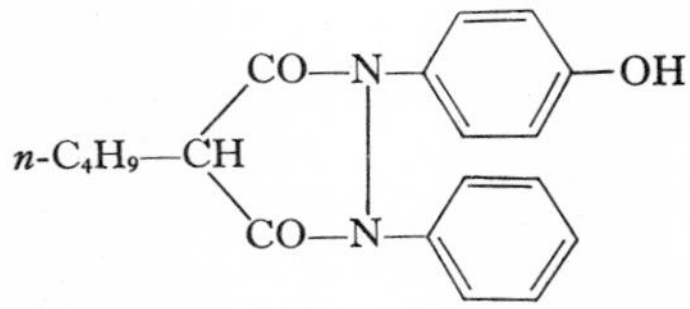

1-*p*-Hydroxyphenyl-2-phenyl-4-*n*-butyl-3,5-pyrazolidinedione

(XLIII)

1. *Synthesis*

After the *p*-hydroxy compound XLIII (see Section III,A,5,*c*) had been isolated in the organism as a metabolite of phenylbutazone and its constitution had been clarified, Pfister and Häfliger worked on its synthesis (*186*) which is outlined in Eq. (22).

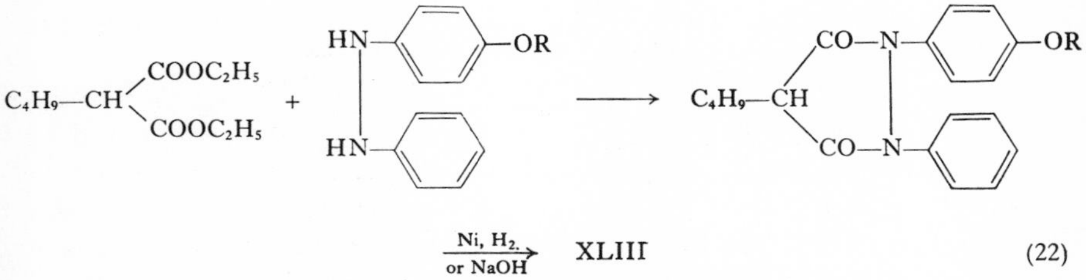

$$\text{XLIII} \qquad (22)$$

(R = C_6H_5—CH_2—; CH_3—CO—)

2. *Properties*

Domenjoz (*187*) subjected Tanderil to a thorough pharmacological examination and also determined its solubility at various pH in comparison

383

to phenylbutazone (Table XII). Tanderil is more toxic than phenylbutazone (Table XIII).

TABLE XII

SOLUBILITY OF TANDERIL AT VARIOUS pH VALUES (IN MG/100 ML)

Solvent	pH	Phenylbutazone	Tanderil
Phosphate buffer, 0.066 M	7.0	188	195
	6.0	34.5	66
Acetoacetate buffer, 0.10 M	4.7	3.6	13.2
	4.1	2.3	9.6
	3.5	1.9	8.1
Distilled water		1.5	13.9

TABLE XIII

LD_{50} OF TANDERIL IN COMPARISON TO PHENYLBUTAZONE (IN MG/KG)

Preparation	Mouse		Rat		Rabbit
	Intravenous	Oral	Intravenous	Oral	Intravenous
Phenylbutazone	112	680	150	1280	146
Tanderil	52	480	68	980	104

The ulcer inducing action of Tanderil on the mucous membrane of the stomach is less than that of phenylbutazone; its frequency is shown in Table XIV.

TABLE XIV

PERCENTAGE FREQUENCY OF GASTRIC ULCERS IN THE RAT, 21 TO 22 HOURS AFTER SUBCUTANEOUS ADMINISTRATION

Dosage (mg/kg)	Phenylbutazone	Tanderil
2×50	10	0
2×75	62	8

The examinations of Domenjoz also revealed that Tanderil is more powerful in its antipyretic action than phenylbutazone, but not in its analgesic action. Its antiphlogistic properties are equal to those of phenylbutazone, whereas it is more effective in comparison to the exudate after air and croto-noline injection. The uricosuric action is practically the same in both pre-parations as are water and sodium retention. Zicha and Bregulla (*188*) made comparative animal experiments on the antagonistic effect of phenylbuta-zone and Tanderil against histamine, serotonin, and acetylcholine. The action of Tanderil is accordingly clearly superior quantitatively to phenyl-butazone in asthma induced in guinea pigs by these three substances.

3. *Fate in the Organism*

According to examinations by Burns *et al.* (*189*), Tanderil is rapidly absorbed in oral administration and decomposed slowly. Its biological half-life period of 3 days is equal to that of phenylbutazone. In oral medica-tion of 600 mg the plasma levels during a period of 4–24 hours were the same as in intravenous injection [Yü *et al.* (*190*)]. In oral administration of 4×200 mg daily for a period of 8 days, the plasma levels rose during the first 3 days and then remained constant. They vary in individual cases from 8 to 16.2 mg%. von Rechenberg and Herrmann (*191*) arrived at the same results. They found a maximum concentration in the blood in single oral adminis-tration after 4–8 hours, while a maximum concentration of 9–10 mg% after repeated daily doses was not reached until several days later because of the slow rate of decomposition. These authors believe that the therapeutic dose lies at 5 mg%.

Tanderil is bound to the plasma protein in a way similar to phenylbuta-zone. Wunderly (*192*) assumes, as a result of experiments on equilibrial dialysis and rediffusion, that, similar to phenylbutazone, Tanderil diffuses into the hydrate envelope of the serum protein when joining with it. This explains its residence time in the organism. Further experiments indicate that the serum albumen is of particular importance for binding and trans-portation within the blood circulation.

4. *Clinical Significance*

In the many clinical trials which Tanderil was subjected to, the fact that it is a good antirheumatic has been demonstrated again and again, and also that it possesses advantages over phenylbutazone in treatment of long duration because of its negligible side effects, although its analgesic action is not as powerful. According to Hart and Burley (*193*) and Mason (*194*) it is suitable as a medium of long-lasting effect in the treatment of chronic rheumatism and, because it causes less gastric trouble, finds application in all cases in which phenylbutazone is not well tolerated. Barczyk and Röth (*195*) also found in their examinations that the antirheumatic properties of Tanderil are equal to those of phenylbutazone. Apart from its outstanding antiphlogistic action (135), it also possesses a reliable antipyretic effect. In virus infections a prompt and lasting improvement was already noted after 2–3 days. Fever disappeared and other inflammatory manifestations such as swellings in thrombophlebitis, headache in meningitis, or sleepiness in encephalitis improved rapidly and noticeably. Its antipyretic effect in neoplastic diseases was remarkable. Its good tolerability was above all expectations: in no case were disorders of the gastrointestinal tract noted which might have made it necessary to discontinue the preparation. Allergic reactions also did not occur on treatment over extended periods.

Strobel (196) tested Tanderil in 220 patients who were suffering from thrombophlebitis of the superficial veins of the leg. Only 21% of the patients treated were not influenced by the medication.

Connell et al. (197) reported on clinical experiences they had with Tanderil in surgery. In 245 cases of surgery they noted a rapid antiphlogistic effect which was also marked by reduced wound edema. In combination with a suitable antibiotic it exerts a powerful effect upon the germs near the wound. The authors suggest therefore that Tanderil should be administered with an antibiotic in all infectious inflammations of wounds.

C. KETAZON

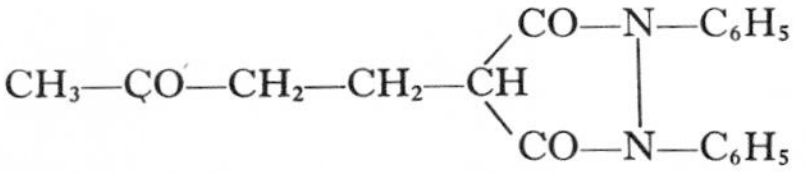

$$CH_3-CO-CH_2-CH_2-CH\begin{smallmatrix} \diagup CO-N-C_6H_5 \\ \diagdown CO-N-C_6H_5 \end{smallmatrix}$$

1.2-Diphenyl-4-γ-ketobutyl-3.5-pyrazolidinedione

(XLVI)

In Eq. (21), Section III,A,5,c, γ-ketophenylbutazone occurs as an intermediate (XLVI). This compound also proved to be a good antirheumatic and was introduced under the name of ketazon.

1. Synthesis

Apart from the reaction in Eq. (21), ketazon can also be obtained by reacting 1,2-diphenyl-3,5-pyrazolidinedione with 1,3-dichlorobutene-(2) and treating the 1,2-diphenyl-4-γ-chlorocrotyl-3,5-pyrazolidinedione (XLVII) with concentrated sulfuric acid (198) (Eq. 23).

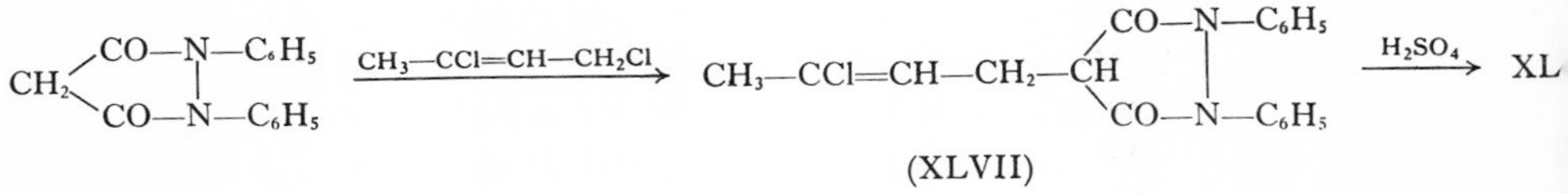

$$CH_2\begin{smallmatrix} \diagup CO-N-C_6H_5 \\ \diagdown CO-N-C_6H_5 \end{smallmatrix} \xrightarrow{CH_3-CCl=CH-CH_2Cl} CH_3-CCl=CH-CH_2-CH\begin{smallmatrix} \diagup CO-N-C_6H_5 \\ \diagdown CO-N-C_6H_5 \end{smallmatrix} \xrightarrow{H_2SO_4} XL$$

(XLVII)

(2

386

2. Properties

According to Horáková et al. (178), ketazon is one-third to one-fourth as toxic as phenylbutazone while its antiphlogistic action is the same and its antipyretic action somewhat less. Administration over longer periods seems to cause more marked changes in the liver and kidneys. Lenfeld et al. (199) found that the intermediate product XLVII in Eq. (23) also possesses antiphlogistic properties similar to phenylbutazone and is less toxic. The LD_{50} of XLVII in mice is 820 mg/kg in oral application as against 660 mg/kg in the case of phenylbutazone.

3. Fate in the Organism

Sibliková et al. (200) examined absorption, excretion, and also the action of ketazon on the uric acid concentration in the blood and urine. It is absorbed at a rate similar to that of phenylbutazone but is excreted more rapidly. Its biological half-life period in man is 27.3 ± 8 hours as against 72 hours in the case of phenylbutazone. After administering 16 mg/kg in rats, the highest concentration of ketazon in the liver, kidneys, and heart was determined after 3 hours. Excretion was determined after 3 hours. Excretion in its unchanged form by way of the urine is slight. After intramuscular application it is on average $3.8 \pm 2.3\%$ after 24 hours. Two metabolites could be detected by paper chromatography, but these have not been identified so far.

4. Clinical Application

It was shown in clinical application that ketazon has the same effect as phenylbutazone on rheumatic and thrombotic diseases but was found to be more tolerable (201). In spite of its short residence time in the organism, ketazon nevertheless has a powerful and protracted effect on the uric acid content of the blood and urine, and is thus a very effective medicament for arthritic therapy.

D. ANTURAN®

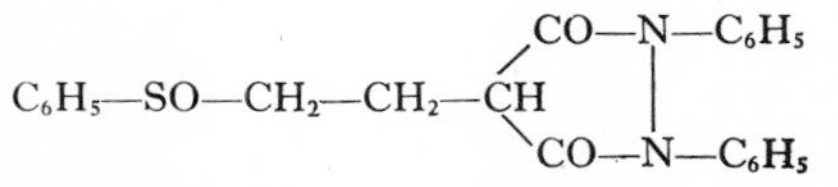

$$C_6H_5-SO-CH_2-CH_2-CH \Big\langle \begin{array}{l} CO-N-C_6H_5 \\ CO-N-C_6H_5 \end{array}$$

1.2-Diphenyl-4-(2'-phenylsulfinylethyl)-3,5-pyrazolidinedione

(XLVIII)

1. Discovery of Its Therapeutic Effect

Anturan (XLVIII) is a further example for the fact that the metabolite of a pyrazolidinedione derivative has better therapeutic properties than the

387

parent substance and it was consequently decided to introduce it as a therapeutic drug in place of the parent substance.

Pharmacological examinations revealed that 1,2-diphenyl-4-phenylthio-ethyl-3,5-pyrazolidinedione (IL) has a powerful uricosuric effect (202)

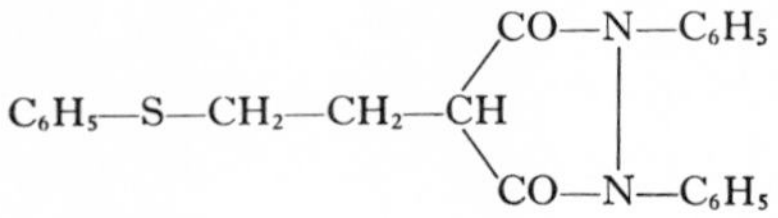

$$C_6H_5-S-CH_2-CH_2-CH \begin{array}{c} CO-N-C_6H_5 \\ | \\ CO-N-C_6H_5 \end{array}$$

(IL)

which exceeds that of phenylbutazone. Clinical trials confirmed the pharmacological results. On searching for the metabolites of IL, compound XLVIII was isolated. Pharmacological tests revealed that this was even more effective uricosurically than IL and after proving itself in clinical trials, it was introduced as a therapeutic agent under the name Anturan.

Although Anturan is not really an analgesic it will nevertheless be dealt with in this chapter because its field of application overlaps that of the other pyrazolidinedione derivatives.

2. Synthesis

It is not possible to obtain Anturan from the corresponding malonic acid ester in a way analogous to the phenylbutazone synthesis because the derivatives of β-phenylsulfinylethylmalonic acid derivatives are decomposed under the conditions prevailing during the reaction. It can, however, be obtained simply by the oxidation at room temperature of IL with perhydrol in glacial acetic acid [Pfister and Häfliger (203)]. Equation 24 depicts the course of the synthesis in which IL is obtained by the classic malonic acid method (204).

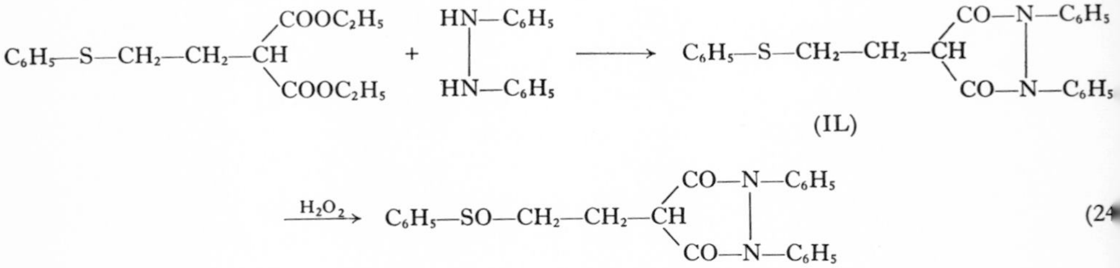

$$C_6H_5-S-CH_2-CH_2-CH\begin{array}{c}COOC_2H_5\\COOC_2H_5\end{array} + \begin{array}{c}HN-C_6H_5\\|\\HN-C_6H_5\end{array} \longrightarrow C_6H_5-S-CH_2-CH_2-CH\begin{array}{c}CO-N-C_6H_5\\|\\CO-N-C_6H_5\end{array}$$

(IL)

$$\xrightarrow{H_2O_2} C_6H_5-SO-CH_2-CH_2-CH\begin{array}{c}CO-N-C_6H_5\\|\\CO-N-C_6H_5\end{array}$$

(XLVIII)

(24)

3. Manufacture of the Optically Active Forms

The sulfoxide XLVIII isolated as a metabolite was optically active, viz., $[\alpha]_D^{24}$ in chloroform is $+11.0°$, while the substance obtained by oxidation was

388

inactive. Pfister *et al.* now sought a method by which they could produce the two enantiomeric forms from the synthetic compound. The direct splitting of the racemic sulfoxide did not succeed, since no crystalline salts could be obtained from optically active bases. The acid salts of phenylsulfinylethylmalonic acids, on the other hand, crystallized readily with (+)-α-phenylethylamine and (−)-α-phenylethylamine, and it was possible to separate them into the diastereomeric salts by repeated crystallization from which the two enantiomeric malonic acids were finally obtained.

Conversion to the corresponding pyrazolidinodione derivatives would, however, require a method by which to close the ring which precludes decomposition and racemization. The carbodiimide process introduced by Sheehan and Hess (*205*) was employed for this purpose. The yields were about 30%. The specific rotations of the substances prepared in this way were +109° and −104°, respectively, in chloroform and are therefore higher than the specific rotations of the sulfoxides isolated as metabolites of the thio compound IL; this may be ascribed to a partial asymmetric synthesis in the organism.

4. *Fate in the Organism*

Burns *et al.* (*202*) examined the fate of Anturan in the human organism. They found that it is transformed completely and swiftly in the body. After intravenous administration of 600 mg, the biological half-life period was 3 hours.

Dayton *et al.* (*206*) found that it is bound to the plasma proteins in a way similar to phenylbutazone and Tanderil. As previously mentioned, the sulfoxide isolated as a metabolite was found to be optically active. In order to study the excretion of its active form, Dayton *et al.* administered the *d*-isomer intravenously and subsequently isolated it in the urine once more. Rotation had only altered negligibly and the authors concluded that marked racemization did not take place in the body and during processing. Inactive Anturan which was injected intravenously was isolated in the urine in its optically inactive form which is proof of the fact that the optically active isomers are excreted in the same way.

Dayton *et al.* were able to isolate 1-*p*-hydroxyphenyl-2-phenyl-4-(2'-phenylsulfinylethyl)-3,5-pyrazolidinedione (L), hydroxysulfinpyrazone, in the urine as a metabolite of Anturan. The transformation of Anturan to hydroxysulfinpyrazone is thus analogous to that of phenylbutazone to Tanderil. The constitution of L was established by comparison with a synthetic preparation which Pfister *et al.* obtained by a method similar to the synthesis of Anturan, by oxidizing 1-*p*-hydroxyphenyl-2-phenyl-4-(2'-phenylthioethyl)-3,5-pyrazolidinedione (LI) with glacial acetic acid and

389

perhydrol. The natural and synthetic preparations had the same ultraviolet and infrared absorption spectra and did not show a depression on determining the mixed melting point. In the ultraviolet in 1 N NaOH, Anturan

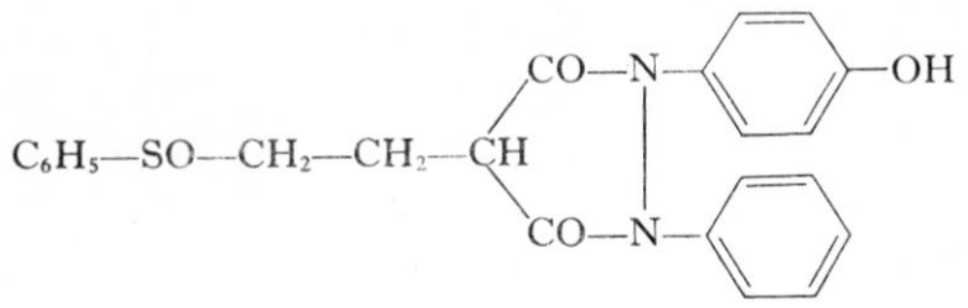

$$C_6H_5—SO—CH_2—CH_2—CH \begin{array}{c} CO—N—\text{〈〉}—OH \\ | \\ CO—N—\text{〈〉} \end{array}$$

(L)

$$C_6H_5—S—CH_2—CH_2—CH \begin{array}{c} CO—N—\text{〈〉}—OH \\ | \\ CO—N—\text{〈〉} \end{array}$$

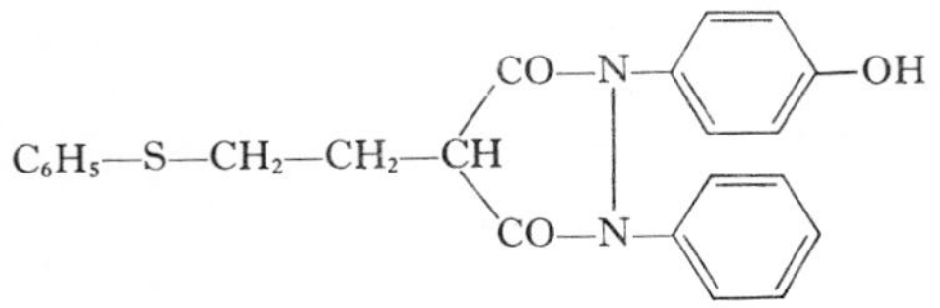

(LI)

possesses a maximum at 260 mμ, and its metabolite hydroxylsulfinpyrazone at 253 mμ.

Dayton *et al.* also investigated the excretion of hydroxysulfinpyrazone in the organism. On intravenous administration of 800 mg they detected a very high rate of excretion, its biological half-life period is 1 hour while that of Anturan is 3 hours. Within 24 hours, about half was excreted in the urine, the fate of the remaining quantity is not known.

Analogous to Anturan, hydroxysulfinpyrazone is bound to the plasma proteins and exhibits an increased uricosuric effect.

5. *Toxicity and Action*

Domenjoz (*187*) conducted the pharmacological analysis of Anturan. The decomposition of the thioethyl compound IL to form Anturan results in a partial reduction of its toxicity (Table XV). The mean lethal dose of Anturan by intravenous application is suprisingly close to its oral LD$_{50}$. This must be ascribed on the one hand to a particularly rapid and quantitative absorption in oral administration in contrast to phenylbutazone and on the other hand to the corresponding solubility conditions as shown in Table XVI.

The action of Anturan is neither analgesic nor antipyretic, but its antiphlogistic effect is superior to that of phenylbutazone so that even the LD$_{50}$ is still sufficient to attain an inhibitive action of 50% on the inflammatory pro-

390

TABLE XV

LD_{50} OF IL AND ANTURAN (IN MG/KG)

| Preparation | Mouse | | Rat | | Rabbit |
	Intravenous	Oral	Intravenous	Oral	Intravenous
IL	178	560	190	450	100
Anturan	240	298	154	375	195

TABLE XVI

SOLUBILITY OF PHENYLBUTAZONE AND ANTURAN AT DIFFERENT pH VALUES
(IN MG/100 ML BUFFER SOLUTION)

Solvent	pH	Phenylbutazone	Anturan
Phosphate buffer, 0.006 M	7.0	188	751
	6.0	34.3	251
Acetoacetate buffer, 0.01 M	4.7	3.6	75.2
	4.1	2.3	35.4
	3.5	1.9	8.6
Distilled water		1.5	12.4

cesses. Its uricosuric effect merits special mention. It is more powerful than that of phenylbutazone or the thionyl compound IL. No significant Na retention was observed when uricosuric dosages were given.

6. Clinical Significance

According to Cubukcu et al. (207), clinical trials of Anturan proved it to be a valuable and only slightly toxic medicament for the treatment of chronic arthritis, either completely eliminating pain in the joints or reducing it. It was possible to maintain continuously the serum levels within normal limits by this treatment.

Even in continuous treatment lasting up to 2 years, Jungbluth and Martin (208) encountered undesirable side effects of a minor nature only in exceptional cases. They did not detect any deleterious effect on the spinal cord, the liver, the kidneys, and the electrolyte balance. They are of the opinion that the use of Anturan is possible without adverse effect even in cases where renal function is disordered.

Kersley *et al.* (*209*) could also not detect any toxic effects after continuous administration over periods of 4–14 weeks.

E. 1-PHENYL-4-*n*-BUTYL-3,5-PYRAZOLIDINEDIONE

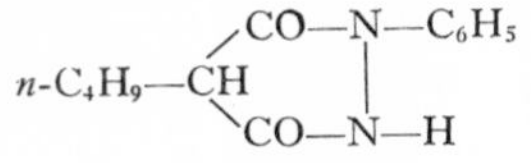

$$n\text{-}C_4H_9\text{---}CH\underset{\displaystyle CO\text{---}N\text{---}H}{\overset{\displaystyle CO\text{---}N\text{---}C_6H_5}{<}}$$

(LII)

Compound LII has recently been introduced into clinical practice. It is obtained by the condensation of butylmalonic ester with phenylhydrazine (*210*). In contrast to phenylbutazone, LII turns violet in color on reaction with $FeCl_3$ in 1:1 alcohol-water mixture (*211*), and in alcoholic solution possesses an absorption maximum at 240 mμ in the ultraviolet which can be used for its determination.

Scarselli (*212*) measured the concentration of LII in the plasma of rabbits after a single intravenous injection. He found that decomposition in the organism was rapid and that its biological half-life period was 28 hours. Under the same conditions, the half-life period of phenylbutazone in rabbits is 48 hours. The rapid decomposition of LII in the body appears to have a bearing on its low toxicity. It is about one-fifth as toxic as phenylbutazone (Table XVII).

TABLE XVII

LD_{50} OF LII (IN MG/KG) IN INTRAPERI-
TONEAL ADMINISTRATION COMPARED TO
PHENYLBUTAZONE

Preparation	Mouse	Rat
Phenylbutazone	172	142
LII	937	848

Investigations conducted by Derouaux *et al.* (*213*) seem to indicate that the antiphlogistic piperazine salts are superior to the straight pyrazolidine-dione derivatives by their more rapid onset of action, lower toxicity, and better gastrointestinal tolerance. Table XVIII compares the toxicity of LII and phenylbutazone with that of their piperazine salts (Table XVIII). LII is equal to phenylbutazone in its analgesic, antipyretic and antiphlogistic properties but on account of its faster rate of decomposition and excretion, its effect wears off more rapidly (*214*). LII is marketed in combination with isopropylphenazone under the name of Butaflex in Germany.

TABLE XVIII

LD$_{50}$ OF LII AND PHENYLBUTAZONE AS WELL AS
THEIR PIPERAZINE SALTS IN INTRAMUSCULAR
ADMINISTRATION IN MICE (IN MG/KG)

Preparation	LII	Phenylbutazone
Compound only	810	215
Piperazine salt	1025	580

F. 1,4-DIPHENYL-3,5-PYRAZOLIDINEDIONE (PHENOPYRAZON®)

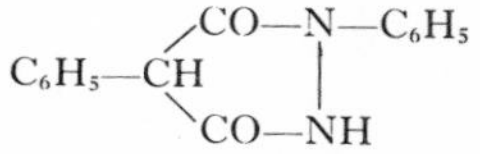

$$C_6H_5-CH \begin{array}{c} CO-N-C_6H_5 \\ | \\ CO-NH \end{array}$$

(LIII)

The last of the pyrazolidinedione derivatives on the market to be mentioned here is Phenopyrazon (LIII). It is prepared by the condensation of phenylmalonic acid ester with phenylhydrazine (*215*). Together with dimethylaminophenazone and procaine hydrochloride or *p*-aminobenzoic acid or their ethyl esters, its diethylaminoethane salt is a component of the combination preparation Osadrin®.

Phenopyrazon is less toxic than dimethylaminophenazone and phenylbutazone (*216*). According to investigations by Theobald (*217*), the antiphlogistic action of Phenopyrazon is less than that of phenylbutazone when applied subcutaneously in the treatment of formalin edema in rats.

TABLE XIX

LD$_{50}$ OF PHENOPYRAZON COMPARED WITH DIMETHYLAMINO-
PHENAZONE AND PHENYLBUTAZONE IN MICE (IN MG/KG)

Preparation	Subcutaneous	Intravenous
Dimethylaminophenazone	263	140
Phenylbutazone	245	148
Phenopyrazon	1003	808

393

Various authors (*218*) point out that clinical trials conducted with Osadrin revealed in particular that it possessed good general and local tolerability. Because of its powerful analgesic, antipyretic, and antiphlogistic action, it has proved to be a valuable therapeutic of low toxicity in the treatment of rheumatic complaints. In addition, it does not promote water retention in the body tissue.

Göbel (*219*) tested Osadrin in rheumatic and degenerative diseases of the spine and joints, comparing the results with those of Irgapyrin and phenylbutazone and found that it was not quite as effective, but that its side effects were not as severe as the previously prepared compounds.

G. Observations on the Constitution and Action of the 3,5-Pyrazolidinedione Derivatives

Various reports are available on the interrelation of chemical constitution and pharmacological action of the 3,5-pyrazolidinedione derivatives.

Büchi *et al.* (*210*) investigated the effect of various substitutions in the 1, 2-, and 4-positions on pharmacological action. The excellent analgesic action of 1-phenyl-3,5-pyrazolidinedione (LIV) substituted in the 4-position un is of interest here. If a second phenyl group is introduced (LV) the low toxicity of LIV is increased and its analgesic action reduced by one half.

$$\begin{array}{ccc}
\underset{\substack{\diagup \text{CO}-\text{N}-\text{C}_6\text{H}_5 \\ \text{CH}_2 \qquad\quad\mid \\ \diagdown \text{CO}-\text{N}-\text{H}}}{} &
\underset{\substack{\diagup \text{CO}-\text{N}-\text{C}_6\text{H}_5 \\ \text{CH}_2 \qquad\quad\mid \\ \diagdown \text{CO}-\text{N}-\text{C}_6\text{H}_5}}{} &
\underset{\substack{\diagup \text{CO}-\text{N}-\text{C}_6\text{H}_5 \\ n\text{-C}_4\text{H}_9-\text{CH} \qquad\mid \\ \diagdown \text{CO}-\text{N}-\text{CH}_2-\text{C}_6\text{H}_5}}{} \\
(\text{LIV}) & (\text{LV}) & (\text{LVI})
\end{array}$$

With monosubstitution in the 4-position, 1-phenyl-4-*n*-butyl-3,5-pyrazolidinedione (LII) and 1-phenyl-2-benzyl-4-*n*-butyl-3,5-pyrazolidinedione (LVI) exhibit the same analgesic action as dimethylaminophenazone; LVI stands out in particular by its low toxicity. The authors came to the conclusion that substitution in the 4-position affects the action more fundamentally than in the 2-position. In the case of an unsubstituted or suitably substituted 4-position, a phenyl group in the 1-position will considerably augment the pharmacological action already present. Substitution also of 2 hydrogen atoms in the 4-position is in agreement with this finding. Introducing 2-methyl groups into the compounds such as 1-phenyl-4,4-dimethyl-3,5-pyrazolidinedione (LVII) and 1-phenyl-2-methyl-4,4-dimethyl-3,5-pyra-

$$\begin{array}{cc}
\underset{(\text{LVII})}{\substack{\text{CH}_3\diagdown \qquad \diagup\text{CO}-\text{N}-\text{C}_6\text{H}_5 \\ \qquad\text{C} \qquad\qquad\mid \\ \text{CH}_3\diagup \quad \diagdown\text{CO}-\text{NH}}} &
\underset{(\text{LVIII})}{\substack{\text{CH}_3\diagdown \qquad \diagup\text{CO}-\text{N}-\text{C}_6\text{H}_5 \\ \qquad\text{C} \qquad\qquad\mid \\ \text{CH}_3\diagup \quad \diagdown\text{CO}-\text{N}-\text{CH}_3}}
\end{array}$$

zolidinedione (LVIII) has an unfavorable effect on the pharmacological properties.

It is not until more weighty substituents such as 2-ethyl groups are introduced that slightly better results are achieved. The exceptionally low toxicity and good analgesic action of 4,4-diethyl-3,5-pyrazolidinedione (LIX) whose nitrogen atoms are unsubstituted is particularly outstanding. It is very similar in structure to 5,5-diethylbarbituric acid (LX), the only difference being that the CO group between the two nitrogen atoms is missing.

$$
\begin{array}{cc}
\underset{C_2H_5}{\overset{C_2H_5}{>}} C \underset{CO-NH}{\overset{CO-NH}{<}} \Big| & \underset{C_2H_5}{\overset{C_2H_5}{>}} C \underset{CO-NH}{\overset{CO-NH}{<}} \hspace{-6pt} > CO \\
(LIX) & (LX)
\end{array}
$$

By introducing a phenyl group into compound LIX, a further slight improvement in the action of 1-phenyl-4,4-diethyl-3,5-pyrazolidinedione (LIX) is achieved, while its toxicity is unchanged. If the second nitrogen atom in LXI is substituted by alkyl groups of increasing length, a great reduction in the pharmacological action and an increase in toxicity results at first in the 2-methyl (LXII) and the 2-ethyl (LXIII) derivative. Yet, LXII does exhibit

$$
\begin{array}{ccc}
\underset{C_2H_5}{\overset{C_2H_5}{>}} C \underset{CO-NH}{\overset{CO-N-C_6H_5}{<}} \Big| & \underset{C_2H_5}{\overset{C_2H_5}{>}} C \underset{CO-N-CH_3}{\overset{CO-N-C_6H_5}{<}} \Big| & \underset{C_2H_5}{\overset{C_2H_5}{>}} C \underset{CO-N-C_2H_5}{\overset{CO-N-C_6H_5}{<}} \Big| \\
(LXI) & (LXII) & (LXIII)
\end{array}
$$

certain antipyretic properties. Surprisingly enough, the 2-*n*-propyl derivative (LXIV) possesses a powerful analgesic action which even surpasses that of dimethylaminophenazone and exhibits a toxicity that is lower than dimethylaminophenazone. The 2-isopropyl (LXV) and 2-allyl (LXVI)

$$
\begin{array}{ccc}
\underset{C_2H_5}{\overset{C_2H_5}{>}} C \underset{CO-N-n-C_3H_7}{\overset{CO-N-C_6H_5}{<}} \Big| & \underset{C_2H_5}{\overset{C_2H_5}{>}} C \underset{CO-N-i-C_3H_7}{\overset{CO-N-C_6H_5}{<}} \Big| & \underset{C_2H_5}{\overset{C_2H_5}{>}} C \underset{CO-N-CH_2-CH=CH_2}{\overset{CO-N-C_6H_5}{<}} \Big| \\
(LXIV) & (LXV) & (LXVI)
\end{array}
$$

derivatives of this series on the other hand have no analgesic effect at all, so that no rule can be enunciated regarding the influence of alkyl groups in the 2-position on pharmacological action.

Substitution in the 2-position of compound LXI revealed further interesting facts. If the ethyl group in the 2-position of the ineffective 2-ethyl derivative (LXIII) is substituted by a β-diethylaminoethyl group (LVIII), the analgesic action is equal to that of dimethylaminophenazone.

395

The 2-benzyl derivative (LXVIII) exhibits the same analgesic action as well as a certain antipyretic action and is at the same time exceptionally non-toxic. Substituting the phenyl group in the 1-position by a benzyl group has a

$$
\begin{array}{l}
C_2H_5 \quad CO-N-C_6H_5 \\
\quad\ \diagdown C \diagup \qquad | \\
C_2H_5 \diagup\quad\diagdown CO-N-C_2H_4-N(C_2H_5)_2 \\
\qquad\qquad (LXVII)
\end{array}
\qquad
\begin{array}{l}
C_2H_5 \quad CO-N-C_6H_5 \\
\quad\ \diagdown C \diagup \qquad | \\
C_2H_5 \diagup\quad\diagdown CO-N-CH_2-C_6H_5 \\
\qquad\qquad (LXVIII)
\end{array}
$$

very unfavorable influence on pharmacological action and toxicity. Enlargement of the alkyl groups in the 4-position does not bring about an improvement of pharmacological properties. While the 4,4-dibutyl and 4-allyl-4-isopropyl derivatives still have an action comparable to the 4,4-diethyl compounds, the 4-ethylisoamyl derivatives are completely ineffective. The introduction on the other hand of a benzyl group, in the 4-position, in conjunction with a *n*-butyl group results in pharmacologically active compounds once more.

Burns *et al.* (*189*) discussed the effect of substitution in the benzene ring of the 3,5-pyrazolidinedione derivatives on the pharmacological properties. It was found that a Cl, CH_3, or NO_2 group in the *para* position of the benzene ring results in increased antirheumatic and sodium-retaining properties and that substitution in the *meta* position of the benzene ring and in the butyl side chain causes the effect to be reduced. According to investigations by Burns *et al.* (*220*), uricosuric action is to a great extent dependent on the acidity of the individual compounds. The uricosuric action of various derivatives was compared in arthritic patients and it was found that the preparations of higher acidity were more effective. 1,2-Diphenyl-4-isopropyl-3,5-pyrazolidinedione (LXIX) and 1,2-di(*p*-tolyl)-4-*n*-butyl-3,5-pyrazolidinedione (LXX) are the least effective.

$$
\begin{array}{l}
\qquad\quad CO-N-C_6H_5 \\
\text{iso-}C_3H_7-CH \qquad\quad | \\
\qquad\quad CO-N-C_6H_5 \\
\qquad\qquad (LXIX)
\end{array}
\qquad
\begin{array}{l}
\qquad\quad CO-N-\!\!\bigcirc\!\!-CH_3 \\
\text{n-}C_4H_9-CH \\
\qquad\quad CO-N-\!\!\bigcirc\!\!-CH_3 \\
\qquad\qquad (LXX)
\end{array}
$$

Phenylbutazone (XLI) and Tanderil (XLIII) were more effective. A considerably enhanced effect is evinced by the more highly acid preparations XLIV and IL. A further considerable increase in uricosuric action is brought about by the even higher acidity of Anturan (XLVIII) and 1-*p*-hydroxyphenyl-2-phenyl-4-(phenylacetyl)-3,5-pyrazolidinedione (LXXI).

By virtue of its substitution and acidity, 1-(*p*-nitrophenyl)-2-phenyl-4-*n*-butyl-3,5-pyrazolidinedione (LXXII) possesses a particularly marked

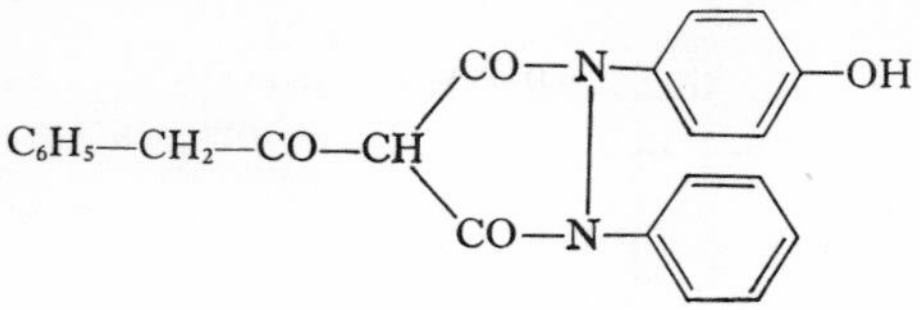

(LXXI)

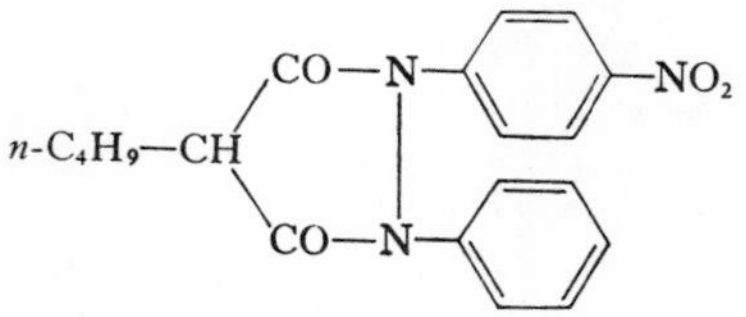

(LXXII)

uricosuric effect in addition to all other pharmacological properties of phenylbutazone.

The derivatives which have the strongest uricosuric action also exhibit a considerably reduced biological half-life period than phenylbutazone (about 3 hours compared to 72 hours). Compound LXXII, on the other hand which, as just mentioned, possesses all the properties of phenylbutazone, has a biological half-life period of 36 hours.

Burns *et al.* conclude from the powerful uricosuric action of the highly acid derivatives that these drugs act in their ionized form and block the reabsorption of uric acid by the renal tubuli. This is probably a clue to the hitherto unknown nature of the complicated transport mechanism of the phenylbutazone derivatives.

REFERENCES

1. L. Knorr, *Chem. Ber.* **16**, 2597 (1883).
2. L. Knorr, *Chem. Ber.* **17**, 546, 2033 (1884).
3. L. Knorr, *Liebigs Ann. Chem.* **238**, 146 (1887).
4. L. Knorr, *Liebigs Ann. Chem.* **238**, 155 (1887).
5. L. Knorr, German Patent 26,429 (1883).
6. L. Knorr, *Liebigs Ann. Chem.* **238**, 161 (1887).
7. A. Michaelis, *Liebigs Ann. Chem.* **320**, 45 (1902).
8. L. Knorr, *Liebigs Ann. Chem.* **293**, 27 (1896).
9. R. Kitamura, *J. Pharm. Soc. Japan* **60**, 3 (1940); *Chem. Zentr.* **II**, 741 (1940).
10. P. Duquénois, *Bull. Soc. Chim. France* [5] **13**, 425 (1946).
11. J. Schwyzer, "Die Fabrikation pharmazeutischer und chemisch-technischer Produkte," p. 167. Springer, Berlin, 1931.
12. Fiat-Final-Report No. 1023.

13. C. Gancia, *Boll. Chim. Farm.* **91**, 49–57 (1952).

14. Farbenfabriken Bayer, British Patent 676,270 (1950).

15. W. Polster, *Tuberkulosearzt* **29**, 594 (1950).

16. K. Unholtz, *Beitr. Klin. Tuberk.* **106**, 44–52 (1951).

17. Alpine Chemische A.G., Austrian Patent 178,164 (1950).

18. Chemiewerk Homburg A.G., German Patent 676,436 (1937); 718,707 (1940); 862,341 (1943).

19. Eggochemia, German Patent 677,152 (1938).

20. I. G. Farben A.G., German Patent 508,334 (1928).

21. Merz & Co., German Patent 649,665 (1932).

22. Riedel de Haën, German Patent 670,089 (1931).

23. L. Knorr, *Chem. Ber.* **17**, 2038 (1884).

24. P. Bourcet, *Bull. Soc. Chim. France* [3] **33**, 572 (1905).

25. M. Hahn, J. Kolšek, and M. Perpar, *Z. Anal. Chem.* **151**, 104–108 (1956).

26. R. Ruggieri, *Boll. Chim. Farm.* **95**, 382 (1956).

27. D. Davidson and J. MacIntyre, *Biochem. J.* **62**, 37 (1956).

28. W. Hale, *Berl. Klin. Wochschr.* **47**, 25 (1910).

29. K. Fromherz, *Arch. Exptl. Pathol. Pharmakol.* **121**, 273–298 (1927).

30. T. Koppányi and A. Liberson, *J. Pharmacol. Exptl. Therap.* **39**, 177–185 (1930).

31. S. Krop, W. Modell, and H. Gold, *J. Am. Pharm. Assoc.* **33**, 10–14 (1944).

32. B. B. Brodie and J. Axelrod, *J. Pharmacol. Exptl. Therap.* **98**, 97 (1950).

33. O. Schweissinger, *Arch. Pharm.* **222**, 693 (1884).

34. R. Soberman, B. B. Brodie, B. B. Levy, J. Axelrod, V. Hollander, and J. M. Steele, *J. Biol. Chem.* **179**, 31–42 (1949).

35. H. Huchard, *Zentr. Klin. Med.* **6**, 344 (1885).

36. J. Halberkann and F. Fretwurst, *Z. Physiol. Chem.* **285**, 123 (1950).

37. J. Zwintz, *Wien. Med. Presse* **45**, 759 (1904).

38. H. Herxheimer and E. Stresemann, *Nature* **192**, 1089–1090 (1961).

39. Hoffmann-La Roche & Co., A.G., German Patent 565,799 (1931).

40. Riedel de Haën, German Patent 962,254 (1954).

41. Hoffman-La Roche & Co., A.G., German Patent 558,473 (1931).

42. O. Jansen, *Pharm. Ind.* **18**, 41 (1956).

43. Hoffmann-La Roche & Co., A.G., German Patent 605,916 (1934).

44. E. Geistlich Söhne, Swiss Patent 275,620 (1948).

45. K. Fromherz, *J. Pharmacol. Exptl. Therap.* **61**, 205–212 (1937).

46. G. Orestano, *Boll. Soc. Ital. Biol. Sper.* **10**, 470 (1935); *Arch. Ital. Sci. Farmacol.* **4**, 419 (1935).

47. G. Bauer, *Arzneimittel-Forsch.* **9**, 401–403 (1959).

48. K. Bodendorf, J. Mildner, and T. Lehmann, *Liebigs Ann. Chem.* **563**, 1 (1949). For further syntheses see W. Krohs and O. Hensel, "Pyrazolone und Dioxopyrazolidine," pp. 42–44. Cantor, Aulendorf, Germany, 1961.

49. A. Béhal and E. Choay, *Ann. Chim.* (*Paris*) [6] **27**, 331 (1892).

50. Dr. Rentschler and Co., German Patent 1,100,029 (1958).

51. Egema, Belgian Patent 578,616 (1959).

52. Farbenfabriken Bayer, Belgian Patent 583,845 (1959).

53. K. Bodendorf and A. Popelak, *Liebigs Ann. Chem.* **566**, 84 (1950).

54. M. Passerini and G. Losco, *Gazz. Chim. Ital.* **69**, 658 (1939); **70**, 410 (1940).

55. J. Ledrut, F. Winternitz, and G. Combes, *Bull. Soc. Chim. France* [5] **28**, 704–706 (1961).

56. Luxema, German Patent 848,954 (1950).
57. H. van Cauwenberge, J. Lecomte, and C. Lapiére, *Compt. Rend. Soc. Biol.* **153**, 1292–1294 (1959).
58. Ravensberg, G.m.b.H., German Patent 1,067,438 (1956); U. S. Patent 2,943,022 (1958).
59. O. Hengen, H. Siemer, and A. Doppstadt, *Arzneimittel-Forsch.* **8**, 421–423 (1958).
60. G. Wilhelmi, *Schweiz. Med. Wochschr.* **79**, 577 (1949).
61. A. Richard, *Medizinische* pp. 81–83 (1959).
62. L. Knorr, *Liebigs Ann. Chem.* **238**, 212 (1887).
63. E. Scheitlin, German Patent 193,632 (1907).
64. Dr. Strunz. u. Körber, O.H.G., German patent 1,005,239 (1952).
65. L. Knorr and Th. Geuter, *Liebigs Ann. Chem.* **293**, 56–57 (1896).
66. S. Pfeifer and O. Manns, *Pharmazie* **12**, 401 (1957).
67. E. Emerson, *J. Org. Chem.* **8**, 417 (1943).
68. C. F. Hiskey and N. Levin, *J. Pharm. Sci.* **50**, 393–395 (1961); *Chem. Zentr.* p. 3693 (1963).
69. C. A. Johnson and R. A. Savidge, *J. Pharm. Pharmacol. Suppl.* **10**, 171–180 (1958); *Chem. Zentr.* p. 8604 (1960).
70. N. P. Yavorskii, *Chem. Abstr.* **56**, 15 608 i (1962).
71. R. Haslinger and W. Strunz, *Arzneimittel-Forsch.* **4**, 299 (1954).
72. M. Strell and S. Reindl, *Arzneimittel-Forsch.* **11**, 552–554 (1961).
73. W. E. Huckabee and G. Walcott, *J. Appl. Physiol.* **15**, 1139–1143 (1960); *Chem. Zentr.* 18 376 (1961).
74. R. Kobert, *Z. Klin. Med.* **62**, 83 (1907).
75. R. Kobert, *Z. Klin. Med.* **62**, 89 (1907).
76. J. Halberkann and F. Fretwurst, *Z. Physiol. Chem.* **285**, 106 (1950).
77. Hoechster Farbwerke, German Patent 90,959; for further procedures see W. Krohs and O. Hensel, "Pyrazolone und Dioxopyrazolone, pp. 51–53. Cantor, Aulendorf, Germany, 1961.
78. R. Kobert, *Z. Klin. Med.* **62**, 70 (1907).
79. K. Jung, *Pharm. Z.* **86**, 542–545 (1950).
80. Thévenon and Rolland, *Ann. Fals.* **10**, 485–486; *Chem. Zentr.* **I**, 877 (1918).
81. C. F. Boehringer and Söhne, German Patent 939,929 (1953).
82. Knoll, A. G., German Patent 738,923 (1938); 835,928 (1950); see also W. Krohs and O. Hensel, "Pyrazolone und Dioxopyrazolidine," pp. 58–60. Cantor, Aulendorf, Germany, 1961.
83. Riedel de Haën, German Patent 936,232 (1952).
84. O. Braun, Austrian Patent 176,949 (1951).
85. G. Madaus and F. Meyer, *Arzneimittel-Forsch.* **1**, 375 (1951).
86. F. Runge, H. J. Engelbrecht, and H. Franke, *Pharmazie* **12**, 11 (1957).
87. E. Oliveri-Mandalà and E. Calderaro, *Gazz. Chim. Ital.* **51**, 324–328 (1921).
88. N. P. Jaworski and J. F. Romanjak, *Chem. Zentr.* p. 8008 (1957).
89. B. Lang and L. Tavaszy, *Z. Anal. Chem.* **158**, 339 (1957); R. Ruggieri, *Boll. Chim. Farm.* **95**, 382 (1956).
90. A. Anastasi, E. Mecarelli, and L. Novacic, *Pharm. Acta Helv.* **30**, 55–61 (1955); L. Domange and A. Pinguet, *Ann. Pharm. Franc.* **9**, 651–657 (1951); W. Groebel and E. Schneider, *Z. Anal. Chem.* **146**, 191–193 (1955); I. Gyenes, *Acta Pharm. Hung.* p. 21 (1954); *Chem. Zentr.* 10 807 (1955); W. Poethke and D. Horn, *Pharm. Zentralhalle* **94**, 41–45 (1955).

 91. R. Pulver, *Arch. Intern. Pharmacodyn.* **81**, 47 (1950).
 92. F. Lohss and E. Kallee, *Arch. Exptl. Pathol. Pharmacol.* **214**, 202 (1952).
 93. R. Haslinger and W. Strunz, *Arzneimittel-Forsch.* **5**, 61 (1955).
 94. E. G. Weirich, *Hautarzt* **8**, 145 (1957).
 95. M. Jaffe, *Chem. Ber.* **35**, 2895 (1902).
 96. R. Kobert, *Z. Klin. Med.* **62**, 92–95 (1907).
 97. J. Halberkann and F. Fretwurst, *Z. Physiol. Chem.* **285**, 126 (1950).
 98. W. Hennig and H. Weiler, *Arzneimittel-Forsch.* **5**, 60 (1955).
 99. E. Brunner and R. Haslinger, *Wien. Med. Wochschr.* **105**, 602–604 (1955).
100. W. Chen, P. A. Vomdten, P. G. Dayton, and J. J. Burns, *Life Sci.* **1**, 35–42 (1962); *Chem. Abstr.* **57**, 1489 (1962).
101. W. Filehne, *Z. Klin. Med.* **32**, 572–573 (1897).
102. H. K. von Rechenberg, *Schweiz. Med. Wochschr.* **83**, 159 (1953).
103. Ch. L. Rühmke, *Acta Physiol. Pharmacol.Neerl.* **8**, 360–363 (1959); *Chem. Zentr.* p. 9893 (1961).
104. Schering-Kahlbaum, German Patent 455,874 (1920); 481,392 (1925). Hoffmann-La Roche & Co., A.G., German Patent 479,669 (1925); P. Pfeiffer, German Patent 464,483 (1925).
105. P. Pfeiffer, "Organische Molekülverbindungen," 2nd ed., p. 322. Enke, Stuttgart, Germany, 1927.
106. E. Starkenstein, *Therap. Monatsh.* **35**, 633 (1921).
107. E. Starkenstein, *Klin. Wochschr.* **4**, 117 (1925).
108. H. Salzer and R. Fischer, *Arch. Exptl. Pathol. Pharmacol.* **179**, 334 (1935).
109. Hoechster Farbwerke, German Patent 150,799 (1903).
110. Schering-Kahlbaum, German Patent 510,066 (1926).
111. Hoffmann-La Roche & Co., A.G., German Patent 471,655 (1921); 474,664 (1924); 479,669 (1925).
112. Riedel de Haën, *Arch. Pharm.* **264**, 464 (1926).
113. Sandoz, A.G., German Patent 690,254 (1935).
114. H. Hofmann, K. H. Boltze, and K. H. Chemnitius, *Arzneimittel-Forsch.* **6**, 208–213 (1956).
115. H. P. Kaufmann, German Patent 652,712 (1932).
116. I. G. Farben, German Patent 442,719 (1925).
117. G. Heinze, *Therap. Gegenwart* **97**, 169 (1958); H. H. Helm and H. Helm, *Med. Klin. (Munich)* **52**, 102 (1957); C. O. von Martius and F. Hünnemeyer, *Ärztl. Praxis* **10**, 356 (1958); K. Schmidt, E. Berger, and P. Pospischil, *Praktische Arzt* **13**, 315 (1959); W. Treiber, *Medizinische* p. 2008 (1958).
118. W. Blumencron, *Praktische Arzt* **13**, 373–378 (1959).
119. W. Treiber, *Z. Rheumaforsch.* **18**, 36 (1959).
120. Th. Kleinschmidt, *Medizinische* p. 1502 (1957).
121. Hoechster Farbwerke, German Patent 254,711 (1911); 259,503 (1911).
122. I. G. Farben, German Patent 476,663 (1922).
123. H. Decker, *Liebigs Ann. Chem.* **395**, 362 (1913).
124. I. G. Farben, German Patent 617,237 (1934).
125. A. Végh, G. Szász, and P. Kertész, *Acta Pharm. Hung.* **29**, 163–164 (1959); *Chem. Zentr.* p. 5180 (1961); *Acta Pharm. Hung.* **31**, 1–7 (1961); *Chem. Abstr.* **55**, 9787 (1961); *Acta Pharm. Hung.* **31**, 49–54 (1961); *Chem. Abstr.* **55**, 12,771 (1961).
126. J. Halberkann and F. Fretwurst, *Z. Physiol. Chem.* **285**, 126 (1950).
127. T. Gordonoff and H. Bosshard, *Arzneimittel-Forsch.* **13**, 314–316 (1963).

128. I. G. Farben, German Patent 679,284 (1937).

129. W. Laubender and A. Schlarb, *Arzneimittel-Forsch.* **12**, 479–485 (1962).

130. A. Skita, F. Keil, and W. Stühmer, *Chem. Ber.* **75**, 1696 (1942).

131. W. Schoetensack, G. Richarz, and P. Bischler, *Arzneimittel-Forsch.* **10**, 665–676 (1960).

132. G. Richarz, W. Schoetensack, and M. Vogel, *Arzneimittel-Forsch.* **10**, 676–683 (1960).

133. B. B. Brodie and J. Axelrod, *J. Pharmacol. Exptl. Therap.* **99**, 171 (1950).

134. W. Heid, German Patent 897,407 (1951).

135. P. Stoltenberg, German Patent 1,046,058 (1957).

136. C. Resta, *Farmaco (Pavia) Ed. Prat.* **16**, 422–427 (1961); *Chem. Abstr.* **56**, 7429 (1962).

137. O. Eichler and I. Staib, *Arzneimittel-Forsch.* **9**, 132–133 (1959).

138. A. Reincke, *Arzneimittel-Forsch.* **9**, 390–391 (1959).

139. W. Eger, *Arzneimittel-Forsch.* **7**, 610 (1957).

140. A. Fleisch and M. Dolivo, *Helv. Physiol. Pharmacol. Acta* **11**, 305 (1953).

141. H. E. Schmitt and H. G. Harwerth, *Arzneimittel-Forsch.* **11**, 1046–1049 (1961).

142. I. Hartert, *Medizinische* **42**, 2003 (1959).

143. F. Ballús y Roca, *Fortschr. Med.* **77**, 615 (1959).

144. E. Zwerenz, *Landarzt* **35**, 278 (1959).

145. W. Schmidt, *Med. Welt.* **18**, 1013 (1960).

146. W. Schmidt and J. Pape, *Med. Welt* **38**, 1942 (1961).

147. H. Eder, P. M. Ansari, G. Presser, and U. Rammner, *Arzneimittel-Forsch.* **11**, 1043–1046 (1961).

148. K. Dziuba, *Arzneimittel-Forsch.* **11**, 1049–1051 (1961).

149. A. Ebnöther, E. Jucker, and A. Lindenmann, *Helv. Chim. Acta* **42**, 1201 (1959); E. Jucker, *Angew. Chem.* **71**, 321 (1959).

150. W. Krohs and O. Hensel, "Pyrazolone and Dioxopyrazolidine," pp. 108–110, Cantor, Aulendorf, Germany, 1961.

151. I. R. Geigy, German Patent 814,150 (1949).

152. I. R. Geigy, Swiss Patent 308,145 (1953).

153. Byk Gulden, Austrian Patent 193,873 (1956).

154. J. Breugelmans and G. Braun, *J. Pharm. Belg.* **11**, 309–337 (1955).

155. N. Deffner and A. I. Deffner, *Chim. Anal. (Paris)* [4] **40**, 460–462 (1958); *Chem. Zentr.* p. 11,661 (1959).

156. R. Pulver, *Schweiz. Med. Wochschr.* **80**, 308 (1950).

157. J. J. Burns, R. K. Rose, T. Chenkin, A. Goldman, A. Schulert, and B. B. Brodie, *J. Pharmacol. Exptl. Therap.* **109**, 346–357 (1953).

158. B. Herrmann, *Med. Exptl.* **1**, 170–178 (1959).

159. W. Fuchs, *Schweiz. Med. Wochschr.* **88**, 686 (1958).

160. E. A. Tophoi, *Acta Med. Scand.* **160**, 197–203 (1958).

161. B. B. Brodie, E. W. Lowman, J. J. Burns, P. R. Lee, T. Chenkin, A. Goldman, M. Weiner, and J. M. Steele, *Am. J. Med.* **16**, 181–190 (1954).

162. H. K. von Rechenberg, *Schweiz. Med. Wochschr.* **83**, 159 (1953); H. K. von Rechenberg and R. Pulver, *Praxis* **41**, 44 (1952).

163. R. Pulver, *Arzneimittel-Forsch.* **5**, 221 (1955).

164. R. Pulver, B. Exer, and B. Herrmann, *Schweiz. Med. Wochschr.* **86**, 1080–1085 (1956).

165. Ch. Wunderly, *Arzneimittel-Forsch.* **6**, 731 (1956).

166. E. R. Heise and K. H. Kimbel, *Arzneimittel-Forsch.* **6**, 722–724 (1956); E. R. Heise, *Arzneimittel-Forsch.* **6**, 724–726 (1956).

167. G. Wilhelmi and R. Pulver, *Arzneimittel-Forsch.* **5**, 221 (1955).

168. H. G. Harwerth and F. Wöhler, *Z. Rheumaforsch.* **16**, 265–275 (1957).

169. E. Leuxner and R. Pulver, *Muench. Med. Wochschr.* **98**, 84–86 (1956).

170. H. K. von Rechenberg, "Phenylbutazon," p. 18. Thieme, Stuttgart, Germany, 1957.

171. J. J. Burns, R. K. Rose, S. Goodwin, J. Reichenthal, E. C. Horning, and B. B. Brodie, *J. Pharmacol. Exptl. Therap.* **113**, 9 (1955); **113**, 481–489 (1955).

172. G. Wilhemi, *Arzneimittel-Forsch.* **10**, 129–133 (1960).

173. R. Denss, F. Häfliger, and S. Goodwin, *Helv. Chim. Acta* **40**, 402 (1957).

174. T. F. Yü, J. J. Burns, B. C. Paton, A. B. Gutman, and B. B. Brodie, *J. Pharmacol. Exptl. Therap.* **123**, 63–69 (1958).

175. G. Wilhelmi and J. P. Currie, *Schweiz. Med. Wochschr.* **84**, 1315–1318 (1954).

176. W. Schoetensack, *Arch. Exptl. Pathol. Pharmacol.* **233**, 365–375 (1958).

177. L. W. Hazleton, T. W. Tusing, and E. G. Holland, *J. Pharmacol. Exptl. Therap.* **109**, 387–392 (1953).

178. Z. Horákowa, O. Némecek, V. Pujmann, J. Mayer, J. Ctortnik, and Z. Voltava, *Arzneimittel-Forsch.* **8**, 228 (1958).

179. E. Adami, *Atti Soc. Lombarda Sci. Med. Biol.* **11**, 49 (1956).

180. H. K. von Rechenberg, "Butazolidin," 2nd ed. Thieme, Stuttgart, Germany, 1961.

181. J. Anders and C. Ritschl, *Med. Klin.* (*Munich*) **52**, 187 (1957); S. Fischer, *Medizinische* pp. 751–752 (1955); F. Lungmuss, *Zentr. Chir.* **80**, 1217–1218 (1955); W. Markgraf, *Therap. Gegenwart* **93**, 303–305 (1954); H. Mergarten, *Zentr. Gynaekol.* **76**, 1878–1881 (1954); C. Münstermann, *Praxis* (*Bern*) **44**, 381–383 (1955); R. von Ondarza and E. Löhr, *Zentr. Chir.* **79**, 1779–1783 (1954); H. K. Schrader, *Schweiz. Monatsschr. Zahnheilk.* **66**, 561–564 (1956); H. Schultze, *Med. Monatsschr.* **9**, 244–246 (1955); E. Wieninger, *Praxis* (*Bern*) **44**, 122–123 (1955).

182. G. Fiegel and H. W. Kelling, *Therap. Gegenwart* **99**, 67–70 (1960).

183. A. Reisenhofer, *Wien. Med. Wochschr.* **111**, 245–247 (1961).

184. J. Ross, T. Til, and E. Mundt, *Ärztl. Wochschr.* **14**, 341–345 (1959).

185. J. Schmid, *Muench. Med. Wochschr.* **101**, 1746–1750 (1959).

186. R. Pfister and F. Häfliger, *Helv. Chim. Acta* **40**, 395 (1957).

187. R. Domenjoz, *Ann. N.Y. Acad. Sci.* **86**, 263–291 (1960).

188. L. Zicha and B. Bregulla, *Arzneimittel-Forsch.* **12**, 474–477 (1962).

189. J. J. Burns, T. F. Yü, P. G. Dayton, A. B. Gutman, and B. B. Brodie, *Ann. N.Y. Acad. Sci.* **86**, 253–262 (1960).

190. T. F. Yü, J. J. Burns, B. C. Paton, A. B. Gutman, and B. B. Brodie, *J. Pharmacol. Exptl. Therap.* **123**, 63–69 (1958).

191. H. K. von Rechenberg and B. Herrmann, *Schweiz. Med. Wochschr.* **91**, 403–405 (1961).

192. Ch. Wunderly, *Arzneimittel-Forsch.* **10**, 910–911 (1960).

193. F. D. Hart and D. Burley, *Brit. Med. J.* pp. 1087–1089 (1959).

194. R. M. Mason, *Brit. Med. J.* p. 1351 (1959).

195. W. Barczyk and G. Röth, *Praxis* **23**, 589–591 (1960).

196. E. Strobel, *Arzneimittel-Forsch.* **10**, 497–500 (1960).

197. J. F. Connell, Jr., R. Wallace, and L. M. Rousselot, *Schweiz. Med. Wochschr.* **91**, 760–764 (1961).

198. Synfarma narodoni podnik, Austrian Patent 198,263 (1955).

199. J. Lenfeld, M. Kroutil, M. Böcek, J. Čtvrtnik, and J. Mayer, *Arzneimittel-Forsch.* **11**, 427–429 (1961).

200. O. Sibliková, J. Lavička, G. Vachek, B. Tesárek, O. Vitulová, M. Černá, *Arzneimittel-Forsch.* **11**, 1106–1108 (1961).

201. Z. Horáková, J. Metys, J. Hladovec, O. Němĕcek, and B. Hoch, *Pharmacotherapeutica Collect Papers 10th Anniv. Res. Inst. Pharm. Biochem., Prague, 1960*, pp. 335–350; *Chem. Abstr.* **55**, 5335 (1962).
202. J. J. Burns, T. F. Yü, A. Ritterband, J, M. Perel, A. Gutman, and B. B. Brodie, *J. Pharmacol. Exptl. Therap.* **119**, 418–426 (1957).
203. R. Pfister and F. Häfliger, *Helv. Chim. Acta* **44**, 232 (1961).
204. J. R. Geigy, Swiss Patent 303,938 (1950).
205. J. C. Sheehan and G. P. Hess, *J. Am. Chem. Soc.* **77**, 1067 (1955).
206. P. G. Dayton, L. E. Sicam, M. Landrau, and J. J. Burns, *J. Pharmacol. Exptl. Therap.* **132**, 287–290 (1961).
207. O. C. Cubukcu, I. Imré, and D. Onel, *Z. Rheumaforsch.* **20**, 351–355 (1961).
208. H. Jungbluth and H. Martin, *Chemotherapia* **3**, 487–494 (1961).
209. G. D. Kersley, E. R. Crook, and D. C. J. Davey, *Lancet* **I**, 774 (1958).
210. J. Büchi, J. Ammann, R. Lieberherr, and E. Eichenberger, *Helv. Chim. Acta* **36**, 75–85 (1953).
211. M. Sahli and H. Ziegler, *Arch. Pharm. Chemi* **68**, 186–197 (1961).
212. V. Scarselli, *Farmaco (Pavia) Ed. Sci.* **14**, 347–351 (1959); *Chem. Zentr.* p. 3899 (1962).
213. Etablissements Marcel du Bled, Belgian Patent 590,756 (1960); G. Derouaux and J. Lecomte, *Compt. Rend. Soc. Biol.* **155**, 1419–1420 (1961).
214. C. Bianchi, *Rass. Med. Sper.* **8**, 88–98 (1961); *Chem. Abstr.* **56**, 10 869 h (1962).
215. Knoll, A.G., Swiss Patent 323,462 (1953).
216. H. Haas and H. Kraft, *Arzneimittel-Forsch.* **4**, 249–257 (1954).
217. W. Theobald, *Arch. Intern. Pharmacodyn.* **103**, 17–25 (1955).
218. R. Bertel and H. Dittrich, *Wien. Med. Wochschr.* **106**, 606 (1956); F. Grühn, *Med. Klin.* (*Munich*) **49**, 705–707 (1954); W. Hussel, *Medizinische* pp. 329–330 (1955); H. Krost and W. Schmidt, *Deut. Med. Wochschr.* **79**, 814–816 (1954); I. Thiery-Steinmetz, *Therap. Gegenwart* **94**, 303–304 (1955).
219. P. Göbel, *Arzneimittel-Forsch.* **8**, 700–706 (1958).
220. J. J. Burns, T. F. Yü, P. G. Dayton, L. Berger, A. B. Gutman, and B. B. Brodie, *Nature* **182**, 1102 (1958).

CHAPTER VIII

General Synthetics

GEORGE deSTEVENS

CIBA PHARMACEUTICAL COMPANY, DIVISION OF CIBA CORPORATION,
SUMMIT, NEW JERSEY

I. Introduction

In the previous chapters on pyrazoles, it was shown that compounds structurally unrelated to morphine or any dissected fragment of morphine were also capable of eliciting an analgetic effect both in animals and in man. Moreover, such substances were also found to be free of some of the disturbing side effects (e.g., addiction liability) associated with morphine and its congeners. In this respect, the alternative approach of the medicinal chemist, that is, the synthesis of a wide variety of different compounds for broad biological evaluation, has been and will continue to be a useful method for uncovering clinically active analgetics. The general theme in this approach has been that compounds unlike the narcotic analgetics could and probably would act by a different mechanism and consequently might offer distinct advantages over known pain relieving substances. Literally, many thousands of synthetic compounds have been prepared in many laboratories throughout the world with this idea in mind. Many of these substances have been reported in the patent literature and in the chemical and biological journals. A substantial number of these synthetics have also been subjected to the fires of clinical trials and it is here where virtually all have met their demise.

It is beyond the scope of this chapter to give an account of the legion of synthetic substances which have shown analgetic effects in animals and thus have warranted clinical evaluation. Instead, a number of compounds have been selected which have unusual structural characteristics and whose analgetic action could not have been predicted *a priori*. Although many of these have not found their way in clinical medicine, still their unique structures and their mode of action may give important clues for the design of new, clinically effective analgetics.

II. Aralkylamines

Although the phenethylamines have been explored most extensively for their pressor and central stimulatory effects, there have been, nevertheless, a substantial number of reports ascribing central depressant properties to these agents. Epinephrine (I) and norepinephrine (II) given by various routes to a variety of animal species have been shown to cause stupor and a relative insensitivity to pain preceded by a period of excitement (*1–6*).

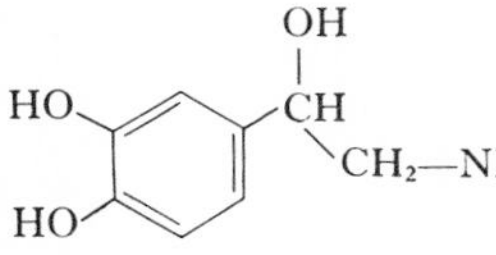

$$\text{(I)} \qquad \text{(II)}$$

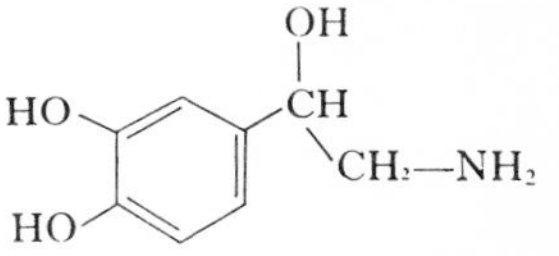

Several of these reports prompted Fellows and Ullyot (*7*) to examine a large number of derivatives of phenethylamines, substituted both in the ring and in the side chain with conventional groups (simple alkyls, OH, OR, etc.), and tested them for analgetic activity. The details of this work are presented by these investigators in an excellent review. However, for historical purposes, several of these compounds exhibiting marked analgesic effects in the cat are listed in Table I. The significant structure-activity relationship to be noted here is that increased activity was observed with α-branched amines in which the amino group is separated from the aromatic nucleus by more than two carbon atoms. However, these compounds are neurotoxic and also have a narrow therapeutic ratio (1:2–3). For this reason they have not attained clinical significance.

406

TABLE I

PHENYLALKYLAMINE AND ANALOGOUS DERIVATIVES EXHIBITING MARKED ANAL-
GESIC ACTIVITY IN CATS (8)

Compound	Dose (mg/kg)	
	Effective	Toxic
$4\text{-}CH_3C_6H_4CH_2CH(CH_3)NH_2$	10	20+
$4\text{-}CH_3OC_6H_4CH_2CH(CH_3)NH_2$	2	6
$4\text{-}CH_3OC_6H_4CH_2CH(CH_3)NHCH_2C_6H_5$	25	35
$4\text{-}CH_3OC_6H_4CH_2CH(CH_3)NHCH(CH_3)_2$	20	50
$4\text{-}HOC_6H_4CH_2CH(CH_3)NH_2$	2	30
$(+)\text{-}4\text{-}HOC_6H_4CH_2CH(CH_3)NH_2$	2	20
$4\text{-}C_6H_5CH_2CO_2C_6H_4CH_2CH(CH_3)NH_2$	20	30
$3,4\text{-}(CH_3O)_2C_6H_3CH_2CH(CH_3)NH_2$	20	75+
$3,4\text{-}(CH_3O)_2C_6H_3CH_2CH(CH_3)NHCH_2CH_2C_6H_5$	35	35
$3,4\text{-}(CH_3O)_2C_6H_3CH_2CH(CH_3)NHCH(CH_3)CH_2C_6H_5$	25	26
$3\text{-}C_6H_5CH_2O\text{-}4\text{-}CH_3OC_6H_3CH_2CH(CH_3)NH_2$	35	35
$3,4\text{-}CH_2O_2C_6H_3CH_2CH(CH_3)_2NH_2$	2.5	7.5
$4\text{-}HOC_6H_4CH_2CH(C_2H_5)NH_2$	10	35
$C_6H_5CH_2CH_2CH(CH_3)NH_2$	15	40
$4\text{-}HOC_6H_4CH_2CH_2CH(CH_3)NHC_4H_9$	20	25
$4\text{-}HOC_6H_4CH_2CH_2CH(C_2H_5)NH_2$	25	50
$3,4\text{-}(CH_3O)_2C_6H_3CH_2CH_2CH(CH_3)NH_2$	25	75
$C_6H_5(CH_2)_3CH(CH_3)NH_2$	6	30
$4\text{-}HOC_6H_4(CH_2)_3CH(CH_3)NH_2$	25	50
$C_6H_5(CH_2)_4CH(CH_3)NH_2$	15	25

Niemann and Hays in 1942 (9) prepared 2-β-pyridylethylamine (III) and found that it was a convulsant and it was believed that this property could be attributed to the ability of this compound to exist in the chelated form. Later, Burger and Ullyot (10) reasoned that a methyl group in the 6-position might interfere with the chelation and thereby reduce the toxicity. Compound IV

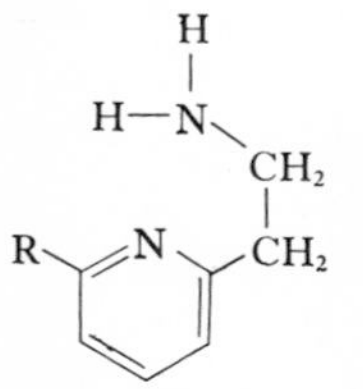

(III) R = H
(IV) R = CH₃

was synthesized and it produced marked analgesia at 7 mg/kg. However, its unfavorable therapeutic ratio (1:3) has militated against its further consideration. Another 2-β-pyridylethylamine derivative which showed excellent analgetic activity is *N*-2(2-pyridylethyl)phthalamide (V). This compound was synthesized by Kirschner *et al.* (*11*) and evaluated pharmacologically by Lewis (*12*).

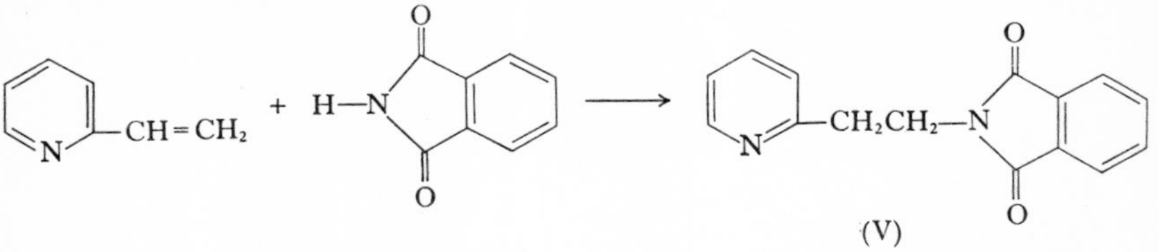

(V)

The Ercoli-Lewis (*13*) method was used for the evaluation of the analgetic activity in rats. It was observed that V was from two to three times more active than aminopyrine and also the effect was of longer duration when the compound was given subcutaneously (approximately 5 hours). However, the maximum analgetic effect of this compound was observed at 60 minutes following subcutaneous administration and at 30 minutes following oral administration.

The effective oral dose in animals was 300 mg/kg. Compound V was submitted for clinical evaluation and the preliminary results proved it to be an effective analgetic in man when administered orally. However, this substance has not been introduced into clinical practice.

III. 2-Aminoindane

The demonstrated analgetic activity of aralkylamines and, in particular the phenethylamines led Huebner and co-workers (*14*) to synthesize a series of 2-amino substituted indanes. These compounds are essentially β-phenethylamine derivatives with the end carbon of the three carbon aliphatic side chain attached back on to the aromatic ring. The synthesis of the parent member of this series follows.

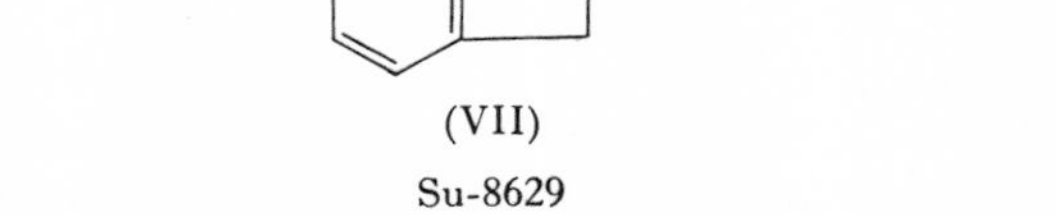

(VII)

Su-8629

SCHEME 1

408

The initial analgetic testing of compounds in this series was done in mice according to the tail flick method of D'Amour and Smith (15). The structure-activity relationship study appeared to be rather straightforward. Substituents on the benzene ring [e.g., 5-F, 5-Cl, 5-CH$_3$, 5-OCH$_3$, 5,6-(OCH$_2$)] did not give compounds with greater analgetic activity than Su-8629. The 5-fluoro derivative was almost as active as the parent substance. Substituents in the 1- or 2-position of VII were not advantageous and mono- and disubstitution of the amino group afforded compounds less active than Su-8629. Therefore, this compound was selected for further pharmacological evaluation (16).

TABLE II

ANALGESIC POTENCY AND THERAPEUTIC INDEX OF SU-8629 AND MORPHINE IN MICE
[METHOD OF D'AMOUR AND SMITH (15)]

Compound	Route	ED$_{50}$ (mg/kg) ± S.E.	24-hr. LD$_{50}$ (mg/kg) ± S.E.	Therapeutic index
Morphine	subcutaneous	2.8 ± 0.1	375 ± 16.4	133.9
Morphine	oral	19.5 ± 1.2	600 ± 44.0	30.8
Su-8629	subcutaneous	15.0 ± 1.8	158 ± 24.6	10.5
Su-8629	oral	21.0 ± 1.9	500 ± 17.3	23.8

TABLE III

ANALGESIC EFFECTS OF SU-8629 AND MORPHINE (HOT PLATE METHOD)[a]

Compound	Dose (mg/kg)	Route	Per cent change reaction time from preinjection control					
			15 min	30 min[b]	45 min	60 min	90 min	120 min
Saline	—	oral	−15.5	−12.6	−4.0	+0.7	+7.1	−11.0
Morphine	25	oral	+100	+130	+95	+80	+35	+17
Su-8629	25	oral	+130	+121	+130	+82	+43	+10

[a] The figures represent the average per cent change using 10 mice/drug.
[b] Time following drug administration.

In Tables II and III are shown the analgetic effects of 2-aminoindane as compared to morphine by two different test methods. Using the tail flick method in mice Su-8629 had about the same analgetic potency and therapeutic ratio as did morphine when given by the same route. Subcutaneously, this substance had about one-fifth the potency and twice the toxicity of morphine. The relative analgetic equivalence of these two compounds by the oral route was substantiated by using the hot plate procedure in which 25 mg/kg of Su-8629 was found to produce the same degree and duration of effects as did 25 mg/kg of morphine. Witkin *et al.* further noted that 2-aminoindane differed from morphine in that it was devoid of nalorphine antagonism, suggesting that it was not liable to cause addiction. Seevers (*17*) also observed that Su-8629 in doses up to 24 mg/kg caused no suppression of abstinence in 8 monkeys which were physically dependent on morphine. It was also found by Witkin *et al.* that Su-8629 caused some stimulation, similar to amphetamine, at high doses.

2-Aminoindane was submitted for clinical evaluation as an analgetic and it was found to be orally effective in man at a dose of 25 mg given three times daily (*18*). However, after extensive studies with this compound in humans, the statistically significant occurrence of stimulation and moderate hypertension precluded its further use in therapy.

IV. Methotrimeprazine

The tremendous success of the 10-substituted phenothiazine derivatives [e.g., chlorpromazine (VIII)] as tranquilizers prompted the further detailed biological evaluation of these compounds. Accordingly, Jackson and Smith in 1956 (*19*) indicated that definite analgesia could be obtained in postoperative patients with the use of 10 to 20 mg of chlorpromazine given by injection. However, these results were open to question on the basis of the statistical clinical studies of Houde and Wallenstein (*20*).

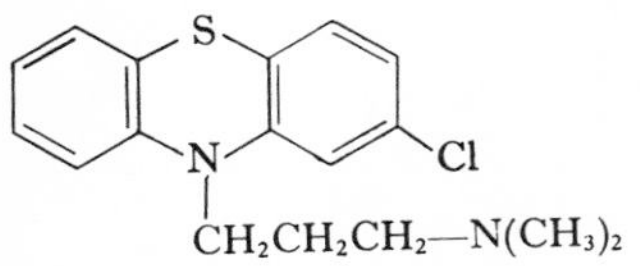

Chlorpromazine
(VIII)

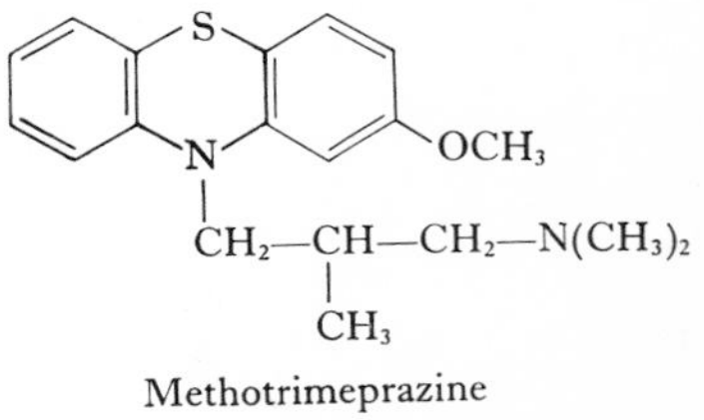

Methotrimeprazine
(IX)

In 1961 Lasagna and DeKornfeld (*21*) carried out a clinical study on the analgetic action of methotrimeprazine (IX) in postoperative and postpartum patients. The results of this work are shown in Figs. 1 and 2.

The postoperative patients were treated by injection, whereas the drug was administered orally to the postpartum patients.

410

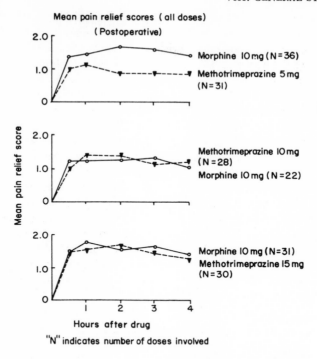

FIG. 1. Mean pain relief scores for post-operative patients.

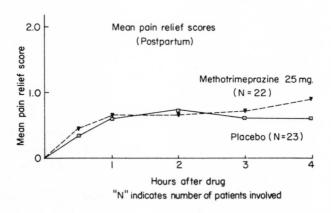

FIG. 2. Mean pain relief scores for post-partum patients.

On the basis of these findings, Lasagna and DeKornfeld concluded that methotrimeprazine when given by injection in doses of 10 to 15 mg is a potent analgetic, at lease as potent as morphine. An additional point of interest is that Deneau and Seevers (22) were unable to demonstrate physical dependence capacity for this compound in monkeys. Because of the possibility of confusing sedation with analgesia, special attention was given to the incidence of sleep. At the three dose levels studied, no evidence of excessive sedation was observed. Since patients were, in addition, routinely awakened for interview, Lasagna and DeKornfeld also observed that there was little opportunity for confusing sedation and analgesia in their experiments.

Doses of 25 mg of this compound when given by mouth for the relief of ambulatory patients with postpartum pain (Fig. 2), however, produced side effects but did not produce analgesia which was superior to that achieved with a placebo. This is not too surprising since morphine, for example, when given in 10 mg doses orally, also cannot be distinguished from placebo.

These results have prompted additional clinical investigations with methotrimeprazine as well as with several other phenothiazine derivatives and these are presently in progress (23).

V. Benzimidazoles

In 1957 Hoffmann and co-workers (Hunger, Kebrle, and Rossi) (24) discovered a new class of analgetics which contained the benzimidazole ring system. One of the first compounds prepared by this group was 1-(β-diethylaminoethyl)-2-benzylbenzimidazole (X) which was found to be about one-tenth as active as morphine when tested in mice according to the method of Gross (25). This finding was of sufficient interest to cause this group to undertake a broad synthetic program to determine the structure-activity relationship of this new and unexplored series.

Two synthetic methods were studied. Firstly, the general scheme for the synthesis of benzimidazole was used (Scheme 2). This involves the condensation of o-phenylenediamine with benzyl cyanide. The resulting 2-benzylbenzimidazole was then alkylated with the desired dialkylamino-alkylene chloride. This procedure was useful for the preparation of compounds without substituents on the benzimidazole benzene ring (26).

However, a more versatile synthesis was developed for the preparation of benzimidazole substituted derivatives (27) (see Scheme 3). This method was particularly useful in the preparation of the 4, 5, 6, or 7-nitrobenzimidazoles The choice of substituted phenylacetic acid imino ether afforded compounds with diverse substituents on the benzene ring at the 2 position.

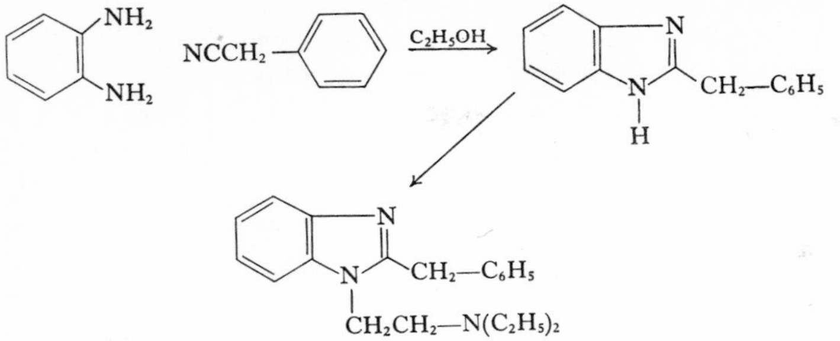

Scheme 2

$$\text{o-diaminobenzene (NH}_2, \text{NH}_2) + \text{NCCH}_2\!-\!\text{C}_6\text{H}_5 \xrightarrow{\text{C}_2\text{H}_5\text{OH}} \text{benzimidazole, N, N-H, CH}_2\!-\!\text{C}_6\text{H}_5$$

(X) 2-benzyl-1-(2-diethylaminoethyl)benzimidazole

N, CH$_2$—C$_6$H$_5$, CH$_2$CH$_2$—N(C$_2$H$_5$)$_2$

SCHEME 2

Scheme 3

$$R\text{—(NO}_2, \text{Cl)} \xrightarrow{\text{H}_2\text{N—CH}_2\text{CH}_2\text{—N(C}_2\text{H}_5)_2} R\text{—(NO}_2, \text{NH—CH}_2\text{CH}_2\text{—N(CH}_3)_2)} \xrightarrow{(\text{NH}_4)_2\text{S}}$$

$$R\text{—(NH}_2, \text{NH—CH}_2\text{CH}_2\text{—N(C}_2\text{H}_5)_2) + \underset{\text{CH}_2,\ \text{C}_6\text{H}_5}{\overset{\text{C}_2\text{H}_5}{\text{O—C=N—H}}} \longrightarrow R\text{—benzimidazole (4,5,6,7; N3, N1, 2-CH}_2\text{—C}_6\text{H}_5, \text{CH}_2\text{CH}_2\text{—N(C}_2\text{H}_5)_2)}$$

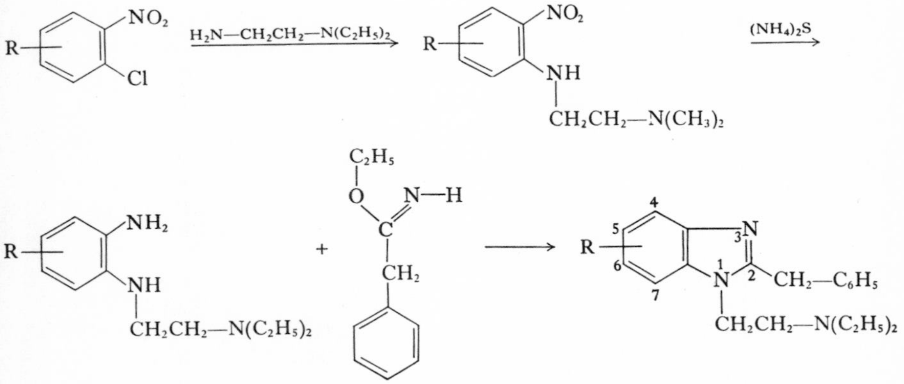

SCHEME 3

The compounds prepared in this series and their analgetic effects as compared to morphine are listed in Tables IV, V, and VI. Out of this list the Hoffmann group were able to deduce a structure-activity relationship which is summarized in Table VII.

(*i*) *Substitution at N1.* Optimum activity is obtained with compounds in which the basic side chain in position 1 of the benzimidazole nucleus is diethylaminoethyl. Substitution with piperidinoethyl also gives good activity. Contrary to the findings in the methadone and propoxyphene series, the diethylaminoethyl compounds are much more potent than the dimethyl-aminoethyl derivatives.

(*ii*) *Effect of nitro group.* A nitro group at the 5 position of the benzimidazole moiety was necessary for maximum activity. A 6-nitro group was also effective but this was only in the case where the other substituents were

413

TABLE IV

SUBSTITUTED BENZIMIDAZOLES

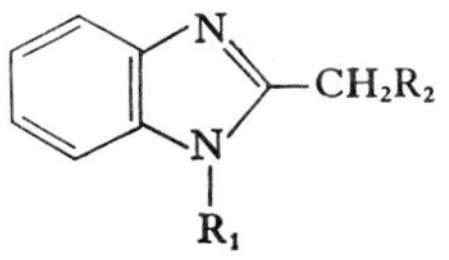

R_1	R_2	Analgetic Activity (Morphine = 1)
—$CH_2CH_2N(CH_3)_2$	—C_6H_5	0
—$CH_2CH_2N(C_2H_5)_2$	—C_6H_5	0.1
—$CH_2CH_2NC_5H_{10}$	—C_6H_5	0
—$CH_2CH(CH_3)N(CH_3)_2$	—C_6H_5	0
—$CH_2CH_2N(CH_3)_2$	—C_6H_4-4'-Cl	0
—$CH_2CH_2N(C_2H_5)_2$	—C_6H_4-4'-Cl	0.1
—$CH_2CH(CH_3)N(CH_3)_2$	—C_6H_4-4'-Cl	0
—$CH_2CH_2NC_5H_{10}$	—C_6H_4-4'-Cl	0
—$CH_2CH_2N(C_2H_4)_2O$	—C_6H_4-4'-Cl	0
—$CH_2CH_2N(C_2H_5)_2$	—C_6H_4-2'-Cl	0
—$CH_2CH_2N(C_2H_5)_2$	—C_6H_5-3'-OH	0
—$CH_2CH_2N(C_2H_5)_2$	—C_6H_5-3'-OCH$_3$	< 0.1
—$CH_2CH_2N(C_2H_5)_2$	—C_6H_3-3',4'-(OH)$_2$	0
—$CH_2CH_2N(C_2H_5)_2$	—C_6H_3-3',4'-(OCH$_3$)$_2$	0.15
—$CH_2CH_2N(C_2H_5)_2$	—C_6H_4-4'-OH	0
—$CH_2CH_2N(C_2H_5)_2$	—C_6H_4-4'-OCH$_3$	1
—$CH_2CH_2N(C_2H_5)_2$	—C_6H_4-4'-OC$_2$H$_5$	70
—$CH_2CH_2N(C_2H_5)_2$	—C_6H_4-4'-O-(n-C$_3$H$_7$)	10
—$CH_2CH_2N(C_2H_5)_2$	—C_6H_4-4'-O-(n-C$_4$H$_9$)	0.5
—$CH_2CH_2N(C_2H_5)_2$	—C_6H_4-2'-CH$_3$	0
—$CH_2CH_2N(C_2H_5)_2$	—C_6H_4-4'-CH$_3$	0.5
—$CH_2CH_2N(C_2H_5)_2$	—C_6H_4-4'-C$_2$H$_5$	0.5
—$CH_2CH_2N(C_2H_5)_2$	—C_6H_4-4'-(n-C$_3$H$_7$)	2
—$CH_2CH_2N(C_2H_5)_2$	—C_6H_4-4'-(n-C$_4$H$_9$)	0.1
—$CH_2CH_2N(C_2H_5)_2$	—C_6H_4-4'-CHOHCH$_3$	0.5
—$CH_2CH_2N(C_2H_5)_2$	—C_6H_4-4'-NO$_2$	0
—$CH_2CH_2N(C_2H_5)_2$	—C_6H_4-4'-NH$_2$	0
—$CH_2CH_2N(CH_3)_2$	—C_6H_4-4'-OC$_2$H$_5$	1.25
—$CH_2CH_2NC_5H_{10}$	—C_6H_4-4'-OC$_2$H$_5$	10
—$CH_2CH_2NC_4H_8$	—C_6H_4-4'-OC$_2$H$_5$	20
—$CH_2CH_2N(C_2H_5)_2O$	—C_6H_4-4'-OC$_2$H$_5$	0.2

TABLE V

SUBSTITUTED BENZIMIDAZOLES

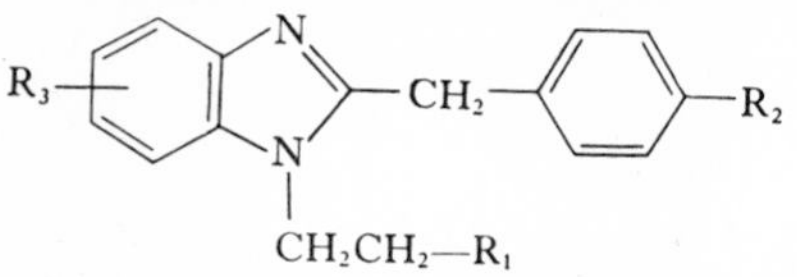

$$R_3 \underset{CH_2CH_2-R_1}{\overline{}} \text{benzimidazole} - CH_2 - \overline{} - R_2$$

R_1	R_2	R_3	Analgetic activity (morphine = 1)
$-N(C_2H_5)_2$	-4'-Cl	-4-NO_2	0
$-N(C_2H_5)_2$	—H	-5-NO_2	2
$-N(CH_3)_2$	-4'-Cl	-5-NO_2	0.3
$-N(C_2H_5)_2$	-4'-Cl	-5-NO_2	3
$-N(C_2H_5)_2$	-4'-F	-5-NO_2	1
$-N(C_2H_5)_2$	-2'-CH_3	-5-NO_2	0.2
$-N(C_2H_5)_2$	-2'-5'-$(CH_3)_2$	-5-NO_2	0
$-N(C_2H_5)_2$	-4'-CH_3	-5-NO_2	10
$-N(C_2H_5)_2$	-4'-CH_2CH_3	-5-NO_2	20
$-N(C_2H_5)_2$	-4'-$(CH_2)_2CH_3$	-5-NO_2	50
$-N(C_2H_5)_2$	-4'-$(CH_2)_3CH_3$	-5-NO_2	1
$-N(C_2H_5)_2$	-4'-$C(CH_3)_3$	-5-NO_2	2
$-N(C_2H_5)_2$	-2'-5'-$(OH)_2$	-5-NO_2	0
$-N(C_2H_5)_2$	-4'-OH	-5-NO_2	1
$-N(C_2H_5)_2$	-3'-OCH_3	-5-NO_2	2
$-N(C_2H_5)_2$	-3'-4'-$(OCH_3)_2$	-5-NO_2	10
$-N(CH_3)_2$	-4'-OCH_3	-5-NO_2	< 5
$-N(C_2H_5)_2$	-4'-OCH_3	-5-NO_2	100
$-N(CH_3)_2$	-4'-OC_2H_5	-5-NO_2	20
$-N(C_2H_5)_2$	-4'-OC_2H_5	-5-NO_2	1000
$-N(C_5H_{10})$	-4'-OC_2H_5	-5-NO_2	100
$-N(CH_2CH_2)_2O$	-4'-OC_2H_5	-5-NO_2	2
$-CH_2N(C_2H_5)_2$	-4'-OC_2H_5	-5-NO_2	0.2
$-N(C_2H_5)_2$	-4'-$OCH(CH_3)_2$	-5-NO_2	500
$-N(C_2H_5)_2$	-4'-$O(CH_2)_2CH_3$	-5-NO_2	200
$-N(C_2H_5)_2$	-4'-$O(CH_2)_3CH_3$	-5-NO_2	5
$-N(C_2H_5)_2$	-4'-$O(CH_2)_2OC_2H_5$	-5-NO_2	50
$-N(C_2H_5)_2$	-4'-$(OCH_2CH_2)_3OCH_3$	-5-NO_2	3
$-N(C_2H_5)_2$	-4'-$(OCH_2CH_2)_9OCH_3$	-5-NO_2	0.1
$-N(C_2H_5)_2$	-4'-$OCOCH_3$	-5-NO_2	5
$-N(C_2H_5)_2$	-4'-SCH_3	-5-NO_2	50
$-N(C_2H_5)_2$	-4'-SC_2H_5	-5-NO_2	30
$-N(C_2H_5)_2$	-4'-$S(CH_2)_2CH_3$	-5-NO_2	2
$-N(C_2H_5)_2$	-4'-$S(CH_2)_3CH_3$	-5-NO_2	0.25
$-N(C_2H_5)_2$	-4'-NO_2	-5-NO_2	0.2

415

TABLE V—*continued*

R_1	R_2	R_3	Analgetic Activity (morphine=1)
—N(CH$_3$)$_2$	—H	-6-NO$_2$	0.07
—N(C$_2$H$_5$)$_2$	—H	-6-NO$_2$	0.3
—CH$_2$N(CH$_3$)$_2$	—H	-6-NO$_2$	0
—N(C$_2$H$_5$)$_2$	-4'-Cl	-6-NO$_2$	0.1
—N(C$_2$H$_5$)$_2$	-2'-CH$_3$	-6-NO$_2$	0.2
—N(C$_2$H$_5$)$_2$	-2'-5'-(CH$_3$)$_2$	-6-NO$_2$	0
—N(C$_2$H$_5$)$_2$	-3'-CH$_3$	-6-NO$_2$	0
—N(C$_2$H$_5$)$_2$	-4'-CH$_3$	-6-NO$_2$	0.5
—N(C$_2$H$_5$)$_2$	-4'-OC$_2$H$_5$	-6-NO$_2$	20
—N(C$_2$H$_5$)$_2$	-4'-Cl	-7-NO$_2$	0
—N(C$_2$H$_5$)$_2$	-4'-OC$_2$H$_5$	-7-NO$_2$	0
—N(C$_2$H$_5$)$_2$	—H	-5-NH$_2$	0
—N(C$_2$H$_5$)$_2$	-4'-Cl	-5-NH$_2$	0
—N(C$_2$H$_5$)$_2$	-4'-CH$_3$	-5-NH$_2$	0
—N(C$_2$H$_5$)$_2$	-4'-OCH$_3$	-5-NH$_2$	0
—N(C$_2$H$_5$)$_2$	-4'-OC$_2$H$_5$	-5-NH$_2$	2
—N(C$_2$H$_5$)$_2$	—H	-6-NH$_2$	0
—N(C$_2$H$_5$)$_2$	-4'-Cl	-7-NH$_2$	0

TABLE VI

SUBSTITUTED BENZIMIDAZOLES

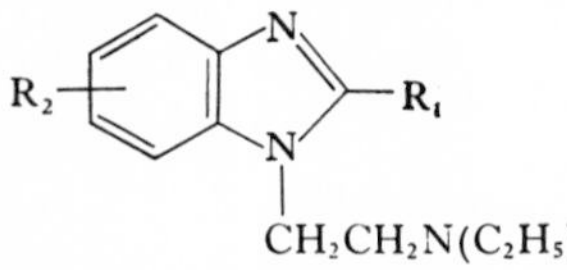

$CH_2CH_2N(C_2H_5)_2$

R_1	R_2	Analgetic activity (morphine = 1)
—CH(CH$_3$)C$_6$H$_5$	-5-NO$_2$	2
—CH(C$_2$H$_5$)C$_6$H$_5$	-5-NO$_2$	0.5
—C(CH$_3$)$_2$C$_6$H$_5$	-5-NO$_2$	0.7
—CH(CH$_3$)C$_6$H$_4$-4'-OCH$_3$	-5-NO$_2$	50
—CH=CH—C$_6$H$_5$	-5-NO$_2$	0
—CH$_2$CH$_2$C$_6$H$_5$	-5-NO$_2$	0
—CH$_2$CH$_2$C$_6$H$_4$-4'-OC$_2$H$_5$	-5-NO$_2$	50
—CH$_2$(α-naphthyl)	-5-NO$_2$	0.5
—CH$_2$-2'-C$_5$H$_4$N	-5-NO$_2$	0.2
—CH$_2$-2'-C$_4$H$_3$S	-5-NO$_2$	1
—CH$_2$-(α-naphthyl)	-6-NO$_2$	0

TABLE VII

ANALGETIC ACTIVITIES IN MICE OF BENZIMIDAZOLE DERIVATIVES
(RELATIVE TO MORPHINE = 1)

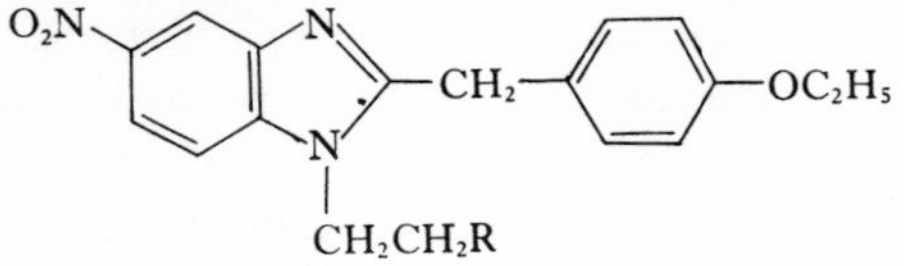

R =	$-N(CH_3)_2$	$-N(C_2H_5)_2$	$-NC_5H_{10}$	$-N(C_2H_4)_2O$	$-CH_2N(C_2H_5)_2$
Activity	20	1000	100	2	0.2

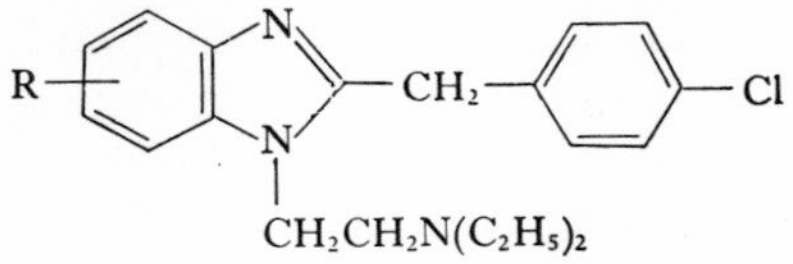

R =	$-H$	$4-NO_2$	$5-NO_2$	$6-NO_2$	$7-NO_2$
Activity	0.1	0	3	0.1	0

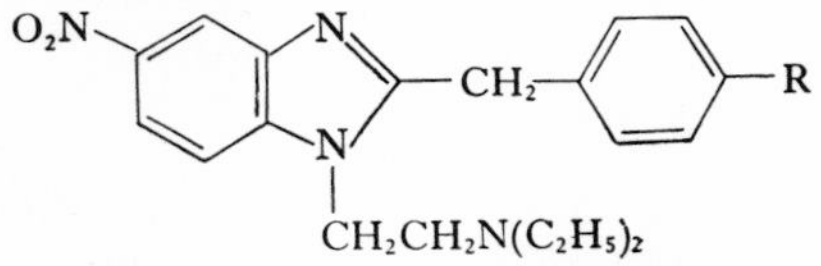

R =	$-H$	$-OCH_3$	$-OC_2H_5$	$-OCH(CH_3)_2$	$-OCH_2)_2CH_3$	$-O(CH_2)_3CH_3$
Activity	2	100	1000	500	200	5
R =	$-H$	$-SCH_3$	$-SC_2H_5$		$-S(CH_2)_2CH_3$	$-S(CH_2)_3CH_3$
Activity	2	50	30		2	0.25
R =	$-H$	$-CH_3$	$-CH_2CH_3$		$-(CH_2)_2CH_3$	$-(CH_2)_3CH_3$
Activity	2	10	20		50	1

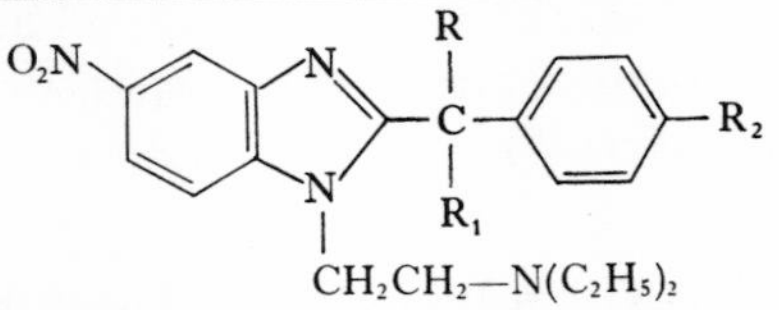

R =	$-H$	$-CH_3$	$-C_2H_5$	$-CH_3$	$-CONH_2$	$-H$	$-CH_3$	$-CONH_2$
$R_1 =$	$-H$	$-H$	$-H$	$-CH_3$	$-H$	$-H$	$-H$	$-H$
$R_2 =$	$-H$	$-H$	$-H$	$-H$	$-H$	$4-OC_2H_5$	$4-OC_2H_5$	$4-OC_2H_5$
Activity	2	2	2	0.7	2.5	1000	100	200

present for maximum activity. Thus, 1-(β-diethylaminoethyl)-2-(4'-ethoxybenzyl)-6-nitrobenzimidazole was one fiftieth as active as an analgetic as its corresponding 5-nitro derivative. The 4- nitro and 7-nitro analogs were inactive.

(*iii*) *Benzyl group substitutions.* Substitutions at the 2 or 3 position of the benzyl group did not give compounds with pronounced analgetic effects. However, substitution at the 4 position, in general, afforded active substances. This was especially so with alkoxy groups. The thioethers also gave potent compounds. Substitution of the methylene group joining phenyl and benzimidazole gave compounds with varying activity. The intensity of activity of such substituted compounds was dependent on the substituent at the 4 position of the benzyl group.

In summary, the structure-activity relationship study in animals revealed that compound XI gave maximum analgetic activity (i.e., 1000 times more active than morphine). Any deviation from this structure gave less active substances, the activity varying from zero to 500 times that of morphine.

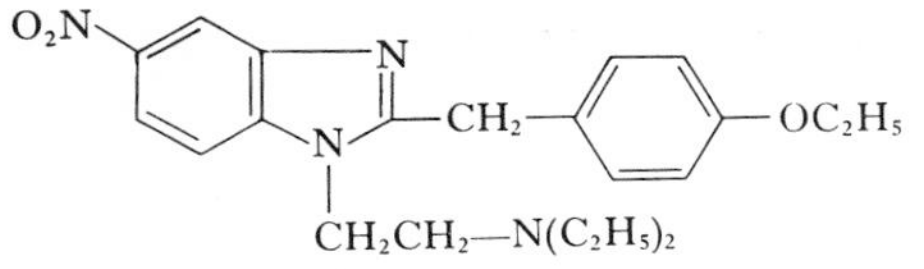

(XI)

Several of the most active compounds were submitted for clinical evaluation. The same order of activity was observed in humans when these compounds were given by injection. However, these substances all caused respiratory depression to a greater or lesser degree. As a matter of fact, when they were given by injection the therapeutic ratio between analgetic and respiratory depression activity was quite narrow and thus offered no advantage over morphine. The analgetic effect of these benzimidazoles when administered orally was weak and irregular. Finally, the most active compound was reported by Fraser *et al.* (*28*) to have addiction potential comparable to morphine. All of these factors were responsible for the discontinuation of further clinical trials (*29*).

VI. 3,8-Diazabicyclo[3.2.1]octanes

Within the past five years Cignarella and co-workers (*30, 31*) at Lepetit have focused their attention on the synthesis and biological evaluation of 3,8-diazabicyclo[3.2.1]octanes. These compounds have been prepared because they bear some resemblance to piperazine if one considers them as bicyclic analogs of this nitrogen-containing heterocycle. Since the pharmacological activity of substituted piperazines is well documented, it seemed of interest to the Lepetit scientists to compare the compounds of both groups in order to assess the influence of the endoethylenic bridge in this structure. A further reason for investigation was given by the structural analogy of 8-methyl-3,8-diazabicyclo[3.2.1]octane (XII) with tropane, whose derivatives are known to possess interesting pharmacological properties. In addition, it was of interest to synthesize derivatives of 3-methyl-3,8-diazabicyclo[3.2.1]octane (XIII).

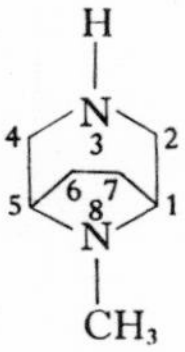

(XII)

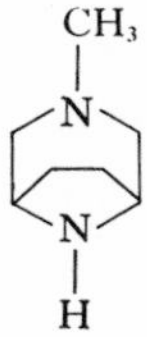

(XIII)

A. 8-METHYL-3,8-DIAZABICYCLO[3.2.1]OCTANE (31)

The synthesis of this heterocycle is outlined in scheme 4. 2,5-Dicarbethoxypyrrolidine was allowed to react with benzylamine to afford 2-benzylcarbamyl-5-carbethoxypyrrolidine. Heating of this substance to 200° yielded the cyclic 2,4-dione derivative which was then reduced with lithium aluminium hydride to give 3-benzyl-3,8-diazabicyclo[3.2.1]octane. Methylation of the 3-benzyl intermediate with formic acid and formaldehyde

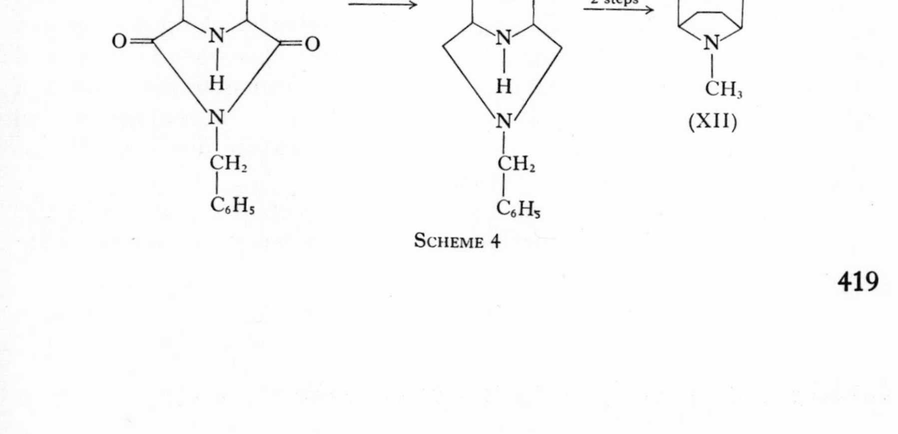

SCHEME 4

followed by hydrogenolysis yielded 8-methyl-3,8-diazabicyclo[3.2.1]octane (XII). The 3-substituted derivatives of this compound were prepared by the usual methods.

B. 3-METHYL-3,8-DIAZABICYCLO[3.2.1]octane (*32*)

The synthesis of this compound is formulated in Scheme 5.

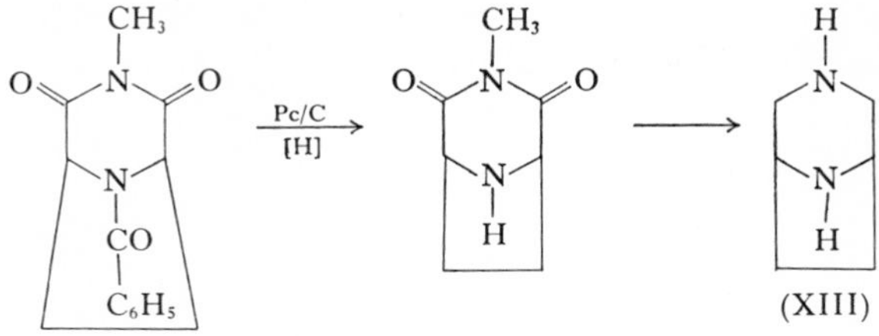

SCHEME 5

As pointed out previously, the configuration of the N—R group at position 8 is such that the endoethylene bridge 1–5 repels the 8-substituent toward the piperazine ring; by contrast the 3-substituent is not deflected in any particular direction. With this consideration in mind, Cignarella and co-workers (*33*) evaluated these compounds for their biological effects. It was noted initially that the 3-methyl-3,8-bicyclo[3.2.1]octane derivatives exhibited some analgetic action when tested by the method of Randall and Selitto (*34*). A more detailed biological study further indicated that this activity is shown primarily by the 3-methyl-8-acyl-3,8-diazabicyclo[3.2.1]-octanes. Some of the compounds initially evaluated are shown in Table VIII. The 8-propionyl derivative (XIV) when injected intraperitoneally in rats or when given orally is the most effective of this group of compounds. Replacement of the propionyl group by other acyl groups led to a diminution in analgetic activity; the replacement also with carbomethoxy, carbethoxy, and phenylcarbamoyl gave products which were scarcely active.

On the basis of these results, it was concluded that any modification of the 8-propionyl group did not lead to substances with improved analgetic effects. Thus, a group of compounds were prepared in which the 8-propionyl group was left intact and changes were made at the 3-position. The choice of the 3-substituent was based on similar studies concerning the substitution of the methyl group bonded to the nitrogen in analgetics such as morphine and meperidine (See Chapters IV and V). In Table IX are listed these compounds and their analgetic activities.

The 3-cinnamyl-8-propionyl-3,8-bicyclo[3.2.1]octane was the most active compound in this series. It showed an analgetic potency approximately 25-

420

TABLE VIII

ANALGETIC ACTIVITY OF 8-SUBSTITUTED -3-METHYL-3,8-BICYCLO[3.2.1]-
OCTANES

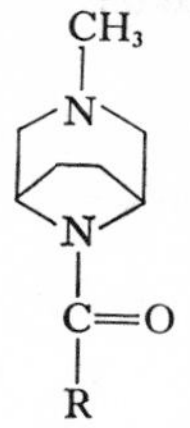

$$\begin{array}{c} CH_3 \\ | \\ N \\ \diagup\diagdown \\ N \\ | \\ C=O \\ | \\ R \end{array}$$

R	Dose (mg/kg)	Increase of pain threshold in rats (%)		Approximate LD_{50} (mg/kg) intraperitoneally in mice
		Intraperitoneally	Orally	
—CH$_3$	50	58	—	
	25	9	—	500
—C$_2$H$_5$	25	327	235	
	10	139	139	
	5	25	22.6	282
—C$_3$H$_7$	25	100	—	
	15	52.8	—	200
C$_6$H$_5$CH=CH—	10	52	—	
	5	19	—	50
—COOCH$_3$	25	10.4	—	200
—COOC$_2$H$_5$	25	48	—	
	15	7	—	200
C$_6$H$_5$NHCO—	10	12	—	50
Morphine HCl	5	186	—	
	3	90	—	410

fold that of the 3-methyl derivative and 10-fold that of morphine hydrochloride. The LD_{50} of this compound is at least 200 times higher than the
dose able to increase the pain threshold by 100%. The 8-benzoylethyl and
8-phenylpropyl derivatives were slightly less active. It is noteworthy that
these compounds are characterized by a rapid onset and short duration of
action. In analogy to the known narcotic analgetics, sublethal doses of the
active compounds in this series produce excitation, stereotyped movements,

421

TABLE IX

ANALGETIC ACTIVITY OF 3-SUBSTITUTED 8-PROPIONYL-3,8-DIAZABICYCLO[3.2.1]OCTANES IN
THE RAT, AND ACUTE TOXICITY IN THE MOUSE

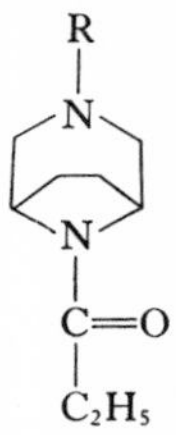

R
|
N
⟨ ⟩
N
|
C=O
|
C_2H_5

Compound	Dose (mg/kg) intraperitoneally	Increase of Pain Threshold (%)	Average duration of action (minutes)	Approximate LD_{50} (mg/kg) intraperitoneally (mouse)
H	25	10	—	300
C_2H_5	25	24	90	300
—C_3H_7	25	32	60	200
n-C_4H_9	10	36	60	300
	25	47.7	60	
	50	46.5	60	
$C_5H_9CH_2$[a]	25	26		200
$C_5H_9CH_2CH_2$[b]	5	23		200
	10	60	45	
C_6H_5	25	36.9		
$C_6H_5CH_2$	25	32	60	200
$C_6H_5CH_2CH_2$	3	32	90	600
	5	41.5	45	
$C_6H_5CH_2CH_2CH_2$	0.5	28	45	400
	1	99	45	
	2	142	60	
$C_6H_5CH{=}CH{—}CH_2$	0.1	46.5	60	73.01
	0.2	75.8	60	
	0.4	143	45	
$C_6H_5COCH_2CH_2$	0.1	11		185
	0.3	76	60	
	0.5	81	30	
	1	330	30	
$(C_6H_5)_2CH$	10	14.2		200
$HOCH_2CH_2$	50			1000
p-$H_2NC_6H_4COOCH_2CH_2$	50	25	30	600
$ClCH_2CH_2$	1	36	45	20
$(C_2H_5)_2NCH_2CH_2$	10	19	30	200
$C_6H_5NHCH_2CH_2$	1	48	45	400
	2	46	60	
C_2H_5CO	50	20		600
Morphine HCl	1.5	31.5	60	410[a]
	3	91	90	
	5	>170	120	
3-Methyl-8-propionyl-3,8-diazabicyclo[3.2.1]octane (XIV)	25	327	130	282
	10	139	90	
	5	25	90	

[a] Cyclopentylmethyl.   [b] Cyclopentylethyl.

and Straub-tail in mice. No clinical data are as yet available on this new group of analgetics.

By comparison, all the tested 3-acyl-8-methyl isomers were inactive as analgetics.

VII. Thiazolin-2-ones

Early in 1955, deStevens and co-workers embarked on a program involving the synthesis of thiazolin-2-ones which were to be submitted for broad biological testing. At the time the work was commenced, very little had been reported on the chemistry of this heterocycle with the exception of the classic work of Hantzsch (*35*) on the parent compound and its 4-methyl substituted derivative.

The initial efforts of the CIBA group were confined to thiazolin-2-ones fused to cycloalkeno moieties at the *d*-position of the heterocycle. Several methods were employed for the preparation of these heterocycles but the two methods shown in Scheme 6 proved to be the most useful (*36, 37*).

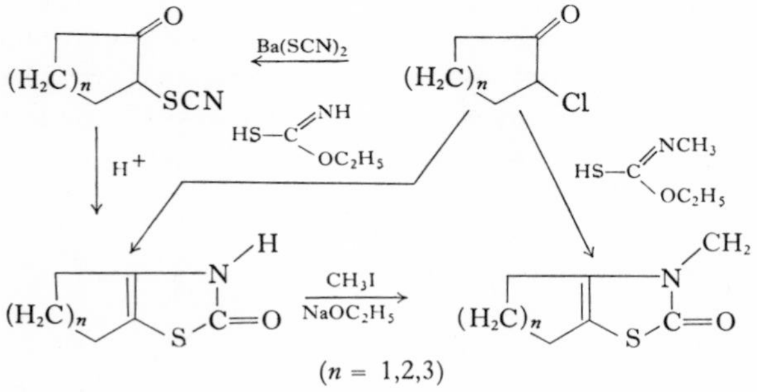

(n = 1,2,3)

SCHEME 6

A variety of cyclic ketones were used but only cyclopentanone will be considered describing the transformations in Scheme 6. α-Chlorocyclopentanone was converted to the α-thiocyano derivative which under hydrolytic conditions undergoes ring closure to the desired thiazolin-2-one. Alternatively, condensation of α-chlorocyclopentanone with ethyl xanthamidate gives rise to the same heterocycle. Methylation of 2,3,5,6-tetrahydro-4*H*-cyclopentathiazolin-2-one afforded the 3-methyl derivative which could also be obtained directly from condensation α-chlorocyclopentanone with ethyl-N-methylxanthamidate. Other 3-substituted thiazolin-2-ones were prepared by similar methods. A wide variety of cycloalkeno[*d*]thiazolin-2-ones and their 3-substituted derivatives were tested for analgetic activity according to the Wolff-Hardy principle as described by Gross. The

423

compound showing the most effective analgetic activity in experimental animals was 2,3,5,6-tetrahydro-3-methyl-4H-cyclopentathiazolin-2-one (XV) ($n = 1$). This compound was active by the oral and parenteral route and was characterized by a rapid onset of action (within 5 to 10 minutes after administration) and a maintenance of analgesia for several hours. It was approximately 5 times more potent than aminopyrine when tested in experimental animals. All substituents (e.g., alkyl, aryl, and aralkyl) at position 3 other than methyl resulted in a diminution in activity. Surprisingly, 2,3,4,5,6,7-hexahydrobenzothiazolin-2-one (XVI) was almost as active as XV and more active than its N-methyl derivative.

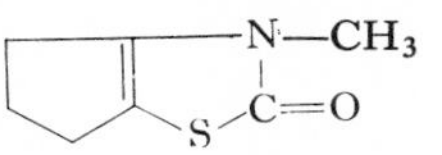

(XV) 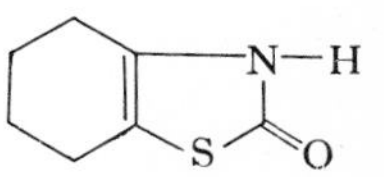   (XVI)

In addition, compound XV showed a better therapeutic ratio (4:1) than XVI (3:1). Encouraged by these results, the search for a more potent compound with a more favorable therapeutic ratio was then turned to compounds with substituents on the alicyclic portion of compounds XV and XVI. A facile approach to compounds of this type was through the Mannich reaction. The sequence of reactions leading to Su-4432, the most important compound in this series, is shown in Scheme 7 (*38*).

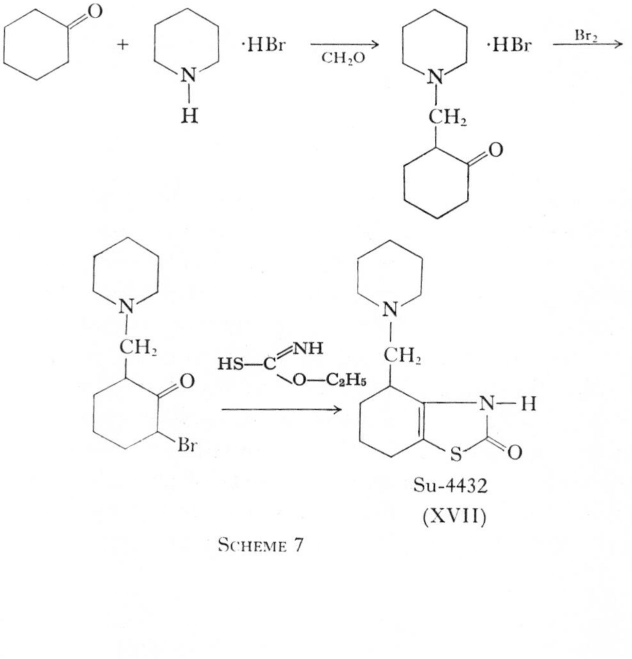

Su-4432

(XVII)

SCHEME 7

The Mannich base was brominated to the α-bromoketone which was allowed to react with ethyl xanthamidate to yield Su-4432. In experimental animals, this substance was found to be as potent as codeine with a rapid onset of action (5 minutes). The N-methyl derivative was slightly less active. The related compound and its N-methyl derivative in the cyclopenta-thiazolin-2-one series were less active and quite toxic. In Table X is listed

TABLE X

CYCLOALKENO[d]THIAZOLIN-2-ONES

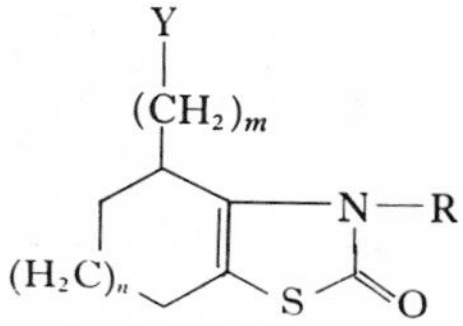

n	m	R	Y	Analgetic effect (codeine = 10)
1	0	H	$N(CH_3)_2$	0
1	0	H	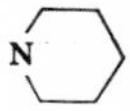 (piperidino)	0
1	0	CH_3	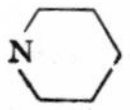 (piperidino)	0
0	1	H	$N(CH_3)_2$	5
0	1	H	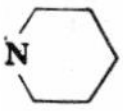 (piperidino)	5
0	1	CH_3	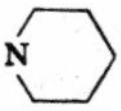 (piperidino)	3
0	1	H	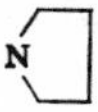 (pyrrolidino)	5
0	1	H	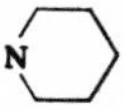 (piperidino)	5
1	1	H	$N(CH_3)_2$	6
1	1	H	$N(C_2H_5)_2$	6
1	1	H	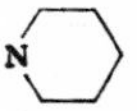 (piperidino)	10

TABLE X—*continued*

n	m	R	Y	Analgetic effect (codeine = 10)
1	1	CH_3	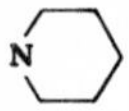 (N-piperidino ring)	5
1	1	H	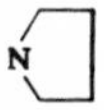 (N-pyrrolidino ring)	6
1	1	H	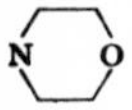 (N-morpholino ring)	6
1	1	H	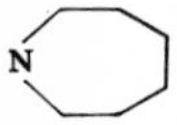 (N-azepanyl, 7-membered ring)	5
1	1	H	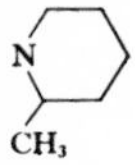 (N-(2-methyl)piperidino, CH_3)	10
1	1	H	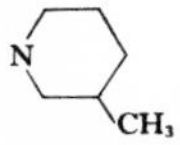 (N-(3-methyl)piperidino, CH_3)	10
1	1	H	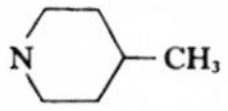 (N-(4-methyl)piperidino, CH_3)	10

some of the compounds prepared and their analgetic activities. Noticeable decrease in activity was observed when the piperidino moiety was exchanged for the dimethylamino, the pyrrolidino, or the morpholino group. Compounds containing ring-substituted piperidino groups were as effective as Su-4432.

The synthesis of compounds in which the tertiary amino group is attached directly to the cyclohexene moiety is outlined in Scheme 8.

These substances were devoid of analgetic effects. Finally, to round out

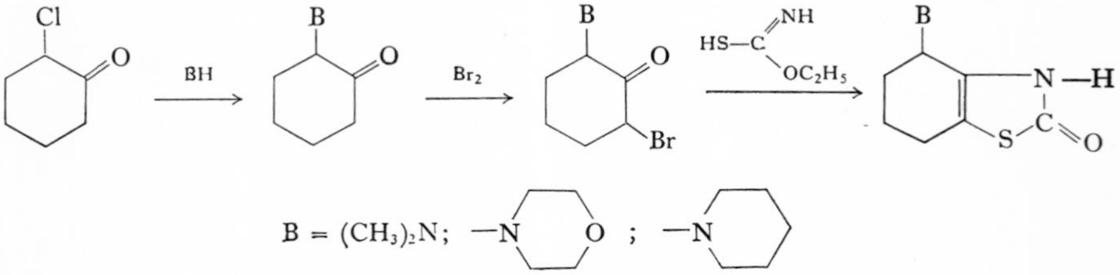

$$B = (CH_3)_2N; \quad -N\diagdown O \; ; \quad -N\diagdown$$

SCHEME 8

the structure-activity relationship study, compounds XVIII–XXI were synthesized.

(XVIII)

(XIX)

(XX)

(XXI)

Compounds XVIII and XIX were weakly active, XX was inactive, and XXI was about one-half as active as Su-4432 but more toxic.

As indicated earlier, Su-4432 proved to be the most effective analgetic of this series when tested by the tail flick method in unanesthetized mice. This effect is shown in Fig. 3.

Doses as low as 10 mg/kg subcutaneously showed threshold effects while

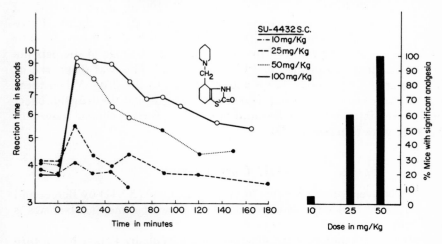

FIG. 3. Analgetic effect (subcutaneously) of Su-4432.

427

doses of 25 mg/kg produced statistically significant effects in over 50% of the mice tested. Since the LD_{50} of this compound in mice was around 225 mg/kg subcutaneously, a therapeutic ratio of more than 10:1 could be established.

When given orally (see Fig. 4) Su-4432 showed definite analgetic effects in doses of 75 mg/kg, whereas threshold effects could be observed with doses as low as 50 mg/kg. The onset of action was rapid (5–10 minutes) and the effect was sustained for approximately 90–100 minutes.

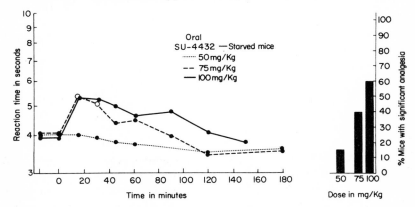

FIG. 4. Analgetic effect (orally) of Su-4432.

Clinical evaluation of Su-4432 in doses of 50–100 mg given orally three times daily established this compound to be an effective analgetic. These studies were carried out in over 100 patients for a period of 6 months with significant promising results. However, a small percentage of the patients taking the drug complained of "blurred vision." This was diagnosed as inflammation of the optic nerve and attributed to the drug. When these patients were taken off the drug vision returned to normal, the drug side effect being reversible. Because of this undesired effect, further clinical trials with Su-4432 were terminated (*39*).

VIII. Carisoprodol

The discovery and development of meprobamate (XXII) by Berger and co-workers has led to the widespread use of carbamates and dicarbamates as tranquilizers and muscle relaxants.

Further exploitation of the dicarbamate molecule by Berger has in turn resulted in the preparation of substances that appear to have a slightly different mode of action from meprobamate. One such substance is N-iso-propyl-2-methyl-2-propyl-1,3-propanedioldicarbamate (XXIII), generically known as carisoprodol (40).

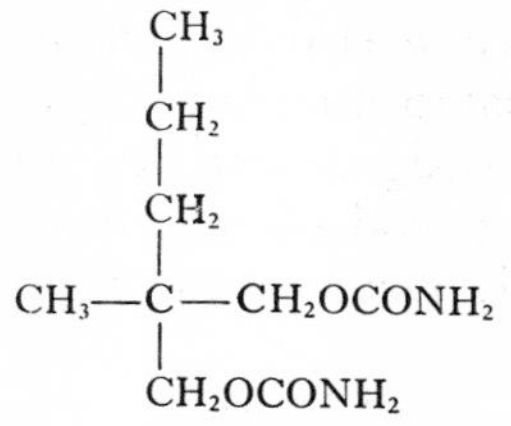

$$CH_3$$
$$|$$
$$CH_2$$
$$|$$
$$CH_2$$
$$|$$
$$CH_3-C-CH_2OCONH_2$$
$$|$$
$$CH_2OCONH_2$$

Meprobamate

(XXII)

$$CH_3$$
$$|$$
$$CH_2$$
$$|$$
$$CH_2 \qquad O \qquad CH_3$$
$$| \qquad \parallel \qquad CH$$
$$CH_3-C-CH_2-O-C-N \qquad CH_3$$
$$| \qquad \qquad H$$
$$CH_2-O-C-NH_2$$
$$\parallel$$
$$O$$

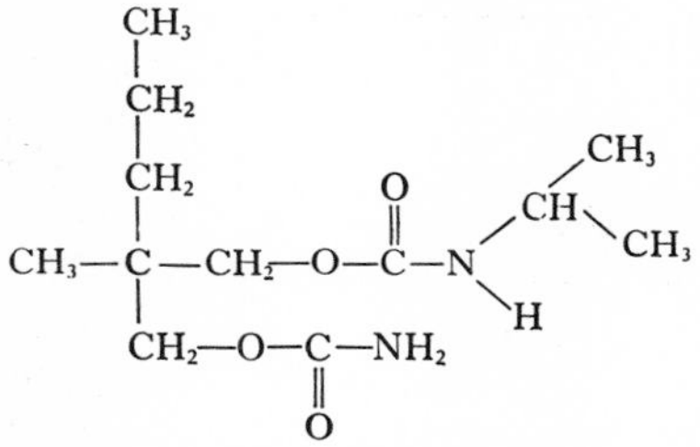

Carisoprodol

(XXIII)

Carisoprodol was compared primarily with mephenesin and meprobamate for its muscle relaxant effects. These compounds were evaluated according to four pharmacological actions: the paralysis of intact animals, the depression of spinal reflexes, the anticonvulsant effect, and the relief of decerebrate rigidity. In these tests carisoprodol was found to resemble other relaxants in producing reversible paralysis of skeletal muscles and depressing multineuronal reflexes to a greater extent than it depresses simple ones. However, it differs from other compounds in that it is a poor strychnine antagonist and it is much more effective in alleviating decerebrate rigidity. Thus, Berger et al. concluded that carisoprodol may have a different mode of action or act at different sites other than centrally acting skeletal muscle relaxants.

Carisoprodol was then evaluated by these investigators for its analgetic effects. The writing test method was used in one study and the substance was found to be devoid of analgetic effects. The effect of carisoprodol on the withdrawal reaction produced in mice placed on a hot plate was investigated according to the method of Woolfe and MacDonald (41). This compound

429

did not produce analgesia in any of the animals receiving 50 to 100 mg/kg. On the contrary, Berger *et al.* noted that the mice receiving the drug appeared to react to the heat somewhat more rapidly than the untreated control animals. They suggested that this increased reactivity indicates that muscular relaxation at this dose level does not interfere in any way with the responsiveness of the animal to stimulation.

To uncover any latent analgetic activity, Berger studied the effect of carisprodol given jointly with codeine which is known to produce analgesia with this test procedure. The results of this study are shown in Table XI.

TABLE XI

EFFECT OF CODEINE SULFATE GIVEN ALONE OR JOINTLY WITH CARISOPRODOL OR MEPRO-
BAMATE ON THE REACTION OF MICE TO HEAT

Preparation/Dose	$\left[\dfrac{\text{No. of mice with analgesia}}{\text{No. of mice used}}\right]$	Mean analgesic dose ± S.C.
Codeine, 10 mg/kg	0/30 ⎤	
Codeine, 16 mg/kg	12/30 ⎬	19.0 ± 0.96
Codeine, 24 mg/kg	20/30 ⎦	
Carisoprodol, 50 mg/kg	0/10	—
Meprobamate, 50 mg/kg	0/10	—
Codeine, 7 mg/kg, + carisoprodol, 50 mg/kg	1/30 ⎤	
Codeine, 10 mg/kg, + carisoprodol, 50 mg/kg	6/30 ⎬	13.9 ± 0.93
Codeine, 16 mg/kg, + carisoprodol, 50 mg/kg	19/30 ⎦	
Codeine, 10 mg/kg, + meprobamate, 50 mg/kg	4/30 ⎤	
Codeine, 16 mg/kg, + meprobamate, 50 mg/kg	12/30 ⎬	19.3 ± 1.79
Codeine, 24 mg/kg, + meprobamate, 50 mg/kg	19/30 ⎦	

At 50 mg/kg carisoprodol appears to increase the analgetic action of codeine. Meprobamate does not possess such synergistic effects.

Carisoprodol was compared with acetylsalicylic acid (aspirin) and with codeine in its ability to alleviate pain due to the electrical stimulation of tooth pulp. The results of this study are shown in Table XII.

The subjects were 19 healthy men and women, 22 to 52 years of age. Carisoprodol, in doses of 700 mg, showed a significant analgetic effect at 1 and 2 hours after drug administration. Codeine phosphate, 30 mg, had a similar effect, but appeared somewhat more effective in elevating the threshold to painful stimulation of the tooth pulp after 1 hour and less effective

TABLE XII

Preparation	Dose	Pain threshold					
		After 60 minutes (%)		t	After 120 minutes (%)		t
Carisoprodol	700 mg (tablets)	113	9.4^a	2.15	151	20.5^a	2.33
Placebo (lactose)	2 tablets	87	7.8^b	—	99	8.8	—
Placebo (lactose)	2 capsules	99	5.8	—	103	7.2	—
Codeine phosphate	30 mg (capsules)	128	8.3^a	2.48	130	10.1^b	2.21
Acetylsalicylic acid	600 mg (capsules)	108	7.2	0.98	109	9.2	0.51
Meprobamate	800 mg (capsules)	87	6.1	1.38	100	7.4	0.29

^{a} Differs significantly from appropriate placebo: $p \leqq 0.05$.

^{b} Not significantly different from capsule placebo: $t = 1.23, p > 0.2$.

than carisoprodol 2 hours after administration. Aspirin, 600 mg, produced a small increase in threshold that was not statistically significant. Meprobamate, 800 mg, did not increase the pain threshold. Thus, Berger concluded that carisoprodol exerts its analgetic action in humans independently of its muscle relaxant action. He was also able to show that this drug is free of addiction liability.

IX. Phenyramidol

Phenyramidol (XXIV) was synthesized by Gray (42) according to the method outlined in Scheme 9.

This compound was evaluated for its analgetic properties in experimental animals by O'Dell (43) and was found to be significantly effective. It was then compared with codeine, d-propoxyphene, carisoprodol, and aspirin in mice according to the radiant-heat stimulus method. As an analgetic, phenyramidol appeared to be comparable to codeine and was superior to the other drugs listed. When these compounds were tested by O'Dell for analgesia in rabbits by the tooth pulp stimulation method, phenyramidol compared favorably with codeine and was superior to d-propoxyphene and carisoprodol. In addition, it was found that this compound induced skeletal relaxation by means of interneuronal blockade.

These desirable properties prompted clinical investigation. Batterman (44) studied the analgetic effects of phenyramidol for almost two years and observed that this drug indeed was clinically effective as a moderately

431

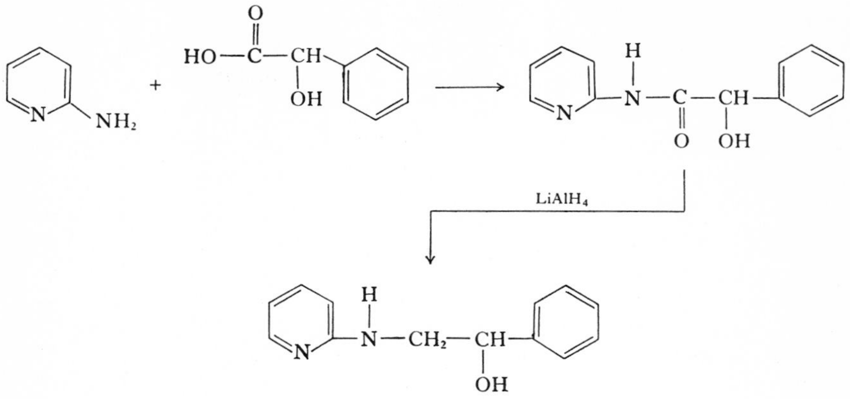

Phenyramidol
(XXIV)
SCHEME 9

potent analgetic agent. The effective dose for satisfactory relief of chronic pain was 100 mg, four times daily. The resultant analgesia occurred promptly and persisted for at least 3 to 4 hours. Untoward reactions were reported to be of no significance. It was also noted by Batterman that phenyramidol did not have any antiinflammatory properties.

Wainer (45) carried out extensive clinical studies on the use of phenyramidol in obstetrics and gynecology. Two hundred cases were studied and with the majority of the patients excellent control of pain due to premenstrual tension, dysmenorrhea, or postpartum effects was maintained with doses of 200 to 400 mg. Since phenyramidol is nonaddicting, it was suggested by Wainer that this substance could be used in place of codeine under the clinical circumstances described.

X. Salicylic Acid and Derivatives

Salicylic acid (XXV) and its derivatives represent a group of compounds which have been in clinical use for over a century. They have been primarily used for the relief of mild to moderate pain. The pain-relieving properties of salicylic acid were first noted in 1876 by Stricker, who observed that this

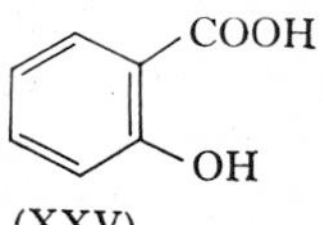

(XXV)

substance caused a specific antipyretic action in rheumatic fever. This effect has been clinically confirmed many times now and, with the exception of hydrocortisone and related substances, salicylic acid in the form of its sodium salt is probably the most widely used drug for the treatment of rheumatoid arthritis despite is disagreeable taste and irritating properties. A considerable amount of work has been carried out to find more effective and less toxic derivatives. In this respect, gentisic acid (XXVI) and 2,3,5-trihydroxybenzoic acid (XXVII), both metabolites of salicylic acid, have

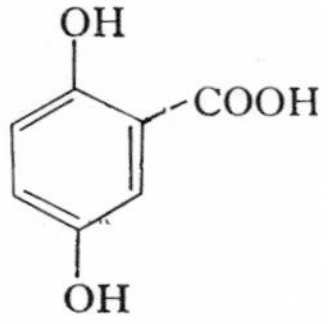

OH
-COOH
OH
(XXVI)

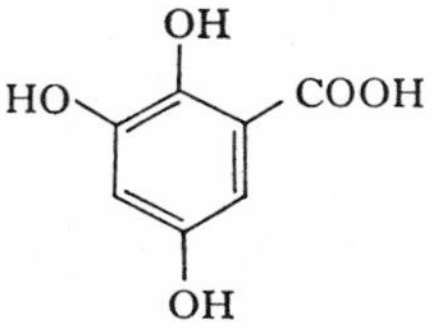

OH
HO   COOH
OH
(XXVII)

been clinically evaluated but have not been found to be superior. Gentisic acid appears to be as potent as salicylic acid and seems to be well tolerated. γ-Resorcylic acid (XXVIII) also has been found to be about as effective as salicylic acid in the treatment of rheumatic heart disease. The daily dose of

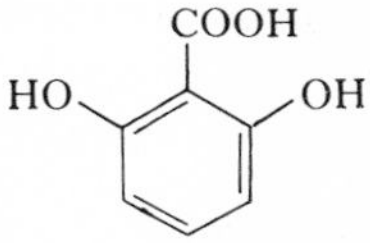

COOH
HO   OH
(XXVIII)

this drug is 1 gm. These derivatives of salicylic acid have been used as their sodium salts.

Acetylsalicylic acid (XXIX) first prepared by Gilm (46) in 1859, is a drug

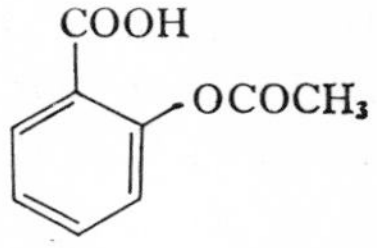

COOH
-OCOCH₃
(XXIX)

which has enjoyed the greatest success for the longest period of time in the history of medicinal chemistry. Since it was first introduced as a therapeutic in 1899 by Dreser (47) under the name of Aspirin it has become the drug of choice for mild aches and pains, and to overcome the effects (e.g. headaches)

433

of neuralgia. It is especially effective as an antipyretic and it also has a mild sedative action. In fact, acetylsalicylic acid is used for many real and imagined painful conditions. All in all, the pharmaceutical industry in the United States alone now manufactures 27 million lb of aspirin a year. Its remarkably low price (about half a cent per tablet) also makes it the cheapest drug available. In spite of its extensive use and the tremendous amount of research carried out with this compound, its mode of action is, as yet, not clearly defined.

Alkyl and aryl esters of salicylic acid have been prepared and some do show some degree of analgetic effect. Salol (XXX) has been recommended by Nencki (48) as an antineuralgic and analgetic drug, whereas methyl-

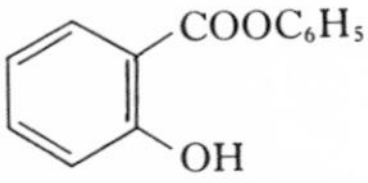

$$\text{(XXX)} \quad \overset{COOC_6H_5}{\underset{OH}{\bigcirc}} \qquad \text{(XXXI)} \quad \overset{COOCH_3}{\underset{OH}{\bigcirc}}$$

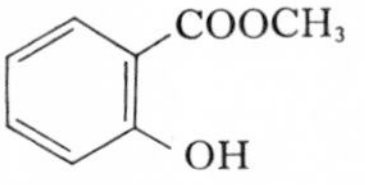

salicylate (XXXI), more commonly known as oil of wintergreen, is widely used for the treatment of muscular pains by topical application. Other alkyl esters of salicylic acid have been used similarly.

Finally, salicylamide (XXXII) has been used clinically as a mild analgetic.

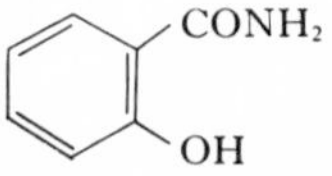

$$\text{(XXXII)} \quad \overset{CONH_2}{\underset{OH}{\bigcirc}}$$

It is reported to be more potent than aspirin and also to have good antipyretic activity. In man, oral doses of 2 gm, three to six times daily, have been reported to produce satisfactory analgesia in approximately 75% of patients with acute rheumatic fever and other rheumatoid conditions. This substance has not gained the favorable position that aspirin has as an analgetic and antipyretic (49, 50).

However, salicylamide has proved to be a useful intermediate in the synthesis of a new group of compounds (1,3-benzoxazines) which have been shown to be analgetics. The most effective compound in this class is chlorthenoxazin (XXXIII) which is prepared by condensing salicylamide with β-chloropropionaldehyde (51).

Using the hot plate method Kadaty (52) showed that a dose of 152.4 mg/kg was capable of eliminating the pain reaction in 50% of a group of 30 mice. This compares with a comparable dose of acetylsalicylic acid of

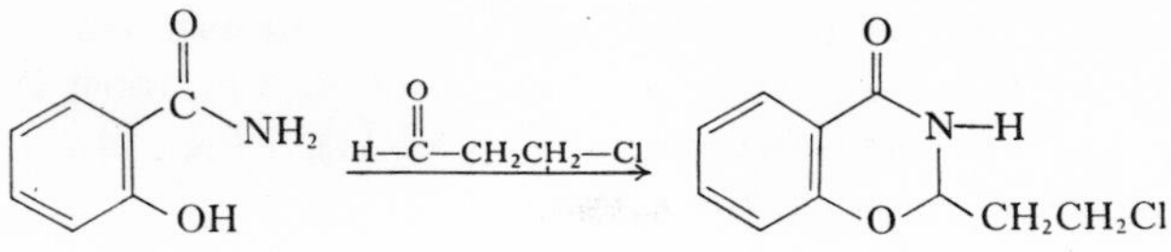

(XXXIII)

nearly 300 mg/kg. It was also shown to possess antipyretic and antiinflammatory activity.

The LD$_{50}$ for rats was shown to be 730 mg/kg by intraperitoneal injection and 10 gm/kg by mouth. Toxic doses produce central depression with respiratory failure. High individual doses of 3 gm by mouth were given to dogs without ill effect (weight of animals 9–14 kg). The long-term toxicity studies in dogs showed no harmful effects after 6 months on a dose of 200 mg/kg daily by mouth. The treated animals remained normal as regards growth and behavior, and their blood picture, coagulation time, and prothrombin time were normal at the end of the test period.

In the rat a dose of 100 mg/kg was completely absorbed after 15 hours and none appeared in the feces. In man 75% of an oral dose appears as metabolites in the urine within 33 hours and complete excretion takes at least 40 hours. By comparison 4 gm of salicylic acid is completely excreted in the urine within 15 hours.

Chlorthenoxazine was tested in humans and found to have an analgetic action up to 50% longer than aspirin or codeine (53). The drug was reported to be free of side effects such as gastrointestinal irritation and intestinal bleeding which are sometimes associated with the salicylates. Use of the drug in a few cases for as long as 18 months, revealed no diminution in hemoglobin levels. Chlorthenoxazine is presently available in Europe but has not been introduced in the United States.

XI. Aniline Derivatives

The stepwise path leading to a useful drug in this series began in 1886 when the pharmacists Cahn and Hepp (54) mistakenly filled a prescription with acetanilide (XXXIV) and discovered that it had antipyretic effects. This accounts for the name Antifebrin which they assigned to it. However, acetanilide is quite a toxic substance since it is readily hydrolyzed to aniline which in turn produces methemoglobin in the blood. Aniline also is oxidized to p-aminophenol (XXXV) which is also quite toxic. Thus, in the course of search for better drugs in this group, it was anticipated that p-acetamidophenol (XXXVI) should be less toxic. This was ultimately borne out, and in addition the ethers and esters of p-aminophenol were found to be less toxic.

435

These findings in turn led to the synthesis of compounds in which both functional groups of *p*-aminophenol were substituted. The most successful of these compounds is acetophenetidine (XXXVII), which is recommended as a strong antipyretic and antineuralgic.

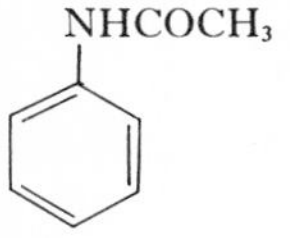

NHCOCH₃   NH₂   NHCOCH₃   NHCOCH₃

           OH   OH   OC₂H₅

(XXXIV) 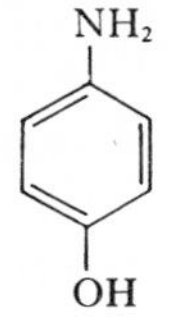   (XXXV) 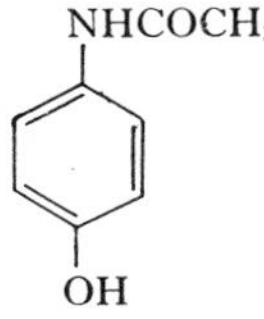   (XXXVI) 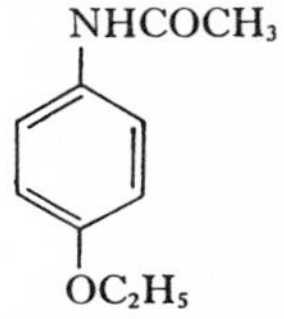   (XXXVII)

The analgetic action of acetophenetidine appears to be similar to that of the salicylates. The type of pain relieved is that which usually occurs in headache, dysenmorrhea, and muscle, joint, and nerve affections. Brodie and Axelrod (*55*) have demonstrated that in man the drug is metabolized to *p*-acetamidophenol, which is then excreted as the glucuronide.

Acetophenetidine is more potent than acetanilide and acetylsalicyclic acid. When the three drugs are combined in equal doses (300 mg), the threshold-raising action of the mixture is no greater than that of any single component alone, but the duration of analgesia is prolonged (*56*). The combination of acetophenetidine, acetylsalicylic acid, and caffeine has gained wide acceptance as a mild analgetic. The combination of such drugs of course leads to less side reactions since the total amount of each drug used is less than that used alone. However, there is probably no other field in which commercial drug exploitation is so extensive as in the manufacture and over-the-counter sale of these headache nostrums. Their indiscriminate use has led to unfortunate cases of drug intoxication, some of which have been fatal. Drugs made up of *p*-aminophenol derivatives should be used with caution and not habitually.

Addendum

Recently, two new series of compounds have been reported to have analgetic effects. The analgetic properties of these substances were discovered while evaluating their anti-inflammatory effects.

Scherrer, Winder, and Short (*57*) have reported on a group of *N*-aryl anthranilic acids showing anti-inflammatory effects. Mefenamic acid (CI-473) (XXXVIII), which showed good anti-inflammatory activity, was also shown by Cass and Frederick (*58*) to have analgetic effects equal to aminopyrine. Another compound in this series (CI-583) (XXXIX), has now been reported to be 150 times more active than aspirin. This brings it into the same order of activity of morphine.

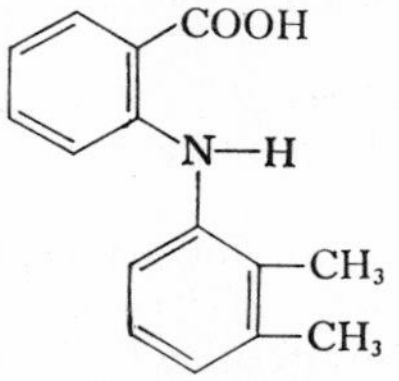

Mefenamic acid
(CI-473)
(XXXVIII)

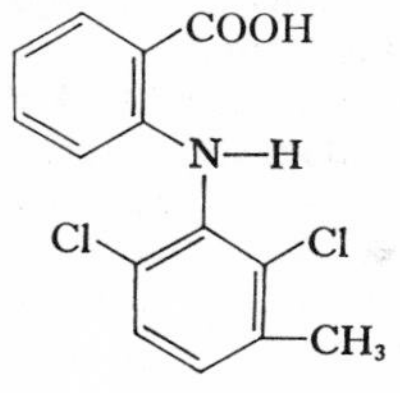

(CI-583)
(XXXIX)

Indomethacin (XL), a new potent anti-inflammatory agent, has also been reported by Winter (*59*) to be about 10 times more potent than aspirin as an analgetic. At present, this substance is undergoing extensive clinical trials and additional reports will be forthcoming on its analgetic action.

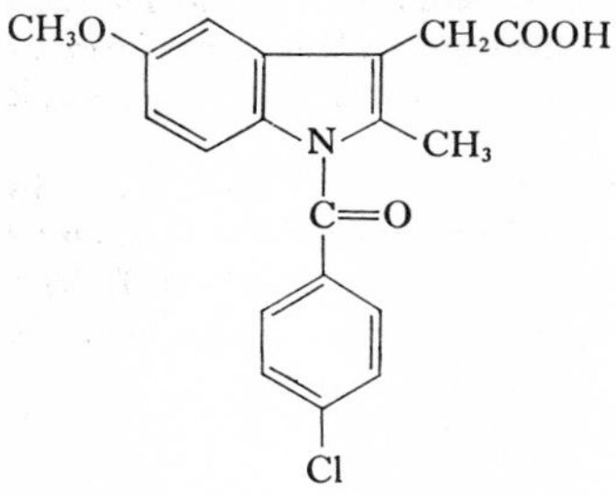

Indomethacin
(XL)

REFERENCES

1. H. Weber, *Verhl. Deut. Ges. Inn. Med.* **21**, 616 (1904).
2. A. Bass, *Z. Ges. Neurol. Psychiat.* **26**, 600 (1914).
3. A. Leimdorfer and W. R. T. Metzner, *Am. J. Physiol.* **157**, 116 (1949).
4. W. Feldberg and S. J. Sherwood, *J. Physiol. (London)* **123**, 148 (1954).
5. T. J. Haley and W. G. McCormick, *Brit. J. Pharmacol.* **12**, 12 (1957).
6. A. B. Rothballer, *Pharmacol. Rev.* **11**, 494 (1959).
7. E. J. Fellows and G. E. Ullyot, *in* "Medicinal Chemistry" (C. M. Suter, ed.), Vol. I, p. 390. Wiley, New York, 1954.
8. R. A. McLean, in "Medicinal Chemistry" (A. Burger, ed.), 2nd ed., p. 611. Wiley, New York, 1960.
9. C. Niemann and J. T. Hays, *J. Am. Chem. Soc.* **64**, 2288 (1942).
10. A. Burger and G. E. Ullyot, *J. Org. Chem.* **12**, 342 (1947).

11. F. K. Kirschner, J. R. McCormick, and C. J. Cavallito, *J. Org. Chem.* **14**, 388 (1949).
12. J. R. Lewis, *Arch. Intern. Pharmacodyn.* **88**, No. 2, 142 (1951).
13. N. Ercoli and M. N. Lewis, *J. Pharmacol. Exptl. Therap.* **84**, 301 (1945).
14. C. F. Huebner, E. Donoghue, P. W. Strachan, P. Beak, and E. Wenkert, *J. Org. Chem.* **27**, 4465 (1962).
15. F. E. D'Amour and D. J. Smith, *J. Pharmacol. Exptl. Therap.* **72**, 74 (1941).
16. L. B. Witkin, C. F. Huebner, F. Galdi, E. O'Keefe, P. Spitaletta, and A. J. Plummer, *J. Pharmacol. Exptl. Therap.* **133**, 400 (1961).
17. M. H. Seevers, personal communication to Dr. A. J. Plummer, Pharmacology Division, CIBA Pharmaceutical Company, Summit, New Jersey.
18. R. C. Batterman, personal communication to Clinical Investigation Division of CIBA Pharmaceutical Company, Summit, New Jersey.
19. G. J. Jackson and D. A. Smith. *Ann. Internal Med.* **45**, 640 (1956).
20. R. W. Houde and S. L. Wallenstein, *Federation Proc.* **14**, 353 (1955).
21. L. Lasagna and T. J. DeKornfeld, *J. Am. Med. Assoc.* **178**, No. 9, 887 (1961).
22. G. A. Deneau and M. H. Seevers, Addendum I to Minutes of 21st Meeting of Committee on Drug Addiction and Narcotics, University of Michigan, January, 1960.
23. L. B. Mellett and J. A. Woods, *in* "Progress in Drug Research" (E. Jucker, ed.), pp. 245–250. Birkhäuser, Basel, Switzerland, 1963.
24. A. Hunger, J. Kebrle, A. Rossi, and K. Hoffmann, *Experientia* **13**, 400 (1957).
25. F. Gross, *Helv. Physiol. Acta* **C31**, V5 (1947).
26. A. Hunger, J. Kebrle, A. Rossi, and K. Hoffmann, *Helv. Chim. Acta* **43**, 800 (1960).
27. A. Hunger, J. Kebrle, A. Rossi and K. Hoffmann, *Helv. Chim. Acta* **43**, 1032 (1960).
28. H. F. Fraser, H. Isbell, and R. Wolback, Bull. Drug Addiction and Narcotics, Addendum 2, p. 35 (1960).
29. F. Gross, Clinical Investigation Reports, CIBA, Basel, Switzerland.
30. G. Cignarella, G. C. Nathansohn, and E. Occelli, *J. Org. Chem.* **26**, 2747 (1961).
31. G. Cignarella, E. Occelli, G. Maffii, and E. Testa, *J. Med. Chem.* **6**, 29 (1961).
32. G. Cignarella, E. Occelli, and E. Testa, *Ann. Chim. (Rome)* **53**, No. 7, 944 (1963); *Chem. Abstr.* **59**, 13,979 (1963).
33. G. Cignarella, E. Occelli, G. Cristiani, L. Paduano, and E. Testa, *J. Med. Chem.* **6**, 764 (1963).
34. L. O. Randall and J. J. Selitto, *Arch. Intern. Pharmacodyn.* **111**, 409 (1957).
35. A. Hantzsch and J. A. Weber, *Ber.* **20**, 3118, 3336 (1887).
36. G. deStevens, H. A. Luts, and J. A. Schneider, *J. Am. Chem. Soc.* **79**, 5263 (1957).
37. G. deStevens, A. Frutchey, A. Halamandaris, and H. A. Luts, *J. Am. Chem. Soc.* **79**, 5263 (1957).
38. G. deStevens, A. F. Hopkinson, M. A. Connelly, P. Oke, and D. C. Schroeder, *J. Am. Chem. Soc.* **80**, 2201 (1958).
39. F. Mohr, CIBA Clinical Investigation Division, Summit, New Jersey.
40. F. M. Berger, M. Kletzkin, B. J. Ludwig, and S. Margolin, *Ann. N.Y. Acad. Sci.* **86**, Art. 1, 90 (1960).
41. G. Woolfe and A. D. MacDonald, *J. Pharmacol. Exptl. Therap.* **80**, 300 (1944).
42. A. P. Gray, U. S. Patent 3,039,930 (June 19, 1962).
43. T. B. O'Dell, *Ann. N.Y. Acad. Sci.* **86**, Art 1, 191 (1960).
44. R. C. Batterman, *Ann. N.Y. Acad. Sci.* **86**, Art. 1, 203 (1960).
45. A. S. Wainer, *Ann. N.Y. Acad. Sci.* **86**, Art. 1, 250 (1960).
46. H. V. Gilm, *Ann.*, **112**, 180 (1859).
47. H. Dreser, *Arch. Ges. Physiol.* **76**, 306 (1899).

48. M. Nencki, *Arch. Exptl. Pathol. Pharmacol.* **20**, 396 (1886).
49. E. M. Bavin, *J. Pharm. Pharmacol.* **4**, 872 (1952).
50. R. C. Batterman and A. J. Grossman, *J. Am. Med. Assoc.* **159**, 1619 (1955).
51. Karl Thomae Company, British Patent 806,729 (December 21, 1958).
52. R. Kadaty, *Arzneimittel-Forsch.* **7**, 651 (1957).
53. D. Wilson, P. H. Kendall, and P. M. Pawsey, *Brit. Med. J.* p. 36 (1960).
54. A. Cahn and P. Hepp, *Centr. Klin. Med.* **7**, 561 (1886).
55. B. B. Brodie and J. Axelrod, *J. Pharmacol. Exptl. Therap.* **97**, 58 (1949).
56. H. G. Wolff, J. D. Hardy, and H. Goodel, *J. Clin. Invest.* **20**, 63 (1941).
57. R. A. Scherrer, C. V. Winder, and F. W. Short, Ninth National Medicinal Chemistry Symposium of the American Chemical Society, Division of Medicinal Chemistry, June 21–24, 1964. University of Minnesota, Minneapolis, Minnesota.
58. J. J. Cass and W. S. Frederick, *J. Pharmacol. Exptl. Therap.* p. 172 (1963).
59. C. A. Winter, Ninth National Medicinal Chemistry Symposium of the American Chemical Society, Division of Medicinal Chemistry, June 21–24, 1964. University of Minnesota, Minneapolis, Minnesota.

Author Index

Numbers in parentheses are reference numbers and are included to assist in locating references in which authors' names are not mentioned in the text. Numbers in italics refer to pages on which the references are listed.

441

447

449

459

461

Subject Index

467

471